HESI

Comprehensive Review for the

NCLEX-RN®
EXAMINATION

EDITION 5

EDITOR

E. Tina Cuellar, PhD, WHNP, PMHCNS, BC
Director of Curriculum
Review and Testing
Elsevier/HESI
Houston, Texas

ELSEVIER

ELSEVIER

3251 Riverport Lane
St. Louis, Missouri 63043

HESI COMPREHENSIVE REVIEW FOR THE NCLEX-RN®
EXAMINATION, FIFTH EDITION

ISBN: 978-0-323-39462-8

Previous editions copyrighted 2014, 2011 and 2008.
International Standard Book Number: 978-0-323-39462-8

NANDA International Nursing Diagnoses: Definitions and Classifications 2015-2017; Herdman T.H. (Ed); copyright 2014, 1994-2014 NANDA International, published by John Wiley & Sons Limited.

NCLEX®, NCLEX-RN®, and NCLEX-PN® are registered trademarks and service marks of the National Council of State Boards of Nursing, Inc.

Senior Content Strategist: Jamie Randall
Content Development Manager: Jean Sims Fornango
Senior Content Development Specialist: Danielle M. Frazier
Publishing Services Manager: Jeff Patterson
Book Production Specialist: Bill Drone
Design Direction: Ryan Cook

Printed in China

Last digit is the print number: 9 8 7 6 5 4 3 2

Working together
to grow libraries in
developing countries

www.elsevier.com • www.bookaid.org

CONTRIBUTING AUTHORS

Safa'a Al-Arabi, PhD, RN, MSN, MPH
Associate Professor and Accelerated BSN Track
  Administrator
University of Texas Medical Branch
School of Nursing
Galveston, Texas

E. Tina Cuellar, PhD, WHNP, PMHCNS, BC
Director of Curriculum
Review and Testing
Elsevier/Education/HESI
Houston, Texas

Claudine Dufrene, PhD, RN-BC, GNP-BC, CNE
Assistant Professor
University of St. Thomas
Carol and Odis Peavy School of Nursing
Houston, Texas

Shelby L. Garner, PhD, RN, CNE
Assistant Professor and Fulbright Scholar
Baylor University
Louise Herrington School of Nursing
Dallas, Texas

Sandy Jemison, MSN, RN
Assistant Professor
Cox College of Nursing and Health Sciences
Springfield, Missouri

Lucindra Campbell-Law, PhD, ANP, PMHNP, BC
Professor
Carol and Odis Peavy School of Nursing
University of St. Thomas
Houston, Texas

Necole Leland, MSN, RN, PNP, CPN
Instructor
University of Nevada, Las Vegas
School of Nursing
Las Vegas, Nevada

Rosemary Pine, PhD, RN, BC, CDE
Review Course Director
Review and Testing
Elsevier/Education/HESI
Houston, Texas

Katherine Ralph, MSN, RN
Nurse Manager Curriculum
Review and Testing
Elsevier/Education/HESI
Houston, Texas

CONTRIBUTING AUTHORS

Safak Al-Arabi, PhD, RN, MSN, MPH
Assistant Professor and Accelerated BSN Track
Coordinator
University of Texas Medical Branch
School of Nursing
Galveston, Texas

E. Tina Cuellar, PhD, WHNP, PMHCNS, BC
Director of Curriculum
Review and Testing
Elsevier/HealthStream (EST)
Houston, Texas

Claudine Dufrene, PhD, RN-BC, CNP-BC, CNE
Assistant Professor
University of St. Thomas
Carol and Odis Peavy School of Nursing
Houston, Texas

Shelby L. Garner, PhD, RN, CNE
Assistant Professor and Fulbright Scholar
Baylor University
Louise Herrington School of Nursing
Dallas, Texas

Sandy Jamison, MSN, RN
Assistant Professor
Cox College of Nursing and Health Sciences
Springfield, Missouri

Luctadia Campbell-Law, PhD, ANP, PMHNP, BC
Professor
Carol and Odis Peavy School of Nursing
University of St. Thomas
Houston, Texas

Necole Leland, MSN, RN, PNP, CPN
Lecturer
University of Nevada Las Vegas
School of Nursing
Las Vegas, Nevada

Rosemary Pine, PhD, RN, BC, CDE
Review Course Director
Review and Testing
Elsevier/Education (HESI)
Houston, Texas

Katherine Ralph, MSN, RN
Course Manager Curriculum
Review and Testing
Elsevier/HealthStream (EST)
Houston, Texas

REVIEWERS

Judy Carlyle, MNSc, RN
ARNEC Program Director
Arkansas Rural Nursing Education
    Consortium (ARNEC)
Nashville, Arkansas

Susan Golden, MSN, RN
Dean of Health
Division of Health
Eastern New Mexico University-Roswell
Roswell, New Mexico

Rose A. Harding, MSN, RN
Instructor, Coordinator of Standardization
    Test Evaluation Committee
JoAnne Gay Dishman
Department of Nursing
Lamar University
Beaumont, Texas

Rosanna M. Henry, MSN, RN
Instructor and Director
Irene Fritzky Lab
School of Nursing
Duquesne University
Pittsburgh, Pennsylvania

Donna Walker Hubbard, MSN, RN, CNNe
Retired Assistant Professor
University of Mary Hardin–Baylor
Belton, Texas

Paula Celeste Hughes, MSN, RN
Nursing Faculty
Practical Nursing
Georgia Northwestern Technical College
Rome, Georgia

Cheryl A. Lehman, PhD, RN, CNS-BC, RN-BC, CRRN
Retired Clinical Professor
School of Nursing
University of Texas Health Science Center at San Antonio
Nursing Consultant
Lehman Consulting LLC
San Antonio, Texas

Donna Wilsker, MSN, RN
Assistant Professor
Dishman Department of Nursing
Lamar University
Beaumont, Texas

Nancee Wozney, PhD, RN
Dean of Nursing and Allied Health/Human Services
Nursing Department
Minnesota State College–Southeast Technical
Winona, Minnesota

PREFACE

Welcome to *HESI Comprehensive Review for the NCLEX-RN® Examination* with online study exams by HESI.

Congratulations! This outstanding review manual with online study exams is designed to prepare nursing students for what is very likely the most important examination they will ever take—the NCLEX-RN Licensing Examination. As a graduate of an RN nursing program, the student has the basic knowledge required to pass tests and perform safely and successfully in the clinical area. *HESI Comprehensive Review for the NCLEX-RN® Examination* allows the nursing student to prepare for the NCLEX-RN licensure examination in a structured way.

- Organize nursing basic knowledge previously learned.
- Review content learned during basic nursing curriculum.
- Identify weaknesses in content knowledge so study effort can be focused appropriately.
- Develop test-taking skills so application of safe nursing practice from knowledge previously learned can be demonstrated.
- Reduce anxiety level by increasing predictability of ability to correctly answer NCLEX-type questions.
- Boost test-taking confidence by being well prepared and knowing what to expect.

Organization

Chapter 1, Introduction to Testing and the NCLEX-RN® Examination, gives an overview of the NCLEX-RN licensing exam history and test plan for the examination. A review of the nursing process, updated with the latest NANDA-approved nursing diagnoses, client needs, and prioritizing nursing care, is also presented.

Chapter 2, Leadership and Management, reviews the legal aspects of nursing, leadership and management, and disaster nursing.

Chapter 3, Advanced Clinical Concepts, presents nursing assessment, analysis (nursing diagnoses), and planning and intervention at the highest level of practice. Topics reviewed include respiratory failure, shock, disseminated intravascular coagulation (DIC), resuscitation, fluid and electrolyte balance, IV therapy, acid–base balance, electrocardiogram (ECG), perioperative care, HIV, pain, and death and grief.

Chapters 4 through 8, Medical-Surgical Nursing, Pediatric Nursing, Maternity Nursing, Psychiatric Nursing, and

Gerontologic Nursing, are presented in traditional clinical areas. Each clinical area is divided into physiologic components, with essential knowledge about basic anatomy, growth and development, pharmacology and medication calculation, nutrition, communication, client and family education, acute and chronic care, leadership and management, complimentary and alternative interventions, cultural and spiritual diversity, and clinical decision making threaded throughout the different components.

Open-ended–style questions with the answers appear at the end of each chapter, which encourage the student to think in depth about the content that is presented throughout the particular chapter. When a variety of learning mechanisms is used, students have the opportunity to comprehensively prepare for the NCLEX exam; these strategies include:

- Reading the manual.
- Discussing content with others.
- Answering open-ended questions.
- Practicing with study exams that simulate the licensure examination.

These learning experiences are all different ways that students should use to prepare for the NCLEX exam. The purpose of the open-ended questions appearing at the end of the chapter is not a focused practice session on managing NCLEX-style multiple-choice questions, but rather a learning approach that allows for more in-depth thinking about specific topics in the chapter. Practice with multiple-choice questions alone cannot provide the depth of critical thinking and analysis possible with the short-answer questions at the end of the chapter. In addition, the open-ended questions presented at the end of the chapter provide a summary experience that helps students focus on the main topics that were covered in the chapter. Teachers use open-ended questions to stimulate the critical thinking process, and *HESI Comprehensive Review for the NCLEX-RN® Examination* facilitates the critical thinking process by posing the same type of questions the teacher might ask.

When students need to practice multiple-choice questions, the online study exams on Evolve offer extensive opportunities for practice and skill building to improve their test-taking abilities. The online study exams include six content-specific exams (Medical-Surgical Nursing, Pharmacology, Pediatrics, Fundamentals, Maternity, and Psychiatric-Mental Health Nursing) and two comprehensive exams patterned after categories on the NCLEX-RN exam. The online study exams on Evolve can be accessed as many times as necessary, and the questions from one study exam are not contained on another study exam. For instance, the Medical-Surgical study exam does not contain questions that are on the Pediatrics study exam. The purpose of the study exams is to provide practice and exposure to the critical thinking–style questions that students will encounter on the NCLEX-RN exam. However, the study exams should not be used to predict performance on the actual NCLEX exam. Only the HESI Exit Exam, a secure, computerized exam that simulates the NCLEX test plan and has evidence-based results from numerous research studies indicating a high level of accuracy in predicting NCLEX success, is offered as a true predictor exam. Students are allowed unlimited practice on each online study exam so that they can be sure to have the opportunity to review all of the rationales for the questions.

Here is a plan for a student to use with the online study exams:

- Step 1: Take the RN study exam without studying for it to see where your strengths and weaknesses are.
- Step 2: After going over the content that relates to the study questions on a particular clinical area (e.g., Pediatrics, Medical-Surgical, or Maternity), review that section of the manual, and take the test again to determine if you have been able to improve your scores.
- Step 3: Purposely miss every question on the exam so that you can view the rationales for every question.
- Step 4: Take the exam again under timed conditions at the pace that you would have to progress in order to complete the NCLEX exam in the time allowed (approximately 1 minute per question.) See if being placed under time constraints affects your performance.
- Step 5: Put the exam away for a while, and continue review and remediation with other textbooks, other resources, and the results of any HESI secure exams that you have taken at your school. Then, take the study exams again to see if your performance improves after in-depth study and following a few weeks' break from these questions.

Step 5 represents a good activity in preparation for the HESI Exit Exam presented in your final semester of the nursing program, especially if you have not used the online study exams for several weeks. Repeated exposure to the questions, however, will make them less useful over time because students tend to memorize the answers. For this reason, these tests are useful only for practice and not prediction of NCLEX-RN success. The tendency to memorize the questions after viewing them multiple times falsely elevates a student's score on the study exams.

Additional assistance for students studying for the NCLEX-RN Licensing Examination can be obtained from a variety of online products in the Elsevier family. Many nursing schools have also adopted the following:

- *HESI Examinations*—A comprehensive set of examinations designed to prepare nursing students for the NCLEX exam. They include customized electronic remediation from current Elsevier textbooks and multimedia, as well as additional practice questions. Each student is given an individualized report detailing exam results and is allowed to view questions and rationales for items that were answered incorrectly. The electronic remediation, a complementary feature of the specialty and exit exams, can be filed by the student for later study.
- *HESI Practice Test*—This is the ideal way to practice for the NCLEX exam. With more than 1200 practice questions included in this online test bank, nursing students can access practice exams 24 hours a day, 7 days a week. *HESI Practice Test* questions are written at the critical thinking level so that students are tested not for memorization but for their skills in clinical application. Students select a test option (either a clinical specialty or a comprehensive exam), and *HESI Practice Test* automatically supplies a series of critical-thinking practice questions. NCLEX exam–style questions include multiple-choice and alternate-item formats and are accompanied by correct answers and rationales.
- *HESI RN Case Studies*—These prepare students to manage complex patient conditions and to make sound clinical judgments. These online case studies cover a broad range of physiologic and psychosocial alterations, plus related management, pharmacology, and therapeutic concepts.
- *HESI Patient Reviews*—These are designed to teach and assess students' retention of core nursing content. These online interactive reviews provide a firsthand look at safe and effective nursing care.
- *HESI Live Review* —A live review course is presented by an expert faculty member who has additional instruction in working with students who are preparing to take the NCLEX exam. Students are presented with a workbook and practice NCLEX-style questions that are used during the course.
- *Evolve eBooks*—Online versions of all of the Mosby, Saunders, and Elsevier textbooks used in the student's nursing curriculum are presented. Search across titles, highlight, make notes, and more—all on your computer.
- *Elsevier Simulations*—Virtual versions simulate the clinical environment. These multilayered, complex, supplemental simulations enable students to experience clinical assignments without the need for actual clinical space.
- *Elsevier Courses*—These are created by experts using instructional design principles. This interactive content engages students with reading, animation, video, audio, interactive exercises, and assessments.

CONTENTS

1 INTRODUCTION TO TESTING AND THE NCLEX-RN® EXAMINATION

Three cheers for you! You have made the wise decision to prepare, in a structured way, for the NCLEX-RN®.

A. You have already successfully completed a basic nursing program and are well acquainted with your ability to take and pass tests and to perform successfully in the clinical area.

B. You have the basic knowledge required to pass the licensing examination. However, it is wise to:
1. Organize your knowledge.
2. Review content learned during the years of your basic nursing curriculum.
3. Identify weaknesses in content knowledge so that you can focus your study time appropriately.
4. Develop test-taking skills so you can demonstrate the knowledge you have.
5. Reduce your level of anxiety by increasing your predictability.
6. Know what to expect. Remember: knowledge is power. You are powerful when you are well prepared and know what to expect.

Test-Taking Tips

There are no absolute ways to ensure that examination questions will always be answered correctly. These test-taking tips are guidelines to help the student study and understand the examination questions. On the NCLEX-RN examination, many different areas are tested with each question. For example, a question may on the surface be a medical/surgical or pediatric question, but included in the question can be such topics as communication, nutrition, growth and development, medication, client and family education, and safety.

> **HESI Hint** • The most essential element of nursing care is client safety. Caring is the hallmark of nursing. Nursing practice includes the nursing process integrated with fundamental components, including but not limited to, caring, communication, culture and spirituality, teaching, and learning, as well as documentation of the integration of each of these elements.

A. Understanding the question
1. Determine whether the question is written in a positive or negative style.
   a. A *positive* style may ask what the nurse should do or ask for the best or first action to implement.

> **HESI Hint** • Most questions are written in a positive style.

   b. A *negative* style may ask what the nurse should avoid, which prescription the nurse should question, or which behavior indicates the need for reteaching the client.

> **HESI Hint** • Negative-style questions will contain key words that denote the negative style.
>
> **EXAMPLES**
> 1. "Which response indicates to the nurse a need to *reteach* the client about...?" (Which information/understanding by the client is incorrect?)
> 2. "Which prescription (order) should the nurse *question?*" (Which prescription is unsafe, not beneficial, inappropriate to this client situation, etc...?)

2. Find the key words in the question.
   a. Ask yourself which words or phrases provide the critical information.
   b. This information may be the age of the client, the setting, the timing, a set of symptoms or behaviors, or any number of other factors.
   c. For example, the nursing actions for a 10-year-old 1-day postop are different from those for a 70-year-old 1-hour postop.
3. Rephrase the question in your own words.
   a. This will help you eliminate nonessential information in the question and help you determine the correct answer.
   b. Ask yourself, "What is this question *really* asking?"
   c. While keeping the options covered, rephrase the question in your own words.

    4. Rule out options.
       a. Based on your knowledge, you can probably identify one or two options that are clearly incorrect.
       b. Physically mark through those options on the test booklet if allowed. Mentally mark through those options in your head if using a computer.
       c. Now differentiate between the remaining options, considering your knowledge of the subject and related nursing principles, such as roles of the nurse, the nursing process, the ABCs (airway, breathing, and circulation), CAB (circulation, airway, and breathing for cardiopulmonary resuscitation [CPR]), and Maslow's hierarchy of needs.

B. General guidelines about test taking
    1. Consider the content of the question and what the question is asking.
    2. Generally, an assessment of the client occurs before an action is taken.
    3. Identify the least invasive intervention before taking action.
    4. Have all the necessary information and take all possible relevant actions before calling the physician or health care provider.
    5. Determine which client to assess first (e.g., most at risk, most physiologically unstable).
    6. Identify opposites in the answers.
       a. Example: prone/supine; elevated/decreased
       b. Read *VERY* carefully; one is likely to be the answer, BUT not always.
       c. If you do not know the answer, choose the most likely of the "opposites" and move on.
    7. Take into account a client's lifestyle, culture, and spiritual beliefs when answering a question.

C. Use CRITICAL THINKING, reasoning, and common sense to answer questions.
    1. DO respond based on…
       a. Client safety
       b. ABCs
       c. CAB for CPR
       d. Caring
       e. Incorporation of culture and spiritual practices
       f. Scientific, behavioral, and sociologic principles
       g. Communication (spoken and written, e.g., documentation) with client, family, and colleagues and other health care professionals
       h. Principles of teaching/learning
       i. Maslow's hierarchy of needs
       j. Nursing process
       k. What's in the stem: no more, no less (do not read more into the question than is already there).
       l. NCLEX-RN ideal hospital
       m. Basic anatomy and physiology
    2. DON'T respond based on…
       a. *YOUR* past client care experiences or agency

       b. A familiar phrase or term
       c. "Of course, I would have already…"
       d. What YOU think is *REALISTIC*
       e. *YOUR* children, pregnancies, parents, elders, personal response to a drug, etc.
       f. The "what-ifs"

D. Keep memorizing to a minimum.
    1. Growth and developmental milestones
    2. Death and dying stages
    3. Crisis intervention
    4. Immunizations schedule
    5. Principles of teaching/learning
    6. Stages of pregnancy and fetal growth
    7. Nurse Practice Act: Standards of Practice and Delegation
    8. Ethical practices and standards

E. Know commonly used laboratory ranges (Appendix A), what variations mean, and the BEST nursing actions.
    1. Hemoglobin and hematocrit (H&H)
    2. White blood cells (WBCs), red blood cells (RBCs), platelets
    3. Electrolytes: K^+, Na^+, Ca^{++}, Mg^{++}, Cl^-, PO_4^-
    4. Blood urea nitrogen (BUN) and creatinine
    5. Relationship of Ca^{++} and PO_4^-
    6. Arterial blood gases (ABGs);
    7. SED rate, erythrocyte sedimentation rate (ESR), prothrombin time (PT), international normalized ratio (INR), partial thromboplastin time (PTT; see aPTT), activated partial thromboplastin time: seconds (aPTT) (don't get them confused)

F. Nutrition
    1. Know commonly used nutrition information.
       a. High or low Na^+
       b. High or low K^+
       c. High PO_4^-
       d. Iron
       e. Vitamin K
       f. Proteins
       g. Carbohydrates
       h. Fats
    2. Foods and diets related to
       a. Gastrointestinal/genitourinary disturbances
       b. Chemotherapy diets and restrictions
       c. Pregnancy and fetal growth needs
       d. Dialysis
       e. Burns
    3. Remember concepts
       a. Introducing one food at a time (infants, allergies)
       b. Progression "AS TOLERATED" (What nursing assessment guides decisions regarding progression?)

G. Medications—SAFE medication administration is more than just knowing the name, classification, and action of the medication.
    1. "Six Rights," including techniques of skill execution
    2. Drug interactions

3. Vulnerable organs
   a. What to assess
   b. Which laboratory values relate to specific organs
4. Allergies
5. Presence of suprainfections
6. Concepts of *peak* and *trough*
7. How you would know
   a. The drug is working
   b. There's a problem
8. Nursing actions
9. Client education should include
   a. Safety
   b. Empowerment
   c. Compliance

The NCLEX-RN Licensing Examination

A. The main purpose of a licensing examination like the NCLEX-RN is to protect the public.
B. The NCLEX-RN
   1. Was developed by the National Council of State Boards of Nursing (the Council; this abbreviation is used to refer to the NCSBN throughout this book)
   2. Is administered by the State Board of Nurse Examiners
   3. Is designed to test candidates'
      a. Capabilities for safe and effective nursing practice
      b. Essential entry-level nursing knowledge

Job Analysis Studies

A. Essential knowledge is determined by job analysis studies.

> **HESI Hint** • The Council wants to ensure that the licensing examination measures current entry-level nursing behaviors. For this reason, job analysis studies are conducted every 3 years. These studies determine how frequently various types of nursing activities are performed, how often they are delegated, and how critical they are to client safety, with criticality given more value than frequency.

B. Job analysis studies indicate that newly licensed registered nurses are using all five categories of the nursing process and that such use is evenly distributed throughout the five nursing process areas. Therefore equal attention is given to each part of the nursing process in selecting test items (Table 1-1).

Nursing Diagnoses

A. Nursing diagnoses are formulated during the analysis portion of the nursing process. They give form and direction to the nursing process, promote priority setting, and guide nursing actions (Table 1-2).
B. To qualify as a nursing diagnosis, the primary responsibility and accountability for recognition and treatment rest with the nurse.
C. The National Conference of the North American Nursing Diagnosis Association (NANDA) provided the following

TABLE 1-1 The Nursing Process

Category	Activities Associated with Nursing Process
Assessment	• Gather objective and subjective data. • Verify data.
Analysis	• Interpret data. • Collect additional data when necessary. • Identify and communicate nursing diagnoses. • Determine health team's ability to meet client's needs.
Planning	• Determine and prioritize outcomes of care. Include client, significant others, and health team in setting outcomes. • Develop and modify plan for delivery of client's care.
Implementation	• Organize and manage the client's care, including safety, caring, cultural and spiritual domains, interprofessional collaboration and communication, and assignment and delegation of tasks. • Perform or assist in performance of client's care. • Counsel and teach client, significant others, and health team. • Provide care specifically directed toward achieving outcomes.
Evaluation	• Compare actual outcomes with expected outcomes. • Evaluate compliance with the established regimen or plan. • Record and describe client's response to plan. • Modify plan as indicated and set priorities.

TABLE 1-2 Components of a Nursing Diagnosis

Component	Explanation
Response	• Includes potential or actual health response • Describes measurable outcomes that can be derived • Cites potential for changes based on nursing actions • *Example:* Alteration in comfort, pain
Etiology	• Includes potential or actual health response • Addresses independent, interdependent, and dependent nursing functions • *Example:* Related to fractured left ankle

definition of a nursing diagnosis: "Nursing diagnosis is a clinical judgment about individual, family, or community responses to actual and potential health problems/life processes. Nursing diagnoses provide the basis for selection of nursing interventions to achieve outcomes for which the nurse is accountable" (Box 1-1). NCLEX-RN does not use NANDA; however, NANDA is used in this book to provide a guide in the formulation and development of the nursing process.

D. NCLEX-RN questions regarding nursing diagnosis can take several forms:
  1. You may be given the nursing diagnosis in the stem and asked to select an appropriate nursing intervention based on the stated nursing diagnosis.
  2. You may be asked to select, from among the choices provided, the most appropriate nursing diagnosis(es) for the described case.

BOX 1-1 *NANDA-Approved Nursing Diagnoses*

A
Activity/Risk for activity intolerance
Ineffective airway clearance
Risk for allergy response
Anxiety
Risk for aspiration
Risk for impaired attachment

B
Disorganized infant behavior (Risk for)
Risk for bleeding
Risk for unstable blood glucose level
Disturbed body image
Risk for imbalanced body temperature
Ineffective breastfeeding
Ineffective breathing pattern

C
Decreased cardiac output
Caregiver role strain (risk for)
Ineffective childbearing process
Impaired comfort
Impaired verbal communication
Acute confusion (risk for)
Chronic confusion
Risk for contamination
Ineffective coping
Compromised family coping

D
Death anxiety
Risk for Sudden Infant Death Syndrome
Decisional conflict
Risk for delayed development

E
Risk for electrolyte imbalance
Disturbed energy field
Impaired environmental interpretation

F
Adult failure to thrive
Dysfunctional family process
Fluid volume deficit (risk for)
Excess fluid volume

G
Impaired gas exchange
Dysfunctional gastrointestinal motility
Grieving/risk for complicated grieving
Delayed growth and development

H
Risk-prone health behavior
Ineffective health maintenance
Hopelessness
Hypothermia/Hyperthermia

I
Ineffective impulse control
Bowel incontinence
Urinary incontinence
Risk for infection
Decreased intracranial adaptive capacity

J
Neonatal jaundice (risk for)

K
Deficient knowledge

M
Risk for disturber maternal-fetal dyad
Impaired memory
Impaired physical mobility
Moral distress

N
Nausea

BOX 1-1 *NANDA-Approved Nursing Diagnoses—cont'd*

Unilateral neglect
Imbalanced nutrition: less than body requirements

O
Impaired oral mucous membrane

P
Acute/Chronic pain
Impaired parenting
Disturbed personal identity
Risk for poisoning
Posttrauma syndrome (risk for)
Powerlessness (risk for)

R
Rape-trauma syndrome
Impaired religiosity
Risk for ineffective renal perfusion
Impaired individual resilience
Parental role conflict
Ineffective role performance

S
Chronic low self esteem
Self-mutilation

Sexual dysfunction
Social isolation
Risk for suicide

T
Ineffective thermal regulation
Impaired tissue integrity
Ineffective peripheral tissue perfusion
Risk for decreased cardiac tissue perfusion
Risk for ineffective cerebral tissue perfusion
Risk for trauma

U
Impaired urinary elimination
Urinary retention

V
Risk for vascular trauma
Impaired spontaneous ventilation
Dysfunctional ventilatory weaning response
Risk for other directed violence

W
Impaired walking
Wandering

3. You may be asked to choose, from four nursing diagnoses, the one that should have priority based on the data in the stem.

HESI Hint • A nursing diagnosis must be subject to oversight by nursing management. It is not a medical diagnosis.
The cause may or may not arise from a medical diagnosis.

Client Needs

A. Job analysis studies have identified categories of care provided by nurses called *client needs*. The test plan is structured according to these categories (Table 1-3).

Prioritizing Nursing Care

A. Many NCLEX-RN test items are designed to test your ability to set priorities—for example:
   1. Identify the *most important* client needs.
   2. Which nursing intervention is *most important?*
   3. Which nursing action should be done *first?*
   4. Which response is *best?*
B. Setting priorities
   1. What should be done first or next? Remember, client safety is paramount.
   2. Those taking the NCLEX-RN should "remember Maslow" (Table 1-4).
   3. The Five Rights of Delegation (see Chapter 2, p. 16)

HESI Hint • Answering NCLEX-RN questions correctly often depends on setting priorities properly, on making judgments about priorities, and on analyzing the case and formulating a decision about care (or the correct response) based on priorities. Using Maslow's hierarchy of needs can help you to set priorities.

The NCLEX-RN Computer Adaptive Testing

A. Computer adaptive testing (CAT) is used for implementation of the NCLEX-RN.
B. The CAT is administered at a testing center selected by the Council.
C. Pearson VUE is responsible for adapting the NCLEX-RN to the CAT format, processing candidate applications, and transmitting test results to its data center for scoring.
D. The testing centers are located throughout the United States.
E. The Council generates the NCLEX-RN test items.

The Way It Works

A. The NCLEX-RN consists of 75 to 265 multiple-choice or alternative-format questions (15 of which are "pilot items") presented on a computer screen.

TABLE 1-3 Components of the NCLEX-RN® Test Plan

NCSBN defines five processes that are essential to nursing and are therefore incorporated throughout the Client Needs categories. Those categories and subcategories are identified as:

- Nursing Process: providing client care using a scientific clinical reasoning approach.
- Caring: Use of mutual trust and respect to meet client needs with compassion and support
- Communication and Documentation: Reciprocal communication among the nurse, client, client's significant others, and interprofessional members of the health care team. Documentation of information related to client care that validates accountability.
- Teaching and Learning: Promoting health by facilitating client's acquisition knowledge.
- Culture and Spirituality: Recognizing and considering the distinctive preferences for care identified by the client that are applicable to standards of care.

Client needs, including percentage of items from each category/subcategory

Safe and Effective Care Environment
- Management of Care 17%-23%
- Safety and Infection Control 9%-15%

Health Promotion and Maintenance 6%-12%

Psychosocial Integrity 6%-12%

Physiologic Integrity 6%-12%
- Basic Care and Comfort 6%-12% (caring interventions, including cultural and spiritual needs)
- Pharmacological and Parental Therapies 12%-18% (includes alternative medicine and modalities)
- Reduction of Risk Potential 9%-15% (client safety)
- Physiologic Adaptation 11%-17%

Category of Client Needs	NCLEX-RN (%)	Activities
Safe and Effective Care Environment Management of Care Provides and directs nursing care that enhances the care delivery setting in order to protect clients and health care personnel	17%-23%	Client safety; Advance directives; Advocacy; Assignment, delegation, and supervision; Case management; Client rights; Collaboration with interdisciplinary team; Concepts of management; Confidentiality/information security; Continuity of care; Establishing priorities; Ethical practice; Informed consent; Information technology; Legal rights and responsibilities; Performance improvement (quality improvement); Referrals
Psychosocial Integrity Directs nursing care, promoting and supporting the emotional, mental, and social well-being of the client experiencing stressful events, as well as clients with acute or chronic mental illness	6%-12%	Client safety; Abuse and neglect; Behavioral interventions; Chemical and other dependencies/substance use disorders; Coping mechanisms; Crisis intervention; Cultural awareness/cultural influences on health; Religious and spiritual influences on health; End-of-life care; Family dynamics; Grief and loss; Sensory perceptual alterations; Stress management; Support systems; Therapeutic communication; Therapeutic environment

Client Needs Category	Percentage	Related Content
Physiologic Integrity — Basic care and comfort: Comfort and assistance in the performance of activities of daily living	11%-17%	• Assistive devices • Elimination • Mobility/immobility • Nonpharmacological comfort interventions • Nutrition and oral hydration • Personal hygiene • Rest and sleep
Physiologic Integrity — Manage and provide care for clients with acute, chronic, or life-threatening physical health conditions	11%-17%	• Alterations in body systems • Fluid and electrolyte imbalances • Hemodynamics • Illness management • Medical emergencies • Pathophysiology • Unexpected response to therapy
Pharmacological and parental therapies — Care related to administration of medications and parental	12%-18%	• Client safety • Adverse effects/contraindications/side effects/interactions • Blood and blood products • Alternative medications adverse effects, contraindications; side effects, interactions, adverse effects • Central venous access devices • Dosage calculation • Expected actions/outcomes • Medication administration • Parental/intravenous therapies • Pharmacological pain management • Total parental nutrition
Reduction of risk potential — Reduction in likelihood that clients develop complications or health problems related to existing conditions, treatments, or procedures	9%-15%	• Client safety • Changes/abnormalities in vital signs • Diagnostic tests • Laboratory values • Potential for alterations in body systems • Potential for complications of diagnostic tests/treatments/procedures • Potential for complications from surgical procedures and health alterations • System-specific assessments • Therapeutic procedures • Alternative procedures (e.g, acupressure)
Safety and Infection Control — Protecting clients and health care personnel from health and environmental hazards	9%-15%	• Promote client safety • Accident/error/injury prevention • Emergency response plan • Ergonomic principles • Handling hazardous and infectious materials • Home safety • Reporting of incident/event/irregular occurrence/variance • Safe use of equipment • Security plan • Standard precautions/transmission-based precautions/surgical asepsis • Use of restraints/safety devices
Health Promotion and Maintenance — Provides and directs nursing care of the client that incorporates: Knowledge of expected growth and development; Prevention and/or early detection of health problems; Strategies to achieve optimal health	6%-12%	• Aging process • Ante/intra/postpartum and newborn care • Developmental stages and transitions • Health promotion/disease prevention • Health screening • High-risk behaviors • Lifestyle choices • Self-care • Techniques of physical assessments • Cultural awareness/cultural influences on health • Religious and spiritual influences on health

TABLE 1-4 Maslow's Hierarchy of Needs

Need	Definition	Nursing Implications
Physiologic	Biologic needs for food, shelter, water, sleep, oxygen, sexual expression	The priority biologic need is breathing (i.e., an open airway). Review Table 1-3, which lists activities associated with physiologic integrity. If you were asked to identify the *most important* action, you would identify needs associated with physiologic integrity (e.g., providing an open airway) as the most important nursing action.
Safety	Avoiding harm; attaining security, order, and physical safety	Review Table 1-3, which lists the activities associated with a safe and effective care environment. Ensuring that the client's environment is safe is a priority (e.g., teaching an older client to remove throw rugs that pose a safety hazard when ambulating would have a greater priority than teaching him or her how to use a walker). The first priority is safety, then coping skills.
Love and belonging Esteem and recognition	Giving and receiving affection; companionship; and identification with a group Self-esteem and respect of others; success in work; prestige	Although these needs are important (described in Table 1-3), they are less important than physiologic or safety needs. For example, it is more important for a client to have an open airway and a safe environment for ambulating than it is to assist him or her to become part of a support group. However, assisting the client in becoming a part of a support group would have higher priority than assisting him or her in developing self-esteem. The sense of belonging would come first, and such a sense might help in developing self-esteem.
Self-actualization Aesthetic	Fulfillment of unique potential Search for beauty and spiritual goals	It is important to understand the last two needs in Maslow's hierarchy. They could deal with client needs associated with health promotion and maintenance, such as continued growth and development and self-care, as well as those associated with psychosocial integrity. However, you will probably not be asked to prioritize needs at this level. Remember, it is the goal of the Council to ensure *safe* nursing practice, and such practice does not usually deal with the client's self-actualization or aesthetic needs.

B. The candidate is presented with a test item and possible answers.

C. If the candidate answers the question correctly, a slightly more difficult item will follow, and the level of difficulty will increase with each item until the candidate misses an item.

D. If the candidate misses an item, a slightly less difficult item will follow, and the level of difficulty will decrease with each item until the candidate has answered an item correctly.

E. This process will continue until the candidate has achieved a definite pass or a definite fail score. There will be no borderline pass or fail scores because the adaptive testing method determines the candidate's level of performance before she or he has finished the examination.

F. The fewest number of items a candidate can answer to complete the examination is 75; 15 of them will be pilot items and will not count toward the pass or fail score; 60 of them will determine the candidate's score.

G. The number of the item the candidate is currently answering will appear on the upper-right area of the screen.

H. When the candidate has answered enough items to determine a definite pass or fail score, a message will appear on the screen notifying the candidate that he or she has completed the examination.

I. The most number of items a candidate can answer is 265, and the longest amount of time the candidate can take to complete the examination is 6 hours.

J. Candidates will have up to 6 hours to complete the NCLEX-RN examination; total examination time includes a short tutorial, two preprogrammed optional breaks, and any unscheduled breaks they may take. The first optional break is offered after 2 hours of testing. The second optional break is offered after 3.5 hours of testing. The computer will automatically tell candidates when these scheduled breaks begin.
1. All breaks count against testing time.
2. When candidates take breaks, they must leave the testing room, and they will be required to provide a palm vein scan before and after the breaks.

K. If a candidate has not obtained a pass/fail score at the end of the 6 hours and has not completed all 265 items in the 6-hour limit but has answered all of the last 60 questions presented correctly, he or she will pass the examination.

L. If a candidate has not obtained a pass/fail score at the end of the 6 hours, has not completed all 265 items in the 6-hour limit, and has not answered correctly all of the last 60 questions presented, he or she will fail the examination.

M. A specific passing score is recommended by the Council. All states require the same score to pass, so that if you pass in one state, you are eligible to practice nursing in any other state. However, states do differ in their requirements regarding the number of times a candidate can take the NCLEX-RN.

N. Although the Council has the ability to determine a candidate's score at the time of completion of the examination, it has been decided that it would be best for candidates to receive their scores from their individual Board of Nurse Examiners. The Council does not want the testing center to be in a position of having to deal with candidates' reactions to scores, nor does the Council want those waiting to take their examinations to be influenced by such reactions.

O. You must answer each question in order to proceed. You cannot omit a question or return to an item presented earlier. There is no going back; this works in your favor!

P. The examination is written at a tenth-grade reading level.

Q. There is no penalty for guessing; with four choices, you have a 25% chance of guessing the correct answer.

HESI Hint • One or more of the choices are likely to be very wrong. You usually will be able to rule out two of the four choices rather quickly. Reread the question and choices again if necessary. Ask yourself which choice answers the question being asked. Even if you have absolutely no idea what the correct answer is, you will have a 50/50 chance of guessing the right answer if you follow this process. Your first response will provide an educated guess and will usually be the correct answer. Go with your gut response!

Pace yourself from the beginning of the test. Allow approximately 1.5 minutes per question.

The NCSBN Candidate Bulletin is available at http://www.ncsbn.org.

Then select: Examinations/Candidates/Basic Information/Bulletin.

Examination Item Formats

A. A number of different types of examination items are presented on the NCLEX-RN examination. The majority of the questions are multiple-choice items with four answers from which the candidate is asked to choose one correct answer. Other format (item types) include:
   1. Multiple-response items require the candidate to select one or more responses. The item will instruct the candidate to choose/select all that apply.
   2. Fill-in-the-blank questions require the candidate to calculate the answer and type in numbers. A drop-down calculator is provided.
   3. Hot-spot items require the candidate to identify an area on a picture or graph and click on the area.
   4. Chart or exhibit formats present a chart or exhibit that the candidate must read to be able to solve the problem.
   5. Drag-and-drop items require a candidate to rank order or move options to provide the correct order of actions or events.
   6. Audio format items require the candidate to listen to an audio clip using headphones and then select the correct option that applies to the audio clip.
   7. Graphic format items require the candidate to choose the correct graphic option in response to the question.

B. There is no set percentage of alternative items on the NCLEX-RN examination. All examination items are scored either right or wrong. There is no partial credit in scoring any examination questions.

Gentle Reminders of General Principles

Take care of yourself. Follow these golden rules for NCLEX-RN success.

A. Eat well: Consume lots of fresh fruits, vegetables, and lean protein and avoid high-fat foods.

B. Sleep well: Get a good night's sleep the night before the test. This is not the time to cram or to party. You have done your job. Now enjoy the process.

C. Eliminate alcohol and other mind-altering drugs: It goes without saying that such substances can inhibit your performance on the examination.

D. Schedule study time: Between now and the examination, review nursing content, focusing on areas that you have identified as your weak points when taking the practice tests (review your computer scoring sheets). Use a study schedule to block out the time needed for study. Then be good to yourself, and use that blocked time for yourself: study.

E. Be prepared: Assemble all necessary materials the night before the examination (admission ticket, directions to the testing center, identification, money for lunch, glasses or contacts).
   1. Approved items: Candidates are allowed to bring only identification forms into the testing room. Watches, candy, chewing gum, food, drinks, purses, wallets, pens, pencils, beepers, cellular phones, Post-It notes, study materials or aids, and calculators are not allowed. A test administrator will provide each candidate with an erasable note board that may be replaced as needed while testing. Candidates may not take their own note boards, scratch paper, or writing instruments into the examination. A calculator on the computer screen will be available for use.
   2. Allow plenty of time: Arrive early; it is better to be early than late. Allow for traffic jams and so forth. The candidate may want to consider spending the night in a hotel or motel near the testing center the night before the examination.
   3. Dress comfortably: Dress in layers so that you can take off a sweater or jacket if you become too warm or wear it if you become too cold.

F. Avoid negative people: From now until you have completed the examination, stay away from those who share their anxieties with you or project their insecurities onto you. Sometimes this is a fellow classmate or even your best friend. The person will still be there when the examination is over. Right now you need to take care of yourself. Avoid the negative; look for the positive.

G. Do not discuss the examination: Avoid talking about the examination during breaks and while waiting to take the examination.

H. Avoid distractions: Take earplugs with you and use them if you find that those around you are distracting you, such as, rattling paper or getting up to leave the examination.

I. Think positively: Use the affirmation "I am successful." Obtain a relaxation and affirmation tape and use it at your hour of sleep PRN (as needed) from now until you take the examination. Use the relaxation tape at night (not on the way to the examination or during breaks while taking the examination; you might fall asleep!). Use the affirmation on the way to the examination or any time you feel the need to boost your confidence. Think, "I have the knowledge to successfully complete the NCLEX-RN."

> **HESI Hint** • The night before taking the NCLEX-RN, allow only 30 minutes of study time. This 30-minute period should be designated for review of test-taking strategies only. Practice these strategies with various practice test items if you wish (for 30 minutes only; do not take an entire test). Spend the night before the examination doing something you enjoy, something that promotes stress reduction, something that does not involve alcohol or other mind-altering drugs. Only you can identify the special something that will work for you. Remember, you can be successful!

For more review, go to **http://evolve.elsevier.com/ HESI/RN** for HESI's online study examinations.

2 LEADERSHIP AND MANAGEMENT

Legal Aspects of Nursing

Laws Governing Nursing

A. Nurse Practice Acts provide the laws that control and regulate the nursing practice in each state to protect the public from harm. Mandatory Nurse Practice Acts authorize that, under the law, only licensed professionals can practice nursing. All states now have mandatory Nurse Practice Acts. Laws affecting nursing practice vary from state to state.

B. Nurse Practice Acts govern the nurse's responsibility in making assignments. Each state sets its own educational and examination requirements.
1. Assignments should be commensurate with the nursing personnel's educational preparation, skills, experience, and knowledge.
2. The nurse should supervise the care provided by nursing personnel for which he or she is administratively responsible.
3. Sterile or invasive procedures should be assigned to or supervised by a registered nurse (RN).
4. Documentation is a legal and professional requirement that includes electronic medical records and other notations placed in a client's medical record.

Torts (Violation of Client's Private Right)

Description: An act involving injury or damage to another (except breach of contract) resulting in civil liability (i.e., the victim can sue) instead of criminal liability (see Crime).

Unintentional Torts

A. Negligence and malpractice
1. Negligence: Performing an act that a reasonable and prudent person would not perform. The measure of negligence is "reasonableness" (i.e., would a reasonable and prudent nurse act in the same manner under the same circumstances?). That is, did the nurse provide care that did not meet the standard?
2. Malpractice: Negligence by professional personnel (e.g., professional misconduct or unreasonable lack of skill in carrying out professional duties). Malpractice is a negligent act performed by an individual in a professional role that results in an INJURY.

B. Four elements are necessary to prove malpractice; if any one element is missing, malpractice cannot be proved.
1. Duty: Obligation to use due care (what a reasonable, prudent nurse would do); failure to care for and/or to protect others against unreasonable risk. The nurse must *anticipate* foreseeable risks. Example: If a floor has water on it, the nurse is responsible for anticipating the risk for a client's falling.
2. Breach of duty: Failure to perform according to the established standard of conduct in providing nursing care.
3. Injury/damages: Failure to meet the standard of care, which causes actual injury or damage to the client (physical injury). Neither emotional nor mental injury is enough to prove malpractice, either physical or mental.
4. Causation: A connection exists between conduct and the resulting injury, referred to as *proximate cause* or *remoteness of damage.*

C. Hospital policies provide a guide for nursing actions. They are not laws, but courts generally rule against nurses who have violated the employer's policies. Hospitals can be liable for poorly formulated or poorly implemented policies. Nurses can avoid negligence and malpractice by following the organization policies and procedures.

D. Incident reports alert administration to possible liability claims and the need for investigation; they do not protect against legal action being taken for negligence or malpractice.

E. Examples of negligence or malpractice:
1. Burning a client with a heating pad
2. Leaving sponges or instruments in a client's body after surgery
3. Performing incompetent assessments
4. Failing to heed warning signs of shock or impending myocardial infarction
5. Ignoring signs and symptoms of bleeding
6. Forgetting to give a medication or giving the wrong medication

Intentional Torts

A. Assault and battery
1. Assault: Mental or physical threat (e.g., forcing [without touching] a client to take a medication or treatment)
2. Battery: Actual and intentional touching of one another, with or without the intent to do harm (e.g., hitting or striking a client). If a mentally competent adult is forced to have a treatment he or she has refused, battery occurs.
B. Invasion of privacy: Encroachment or trespassing on another's body or personality
1. False imprisonment: Confinement without authorization
2. Exposure of a person: Exposure or discussion of a client's case. After death, a client has the right to be unobserved, excluded from unwarranted operations, and protected from unauthorized touching of the body.
3. Defamation: Divulgence of privileged information or communication (e.g., through charts, conversations, or observations)
C. Fraud: Illegal activity and willful and purposeful misrepresentation that could cause, or has caused, loss or harm to a person or property. Examples of fraud include:
1. Presenting false credentials for the purpose of entering nursing school, obtaining a license, or obtaining employment (e.g., falsification of records)
2. Describing a myth regarding a treatment (e.g., telling a client that a placebo has no side effects and will cure the disease, or telling a client that a treatment or diagnostic test will not hurt, when indeed pain is involved in the procedure)

Crime

A. An act contrary to a criminal statute. Crimes are wrongs punishable by the state and committed against the state, with intent usually present. The nurse remains bound by all criminal laws.
B. Commission of a crime involves the following behaviors:
1. A person commits a deed contrary to criminal law.
2. A person omits an act when there is a legal obligation to perform such an act (e.g., refusing to assist with the birth of a child if such a refusal results in injury to the child).
3. Criminal conspiracy occurs when two or more persons agree to commit a crime.
4. Assisting or giving aid to a person in the commission of a crime makes that person equally guilty of the offense (awareness must be present that the crime is being committed).
5. Ignoring a law is not usually an adequate defense against the commission of a crime (e.g., a nurse who sees another nurse taking narcotics from the unit supply and ignores this observation is not adequately defended against committing a crime).

6. Assault is justified for self-defense. However, to be justified, only enough force can be used to maintain self-protection.
7. Search warrants are required before searching a person's property.
8. It is a crime *not* to report suspected child abuse (i.e., the nurse's legal responsibility is to report suspected child abuse).

Nursing Practice and the Law

Psychiatric Nursing

A. Civil procedures: Methods used to protect the rights of psychiatric clients.
B. Voluntary admission: Client admits himself or herself to an institution for treatment and retains civil rights.
C. Involuntary admission: Someone other than the client applies for the client's admission to an institution.
1. This requires certification by a health care provider that the person is a danger to self or others. (Depending on the state, one or two health care provider certifications are required.)
2. Individuals have the right to a legal hearing within a certain number of hours or days.
3. Most states limit commitment to 90 days.
4. Extended commitment is usually no longer than 1 year.
D. Emergency admission: Any adult may apply for emergency detention of another. However, medical or judicial approval is required to detain anyone for observation, diagnosis and treatment for those clients whose behavior is indicative of mental illness manifested in behavior that poses a danger to themselves or others. Length of admission time is based on state laws.
1. A person held against his or her will can file a writ of habeas corpus to try to get the court to hear the case and release the person.
2. The court determines the sanity and alleged unlawful restraint of a person.
E. Legal and civil rights of hospitalized clients
1. The right to wear their own clothes and to keep personal items and a reasonable amount of cash for small purchases
2. The right to have individual storage space for one's own use
3. The right to see visitors daily
4. The right to have reasonable access to a telephone and the opportunity to have private conversations by telephone
5. The right to receive and send mail (unopened)
6. The right to refuse shock treatments and lobotomy
F. Competency hearing: Legal hearing that is held to determine a person's ability to make responsible decisions about self, dependents, or property
1. Persons declared incompetent have the legal status of a minor—they cannot:
a. Vote
b. Make contracts or wills

c. Drive a car

d. Sue or be sued

e. Hold a professional license

2. A guardian is appointed by the court for an incompetent person. Declaring a person incompetent can be initiated by the state or the family.

G. Insanity: Legal term meaning the accused is not criminally responsible for the unlawful act committed because he or she is mentally ill.

H. Inability to stand trial: Person accused of committing a crime is not mentally capable of standing trial. He or she:

1. Cannot understand the charge against himself or herself

2. Must be sent to the psychiatric unit until legally determined to be competent for trial

3. Once mentally fit, must stand trial and serve any sentence, if convicted

---

HESI Hint • Often an NCLEX-RN® question asks who should explain and describe a surgical procedure to the client, including both complications and the expected results of the procedure. The answer is the health care provider. Remember that it is the nurse's responsibility to be sure that the operative permit is signed and is on the chart. It is not the nurse's responsibility to explain the procedure to the client. The nurse must document that the client was given the information and agreed to it.

Patient Identification

A. The Joint Commission has implemented new patient identification requirements to meet safety goals (http://www.jointcommission.org/standards_information/npsgs.aspx).

B. Use at least two patient identifiers. Ask the client to tell you his or her name and date of birth (DOB) whenever taking blood samples, administering medications, or administering blood products.

C. The patient room number may *not* be used as a form of identification.

Surgical Permit

A. Consent to operate (surgical permit) must be obtained before any surgical procedure, however minor it might be.

B. Legally, the surgical permit must be:

1. Written

2. Obtained voluntarily

3. Explained to the client (i.e., informed consent must be obtained)

C. Informed consent means the procedure and treatment or operation has been fully explained to the client, including:

1. Possible complications, risks, and disfigurements

2. Removal of any organs or parts of the body

3. Benefits and expected results

D. Surgery permits must be obtained as follows:

1. They must be witnessed by an authorized person, such as the health care provider or a nurse.

2. They protect the client against unsanctioned surgery, and they protect the health care provider and surgeon, hospital, and hospital staff against possible claims of unauthorized operations.

3. Adults and emancipated minors may sign their own operative permits if they are mentally competent.

4. Permission to operate on a minor child or an incompetent or unconscious adult must be obtained from a legally responsible parent or guardian. The person granting permission to operate on an adult who lacks capacity (e.g., advanced Alzheimer disease or unconscious adult) to understand information about the proposed treatment must be identified in a Durable Power of Attorney or an Advance Health Directive.

Consent

A. The law does not *require* written consent to perform medical treatment.

1. Treatment can be performed if the client has been fully informed about the procedure.

2. Treatment can be performed if the client voluntarily consents to the procedure.

3. If informed consent cannot be obtained (e.g., client is unconscious) and immediate treatment is required to save life or limb, the emergency laws can be applied. (See the subsequent section, Good Samaritan Act.)

B. Verbal or written consent

1. When verbal consent is obtained, a notation should be made.

a. It describes in detail how and why verbal consent was obtained.

b. It is placed in the client's record or chart.

c. It is witnessed and signed by two persons.

2. Verbal or written consent can be given by:

a. Alert, coherent, or otherwise competent adults

b. A parent or legal guardian

c. A person in loco parentis (a person standing in for a parent with a parent's rights, duties, and responsibilities) in cases of minors or incompetent adults

C. Consent of minors

1. Minors 14 years of age and older must agree to treatment along with their parents or guardians.

2. Emancipated minors can consent to treatment themselves. Be aware that the definition of an emancipated minor may change from state to state.

Emergency Care

A. Good Samaritan Act: Protects health care providers against malpractice claims for care provided in emergency situations (e.g., the nurse gives aid at the scene to an automobile accident victim).

B. A nurse is required to perform in a "reasonable and prudent manner."

HESI Hint • Often questions are asked regarding the Good Samaritan Act, which is the means of protecting a nurse when she or he is performing emergency care.

Prescriptions and Health Care Providers

A. A nurse is required to obtain a prescription (order) to carry out medical procedures from a health care provider.
B. Although verbal telephone prescriptions should be avoided, the nurse should follow the agency's policy and procedures. Failure to follow such rules could be considered negligence. The Joint Commission requires that organizations implement a process for taking verbal or telephone orders that includes a read-back of critical values. The employee receiving the prescription should write the verbal order or critical value on the chart or record it in the computer and then read back the order or value to the health care provider.
C. If a nurse questions a health care provider's (e.g., physician, advanced practice RN, physician's assistant, dentist) prescription because he or she believes that it is wrong (e.g., the wrong dosage was prescribed for a medication), the nurse should do the following:
   1. Inform the health care provider.
   2. Record that the health care provider was informed and record the health care provider's response to such information.
   3. Inform the nursing supervisor.
   4. Refuse to carry out the prescription.
D. If the nurse believes that a health care provider's prescription was made with poor judgment (e.g., the nurse believes the client does not need as many tranquilizers as the health care provider prescribed), the nurse should:
   1. Record that the health care provider was notified and that the prescription was questioned
   2. Carry out the prescription because nursing judgment cannot be substituted for a health care provider's judgment
E. If a nurse is asked to perform a task for which he or she has not been prepared educationally (e.g., obtain a urine specimen from a premature infant by needle aspiration of the bladder) or does not have the necessary experience (e.g., a nurse who has never worked in labor and delivery is asked to perform a vaginal examination and determine cervical dilation), the nurse should do the following:
   1. Inform the health care provider that he or she does not have the education or experience necessary to carry out the prescription.
   2. Refuse to carry out the prescription.

> **HESI Hint** • If the nurse carries out a health care provider's prescription for which he or she is not prepared and does not inform the health care provider of his or her lack of preparation, the nurse is solely liable for any damages.
>
> If the nurse informs the health care provider of his or her lack of preparation in carrying out a prescription and carries out the prescription anyway, the nurse *and* the health care provider are liable for any damages.

F. The nurse cannot, without a health care provider's prescription, alter the amount of drug given to a client. For example, if a health care provider has prescribed pain medication in a certain amount and the client's pain is not, in the nurse's judgment, severe enough to warrant the dosage prescribed, the nurse cannot reduce the amount without first checking with the health care provider. Remember, nursing judgment cannot be substituted for medical judgment.

> **HESI Hint** • Assignments are often tested on the NCLEX-RN. The Nurse Practice Acts of each state govern policies related to making assignments. Usually, when determining who should be assigned to do a sterile dressing change, for example, a licensed nurse should be chosen—that is, an RN or licensed practical nurse (LPN) who has been checked off on this procedure.

Restraints

A. Clients may be restrained only under the following circumstances:
   1. In an emergency
   2. For a limited time
   3. For the purpose of protecting the client or others from injury or from harm
B. Nursing responsibilities with regard to restraints
   1. The nurse must notify the health care provider immediately that the client has been restrained.
   2. It is required and imperative that the nurse accurately document the facts and the client's behavior leading to restraint.
C. When restraining a client, the nurse should do the following:
   1. Use restraints (physical or chemical) after exhausting all reasonable alternatives.
   2. Apply the restraints correctly and in accordance with facility policies and procedures.
   3. Check frequently to see that the restraints do not impair circulation or cause pressure sores or other injuries.
   4. Allow for nutrition, hydration, and stimulation at frequent intervals.
   5. Remove restraints as soon as possible.
   6. Document the need for and application, monitoring, and removal of restraints.
   7. Never leave a restrained person alone.

> **HESI Hint** • Restraints of any kind may constitute false imprisonment. Especially if there is no documentation indicating specific reasons to prevent harm to the client or others.
>
> Freedom from unlawful restraint is a basic human right and is protected by law.
>
> Use of restraints must fall within guidelines specified by state law and hospital policy.

Health Insurance Portability and Accountability Act of 1996

Congress passed the Health Insurance Portability and Accountability Act of 1996 (HIPAA) to create a national patient-record privacy standard.

A. HIPAA privacy rules pertain to health care providers, health plans, and health clearinghouses and their business partners who engage in computer-to-computer transmission of health care claims, payment and remittance, benefit information, and health plan eligibility information and who disclose personal health information that specifically identifies an individual and is transmitted electronically, in writing, or verbally.

B. Patient privacy rights are of key importance. Patients must provide written approval of the disclosure of any of their health information for almost any purpose. Health care providers must offer specific information to patients that explains how their personal health information will be used. Patients must have access to their medical records, and they can receive copies of them and request that changes be made if they identify inaccuracies.

C. Health care providers who do not comply with HIPAA regulations or make unauthorized disclosures risk civil and criminal liability.

D. For further information, use this link to the Department of Health and Human Services (DHHS) website, Office of Civil Rights, which contains frequently asked questions about HIPAA standards for privacy of individually identifiable health information: http://aspe.hhs.gov/admnsimp/final/pvcguide1.htm.

Review of Legal Aspects of Nursing

1. What types of procedures should be assigned to professional nurses?
2. Negligence is measured by reasonableness. What question might the nurse ask when determining such reasonableness?
3. List the four elements that are necessary to prove malpractice (professional negligence).
4. Define an *intentional tort*, and give one example.
5. Differentiate between voluntary and involuntary admission.
6. List five activities a person who is declared incompetent cannot perform.
7. Name three legal requirements of a surgical permit.
8. Who may give consent for medical treatment?
9. What law protects the nurse who provides care or gives aid in an emergency situation?
10. What actions should the nurse take if he or she questions a health care provider's prescription—that is, believes the prescription is wrong?
11. Describe the nurse's legal responsibility when asked to perform a task for which he or she is unprepared.
12. Describe nursing care of the restrained client.
13. Describe six patient rights guaranteed under HIPAA regulations that nurses must be aware of in practice.

Answers to Review

1. Sterile or invasive procedures
2. Would a reasonable and prudent nurse act in the same manner under the same circumstances?
3. Duty: Failure to protect client against unreasonable risk. Breach of duty: Failure to perform according to established standards. Causation: A connection exists between conduct of the nurse and the resulting damage. Damages: Damage is done to the client, whether physical or mental.
4. Conduct causing damage to another person in a *willful* or *intentional* way *without* just cause. Example: Hitting a client out of anger, not in a manner of self-protection.
5. Voluntary: Client admits self to an institution for treatment and retains his or her civil rights; he or she may leave at any time. Involuntary: Someone other than the client applies for the client's admission to an institution (a relative, a friend, or the state); requires certification by one or two health care providers that the person is a danger to self or others; the person has a right to a legal hearing (habeas corpus) to try to be released, and the court determines the justification for holding the person.
6. Vote, make contracts or wills, drive a car, sue or be sued, hold a professional license
7. Voluntary, informed, written
8. Alert, coherent, or otherwise competent adults; a parent or legal guardian; a person in loco parentis of minors or incompetent adults
9. The Good Samaritan Act
10. Inform the health care provider; record that the health care provider was informed and the health care provider's response to such information; inform the nursing supervisor; refuse to carry out the prescription.

Continued

Answers to Review—cont'd

11. Inform the health care provider or person asking the nurse to perform the task that he or she is unprepared to carry out the task; refuse to perform the task.
12. Apply restraints properly; check restraints frequently to see that they are not causing injury and *record* such monitoring; remove restraints as soon as possible; use restraints *only* as a last resort.
13. A patient must give written consent before health care providers can use or disclose personal health information; health care providers must give patients notice about providers' responsibilities regarding patient con-

fidentiality; patients must have access to their medical records; providers who restrict access must explain why and must offer patients a description of the complaint process; patients have the right to request that changes be made in their medical records to correct inaccuracies; health care providers must follow specific tracking procedures for any disclosures made that ensure accountability for maintenance of patient confidentiality; patients have the right to request that health care providers restrict the use and disclosure of their personal health information, although the provider may decline to do so.

Leadership and Management

Description: Nurses act in both leadership and management roles.
A. A leader is an individual who influences people to accomplish goals.
B. A manager is an individual who works to accomplish the goals of the organization.
C. A nurse manager acts to achieve the goals of safe, effective client care within the overall goals of a health care facility.

Skills of the Nurse Manager

Refer to Box 2-1.

Communication Skills

Assertive communication:
A. Includes clearly defined goals and expectations
B. Includes verbal and nonverbal messages that are congruent
C. Is critical to the directing aspect of management

> **HESI Hint** • Assertive communication starts with "I need" rather than with "You must."

> **HESI Hint** • Motivation comes from within an individual. A nurse leader can provide an environment that will promote motivation through positive feedback, respect, and seeking input. Look for responses that demonstrate these behaviors.

> **HESI Hint** • Workplace violence, substance abuse, bullying, social media, and inappropriate nurse–client relationships are areas of concern that nurse managers must provide systems in place to educate staff for heightened awareness of common behaviors associated with the items comentioned, as well as providing mechanisms for reporting any of these items.

BOX 2-1 *Skills and Characteristics of the Nurse Manager*

Skills of the Nurse Manager	Characteristics of the Nurse Manager
Communication Act as a liaison between clients and others. Engage in conflict resolution as needed with staff.	Authority
Organization Plan overall strategies to address client problems. Review management outcomes.	Accountability
Delegation Identify roles/responsibilities of health care team members.	Responsibility
Supervision Supervise care provided by others (e.g., LPN/VN [vocational nurse], assistive personnel, other RNs).	Leadership
Critical Thinking Serve as resource person to other staff.	Commitment to quality

> **HESI Hint** • NCLEX-RN questions often include examples of nursing interventions that do or do not demonstrate these skills and characteristics.

Classic Leadership Styles	Behavior Associated with Leadership Styles
Democratic (participative)	Assertive
Authoritarian (autocratic)	Aggressive
Laissez-faire (permissive)	Passive

> **HESI Hint** • Effective leadership involves assertive management skills. Look for responses that demonstrate that the nurse is using assertive communication skills.

Organizational Skills

Organizational skills encompass management of:
A. People
B. Time
C. Supplies

Delegation Skills

A. The authority, accountability, and responsibility of the RN are based on the state Nurse Practice Act, standards of professional practice, the policies of the health care organization, and ethical-legal models of behavior.
B. Definitions
   1. *Delegation* is the process by which duties, tasks, and coordination of care are transferred to ancillary and assistive personnel, as well as other nurses. The nurse maintains responsibility and accountability for the quality and quantity of supervision in regard to delegated assignments.
   2. *Responsibility* is the obligation to complete a task.
   3. *Authority* is the right to act or command the actions of others.
   4. *Accountability* is the ability and willingness to assume responsibility for actions and related consequences.
C. The nurse transfers responsibility and authority for the completion of delegated tasks, but the nurse retains accountability for the delegation process. This accountability involves ensuring that the Five Rights of Delegation have been achieved.
D. Five Rights of Delegation (as defined by the National Council of State Boards of Nursing)
   1. Right task: Is this a task that can be delegated by a nurse?
   2. Right circumstance: Considering the setting and available resources, should delegation take place?
   3. Right person: Is the task being delegated by the right person to the right individual?
   4. Right direction/communication: Is the nurse providing a clear, concise description of the task, including limits and expectations?
   5. Right supervision: Once the task has been delegated, is appropriate supervision maintained?

> **HESI Hint** • Delegating to the right person requires that the nurse be aware of the qualifications of the delegatee: appropriate education, training, skills, experience, and demonstrated and documented competence.

> **HESI Hint** • Unlicensed assistive personnel (UAP) generally do not perform invasive or sterile procedures.

> **HESI Hint** • RNs should give clear instructions—be specific, communicating the objectives of the delegated task and the expected results.
> Remember that even though a task may be delegated under law and facility policy, you, the nurse, are responsible for its outcome.

Supervision Skills

A. Direction/guidance
   1. Clear, concise, specific directions
   2. Expected outcome
   3. Time frame
   4. Limitations
   5. Verification of assignment
B. Evaluation/monitoring
   1. Frequent check-in
   2. Open communication lines
   3. Achievement of outcome
C. Follow-up
   1. Communication of evaluation findings to the LPN or UAP and other appropriate personnel
   2. Need for teaching or guidance

> **HESI Hint** • The RN is accountable for adhering to the three basic aspects of supervision when delegating to other health care personnel, such as LPNs, graduate nurses, inexperienced nurses, student nurses, and UAP.

> **HESI Hint** • Remember the nursing process: Assessments, analysis, diagnosis, planning, and evaluation (any activity requiring nursing judgment) may not be delegated to UAP. Delegated activities fall within the implementation phase of the nursing process.

Critical Thinking Skills

A. Nurses are accustomed to using the nursing process as the model for problem solving in client care situations.
B. Use this model to think critically in leadership and management situations.
   1. Assessment: What are the needs or problems?
   2. Analysis: What has the highest priority?
   3. Planning
      a. What outcomes and goals must be accomplished?
      b. What are the available resources?
         1. Nursing staff
         2. Interdisciplinary team members
         3. Time
         4. Equipment and supplies
         5. Space (client rooms, home environment, etc.)
   4. Implementation
      a. Communicating expectations
      b. Is documentation complete?
   5. Evaluation
      a. Were the desired outcomes achieved?
      b. Was safe, effective care provided?

> **HESI Hint** • Priorities often center on which client the nurse should assess first. Ask yourself: Which client is the most critically ill and unstable? Which client is most likely to experience a significant change in condition? Which client requires assessment by an RN?

HESI Hint • The nurse manager must analyze all the desired outcomes involved when assigning rooms for clients or assigning client care responsibilities. A client with an infection should not be assigned to share a room with a surgical or immunocompromised client. A nurse's client care management should be based on the nurse's abilities, the individual client's needs, and the needs of the entire group of assigned clients. Safety and infection control are high priorities.

Skills Needed by Change Agents

A. Problem solving
B. Decision making
C. Interpersonal relationships (Table 2-1)

Nurse Leaders and Managers as Collaborators

A. Interprofessional health care teams require:
  1. Shared goals, commitment, and accountability
  2. Open and clear communication
  3. Respect for the expertise of all team members

TABLE 2-1 Nurse Leaders and Managers as Change Agents

Lewin's Change Theory	Nurses Act as Change Agents, which Involves:
Unfreezing	Initiation of a change
Moving	Motivation toward a change
Refreezing	Implementation of a change

B. Critical pathways:
  1. Are interprofessional plans of care
  2. Are used for diagnoses and care that can be standardized
  3. Are guides to track client progress
  4. Do *not* replace individualized care
C. Case management:
  1. Coordinates care provided by an interprofessional team
  2. Manages resources effectively
  3. Uses critical pathways to organize care
D. Quality assurance:
  1. Involves continuous quality improvement (CQI)/total quality management (TQM)
  2. Is an organized approach to the improvement of:
    a. Outcome achievement
    b. Quality of care provided

HESI Hint • Change causes anxiety. An effective nurse change agent uses problem-solving skills to recognize factors such as anxiety that contribute to resistance to change and uses decision making and interpersonal skills to overcome that resistance. Interventions that demonstrate these skills include seeking input, showing respect, valuing opinions, and building trust.

HESI Hint • The Interprofessional Education Collaborative Expert Panel (IPEC) recommended development of four core competencies for interprofessional collaborative practice. Those competency domains among health care professionals include 1. values/ethics for interprofessional practice; 2. roles/responsibilities; 3. interprofessional communication; and 4. teams and teamwork.

Review of Leadership and Management

1. By what authority may RNs delegate nursing care to others?
2. A UAP may perform care that falls within which component of the nursing process?
3. Which type of communication is necessary to implement a democratic leadership style?
4. What are the five rights of delegation?
5. Which tasks can be delegated to a UAP?
   A. Inserting a Foley catheter
   B. Measuring and recording the client's output through a Foley catheter
   C. Teaching a client how to care for a catheter after discharge
   D. Assessing for symptoms of a urinary tract infection
6. What are the essential steps of effective supervision?
7. Which of the following is an example of assertive communication?
   A. "You need to improve the way you spend your time so that all of your care gets performed."
   B. "I've noticed that many of your clients did not get their care today."
8. Common signs of substance abuse are clients complaining that pain medication does not relieve pain when administered by a certain nurse, frequent inaccuracies of controlled medication counts for a specific nurse, and client reports not taking pain medications but several doses are signed out for that client.
9. Common characteristics of bullying are refusing to work with others, yelling or cursing at peers, making degrading comments, and verbal abuse.
10. Workplace violence contributes to a high staff turnover rate and decline in client care.

Answers to Review

1. State Nurse Practice Act
2. Implementation
3. Assertive communication skills
4. Right task, right circumstance, right person, right direction or communication, and right supervision
5. Delegation is as follows:
    A. Is a sterile invasive procedure and should not be delegated to a UAP
    B. Falls within the implementation phase of the nursing process and does not require nursing judgment. Evaluation of the intake and output (I&O) must be done by the nurse.
    C. Client teaching requires the abilities of a nurse and should not be delegated. The UAP may be instructed to report anything unusual that is observed and any symptoms reported by the client, but this does not replace assessment by the nurse.
    D. Assessment must be performed by the nurse and should not be delegated. The UAP may be instructed to report anything unusual that is observed or any symptoms reported by the client, but this does not replace assessment by the nurse.
6. Direction, evaluation, and follow-up
7. Examples:
    A. This is an aggressive communication, which causes anger, hostility, and a defensive attitude.
    B. Assertive communication begins with "I" rather than "you" and clearly states the problem.

Disaster Nursing

A. The role of the nurse takes place at all three levels of disaster management:
    1. Disaster preparedness
    2. Disaster response
    3. Disaster recovery
B. To achieve effective disaster management:
    1. Organization is the key.
    2. All personnel must be trained.
    3. All personnel must know their roles.

Levels of Prevention in Disaster Management

A. Primary prevention
    1. Participate in the development of a disaster plan.
    2. Train rescue workers in triage and basic first aid.
    3. Educate personnel about shelter management.
    4. Educate the public about the disaster plan and personal preparation for disaster.
B. Secondary prevention
    1. Triage
    2. Treatment of injuries
    3. Treatment of other conditions, including mental health
    4. Shelter supervision
C. Tertiary prevention
    1. Follow-up care for injuries
    2. Follow-up care for psychological problems
    3. Recovery assistance
    4. Prevention of future disasters and their consequences

Triage

A. A French word meaning "to sort or categorize"
B. Goal: Maximize the number of survivors by sorting the injured according to treatable and untreatable victims (Table 2-2).
C. Primary criteria used
    1. Potential for survival
    2. Availability of resources

Nursing Interventions and Roles in Triage

A. Triage duties using a systematic approach such as the simple triage and rapid treatment (START) method (Fig. 2-1)
B. Treatment of injuries
    1. Render first aid for injuries.
    2. Provide additional treatment as needed in definitive care areas.
C. Treatment of other conditions, including mental health
    1. Determine health needs other than injury.
    2. Refer for medical treatment as required.
    3. Provide treatment for other conditions based on medically approved protocols.

Shelter Supervision

A. Coordinate activities of shelter workers.
B. Oversee records of victims admitted and discharged from shelter.
C. Promote effective interpersonal and group interactions among victims in shelter.
D. Promote independence and involvement of victims housed in the shelter.

Bioterrorism

A. Learn the symptoms of illnesses that are associated with exposure to likely biologic and chemical agents.

TABLE 2-2 **Triage Color Code System**

	Red	Yellow	Green	Black
Urgency	Most urgent, first priority	Urgent, second priority	Third priority	Dying or dead
Injury type	Life-threatening injuries	Injuries with systemic effects and complications	Minimal injuries with no systemic complications	Catastrophic injuries
May delay treatment?	No	For 30-60 mins	Several hours	No hope for survival, no treatment

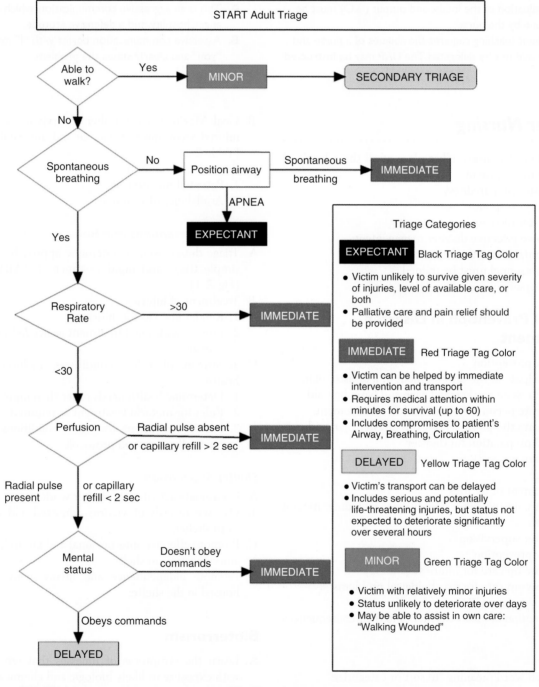

FIGURE 2-1 Simple triage and rapid treatment (START) method for triage. https://chemm.nlm.nih.gov/startadult.htm.

B. Understand that they could appear days or weeks after exposure.

C. Nurses and other health care providers would be the first responders when victims seek medical evaluation after symptoms manifest. First responders are critical in identifying an outbreak, determining the cause of the outbreak, identifying risk factors, and implementing measures to control and minimize the outbreak.

D. Possible agents (Table 2-3)
   1. Biologic agents
      a. Anthrax
      b. Pneumonic plague
      c. Botulism
      d. Smallpox
      e. Inhalation tularemia
      f. Viral hemorrhagic fever
   2. Chemical agents
      a. Biotoxin agents: ricin
      b. Nerve agents: sarin
   3. Radiation

> **HESI Hint** • In a disaster the nurse must consider both the individual and the community.

Nursing Assessment

A. Community-disaster risk assessment
B. Measures to mitigate disaster effect
C. Exposure symptom identification

Analysis (Nursing Diagnosis)

A. *Deficient knowledge (specify)* related to…
B. *Risk for poisoning* related to…
C. *Risk for trauma* related to…
D. *Anxiety* related to…
E. *Fear* related to…
F. *Ineffective community coping* related to…
G. *Risk for posttrauma syndrome* related to…

Nursing Plans and Interventions

A. Participate in development of disaster plan.
B. Educate the public on the disaster plan and personal preparation for disaster.
C. Train rescue workers in triage and basic first aid.
D. Educate personnel on shelter management.
E. Practice triage.
F. Treat injuries and illness.
G. Treat other conditions, including mental health.
H. Supervise shelters.
I. Arrange for follow-up care for injuries.
J. Arrange for follow-up care for psychological problems.
K. Assist in recovery.
L. Work to prevent future disasters and their consequences.

Nursing Management for Ebola

Client Evaluation for Ebola

Recommendations to Health Care Providers

The risk of getting Ebola in the United States is very low, even when working with West African communities in the United States. Ebola is spread by direct contact with blood or body fluids of a person ill with or who has died from Ebola, or a person who has contact with objects like needles that have been contaminated with the virus. It is also possible that Ebola virus can be transmitted through the semen of men who have survived infection.

The Centers for Disease Control and Prevention (CDC) implemented entry screening at five U.S. airports for travelers arriving from Guinea, Liberia, and Sierra Leone. The CDC strongly recommends that travelers from these countries be actively monitored for symptoms by state or local health departments for 21 days after returning from any of these countries.

Recommended Infection Control Measures

Even if travelers were exposed, they are only contagious after they start to have symptoms (for example, fever, severe headache, muscle pain, diarrhea, vomiting, and unexplained bleeding).

Nursing Interventions

Obtain a thorough history, including recent travel from areas where the virus is present. Use personal protective equipment (PPE). Monitor vital signs

Place client in strict isolation for 21 days using special precautions identified by the CDC and state.

People of West African descent are not at more risk than other Americans if they have not recently traveled to the region. Neither ethnic nor racial backgrounds have anything to do with becoming infected with the Ebola virus.

Zika Virus

Transmission of the Zika virus has been reported in many countries making it difficult to determine where the virus is spreading. There have been reports of microcephaly in babies of mothers who had Zika virus while pregnant. As a result, the CDC recommends special precautions for pregnant women. Travel to areas where Zika is spreading is not recommended for pregnant women in any trimester. It is strongly recommended that women who are trying to get pregnant and their male partners discuss travel with their

TABLE 2-3 **Signs, Symptoms, and Treatments of Biologic and Chemical Agents and Radiation**

BIOLOGIC AGENTS

	Anthrax	Pneumonic Plague	Botulism

Agent	• *Bacillus anthracis*
	 • Bacterium that forms spores
	 • Three types:
	  • Cutaneous
	  • Inhalation
	  • Digestive
		• *Yersinia pestis*
		 • Bacterium found in rodents and their fleas
			• *Clostridium botulinum*
			 • Toxin made by a bacterium

Transmission	• Inhalation of powder form • Inhalation of spores from infected animal products (e.g., wool) • Handling of infected animals • Eating undercooked meat from infected animals • Not spreadable from person to person	• Aerosol release into the environment • Respiratory droplets from an infected person (6-ft range) • Untreated bubonic plague sequelae	• Food: a person ingests preformed toxin • Wound: infection by *C. botulinum* that secretes the toxin • Not spreadable from person to person
Incubation period	• Within 7 days (all types) • Inhalation incubation: period extends to 42 days	• 1-6 days	• A few hours to a few days • Foodborne: most commonly 12-36 hrs, but range is 6 hrs to 2 wks
Signs and symptoms	• Cutaneous: sores that develop into painless blisters, then ulcers with black centers • Gastrointestinal: nausea, anorexia, bloody diarrhea, fever, severe stomach pain • Inhalation: cold and flu symptoms, including sore throat, mild fever; muscle aches, cough, chest discomfort, shortness of breath, tiredness, muscle aches	• Fever • Weakness • Rapidly developing pneumonia • Bloody or watery sputum • Nausea, vomiting • Abdominal pain • Without early treatment, will see shock, respiratory failure, and rapid death	• Double and/or blurred vision • Drooping eyelids • Slurred speech • Difficulty swallowing • Descending muscle weakness
Treatment	• Prevention after exposure consists of the use of antibiotics, such as ciprofloxacin, doxycycline, or penicillin, and vaccination • Treatment after infection is usually a 60-day course of antibiotics • Success of treatment after infection depends on the type of anthrax and how soon the treatment begins	• If close contact with infected person and within 7 days of exposure, treatment is with antibiotics prophylactically • Recommended antibiotic treatment within 24 hrs of first symptom; treat for at least 7 days • Oral: tetracyclines, fluoroquinolones • IV: streptomycin or gentamycin	• Antitoxin to reduce severity of disease (most effective when administered early in course of disease) • Supportive care • May require mechanical ventilation
Miscellaneous	• Vaccine available, but not to the general public • Given to those who may be exposed, such as certain members of the U.S. armed forces, laboratory workers, and workers who enter or reenter contaminated areas	• Easily destroyed by sunlight and drying • In air can survive up to 1 hr • No vaccine available	• No vaccine available

	Smallpox	Inhalation Tularemia	Viral Hemorrhagic Fever
Agent	• Variola virus • Orthopoxvirus	• *Francisella tularensis* • Highly infectious bacterium	• Five families of viruses (examples: Ebola, Lassa, dengue, yellow, Marburg) • RNA viruses enveloped in a lipid coating
Transmission	• Aerosol release into the environment • Contact with infected person (direct and prolonged, face to face) • Bodily fluids • Contaminated objects • Air in enclosed settings (rare)	• Insect (usually tick or deerfly) bites • Handling of sick or dead infected animals • Consuming of contaminated food or water • Inhalation of airborne bacterium • Cannot be spread from person to person	• From viral reservoirs such as rodents and arthropods or an animal host; some hosts remain unknown • May be transmitted person to person via close contact or bodily fluids • Objects contaminated by bodily fluids
Incubation period	• 7-17 days	• Most commonly 3-5 days, but may range from 1-14 days	• 2-21 days (varies according to virus)

Signs and symptoms	• High fever
	• Head and body aches
	• Vomiting
	• Rash that progresses to raised bumps and pus-filled blisters that crust and scab, then fall off in about 3 wks; leaving a pitted scar
		• Skin ulcers
		• Swollen and painful lymph glands
		• Sore throat
		• Mouth sores
		• Diarrhea
		• Pneumonia
		• If inhaled: abrupt onset of fever and chills, headache, muscle aches, joint pain, dry cough, and progressive weakness
		• If pneumonia develops: may exhibit chest pain, difficulty breathing, bloody sputum, and respiratory failure
			• Varies by individual virus but common symptoms exist:
			  • Marked fever
			  • Exhaustion
			  • Muscle aches
			  • Loss of strength
			• As disease worsens more severe symptoms emerge:
			  • Bleeding under skin, in internal organs, or from body orifices (mouth, eyes, ears)
			  • Shock
			  • Central nervous system malfunction
			  • Seizures
			  • Coma
			  • Renal failure

Treatment	• No proven treatment • Supportive therapy • Antibiotic treatment for secondary infections • Research being done with antivirals	• Antibiotics for 10-14 days • Oral: tetracyclines, fluoroquinolones • IM or IV: streptomycin, gentamicin	• Supportive therapy • Generally no established cure • May use ribavirin with Lassa fever

Continued

TABLE 2-3 Signs, Symptoms, and Treatments of Biologic and Chemical Agents and Radiation—cont'd

	Smallpox	Inhalation Tularemia	Viral Hemorrhagic Fever
Miscellaneous	• A fragile virus; if aerosolized, dies within 24 hrs (quicker if in sunlight) • Vaccine available	• Can remain alive in water and soil for 2 wks • No vaccine available	• Need a reservoir to survive; humans are not the natural reservoir, but once infected by the host, can transmit to one another • Once geographically restricted to where the host lived; increasing international travel brings outbreaks to places where the viruses have never been seen before • No vaccines available except for Argentine and yellow fever

CHEMICAL AGENTS AND RADIATION

	Ricin	Sarin	Radiation
Agent	• Poison made from waste left over from processing castor beans • Forms include powder, mist, pellet • Dissolved in water or weak acid	• Human-made chemical • Similar to but far more potent than organo-phosphate pesticides • Clear, odorless, and tasteless liquid that can evaporate into a gas and spread into the environment	• Form of energy both human-made and natural
Transmission	• Deliberate act of poisoning by inhalation or injection (need minuscule amount [500 mcg] to kill) • Deliberate act of contamination of food and water supply (requires greater amount to kill) • Cannot be spread from person to person through casual contact	• Agent in air: exposed through skin, eyes, inhalation • Ingested in water or food • Clothing can release sarin for approximately 30 mins after contact	• External exposure comes from the sun or from human-made sources such as x-rays, nuclear bombs, and nuclear disasters (e.g., Chernobyl) • Small quantities in air, water, food, cause internal exposure
Incubation period	• Inhalation: within 8 hrs • Ingestion: <6 hrs	• Vapor: a few seconds • Liquid: a few minutes to 18 hrs	• Exposure is cumulative; low-dose exposure effects may not be seen for several years. • High dose received in a matter of minutes results in acute radiation syndrome (ARS)

Signs and symptoms	• Inhalation: respiratory distress, fever, nausea, tightness in chest, heavy sweating, pulmonary edema, decreased blood pressure, respiratory failure, death • Ingestion: vomiting and diarrhea that becomes bloody, severe dehydration, decreased blood pressure, hallucinations, seizures, hematuria; within several days, liver, spleen, and kidney failure occur • Skin and eyes: redness and pain	• Runny nose • Watery eyes • Pinpoint pupils • Eye pain and blurred vision • Drooling • Excessive sweating • Respiratory symptoms • Diarrhea • Altered level of consciousness (LOC) • Nausea and vomiting • Headache • Decreased or increased blood pressure • In large doses: loss of consciousness, convulsions, paralysis, respiratory failure, death	• ARS: nausea, vomiting, diarrhea; then bone marrow depletion, weight loss, loss of appetite, flulike symptoms, infection, and bleeding • Mild effects include skin reddening • May lead to cancers (with low dose and in those surviving ARS)
Treatment	• Supportive care	• Remove from body as soon as possible • Supportive care • Antidote available: most effective if given as soon as possible after exposure	• Dependent on dose and type of radiation • Supportive care
Miscellaneous	• Stable agent; not affected by very hot or very cold temperatures • Death usually occurs in about 36-72 hrs • If victim survives for 3-5 days, usually recovers • No vaccine available	• A heavy vapor, this agent sinks to low-lying areas • Mildly or moderately exposed people usually recover completely • Severely exposed people usually do not survive • May experience neurologic problems lasting 1-2 wks after exposure	• Survival dependent on dose • Full recovery may take a few weeks to a few years

Note: For further information, go to http://www.bt.cdc.gov/index.asp.
IM, Intramuscular; *IV,* intravenous.

health care provider (HCP) before traveling to areas with Zika since sexual transmission is possible. Men and women should strictly follow steps to prevent mosquito bites while traveling. The Zika virus remains in the blood of an infected person approximately 1 week.

Check the CDC's Zika Travel Information webpage for the most up-to-date travel recommendations.

It is important for a pregnant women to see an HCP if she develops rashes, fever, joint pain or red eyes while traveling or within 2 weeks after traveling to an area with the Zika virus.

Review of Disaster Nursing

1. List the three levels of disaster management.
2. List examples of the three levels of prevention in disaster management.
3. Define *triage*.
4. Identify three bioterrorism agents.
5. Identify three infection control measures for Ebola.
6. Identify the agency to notify when providing care for a client with a suspected diagnosis of Ebola virus.
7. Describe the delayed triage category.
8. Describe travel recommendations for a couple preparing for in vitro fertilization.

Answers to Review

1. Disaster preparedness, disaster response, disaster recovery
2. Primary: Develop plan, train and educate personnel and public; secondary: Triage, treatment-shelter supervision; tertiary: Follow-up, recovery assistance, prevention of future disasters
3. To sort or categorize
4. Anthrax, pneumonic plague, botulism, smallpox, inhalation tularemia, viral hemorrhagic fever, ricin, sarin, radiation
5. Three infection control measures for Ebola include the following:
   A. Place the client in a single-patient room with a private bathroom.
   B. Wear full PPE.
   C. When there are copious amounts of blood and other body fluids, caregivers should wear additional PPE, including double gloves, disposable shoe covers, and leg coverings.
6. Notify appropriate health care providers, supervisors, and the CDC of clients with a suspected diagnosis of Ebola virus.
7. Delayed triage category indicates that the status of a client who has a serious life-threatening injury is not expected to deteriorate significantly in a few hours.
8. Inform couple that the Zika virus is probably transmitted via sexual contact and provide information regarding the possible transmission of the Zika virus resulting in the congenital defect to the fetus. Recommend obtaining information regarding travel from CDC travel line.
   For more review, go to http://evolve.elsevier.com/HESI/RN for HESI's online study examinations.

Client Evaluation Recommendations to Health Care Providers for Management of Clients with Suspected Ebola Virus Infection

Health care providers should be alert for and evaluate suspected clients for Ebola virus infection who have both consistent symptoms and risk factors as follows:

1. Clinical criteria, which include fever of greater than 38.6° C or 101.5° F, and additional symptoms such as severe headache, muscle pain, vomiting, diarrhea, abdominal pain, or unexplained hemorrhage; *and*
2. Epidemiologic risk factors within the pastweeks before the onset of symptoms, such as contact with blood or other body fluids of a client known to have or suspected to have Ebola virus disease (EVD); residence in—or travel to—an area where EVD transmission is active; or direct handling of bats, rodents, or primates from disease-endemic areas. Malaria diagnostics should also be a part of initial testing because it is a common cause of febrile illness in persons with a travel history to the affected countries.

Testing of clients with suspected EVD should be guided by the risk level of exposure, as described here:

CDC recommends testing for all persons with onset of fever within 21 days of having a high-risk exposure. A high-risk exposure includes any of the following:

- Percutaneous or mucous membrane exposure or direct skin contact with body fluids of a person with a confirmed or suspected case of EVD without appropriate PPE
- Laboratory processing of body fluids of suspected or confirmed EVD cases without appropriate PPE or standard biosafety precautions
- Participation in funeral rites or other direct exposure to human remains in the geographic area where the outbreak is occurring without appropriate PPE

For persons with a high-risk exposure but without a fever, testing is recommended only if there are other compatible clinical symptoms present and blood work findings are abnormal (i.e., thrombocytopenia <150,000 cells/μL and/or elevated transaminases) or unknown.

Persons considered to have a low-risk exposure include persons who spent time in a health care facility where EVD clients are being treated (encompassing health care workers who used appropriate PPE, employees not involved in direct client care, or other hospital clients who did not have EVD and their family caretakers), or household members of an EVD client without high-risk exposures as defined earlier. Persons who had direct unprotected contact with bats or primates from EVD-affected countries would also be considered to have a low-risk exposure. Testing is recommended for persons with a low-risk exposure who develop fever with other symptoms and have unknown or abnormal blood work findings. Persons with a low-risk exposure and with fever and abnormal blood work findings in the absence of other symptoms are also recommended for testing. Asymptomatic persons with high- or low-risk exposures should be monitored daily for fever and symptoms for 21 days from the last known exposure and evaluated medically at the first indication of illness.

Persons with no known exposures listed earlier but who have fever with other symptoms and abnormal blood work within 21 days of visiting EVD-affected countries should be considered for testing if no other diagnosis is found. Testing may be indicated in the same clients if fever is present with other symptoms and blood work is abnormal or unknown. Consultation with local and state health departments is recommended.

If testing is indicated, the local or state health department should be immediately notified.

Recommended Infection Control Measures

- **Client placement:** Clients should be placed in a single-client room (containing a private bathroom) with the door closed.
- **Health care provider protection:** Health care providers should wear gloves, gown (fluid resistant or impermeable), shoe covers, eye protection (goggles or face shield), and a facemask. Additional PPE might be required in certain situations (e.g., copious amounts of blood, other body fluids, vomit, or feces present in the environment), including but not limited to double gloving, disposable shoe covers, and leg coverings.
- **Aerosol-generating procedures:** Avoid aerosol-generating procedures. If performing these procedures, PPE should include respiratory protection (N95 filtering face piece respirator or higher), and the procedure should be performed in an airborne isolation room.
- **Environmental infection control:** Diligent environmental cleaning and disinfection and safe handling of potentially contaminated materials is paramount, because blood, sweat, emesis, feces, and other body secretions represent potentially infectious materials. Appropriate disinfectants for Ebola virus and other filo viruses include 10% sodium hypochlorite (bleach) solution or hospital-grade quaternary ammonium or phenolic products. Health care providers performing environmental cleaning and disinfection should wear recommended PPE (described earlier) and consider use of additional barriers (e.g., shoe and leg coverings) if needed. Face protection (face shield or facemask with goggles) should be worn when performing tasks such as liquid waste disposal that can generate splashes. Follow standard procedures per hospital policy and manufacturers' instructions for cleaning and/or disinfection of environmental surfaces, equipment, textiles, laundry, food utensils, and dishware (http://www.cdc.gov/vhf/ebola/hcp/infection-prevention-and-control-recommendations.html).

Respiratory Failure

Acute Respiratory Distress Syndrome (ARDS)

Description: Is a progressive disorder leading to acute respiratory failure. The exchange of oxygen for carbon dioxide in the lungs is inadequate for oxygen consumption and carbon dioxide production within the body's cells. The increased permeability of the alveolar membrane leading to fluid buildup in the alveoli interferes with the the exchange of CO_2 and O_2 at the capillary beds (Figure 3-1).

A. ARDS is characterized by:
1. Hypoxemia that persists even when 100% oxygen is given
2. Decreased pulmonary compliance
3. Dyspnea
4. Non–cardiac-associated bilateral pulmonary edema
5. Dense pulmonary infiltrates on radiography

> **HESI Hint** • ARDS is an unexpected, catastrophic pulmonary complication occurring in a person with no previous pulmonary problems. Clients are critically ill and are managed in an intensive care setting. The mortality rate is high (50%).

There are two categories of acid-base imbalance, respiratory and metabolic. The corrective and compensatory responses to acid-base balance are presented in the following tables and figure. Table 3-1 refers to normal blood gas values while Table 3-2 refers to normal and abnormal compensation. Clinical manifestations of interrupted acid-base balance are presented in Table 3-3.

> **HESI Hint** • Interventions to prevent complications of clients on mechanical ventilation with ARDS:
> • Elevate head of bed (HOB) to at least 30 degrees.
> • Assist with daily awakening ("sedation vacation").
> • Implement a comprehensive oral hygiene program.
> • Implement a comprehensive mobilization program.

B. Clients are initially admitted to the hospital for another illness and are generally critically ill during the process of their hospitalization; the client may develop ARDS as a complication that usually involves mechanical ventilation.

> **HESI Hint** • There appears to be a correlation of an increased risk and mortality rate from ARDS in individuals who have a history of alcohol abuse.

C. No abnormal lung sounds are present on auscultation because the edema of ARDS occurs first in the interstitial spaces, not in the airways.
D. Common causes of respiratory failure include:
1. Exacerbation of chronic obstructive pulmonary disease (COPD)
2. Pneumonia
3. Tuberculosis
4. Contusion
5. Aspiration
6. Inhaled toxins
7. Emboli
8. Drug overdose
9. Fluid overload
10. Disseminated intravascular coagulation (DIC)
11. Shock

Nursing Assessment

A. Dyspnea, hyperpnea, crackles (or rales), wheezing or decreased breath sounds
B. Intercostal retractions or substernal retractions
C. Cyanosis, pallor, mottled skin
D. Hypoxemia: P_{O_2} <50 mm Hg with F_{IO_2} >60%
E. Increasing diminished breath sounds
F. Diffuse pulmonary infiltrates seen on chest radiograph as "white-out" appearance
G. Verbalized anxiety, restlessness, confusion and agitation

Analysis (Nursing Diagnoses)

A. *Impaired gas exchange* related to…
B. *Risk for deficient fluid volume* related to…
C. *Ineffective breathing pattern* related to…

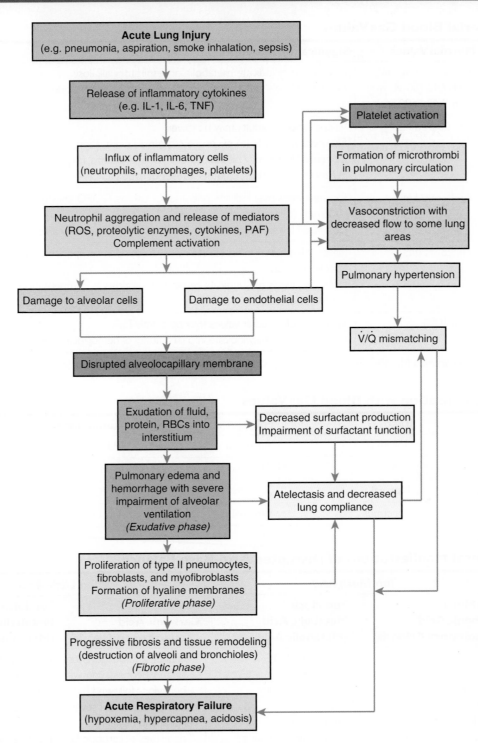

FIGURE 3-1 Clinical Manifestations of Disrupted Acid-Base Balance. (From Giddens JF: *Concepts for nursing practice* (with Pageburst Digital Book Access on VST), ed 2. VitalBook file. St. Louis, 2017, Mosby, 2017. Page 81.)

D. *Risk for injury* related to...
E. *Risk for infection* related to...
F. *Death anxiety* related to ...
G. *Alteration in tissue perfusion* related to...

Nursing Plans and Interventions

A. Position client for maximal lung expansion.
B. Monitor client for signs of hypoxemia and oxygen toxicity

HESI Hint • Suction only when secretions are present.

C. Monitor breath sounds for pneumothorax.
D. Provide emotional support to decrease anxiety and allow ventilator to "work" the lungs.

TABLE 3-1 Arterial Blood Gas Values

Blood Gases	Normal Values	Significant Differences
pH	7.35-7.45 (<age 60) 7.31-7.42 (60-90 y/o) 7.26-7.43 (>90 y/o)	*Elevations may* indicate metabolic or respiratory alkalosis. *Decreased* levels may indicate metabolic or respiratory acidosis.
PaO_2	80-100 mm Hg	Values for older adults may be lower. *Elevations* may indicate excessive oxygen administration. *Decreased* levels may be indicative of asthma, anemia, respiratory distress syndrome, cancer of the lungs, or other causes of hypoxia.
$PaCO_2$	35-45 mm Hg	*Elevated* levels may indicate pneumonia, asthma, COPD, anesthesia effects or use of opioids (respiratory acidosis). *Decreased* levels may indicate hyperventilation/ respiratory alkalosis.
HCO_3	21- 28 mEq/L	*Elevated levels* may indicate respiratory acidosis as compensation for primary metabolic alkalosis. *Decreased* levels may indicate respiratory alkalosis as compensation for primary metabolic acidosis.
SpO_2 Saturation	95%-100%	Values for older adult values may be slightly lower. *Decreased* levels may indicate impaired ability of hemoglobin to release oxygen to tissues.

From Ignatavicius DD, Workman ML: *Medical-surgical nursing: patient-centered collaborative care*, ed 7, St. Louis. 2013, Saunders. Page 557.

TABLE 3-2 Compensation with Blood Gas Values

pH →	Paco₂ →	HCO₃ →	Compensation
Normal	*Abnormal*	*Abnormal*	FULLY
Abnormal	*Abnormal*	*Abnormal*	PARTIAL
Abnormal	Normal	*Abnormal*	UNCOMPENSATED
Abnormal	*Abnormal*	Normal	UNCOMPENSATED

TABLE 3-3 Clinical Manifestations of Disrupted Acid-Base Balance

	Too Much Acid		*Too Little Acid*	
Types of Problem	Too Much Carbonic Acid (Respiratory Acidosis)	Too Much Metabolic Acid (Metabolic Acidosis)	Too Little Carbonic Acid (Respiratory Alkalosis)	Too Little Metabolic Acid (Metabolic Alkalosis)
Common clinical findings	Headache Decreased LOC Hypoventilation (cause of problem) Cardiac dysrhythmias If severe: hypotension	Decreased LOC Hyperventilation (compensatory mechanism) Abdominal pain Nausea and vomiting Cardiac dysrhythmias	Excitation and belligerence, lightheadedness, unusual behaviors; followed by decreased LOC if severe Perioral and digital paresthesias, carpopedal spasm, tetany Diaphoresis Hyperventilation (cause of problem) Cardiac dysrhythmias	Excitation followed by decreased LOC if severe Perioral and digital paresthesias, carpopedal spasm Hypoventilation (compensatory mechanism) Signs of volume depletion and hypokalemia if present
Blood gas findings	Blood gases; pH decreased (or low normal if fully compensated); $PaCO_2$ increased; HCO_3^- increased from compensation	Blood gases; pH decreased (or low normal if fully compensated); $PaCO_2$ decreased from compensation; HCO_3^- decreased	Blood gases; pH increased; $PaCO_2$ decreased; HCO_3^- decreased if compensation	Blood gases; pH increased; $PaCO_2$ increased from compensation; HCO_3^- increased

LOC, Level of consciousness

From Giddens JF: *Concepts for nursing practice* (with Pageburst Digital Book Access on VST), ed 2. VitalBook file. St. Louis, 2017, Mosby. Page 81.

E. Monitor client hemodynamically with essential vital signs and cardiac monitor for alteration in QRS waveforms—peaked T waves (early sign) as seen in hyperkalemia; as potassium levels become higher there is increased P-R intervals, no P waves with ST elevations is indicative of myocardial hypoxia.

F. Monitor arterial blood gases (ABGs) routinely.

G. Monitor vital organ status: central nervous system (CNS), level of consciousness, renal system output, and myocardium (apical pulse, blood pressure [BP]).

H. Monitor fluid and electrolyte balance.

I. Monitor metabolic status through routine laboratory work

J. It is important for the registered nurse to be able to read and interpret what arterial blood gases indicate.
  1. The nurse needs to determine whether the client is in a respiratory or metabolic state.
  2. The respiratory system is the "first responder" if the client's status is not normal, followed by the metabolic "kidneys," which can take up to 24 to 48 hours to compensate for the client's status
  3. Then determine whether the interventions are effective or whether more interventions are needed.
  4. The goal is to get the ABG pH level as close to normal as possible.

> **HESI Hint** • Before drawing a sample for ABGs from the radial artery, perform the Allen test to assess collateral circulation. Make the client's hand blanch by obliterating both the radial and the ulnar pulses. Then release the pressure over the ulnar artery only. If flow through the ulnar artery is good, flushing will be seen immediately. The Allen test is then positive; therefore the radial artery can be used for puncture. If the Allen test is negative, repeat on the other arm. If that test is also negative, seek another site for arterial puncture. The Allen test ensures collateral circulation to the hand if thrombosis of the radial artery should follow the puncture.

Respiratory Failure in Children

Description: Occurs when there is an insufficient exchange of oxygen and carbon dioxide resulting in blood hypoxemia and tissue hypoxia and hypercapnia. Children normally will experience respiratory failure first before cardiac arrest, unless there is a known history of cardiac disease. Obstruction of a major airway such as choking and/or cardiac arrest resulting in respiratory failure is easy to identify. Signs and symptoms of pending respiratory failure in children are not always evident and are more difficult to recognize. Common causes of respiratory failure in children include:

A. Congenital heart disease
B. Respiratory distress syndrome
C. Infection, sepsis
D. Neuromuscular diseases
E. Trauma and burns
F. Aspiration
G. Fluid overload and dehydration
H. Anesthesia and narcotic overdose
I. Structural anomalies resulting in obstruction of the airway.

Nursing Assessment
Refer to Table 3-2.

> **HESI Hint** • Infants and young children grunt during expiration as respiratory distress begins. Grunting is how the body attempts to create a form of "PEEP" (positive end-expiratory pressure) to help keep the alveoli open.

> **HESI Hint**
> • Pco_2 >45 or Po_2 > 60 on 50% O_2 signifies respiratory failure.
> • A child in severe distress should be on 100% O_2.

Review of Respiratory Failure

1. What Pao_2 value indicates respiratory failure in adults?
2. What blood value indicates hypercapnia?
3. Identify the condition that exists when the Pao_2 is less than 50 mm Hg and Fio_2 is greater than 60%.
4. List three symptoms of respiratory failure in adults.
5. List four common causes of respiratory failure in children.
6. What percentage of O_2 should a child in severe respiratory distress receive?

Answers to Review

1. Pao_2 below 60 mm Hg
2. Pco_2 above 45 mm Hg
3. Hypoxemia
4. Dyspnea/tachypnea; intercostal and sternal retractions; cyanosis
5. Congenital heart disease; infection or sepsis; respiratory distress syndrome; aspiration; fluid overload or dehydration
6. 100%

Shock

Description: Widespread, serious reduction of tissue perfusion (lack of O_2 and nutrients) that, if prolonged, leads to generalized impairment of cellular functioning (Box 3-1)

A. Arterial pressure is the driving force of blood flow through all the organs.
1. It is dependent on cardiac output to perfuse the body.
2. It is dependent on peripheral vasomotor tone to return blood and other fluids to the heart.
3. It is dependent on the amount of circulating blood.
4. Marked reduction in either cardiac output or peripheral vasomotor tone, without a compensatory elevation in the other, results in system hypotension.

BOX 3-1	*Clinical Manifestations of Respiratory Distress*		
Respiratory Acidosis	**SEVERE Respiratory Acidosis**	**Respiratory Alkalosis**	**SEVERE Respiratory Alkalosis**
Restlessness	Cyanosis	Lightheadedness	Confusion
Confusion	Dilated facial blood vessels	Anxiety	Syncope
Diaphoresis	Dilated conjunctival vessels	Circumoral numbness	Cardiac dysrhythmias
Tachypnea	Lethargy	Paresthesias	Seizures
Dyspnea	Ventricular dysrhythmias		Tetany
	Coma		

From Potter P, Perry A, Stockert P, Hall A, Peterson V: *Clinical companion for fundamentals of nursing: just the facts*, ed 8. VitalBook file. St. Louis, 2013, Mosby. Page 218; Monahan FD: *Phipps' medical-surgical nursing: health and illness perspectives*, ed 8, St. Louis, 2006, Mosby. Page 364.

5. Those at risk for development of shock include:
a. Very young and very old clients
b. Postmyocardial infarction (MI) clients
c. Clients with severe dysrhythmia
d. Clients with adrenocortical dysfunction
e. Persons with a history of recent hemorrhage or blood loss
f. Clients with burns
g. Clients with massive or overwhelming infection

HESI Hint • Early signs of shock are agitation and restlessness resulting from cerebral hypoxia.

B. Types of shock (Table 3-4)
C. Consequences of shock (Box 3-2)

HESI Hint • All types of shock can lead to systemic inflammatory response syndrome (SIRS) and result in multiple organ dysfunction syndrome (MODS).

HESI Hint • If cardiogenic shock exists in the presence of pulmonary edema (i.e., from pump failure), position client to reduce venous return (high Fowler position with legs down) to decrease further venous return to the left ventricle.

If an intraaortic balloon pump is used to decrease myocardial oxygen demand and improve myocardial perfusion, the nursing responsibilities are to assess that the balloon is inflating during diastole (spike on P wave on electrocardiogram [ECG]) and that blood is not backing up into the tubing. The nurse is also responsible for assessing for potential complications of this device such as limb ischemia, compartment syndrome, aorta dissection, plaque or emboli dislodgement, migration of the catheter, insertion site bleeding, rupture of the balloon, signs and symptoms of infection, and skin breakdown because the client has limited movement.

TABLE 3-4 Types of Shock

Types of Shock →		Cause →	End Result
Hypovolemic (most common)		Loss of **fluid** and/or blood → internal or externally	Refer to Table 3-2
Cardiogenic		Damaged **heart** → ischemia or impairment of tissue perfusion	Decreased cardiac output
Distributive	Anaphylactic	Reaction to an **allergen**	Excessive vasodilation and impaired distribution of blood flow
	Neurogenic	**Spinal cord** injury to descending sympathetic pathways	
	Septic	**Endotoxins** from bacteria	
Obstructive		Physical **obstruction** → tamponade, emboli, compartment syndrome	Impeded filling and outflow of blood resulting in decreased cardiac output

Medical Treatment for Shock

A. Correct decreased tissue perfusion and restore cardiac output
 1. Oxygenation and ventilation
   a. Optimize oxygen delivery and reduce demand on heart.
   b. Increase arterial oxygen saturation with supplemental oxygenation and mechanical ventilation.
   c. Space activities that decrease oxygen consumption.
 2. Fluid resuscitation
   a. Cause of shock dictates the type of treatment. Rapid infusion of volume-expanding fluids is the cornerstone of treatment for hypovolemic shock and anaphylactic shock.
   b. Whole blood, plasma, plasma substitutes (colloid fluids) may be used.
   c. Isotonic, electrolyte intravenous (IV) solutions such as Ringer's lactate solution and normal saline may also be used.
   d. If shock is cardiogenic in nature, the infusion of volume-expanding fluids may result in pulmonary edema.
 3. Drug therapy
   a. Restoration of cardiac function should take priority. Drug selection is based on the effect of the shock on preload, afterload, or contractility.
     (1) Drugs that increase preload (e.g., blood products, crystalloids) or decrease preload (e.g., morphine, nitrates, diuretics)
     (2) Drugs that increase afterload (e.g., vasopressors, dopamine,) or decrease afterload (e.g., nitroprusside, angiotensin-converting enzyme inhibitor [ACE-I], angiotensin II receptor blocker [ARB])
     (3) Drugs that decrease contractility (e.g., beta blockers, calcium channel blockers) or increase contractility (e.g., digoxin dobutamine)

BOX 3-2 *Consequences of Shock*	
Early	**Severe**
Tachycardia	Organ dysfunction
Hypotension	Renal failure
Weakened peripheral pulses	Pleural effusion
Restlessness, agitation, confusion	Respiratory distress
Pale cool, clammy skin	Renal failure
Decreased urine output (M30 mL/hr)	Death

Data from Giddens, JF: *Concepts for nursing practice* (with Pageburst Digital Book Access on VST), ed 2. VitalBook file. St. Louis, 2017, Mosby. Page 233; Harkreader H: *Fundamentals of nursing: caring and clinical judgment*, ed 3. VitalBook file. Philadelphia, 2007, Saunders. Page 957.

 4. Monitoring
   a. Central venous pulmonary artery catheters are inserted in the operating room (OR) and intensive care unit (ICU) to monitor shock.
   b. Serial measurements of cardiopulmonary function (using electrocardiogram, pulse oximetry, end-tidal carbon dioxide monitoring, ABGs, and hemodynamic monitoring via arterial lines and/ or pulmonary artery catheters), urinary output, clinical assessment (i.e., mental status) of the client are taken every 5 to 15 minutes.
   c. After immediate attention to improvement of perfusion, attention is directed toward treating the underlying cause of the condition.
   d. Administration of drugs is usually withheld until circulating volume has been restored.
   e. Medical treatment of shock (see Table 3-4)

Nursing Assessment
Refer to Table 3-5.

> **HESI Hint** • If cardiogenic shock exists in the presence of pulmonary edema (i.e., from pump failure), position client to reduce venous return (high Fowler position with legs down) to decrease further venous return to the left ventricle.

Analysis (Nursing Diagnoses)
A. *Deficient fluid volume* related to…
B. *Decreased cardiac output* related to…
C. *Anxiety (family and individual)* related to…

Nursing Plans and Interventions
A. Monitor arterial pressure by understanding the concepts related to arterial pressure (Table 3-6).
B. Monitor BP, pulse, respirations, and arrhythmias every 15 minutes or more often, depending on stability of client.
C. Assess urine output every hour to maintain at least 30 mL/hr.
D. Notify health care provider if urine output drops below 30 mL/hr (reflects decreased renal perfusion and may result in acute renal failure).
E. Administer fluids as prescribed by provider to improve preload: blood, colloids, or electrolyte solutions until designated central venous pressure (CVP) is reached (Table 3-7).
F. Remember client's bed position is dependent on cause of shock.
G. Administer medications IV (*not* intramuscular [IM] or subcutaneous) until perfusion improves in muscles and subcutaneous tissue.
H. Keep client warm; increase heat in room or put warm blankets (not too hot) on client.
I. Keep side rails up during all procedures; clients in shock experience mental confusion and may easily be injured by falls.

TABLE 3-5 Nursing Assessment for Shock

NURSING ASSESSMENT	CARDIOGENIC	DISTRIBUTIVE			OBSTRUCTIVE		
		Analhpylatic	Neurogenic	Septic	Tamponade	Emboli	Compartment syndrome
Blood pressure	SBP < 90 mm Hg	SBP < 90 mm Hg	SBP < 90 mm Hg	SBP < 90 mm Hg	SBP < 90 mm Hg	Assessment varies dependent upon the locale	
Heart rate	> 100 BPM	> 100 BPM then <60 BPM	<60 BPM	>100 PM			
Pulse	Weak, thready			Full, bounding Widen pulse pressure	JVD Pulse paradoxus		
Heart	Diminished sounds Chest pain Dysrhythmias Decreased CO	Chest pain Decreased CO	Decreased CO	Increase CO initially, but then contractility fails → Decreased CO	Muffled heart sounds Decreased CO	Decreased CO	
Pulmonary	RR >24 Crackles	Throat tightening Cough Dyspnea Stridor Wheezing		>24 (early) <10 (late) Crackles			
Skin	Cool, pale	Warm Pruritus Redness Urticaria	Warm, dry	Pink, warm, flushed			
Mental status	Change in alertness	Apprehensive Dizzy HA Confuse Syncope		Change in alertness			
GI/GU		N,V,D Abdominal cramping incontin		Decreased U.O.			

Table created by Katherine Ralph

TABLE 3-6 **Arterial Pressure**

Concept	Definition
Mean arterial pressure (MAP)	• Level of pressure in the central arterial bed measured indirectly by BP measurement • MAP = cardiac output × total peripheral resistance = systolic BP + 2 (diastolic BP)/3 • In adults, usually approaches 100 mm Hg • Can be measured directly through arterial catheter insertion
Cardiac output (CO)	• Volume of blood ejected by the left ventricle per unit of time • Stroke volume (amount of blood ejected per beat) × heart rate (normal: 4-6 L/min)
Peripheral resistance (PR)	• Resistance to blood flow offered by the vessels in the peripheral vascular bed
Central venous pressure (CVP)	• Pressure within the right atrium; normal CVP/RAP ranges from 2-6 mm Hg

TABLE 3-7 **Administration of Blood Products**

Component therapy has replaced the use of whole blood, which accounts for less than 10% of all transfusions.		
Blood Products		
Description	**Special Considerations**	**Indications for Use**
Packed red blood cells (RBCs)	Less danger of fluid overload	Acute blood loss
Frozen RBCs: prepared from RBCs using glycerol for protection and then frozen	Must be used within 24 hrs of thawing	Auto transfusion: infrequently used because filters remove most of white blood cells
Platelets: pooled—300 mL One unit contains single donor—200 mL	Bag should be agitated periodically.	Bleeding caused by thrombocytopenia
Fresh-frozen plasma (FFP): liquid portion of whole blood separated from cells and frozen	The use of FFP is being replaced by albumin plasma expanders.	Bleeding caused by deficiency in clotting factors
Albumin: prepared from plasma and is available in 5% and 25% solutions	Albumin 25 g/100 mL is osmotically equal to 500 mL of plasma.	Hypovolemic shock, hypoalbuminemia
Cryoprecipitates and commercial concentrates: prepared from fresh-frozen plasma with 10- to 20-mL/bag	Used in treating hemophilia	Replacement of clotting factors, especially factor VIII and fibrinogen
Transfusion Reactions		
Reactions/Complications	**Assessment**	**Nursing Interventions**
Acute hemolytic	Chills, fever, low back pain, flushing, tachycardia, hypotension progressing to acute renal failure, shock, and cardiac arrest	*Stop transfusion.* Change tubing, then continue saline IV. Treat for shock if present. Draw blood samples for serologic testing. Monitor hourly urine output. Give diuretics as prescribed.
Febrile nonhemolytic (most common)	Sudden chills and fever, headaches, flushing, anxiety, and muscle pain	Give antipyretics as prescribed.
Mild allergic	Flushing, itching, urticaria (hives)	Give antihistamine as directed.
Anaphylactic and severe allergic	Anxiety, urticaria, wheezing, progressive cyanosis leading to shock and possible cardiac arrest	Stop transfusion. Initiate CPR.

Continued

TABLE 3-7 Administration of Blood Products—cont'd

Transfusion Reactions		
Reactions/Complications	**Assessment**	**Nursing Interventions**
Circulatory overload	Cough, dyspnea, pulmonary congestion, headache, hypertension	Place client in upright position with feet in dependent position and administer diuretics, oxygen, morphine; slow IV rate.
Sepsis	Rapid onset of chills, high fever, vomiting, marked hypotension, or shock	Ensure a patent airway, obtain blood for culture, administer prescribed antibiotics, take vital signs every 5 minutes until stable.
Nursing Skills		

- Obtain venous access; use central venous catheter or 19-gauge needle.
- Use only blood administration tubing to infuse blood products.
- Run blood products with saline solutions only. Dextrose solutions and Ringer's lactate solution will induce RBC hemolysis.
- Run infusion at prescribed rate, and remain with client for the first 15 to 30 minutes of infusion.
- The blood should be administered as soon as it is brought to the client.
- Check vital signs frequently before, during, and immediately after the infusion; note any increase in temperature.
- Follow agency policy regarding specific timetable for blood infusion.
- Check and double check the product before infusing to see that it is the:
  - Correct product, as prescribed; double check with a second licensed person.
  - Correct blood type and Rh factor, matched with the client, and note expiration date.

J. Obtain blood for laboratory work as prescribed: complete blood count (CBC), electrolytes, blood urea nitrogen (BUN), creatinine (renal damage), lactate (sepsis), and blood gases (oxygenation and ventilation).

K. When administering vasopressors or adrenergic stimulants, such as epinephrine, dopamine, dobutamine, norepinephrine, or isoproterenol:
   1. Administer through volume-controlled pump.
   2. Monitor hemodynamic status every 5 to 15 minutes.
   3. Watch intravenous site carefully for extravasation and tissue damage.
   4. Ask health care provider for target mean systolic BP (usually 80 to 90 mm Hg).

L. When administering vasodilators, such as hydralazine nitroprusside (or labetalol hydrochloride), to counteract effects of vasopressors:
   1. Wait for precipitous decrease or increase in BP if prescribed together.
   2. If drop in BP occurs, decrease vasodilator infusion rate first; then increase vasopressor.
   3. If BP increases precipitously, decrease vasopressor rate first; then increase rate of vasodilator.
   4. Obtain blood work as prescribed: CBC, electrolytes, BUN, creatinine (renal damage), and blood gases (oxygenation).
   5. Glucose levels should be maintained at 140 to 180 mg/dL.

M. Ensure the pulse oximetry probe is placed either on the client's earlobe or forehead, not on a digit because of the client's decreased tissue perfusion.

HESI Hint • All vasopressor and vasodilator drugs are potent and dangerous and require that the client be titrated prudently.

N. Provide family support:
   1. Notify appropriate support persons for families waiting during crisis—call spiritual advisor, other family members, or anyone the family thinks will be supportive.
   2. At intervals, notify family of actions and progress or lack of progress in realistic terms.
   3. Collaborate with health care provider before notifying family of medical interventions.

Disseminated Intravascular Coagulation (DIC)

Description: A coagulation disorder is a rarely seen complication occurring as a result of another severe and/or life-threatening illness. This disorder destroys the client's clotting factors, platelets, and RBCs.

A. Many diseases and conditions can precipitate the development of DIC. Twenty percent of the cases reported have been linked to gram-negative sepsis (Box 3-3).

B. The first phase involves abnormal clotting in the microcirculation, which uses up clotting factors and results in the inability to form clots, so hemorrhage occurs (Fig. 3-2).

BOX 3-3 *Comparison of HELLP Syndrome and Disseminated Intravascular Coagulation (DIC)*

	HELPP Syndrome	DIC
Signs and Symptoms	Nausea with or without vomiting Epigastric pain or pain in right upper abdominal quadrant Hypertension varying from mild to severe Malaise	Obvious signs of bleeding, such as hematuria or hematoma development at venipuncture sites, hemorrhage in the conjunctiva, and petechiae
Laboratory Blood Values	Increased aminotransferase, bilirubin, hemoglobin levels, and increased hematocrit Decreased platelet count	Elevated levels of fibrin degradation products, prothrombin time, and stimulated partial thromboplastin time
Treatment	Delivery of the fetus if the outcome of the mother or fetus is endangered Platelet administration if the cell count is <20,000/mm^3 Monitoring of liver function Observation for organ systems dysfunction	Volume blood and clotting factor replacement Removal of the underlying precipitating factor to reverse the DIC Support for organ systems dysfunction

From Bridges EJ, Womble S, Wallace M, et al: Hemodynamic monitoring in high-risk obstetrics patients: I. Expected hemodynamic changes during pregnancy, *Crit Care Nurse* 23:53-62, 2003; Pourrat O, Pierre F, Magnin G: Le syndrome HELLP: les dix commandements. *La Revue de Médecine Interne* 30(1): 58–64, 2009; Beucher G, Simonet T, Dreyfus M: Point de vue d'expert Prise en charge du HELLP syndrome Management of HELLP syndrome. *Gynecologie Obstetrique Fertilite* 36: 1175–1190, 2008; Alspach, AACN. *Core curriculum for critical care nursing*, ed 6. VitalBook file. St. Louis, Saunders, 2006.

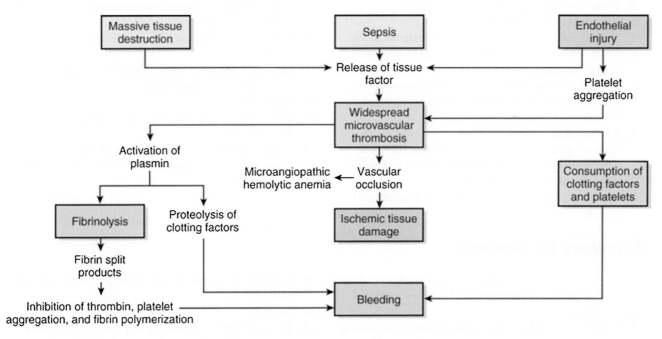

FIGURE 3-2 Pathophysiology of disseminated intravascular coagulation (DIC). (From Urden LD, Stacy KM, Lough ME: *Priorities in critical care nursing*, ed 7, St. Louis, 2016, Mosby.)

C. The diagnosis is based on laboratory findings.
   1. Prothrombin time (PT): prolonged
   2. Partial thromboplastin time (PTT): prolonged
   3. Fibrinogen: decreased
   4. Platelet count: decreased
   5. Fibrin degradation (split) products (FDP): increased

Nursing Assessment

A. Petechiae, purpura, hematomas
B. Oozing from IV sites, drains, gums, and wounds

C. Gastrointestinal and genitourinary bleeding
D. Hemoptysis
E. Mental status change
F. Hypotension, tachycardia
G. Pain

Analysis (Nursing Diagnoses)

A. *Risk for injury* related to…
B. *Ineffective tissue perfusion (specific type)* related to…

Nursing Plans and Interventions

A. Monitor client for bleeding.
B. Monitor vital signs.
C. Monitor PT/INR.
D. Protect client from injury and bleeding.
   1. Provide gentle oral care with mouth swabs.
   2. Minimize needle sticks; use smallest gauge needle possible.
   3. Turn client frequently to eliminate pressure points.
   4. Minimize number of BP measurements taken by cuff.
   5. Use gentle suction to prevent trauma to mucosa.
   6. Apply pressure to any oozing site(s).
E. Administer heparin IV during the first phase to inhibit coagulation.
F. Provide emotional support to decrease anxiety.

HESI Hint • You are caring for a woman who was in a severe automobile accident several days earlier. She has several fractures and internal injuries. The exploratory laparotomy was successful in controlling the bleeding. However, today you find that this client is bleeding from her incision; is short of breath; and has a weak and thready pulse, cold and clammy skin, and hematuria.

What do you think is wrong with the client, and what would you expect to do about it?

These are typical signs and symptoms of DIC crisis. Expect to administer IV heparin to block the formation of thrombin (warfarin does not block thrombin formation). However, the client described is already past the coagulation phase and into the hemorrhagic phase. Her care would include administration of clotting factors, along with palliative treatment of the symptoms as they arise. (Her prognosis is poor.)

Review of Shock and DIC

1. Define *shock*.
2. What is the most common cause of shock?
3. What causes septic shock?
4. What is the goal of treatment for hypovolemic shock?
5. What intervention is used to restore cardiac output when hypovolemic shock exists?
6. It is important to differentiate between hypovolemic and cardiogenic shock. How might the nurse determine the existence of cardiogenic shock?
7. If a client is in cardiogenic shock, what might result from administration of volume-expanding fluids, and what intervention can the nurse expect to perform in the event of such an occurrence?
8. List five assessment findings that occur in most shock victims.
9. Once circulating volume is restored, vasopressors may be prescribed to increase venous return. List the main drugs that are used.
10. What is the established minimum renal output per hour?
11. List four measurable criteria that are the major expected outcomes of a shock crisis.
12. Define *DIC*.
13. What is the effect of DIC on PT, PTT, platelets, and FSPs (FDPs)?
14. What drug is used in the treatment of DIC?
15. Name four nursing interventions to prevent injury in clients with DIC.

Answers to Review

1. Widespread, serious reduction of tissue perfusion, which leads to generalized impairment of cellular function
2. Hypovolemia
3. Release of endotoxins by bacteria, which act on nerves in vascular spaces in the periphery, causing vascular pooling, reduced venous return, and decreased cardiac output and result in poor systemic perfusion
4. Quick restoration of cardiac output and tissue perfusion
5. Rapid infusion of volume-expanding fluids
6. History of MI with left ventricular failure or possible cardiomyopathy, with symptoms of pulmonary edema
7. Pulmonary edema; administer medications to manage preload, contractility, and/or afterload. For example, to decrease afterload, nitroprusside may be administered.
8. Tachycardia; tachypnea; hypotension; cool, clammy skin; decrease in urinary output
9. Epinephrine, dopamine, dobutamine, norepinephrine, or isoproterenol
10. 30 mL/hr
11. BP mean of 80 to 90 mm Hg; Po_2 >50 mm Hg; CVP 2 to 6 mm HG H_2O; urine output at least 30 mL/hr
12. A coagulation disorder in which there is paradoxical thrombosis and hemorrhage
13. PT, prolonged; PTT, prolonged; platelets, decreased; FSPs, increased
14. Heparin
15. Gently provide oral care with mouth swabs. Minimize needle sticks and use the smallest gauge needle possible when injections are necessary. Eliminate pressure by turning the client frequently. Minimize the number of BP measurements taken by cuff. Use gentle suction to prevent trauma to mucosa. Apply pressure to any oozing site.

Resuscitation

Cardiopulmonary Arrest

A. Usually caused by MI; necrosis of the heart muscle caused by inadequate blood supply to heart

B. MIs usually occur at rest or with moderate activity, contrary to the belief that they occur with strenuous activity.

C. Symptoms immediately preceding MI:
1. Chest pain or discomfort at rest or with ordinary activity
2. Change in previous stable anginal pain—an increase in frequency or severity or rest angina occurring for the first time
3. Chest pain in a client with known coronary heart disease that is unrelieved by rest or nitroglycerin

D. O_2 is necessary for survival; all other injuries are secondary except for removal of any source of imminent danger such as a fire.

> **HESI Hint** • NCLEX-RN® questions on cardiopulmonary resuscitation (CPR) often deal with prioritization of actions.
>
> Question: What actions are required for each of the following situations?
> • 24-year-old motorcycle accident victim with a ruptured artery of the leg who is pulseless and apneic
> • 36-year-old first-time pregnant woman who arrests during labor
> • 17-year-old with no pulse or respirations who is trapped in an overturned car that is starting to burn
> • 40-year-old businessman who arrests 2 days after a cervical laminectomy

E. Chest pain in MI:
1. Is usually described as crushing, pressing, constricting, oppressive, or heavy
2. Tends to increase in intensity over a few minutes
3. May be substernal or more diffused
4. May radiate to one or both shoulders and arms or to neck, jaw, or back
5. Atypical symptoms occur with women and patients diagnosed with diabetes. For example, women experience unexpected shortness of breath, breaking out in a cold sweat, or sudden fatigue, nausea, or lightheadedness.

F. Occasions for CPR are often unwitnessed cardiac arrests.

G. Family presence during CPR has sparked controversy among health care professionals. The American Heart Association (AHA) (2010) suggests that family presence is a significant source of support for the client and may be a benefit to the family. Observation of the resuscitation can aid in the grieving process. Family presence during resuscitative measures should be coupled with staff support.

> **HESI Hint** • When to seek emergency medical services (EMS):
> The American Heart Association recommends that those with known angina pectoris activate an emergency medical system if chest pain does NOT go away immediately with rest or is NOT relieved in 5 minutes after taking nitroglycerin or if additional symptoms such as nausea and sweating are also present with the chest pain.
> A person with previously unrecognized coronary disease experiencing chest pain persisting for 2 minutes or longer should seek emergency medical treatment.

Management of Cardiac Arrest

> **HESI Hint** • It is important for the nurse to stay current with the AHA guidelines for basic life support (BLS) by being certified every 2 years, as required. See the AHA website for current CPR Guidelines and to locate a CPR class: http://www.cpr.heartorg/CPR

Major components of BLS consist of immediate recognition of cardiac arrest and activation of the emergency response system, CPR with emphasis on chest compression, and rapid defibrillation if indicated.

The trained layperson is a *hands-only* CPR (chest compressions–only CPR). The focus is on early, high-quality chest compressions. The health care provider includes chest compressions before rescue breaths. "C-A-B" (Chest Compression, Airway, and Breathing) is now used for adults and children, whereas steps for the newborns remain "A-B-C" (Airway, Breathing, and Compressions [Circulation]). Chest compressions are described by the phrase "push hard and push fast." The phrase reflects an increased emphasis on high-quality chest compressions and decreased emphasis on pulse checks. High-quality chest compressions mean the chest in adults is compressed at a rate of at least 100 compressions per minute at a depth of 2 inches/5 cm.

In-Hospital Cardiac Arrest

> **HESI Hint** • Initiate CPR with BLS guidelines immediately; then move on to advanced cardiac life support (ACLS) guidelines.

A. Determine responsiveness of client:
1. If no response occurs, call a "code," or cardiac arrest, in order to initiate response of cardiac arrest team. The nurse remains with the client and tasks someone else to obtain AED or emergency crash cart with defibrillator.

2. Position client on cardiac board or put bed in CPR position. If pulse is not identified in 10 seconds or less, begin chest compressions.
3. Initiate 30 chest compressions—with both hands over the lower half of the sternum at a rate of at least 100 compressions per minute with a depth of 2 inches (5 cm).
4. After 30 compressions, open airway with head tilt–chin lift maneuver and ventilate by mask or bag over 1 second per breath for 2 breaths.

B. Team leader arrives and assesses client, directs team members, and obtains history and precipitating events to arrest.
   1. Without interrupting CPR, apply cardiac portable monitor "quick-look" paddles or AED to determine whether defibrillation is necessary or whether asystole has occurred.
   2. Follow hospital policies and procedures to convert client to a normal sinus rhythm.
   3. Resume CPR, beginning with compressions, immediately after defibrillations.

HESI Hint • When significant arterial acidosis is noted, try to reduce PCO$_2$ by increasing ventilation, which will correct arterial, venous, and tissue acidosis.

   Bicarbonate may exacerbate acidosis by producing CO$_2$. ACLS guidelines recommend that bicarbonate *not* be used unless hyperkalemia, tricyclic antidepressant overdose, or preexisting metabolic acidosis is documented.

Pediatric Resuscitation

See "Maternity Nursing" (Chapter 6) for Newborn Resuscitation.

A. If no response occurs, call a "code," or cardiac arrest, in order to initiate response of cardiac arrest team. Obtain AED or emergency crash cart with defibrillator.
B. Check for pulse.
   1. Infant <1 year old, brachial pulse
   2. Children 1 year to puberty, carotid or femoral
C. Begin compressions within 10 seconds.
   1. Infant compressions cover at least one third of the anterior/posterior diameter of the chest at 1.5-inch depth in most infants.
   2. In children, compressions cover at least one third of the anterior/posterior diameter of the chest at 2-inch depth in most children.
   3. Thirty compressions to 2 breaths with one rescuer; 15 compressions to 1 breath with 2 rescuers.
D. Deliver each breath over 1 second (avoid excess ventilation [gastric inflation]).
E. Minimize interruption in chest compression.
F. Allow full chest recoil.

HESI Hint • In the pulseless arrest algorithm, the search for and treatment of possible contributing factors should include checking for hypovolemia, hypoxia, hydrogen ion acidosis, hypokalemia and hyperkalemia, hypoglycemia, hypothermia, toxins, tamponade (cardiac), tension pneumothorax, thrombosis (cardiac, pulmonary), and trauma.

Management of Foreign Body Airway Obstruction (FBAO)

Adults and Children 1 Year and Older

A. If unable to ventilate the person during CPR, suspect a foreign body in airway.
B. Signs of FBAO that require rescuer intervention include silent cough, inability to speak or breathe, or cyanosis. The victim typically clutches the neck.
C. Ask, "Are you choking?" If patient nods without talking then intervention is required.
D. If person is conscious, stand behind person, grasp around waist with clenched fist (halfway between navel and xiphoid), and exert palmar thrust inward at epigastrium (Heimlich maneuver) in rapid sequence.
E. Chest thrust should be used in obese or pregnant patients.
F. Continue until object is expelled or person falls to ground unconscious; then activate EMS and begin CPR.
G. Use a finger sweep only if the object is seen obstructing the airway.

Infants and Children

A. For a child, perform subdiaphragmatic abdominal thrusts (Heimlich maneuver) until the object is expelled or the victim becomes unresponsive. For an infant, deliver repeated cycles of 5 back blows (slaps) followed by 5 chest compressions until the object is expelled or the victim becomes unresponsive. Abdominal thrusts are not recommended for infants because they may damage the infant's relatively large and unprotected liver. Open a conscious child's mouth and attempt to clear obstruction manually if the object can be seen (no blind sweeps; they may push the foreign object farther down the throat).
B. If the infant is able to cry, cough, or breathe, do *not* interfere.
C. If the infant is conscious and *cannot* cry, cough, or breathe:
   1. Place infant face down, head lower than trunk, with legs straddling your arm and chest supported by your upturned hand.
   2. Give five firm blows to back with heel of hand (compresses rib cage between two hands).
   3. Position face upward and give five chest thrusts as you would for cardiac massage.
   4. Repeat until the object is expelled or the infant becomes unresponsive.
D. If unresponsive, begin CPR.

Review of Resuscitation

1. What is the first priority when a client with an unwitnessed cardiac arrest is found?
2. Define myocardial infarction.
3. What criteria should alert a client with known angina who takes nitroglycerin tablets sublingually to call EMS?
4. After calling out for help and asking someone to dial for emergency services, what is the next action in CPR?
5. True or false? In feeling for presence of a carotid pulse, no more than 5 seconds should be used.
6. During one-rescuer CPR, what is the ratio of compressions to ventilations for an adult? During one-rescuer CPR, what is the ratio of compressions to ventilations for a child?

7. What is the first drug most likely to be used for an in-hospital cardiac arrest?
8. A client in cardiac arrest is noted on bedside monitor to be in pulseless ventricular tachycardia. What is the first action that should be taken?
9. How would the nurse assess the adequacy of compressions during CPR? How would the nurse assess the adequacy of ventilations during CPR?
10. If a person is choking, when should the rescuer intervene?
11. One should never make blind sweeps into the mouth of a choking child or infant. Why?

Answers to Review

1. Begin CPR.
2. Necrosis of the heart muscle due to poor perfusion of the heart
3. Unrelieved chest pain after nitroglycerin
4. For adults check carotid pulse and if no pulse deliver C-A-B.
5. False. Palpate for no more than 10 seconds, recognizing that arrhythmias or bradycardia could be occurring.
6. 30:2; 15:2 for a child or neonate with two rescuers and 30:2 for 1 rescuer.

7. Epinephrine
8. Defibrillation
9. Check for a carotid or femoral pulse. Watch for chest excursion and auscultate bilaterally for breath sounds.
10. When the person points to his or her throat and can no longer cough, talk, or make sounds
11. Because the object might be pushed farther down into the throat

Fluid and Electrolyte Balance

Homeostasis

Description: The process in which the body interacts and adjusts to internal and external stimuli to maintain a relative state of equilibrium. It is a process that is constant and acclimates to the body's needs.

A. Homeostasis occurs in relation to maintenance of the composition of fluids.
B. Fluid composition involves a number of variables (Table 3-8).

HESI Hint • Changes in osmolarity cause shifts in fluid. The osmolarity of the extracellular fluid (ECF) is almost entirely due to sodium. The osmolarity of intracellular fluid (ICF) is related to many particles, with potassium being the primary electrolyte. The pressures in the ECF and the ICF are almost identical. If either ECF or ICF changes in concentration, fluid shifts from the area of lesser concentration to the area of greater concentration.

HESI Hint • Dextrose 10% is a hyperosmolar solution and should be administered IV.

Normal saline is an isotonic solution and is used for irrigations, such as bladder irrigations or IV flush lines with intermittent IV medication.

Use only isotonic (neutral) solutions in irrigations, infusions, etc., unless the specific aim is to shift fluid to intracellular or extracellular spaces.

Organ Function

A. Kidneys
  1. Main function of the kidneys is to filter a person's blood and adjust the amount and composition of fluids in the body. The total blood volume is determined by a client's gender, height, and weight. The average healthy adult has approximately 5.2 to 6 liters of circulating blood in the body.
  2. As a result of this filtration process, the kidney selectively maintains and excretes body fluids, producing approximately 1 to 2 liters of urine.

TABLE 3-8 **Fluid Volume**

Variable	Deficit	Excess
Description	• Occurs when the body loses water and electrolytes isotonically—that is, in the same proportion as exists in the normal body fluid • Serum electrolyte levels remain normal • Dehydration: state in which the body loses water and serum sodium levels increase	• Occurs when the body retains water and electrolytes isotonically • Water intoxication: state in which the body retains water and serum sodium levels decrease
Causes	• Vomiting • Diarrhea • GI suctioning • Sweating • Inadequate fluid intake • Massive edema, as in initial stage of major burns • Ascites • Older adults forgetting to drink	• Heart failure (HF) • Renal failure • Cirrhosis, liver failure • Excessive ingestion of table salt • Overhydration with sodium-containing fluid • Poorly controlled IV therapy, especially in young and old clients
Symptoms	• Weight loss (1 liter of fluid weight loss or gain is approximately equal to 2.2 pounds or 1 kilogram) • Decreased skin turgor • Oliguria (concentrated urine) • Dry and sticky mucous membranes • Postural hypotension or weak, rapid pulse	• Peripheral edema • Increased bounding pulse • Elevated BP • Distended neck and hand veins • Dyspnea; moist crackles heard when lungs auscultated • Attention loss, confusion, aphasia • Altered level of consciousness
Laboratory findings	• Elevated BUN and creatinine • Increased serum osmolarity • Elevated hemoglobin and hematocrit	• Decreased BUN • Decreased hemoglobin and hematocrit • Decreased serum osmolality • Decreased urine osmolality and specific gravity
Treatment and nursing care	• Strict I&O • Replacement of fluids isotonically, preferably orally • *Water is a hypotonic fluid.* • If intravenous hydration is needed, isotonic fluids are used.	• Diuretics • Fluid restriction • Strict I&O • Sodium-restricted diet • Weighed daily • Serum K+ monitored

HESI Hint • *Fluid Volume Deficit: Dehydration*
- Elevated BUN: The BUN measures the amount of urea nitrogen in the blood. Urea is formed in the liver as the end product of protein metabolism. The BUN is directly related to the metabolic function of the liver and the excretory function of the kidneys.
- Creatinine, as with BUN, is excreted entirely by the kidneys and is therefore directly proportional to renal excretory function. However, unlike BUN, the creatinine level is affected very little by dehydration, malnutrition, or hepatic function. The daily production of creatinine depends on muscle mass, which fluctuates very little. Therefore it is a better test of renal function than is the BUN. Creatinine is generally used in conjunction with the BUN test, and they are normally in a 1:20 ratio.
- Serum osmolality measures the concentration of particles in a solution. It refers to the fact that the same amount of solute is present, but the amount of solvent (fluid) is decreased. Therefore the blood can be considered "more concentrated."
- Urine osmolality and specific gravity increase.

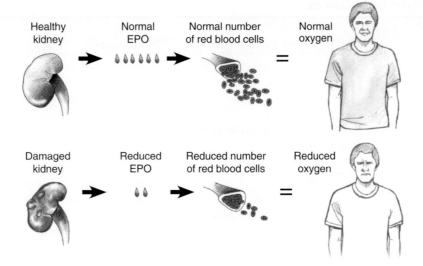

FIGURE 3-3 Top: kidney → normal EPO → normal number RBCs → normal O_2. **Bottom:** Damaged kidney → reduced EPO → less RBCs → reduced O_2. (Brugnara C, Eckardt KU. *Hematologic aspects of kidney disease.* In: Taal MW, ed. *Brenner and Rector's The Kidney.* 9th ed. Saunders; 2011: 2081–2120. National Kidney and Urologic Diseases Information Clearinghouse from National Institute of Diabetes and Digestive and Kidney Diseases.)

3. Regulates sodium and potassium levels and maintains the pH level by excreting or maintaining hydrogen ions and bicarbonate
4. Excretes metabolic wastes and toxic substances.
5. The kidneys are also responsible for manufacturing the hormone erythropoietin (EPO).
B. Lungs (Fig. 3-3)
1. Regulate carbon dioxide concentration as a result of O_2 and CO_2 gas exchange at the alveolar capillary beds, thus influencing the acid-base balance.
2. Rid the body of approximately 300 to 500 mL of fluid daily through the process of inhalation and exhalation.
C. Heart
1. Pumps blood with sufficient force to perfuse the kidneys, allowing the kidneys to work effectively.
2. Potassium, sodium, and calcium electrolyte levels are crucial in maintaining adequate electrical conductivity to help with efficient myocardial pumping action.
D. Adrenal glands
1. Secretes aldosterone, when the body's blood pressure (BP) becomes low, resulting in sodium retention (leading to water retention), thereby increasing BP and potassium excretion to maintain homeostasis.
E. Parathyroid glands
1. Regulates calcium and phosphorus balance levels in blood by increasing or decreasing the manufacture of parathyroid hormone, which influences transference of calcium and phosphorous from the bones.
F. Pituitary gland
1. Secretes antidiuretic hormone (ADH), which causes the body to retain water by signaling the kidneys to increase the water absorption when filtering the blood.

Electrolyte Imbalance

Nursing Assessment
Refer to Table 3-9.

Nursing Plans and Interventions
Refer to Table 3-9.

> **HESI Hint •** Potassium imbalances are potentially life threatening; they must be corrected immediately. A low magnesium level often accompanies a low K^+, especially with the use of diuretics.

Intravenous (IV) Therapy

Description: IV solutions are used to supply electrolytes, nutrients, and water (Table 3-10).

Administration of IV Therapy
A. The purpose and duration of the IV therapy is determined by the needs of the client's condition/situation. This also determines the type of equipment, such as vascular access device, including IV tubing and size of needle.
B. Types of vascular devices for intravenous administration.
1. Peripheral
2. Central
C. Gloves *must* be worn during venipunctures and when discontinuing an IV line.
D. Assess the IV and insertion site frequently (minimum of every 2 hours) for the prescribed rate of infusion and for patency. It is the nurse's legal responsibility to observe the client, to report any reactions, and to take measures necessary to prevent complications.

TABLE 3-9 Electrolyte Imbalances

Abnormalities and Common Causes	Signs and Symptoms	Treatment
Hyponatremia (↓Na) • Diuretics • GI fluid loss • Hypotonic tube feeding • D_5W or hypotonic IV fluids • Diaphoresis	• Anorexia, nausea, vomiting • Weakness • Lethargy • Confusion • Muscle cramps, twitching • Seizures • Na <135 mEq/L	• Restrict fluids (safer). • If IV saline solutions prescribed, administer very slowly; use isotonic saline if fluid restriction not effective.
Hypernatremia (↑Na) • Water deprivation • Hypertonic tube feeding • Diabetes insipidus • Heatstroke • Hyperventilation • Watery diarrhea • Renal failure • Cushing syndrome	• Thirst • Hyperpyrexia • Sticky mucous membranes • Dry mouth • Hallucinations • Lethargy • Irritability • Seizures • Na >145 mEq/L	• Restrict sodium in the diet. • Beware of hidden sodium in foods and medications. • Increase water intake.
Hypokalemia (↓K) • Diuretics • Diarrhea • Vomiting • Gastric suction • Steroid administration • Hyperaldosteronism • Amphotericin B • Bulimia • Cushing syndrome	• Fatigue • Anorexia • Nausea, vomiting • Muscle weakness • Decreased GI motility • Dysrhythmias • Paresthesia • Flat T waves on ECG • K <3.5 mEq/L	• Administer potassium supplements orally or IV. • Oral forms of potassium are unpleasant tasting and are irritating to the GI tract (do not give on empty stomach; dilute). • *Never give IV bolus; must* be well diluted. • Assess renal status (i.e., urinary output) before administering. • Encourage foods high in potassium (e.g., bananas, oranges, cantaloupes, avocados, spinach, potatoes).
Hyperkalemia (↑K) • Hemolyzed serum sample produces pseudohyperkalemia • Oliguria • Acidosis • Renal failure • Addison disease • Multiple blood transfusions	• Muscle weakness • Bradycardia • Dysrhythmias • Flaccid paralysis • Intestinal colic • Tall T waves on ECG • K >5.0 mEq/L	• Eliminate parenteral potassium from IV infusions and medications. • Administer 50% glucose with regular insulin. • Administer cation exchange resin (Kayexalate). • Monitor ECG. • Administer calcium gluconate to protect the heart. • IV loop diuretics may be prescribed. • Renal dialysis may be required.
Hypocalcemia (↓Ca) • Renal failure • Hypoparathyroidism • Malabsorption • Pancreatitis • Alkalosis	• Diarrhea • Numbness • Tingling of extremities • Convulsions • Positive Trousseau sign • Positive sign • Ca <8.5 mEq/L • At risk for tetany	• Administer calcium supplements orally 30 minutes before meals. • Administer calcium IV slowly; infiltration can cause tissue necrosis. • Increase calcium intake (e.g., dairy products, greens).
Hypercalcemia (↑Ca) • Hyperparathyroidism • Malignant bone disease • Prolonged immobilization • Excess calcium supplementation	• Muscle weakness • Constipation • Anorexia • Nausea, vomiting • Polyuria • Polydipsia • Neurosis • Dysrhythmias • Ca >10.5 mEq/L	• Eliminate parenteral calcium. • Administer agents such as calcitonin to reduce calcium. • Avoid calcium-based antacids. • Renal dialysis may be required.

Continued

TABLE 3-9 **Electrolyte Imbalances—cont'd**

Abnormalities and Common Causes	Signs and Symptoms	Treatment
Hypomagnesemia (↓Mg) • Alcoholism • Malabsorption • Diabetic ketoacidosis • Prolonged gastric suction • Diuretics	• Anorexia, distention • Neuromuscular irritability • Depression • Disorientation • Mg <1.5 mEq/L	• Administer $MgSO_4$ IV. • Encourage foods high in magnesium (e.g., meats, nuts, legumes, fish, and vegetables).
Hypermagnesemia (↑Mg) • Renal failure • Adrenal insufficiency • Excess replacement	• Flushing • Hypotension • Drowsiness, lethargy • Hypoactive reflexes • Depressed respirations • Bradycardia • Mg >2.5 mEq/L	• Avoid magnesium-based antacids and laxatives. • Restrict dietary intake of foods high in magnesium.
Hypophosphatemia (↓pH) • Refeeding after starvation • Alcohol withdrawal • Diabetic ketoacidosis • Respiratory alkalosis	• Paresthesias • Muscle weakness • Muscle pain • Mental changes • Cardiomyopathy • Respiratory failure • pH <2.0 mEq/L	• Correct underlying cause. • Administer oral replacement of phosphates with vitamin D.
Hyperphosphatemia (↑pH) • Renal failure • Excess intake of phosphorus	• Short-term: tetany symptoms • Long-term: phosphorus precipitation in nonosseous sites • pH >4.5 mEq/L	• Administer aluminum hydroxide with meals to bind phosphorus. • Dialysis may be required if renal failure is underlying cause.

TABLE 3-10 **Types of IV Solutions**

Isotonic	Hypotonic	Hypertonic

• Have an osmolality close to the extracellular fluid (ECF)
• Do not cause red blood cells to swell or shrink
• Indicated for intravascular dehydration
• Isotonic solutions
  • → Normal saline (0.9% NS)
  • → Lactated Ringer's solution (LR)
  • → 5% dextrose in water (D_5W is on the low end of isotonic; some sources classify it as hypotonic)
• Used to treat intravascular dehydration (not enough fluid in vascular system)
• Common type of dehydration
• Examples: dehydration caused by running, labor, fever, etc.
	• Have an osmolality lower than the ECF
	• Cause fluid to move from ECF to intracellular fluid (ICF)
	• Indicated for cellular dehydration
	• Used in the management of the patient who is both volume-depleted and hyperosmolar (e.g., in cases of hypernatremia or hyperglycemia).
	• Hypotonic solutions
	  • → 0.5% normal saline (HNS or 0.45% NS)
	  • → 2.5% dextrose in 0.45% saline ($D_{2.5}$ 45% NS)
	• Used to treat intracellular dehydration (cells have too many osmoles, need to drive fluid into the cells)
	• Not a common occurrence
	• Examples: dehydration caused by prolonged dehydration (may also see in clients who are on TPN for prolonged periods)
		• Have an osmolality higher than the ECF.
		• Indicated for intravascular dehydration with interstitial or cellular overhydration.
		• To be used with extreme caution.
		• High concentrations of dextrose are given for caloric replacement such as intravenous hyperalimentation into a central vein for rapid dilution.
		• Hypertonic saline solutions are available but used only when serum osmolality is dangerously low.
		• Hypertonic solutions
		  • → 5% dextrose in lactated Ringer's (D_5LR)
		  • → 5% dextrose in 0.45% saline
		  • → 5% dextrose in 0.9% saline (D_5NS)
		  • → 10% dextrose in water ($D_{10}W$)
		• Used to treat intravascular dehydration with cellular or interstitial overhydration.
		• Examples: dehydration resulting from surgery; blood loss causes intravascular dehydration, but the tissue cuts inflame and pull fluid into the area, causing interstitial overhydration; may also see with ascites and third-spacing.

TABLE 3-10 Types of IV Solutions—cont'd

Flow Rate Calculation
Several formulas exist for calculating intravenous flow rates.
Infusion pumps are used when measurement of exact flow is necessary.
Using the following steps for IV calculation will ensure proper calculation:
1. mL/hr: Total mL fluid to be given/Total hours to be administered = mL/hr (rate for IV infusions on a pump)
2. gtts/min: Total mL fluid to be given/Total minutes to be administered × gtts/mL = gtts/min (rate for IV infusions by gravity)

HESI Hint • Check the IV tubing container to determine the drip factor because drip factors vary. The most common drip factors are 10, 12, 15, and 60 drops per milliliter. A microdrip is 60 drops per milliliter.

TABLE 3-11 Occlusion/Catheter Damage

Assess for:	Peripheral	Central	Interventions
Leaks around the insertion site	X	X	Discontinue infusion; either restart peripheral IV or notify physician about central line.
Pinholes, leaks, and tears		X	Discontinue infusion; then notify physician about central line.
Blood return	X	X	Gently flush and attempt to draw back blood
Inability to infuse fluid	X	X	Starting from the insertion site, double check for kinks in tubing or catheter.
Needleless adapter placement, if a port or IV catheter tip lodged against the venous wall	X	X	Reposition the client's extremity for peripheral catheter; for central catheter reposition the client.
Pain in shoulder, neck, or arm		X	Discontinue the infusion and notify physician about central line
Neck or shoulder edema		X	Discontinue the infusion and notify physician about central line
Suture damage		X	Secure with a sterile transparent, self-adhesive dressing and notify physician.
			Do not use syringes less than 5 mL to irrigate because the psi would be too high and possibly damage the catheter Do not irrigate forcefully.

E. Intermittent IV therapy may be given through a saline lock; regular flushing maintains patency.

F. IV tubing and dressing should be changed according to hospital policy (usually every 72 to 96 hours).

G. When the IV catheter is discontinued, apply pressure to the site for 1 to 3 minutes for peripheral lines and 5 to 10 minutes for central lines after the catheter is removed, and inspect the tip of the catheter to ensure it is intact; then document.

Complications Associated with IV Administration

A. Occlusion/catheter damage (Table 3-11)

B. Infection/phlebitis (Table 3-12)

HESI Hint • If an intravenous catheter is suspected as the causative factor of sepsis, ensure that the tip of the removed catheter is placed in a sterile container to be sent down to the laboratory for culture, along with the ordered blood cultures.

C. Dislodgment/migration/incorrect placement (Table 3-13)

D. Skin erosion/hematomas/scar tissue formation over port/infiltration/extravasation (Table 3-14)

E. Pneumothorax/hemothorax/air emboli/hydrothorax (Table 3-15)

TABLE 3-12 **Infection/Phlebitis**

Assess for:	Peripheral	Central	Interventions
Insertion site for redness, drainage, edema, or tenderness	X	X	Peripherally IVs → Use aseptic and antiseptic techniques when starting an IV line and when caring for IV site Central IVs → use sterile technique when inserting and changing central dressings.
Temperature	X	X	Monitor temperature for fever.
Labs		X	Monitor WBC with differential count/ for central lines twice weekly
IV fluids		X	Ensure parental IV fluids bags are changed out every 24 hours or according to institution's policy.
IV tubing	X	X	Change IV tubing according to institution's policy.
IV dressings	X	X	Change according institutions policy; avoid getting wet and/or soiled.
	X		Use a catheter that is smaller than the vein when initiating IV

TABLE 3-13 **Dislodgement/Migration/Incorrect Placement**

Assessment:	Site: Peripheral	Site: Central	Usual Interventions
Length of catheter	X	X	Provide tubing long enough for client movement.
Edema, drainage, and coiling of catheter	X	X	
Neck distention or distended neck veins	X	X	Anchor the catheter to the client.
Client complaints of gurgling sounds	X	X	
Change in patency of catheter	X	X	Measure and record length of catheter.
Chest radiograph	X	X	
Cardiac dysrhythmias Hypotension	X	X	Discontinue the infusion and notify physician about probable dislodged IV line.

TABLE 3-14 **Skin Erosion/Hematomas/Scar Tissue Formation Over Port/Infiltration/Extravasation**

Assess for:	Peripheral	Central	Interventions
Loss of tissue or separation at exit site	X	X	Dilute medications adequately.
Drainage at exit site	X	X	Follow institutional protocol for administration of vesicant drugs.
Erythema and edema at exit site	X	X	Change IV line within the time frame outlined in institutional protocol.
Spongy feeling at exit site	X	X	Provide gentle skin care at exit/insertion site.
Labored breathing	X	X	Avoid selecting site over a joint.
Complaints of pain	X	X	Anchor the catheter well.

TABLE 3-15 **Pneumothorax/Hemothorax/Air Emboli/Hydrothorax**

Assess for:	Peripheral	Central	Interventions
Subcutaneous emphysema	X	X	Use clot filters when infusing blood and blood products.
Chest pain	X	X	Avoid using veins in the lower extremities. Prevent fluid containers from becoming empty.
Dyspnea and hypoxia	X	X	Check valves and micropore filters on vented Y-type infusions
Tachycardia	X	X	or piggyback infusions, which allow solutions to run simultaneously. Air may be introduced into the line if the
Hypotension	X	X	containers become empty.
Confusion	X	X	*If air embolism is suspected, place patient in left lateral Trendelenburg*
Nausea	X	X	*position.*

HESI Hint • Flushing a saline lock efficiently requires approximately 1.5 times the amount of fluid the tubing will hold. Remember to use sterile technique to prevent complications, such as infiltration, emboli, and infection.

Acid-Base Balance

Description: An acid-base balance must be maintained in the body because alterations can result in alkalosis or acidosis.

A. Maintaining the acid-base balance is imperative and involves three systems:
  1. Chemical buffer system
  2. Kidneys
  3. Lungs
B. Acid-base balance is determined by the hydrogen ion concentration in body fluids.
  1. Normal range is 7.35 to 7.45 expressed as the pH (Fig. 3-4).
  2. A pH level below 7.35 indicates acidosis.
  3. A pH level above 7.45 indicates alkalosis.
  4. Measurement is made by examining ABGs (Table 3-16).

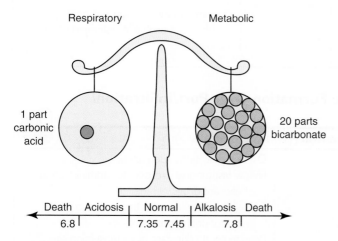

FIGURE 3-4 Relationship of sodium bicarbonate to carbonic acid. (From Potter PA, Perry AG: *Fundamentals of nursing*, ed 7, St. Louis, 2009, Mosby.)

Chemical Buffer System

A. Chemical buffers act quickly to prevent major changes in body fluid pH by removing or releasing hydrogen ions.
B. The main chemical buffer is the bicarbonate–carbonic acid (HCO_3-H_2CO_3) system.
  1. Normally there are 20 parts of bicarbonate to 1 part carbonic acid. If the 20:1 ratio is altered, the pH is changed (ratio is important, not absolute values).
  2. Carbonic acid (H_2CO_3) is formed when carbon dioxide (CO_2) combines with water (H_2O).
  3. Excess CO_2 in the body alters the ratio and creates an imbalance. Other chemical buffers involve:
    a. Phosphate
    b. Protein
    c. Hemoglobin
    d. Plasma

Lungs

A. Control CO_2 content through respirations (carbonic acid content).
B. Control, to a small extent, water balance ($CO_2 + H_2O = H_2CO_3$).
C. Release excess CO_2 by increasing respiratory rate.
D. Retain CO_2 by decreasing respiratory rate.

Kidneys

A. Regulate bicarbonate levels by retaining and reabsorbing bicarbonate as needed.
B. Provide a very slow compensatory mechanism (can require hours or days).
C. Cannot help with compensation when metabolic acidosis is created by renal failure.

Determining Acid-Base Disorders

A. In uncompensated acid-base disturbances, it is easy to determine when a disorder exists. Arrows are used to indicate whether the pH, P_{CO_2}, or HCO_3 is high (↑), low (↓), or within normal limits (WNL) (⟷).
B. When pH is high (↑), alkalosis is present.
C. In respiratory disorders, the HCO_3 is normal, and the arrows for pH and P_{CO_2} point in opposite directions.
D. In metabolic disorders, the P_{CO_2} is normal, and the arrows for pH and HCO_3 point in the same direction or are equal (Table 3-17).

TABLE 3-16 Arterial Blood Gas Comparisons

Acid-Base Conditions	pH	Pco₂ (mm Hg)	Hco₃ (mEq/L)
Normal	7.35-7.45	35-45	21-28
Respiratory acidosis	↓	↑	Normal
Respiratory alkalosis	↑	↓	Normal
Metabolic acidosis	↓	Normal	↓
Metabolic alkalosis	↑	Normal	↑

E. The body will begin to compensate in acid-base disorders to bring the pH back within the normal range of 7.35 to 7.45 (Tables 3-18 and 3-19).

F. Example: For a client with a pH of 7.29 (↓), a P_{CO_2} of 50 (↑), and an HCO_3 of 28 (⟷):
  1. Determine the pH: acidosis.
  2. Determine the P_{CO_2}: respiratory.
  3. Determine HCO_3: not metabolic.

4. Respiratory acidosis is the disorder (Table 3-20).
5. Determine state of compensation: The client's arterial blood gas reflects an uncompensated state → indicating more interventions need to be implemented.

HESI Hint • The acronym ROME can help you remember: respiratory, opposite, metabolic, equal.

TABLE 3-17 Analysis of Arterial Blood Gases

Component	Description	Values
pH	• Measures hydrogen ion (H^+) concentration • ↑ in ions (acidosis) reflects in pH • ↓ in ions (alkalosis) reflects in pH	• 7.35-7.45 • <7.35 • >7.45
P_{CO_2}	• Partial pressure of CO_2 in arteries • Respiratory component of acid-base regulation • Hypercapnia/hypoventilation (respiratory acidosis) • Hypocapnia/hyperventilation (respiratory alkalosis)	• 35-45 mm Hg • >45 mm Hg • <35 mm Hg
HCO_3	• Measures serum bicarbonate • May reflect primary metabolic disorder or compensatory mechanism to respiratory acidosis • Metabolic acidosis • Metabolic alkalosis	• Normal 21-28 mEq/L • <21 mEq/L • >28 mEq/L

TABLE 3-18 Determining Respiratory vs. Metabolic and Acidosis vs. Alkalosis

	(7.35-7.45)	(35-45 mm Hg)	(21-28 mEq/L)
R	(+) pH	(−)P_{aCO_2}	Alkalosis
O	(−)pH	(+)P_{aCO_2}	Acidosis
M	(+)pH	(+)HCO_3	Alkalosis
E	(−)pH	(−)HCO_3	Acidosis

TABLE 3-19 Determining Compensated or Partial Compensated or Uncompensated

pH →	P_{aCO_2} →	HCO_3 →	Compensation
Normal	Abnormal	Abnormal	FULLY
Abnormal	Abnormal	Abnormal	PARTIAL
Abnormal	Normal	Abnormal	UNCOMPENSATED
Abnormal	Abnormal	Normal	UNCOMPENSATED

TABLE 3-20 Potential Causes of Acid-Base Conditions

Condition	Primary Cause	Contributing Causes
Respiratory acidosis	• Hypoventilation	• COPD (primary cause) • Pulmonary disease • Drugs • Obesity • Mechanical asphyxia • Sleep apnea

TABLE 3-20 Potential Causes of Acid-Base Conditions—cont'd

Condition	Primary Cause	Contributing Causes
Metabolic acidosis	• Addition of large amounts of fixed acids to body fluids	• Lactic acidosis (circulatory failure) • Ketoacidosis (diabetes, starvation) • Phosphates and sulfates (renal disease) • Acid ingestion (salicylates) • Secondary to respiratory alkalosis • Adrenal insufficiency
Respiratory alkalosis	• Hyperventilation	• Overventilation on a ventilator • Response to acidosis • Bacteremia • Thyrotoxicosis • Fever • Hepatic failure • Response to hypoxia • Hysteria
Metabolic alkalosis	• Retention of base or removal of acid from body fluids	• Excessive gastric drainage • Vomiting • Potassium depletion (diuretic therapy) • Burns • Excessive $NaHCO_3$ administration

Review of Fluid and Electrolyte Balance

1. List four common causes of fluid volume deficit.
2. List four common causes of fluid volume overload.
3. Identify two examples of isotonic IV fluids.
4. List three systems that maintain acid-base balance.
5. Cite the normal ABGs for the following:
   A. pH
   B. Pco_2
   C. HCO_3
6. Determine the following acid-base disorders:
   A. pH 7.50, Pco_2 30, HCO_3 28
   B. pH 7.30, Pco_2 42, HCO_3 20
   C. pH 7.48, Pco_2 42, HCO_3 32
   D. pH 7.29, Pco_2 55, HCO_3 28

Answers to Review

1. Gastrointestinal (GI) causes: vomiting, diarrhea, GI suctioning; decrease in fluid intake; increase in fluid output such as sweating, massive edema, ascites
2. Heart failure, renal failure; cirrhosis; excess ingestion of table salt or overhydration with sodium-containing fluids
3. Ringer's lactate; normal saline
4. Lungs; kidneys; chemical buffers
5. Normal values
   A. 7.35 to 7.45 pH
   B. 35 to 45 mm Hg Pco_2
   C. 21 to 28 mEq/L HCO_3
6. Disorders
   A. Respiratory alkalosis
   B. Metabolic acidosis
   C. Metabolic alkalosis
   D. Respiratory acidosis

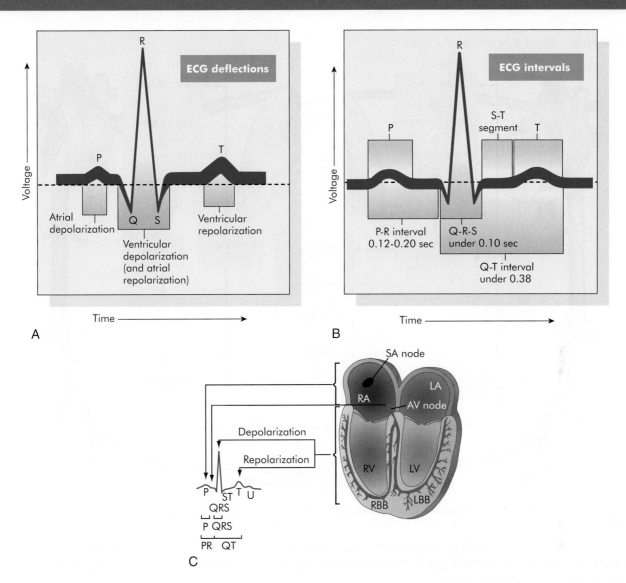

FIGURE 3-5 Electrocardiogram (ECG) and Cardiac Electrical Activity. (From Ignatavicius DD, Workman ML: *Medical surgical nursing: patient-centered collaborative care.* St. Louis: 2013, Saunders. **A** and **B** from Patton KT, Thibodeau GA: *Anatomy and physiology.* St. Louis, 2010, Mosby.

Electrocardiogram (ECG)

Description: The visual representation of the electrical activity of the heart reflected by changes in the electrical potential at the skin surface. It is not a record of the heart's contractions, but of the electrical events that precede them (Fig. 3-5).

A. The visual representation of an ECG can be recorded as a tracing on a strip of graph paper or seen on an oscilloscope.

B. The following conditions can interfere with normal heart functioning:
1. Disturbances of rate or rhythm
2. Disorders of conductivity
3. Enlarged heart chambers
4. Presence of MI
5. Fluid and electrolyte imbalances

C. Each ECG should include identifying information:
1. Client's name and identification number
2. Location, time, and date of recording
3. Client's age, gender, and cardiac and noncardiac medications currently being taken
4. Height, weight, and BP
5. Clinical diagnosis and current clinical status
6. Any unusual position of the client during the recording
7. If present, thoracic deformities, respiratory distress, and muscle tremor

HESI Hint • Blood flow through the heart:

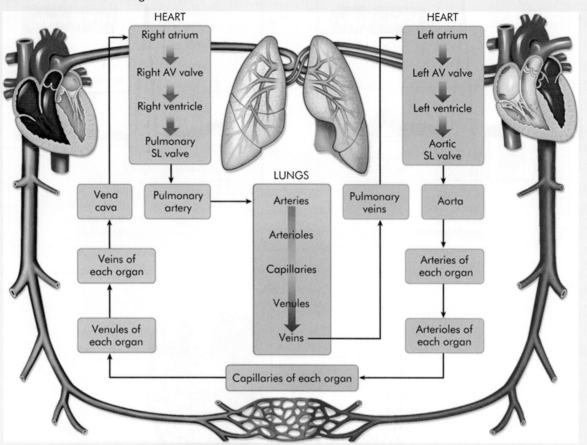

Right-sided heart failure → edema of periorbital, extremities, ascites Left-sided heart failure leads to congestive heart failure → pulmonary edema / muffled heart sounds (From Patton KT, Thibodeau GA: *Anatomy and physiology.* ed 7. St. Louis, 2010, Mosby.)

Superior/inferior VENA CAVA (unoxygenated) → Right ATRIUM → (Tricuspid Valve) → Right VENTRICLE → (Pulmonic Valve) Pulmonary Artery → LUNGS (gas exchanged at alveoli – oxygenated) → Left ATRIUM →(Mitral Valve) → Left VENTRICLE → (Aortic Valve) → Aorta

Review the three structures that control the one-way flow of blood through the heart:
Atrioventricular valves
    Tricuspid (right side)
    Mitral (left side)
Semilunar valves
    Pulmonic (in pulmonary artery)
    Aortic (in aorta)
Chordae tendineae
Papillary muscles

D. The standard ECG is the 12-lead ECG.
E. Bedside monitoring through telemetry is more commonly seen in the clinical setting.
  1. Telemetry uses three or five leads transmitted to an oscilloscope.
  2. Graphic information is printed either on request or at any time the set parameters are transcended.
F. A portable continuous monitor (Holter monitor) can be placed on the client to provide a magnetic tape recording. While wearing a Holter monitor, the client is instructed to keep a diary concerning:

  1. Activity
  2. Medications
  3. Chest pains
G. The ECG graph paper consists of small and large squares (Fig. 3-6).
  1. The small squares represent 0.04 second each; five of these small squares combine to form one large square.
  2. Each large square represents 0.20 second (0.04 second × 5). Five large squares represent 1 second. Calculation of heart rate uses the 6-second rule (Box 3-4):

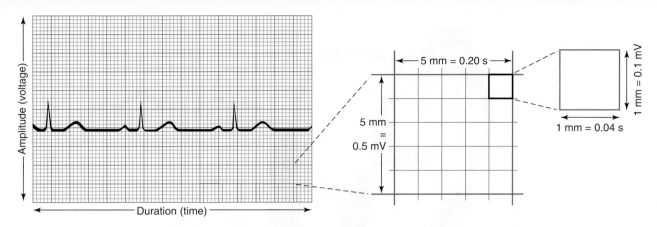

FIGURE 3-6 Composition of ECG paper. The ECG's waveforms are measured in amplitude (voltage) and duration (time). (From Ignatavicius DD, Workman ML: *Medical-surgical nursing: patient-centered collaborative care*, ed 7. St. Louis, 2013, Saunders.)

BOX 3-4 *Methods of Estimating Heart Rate Using an Electrocardiogram Tracing*

1. Measure the interval between consecutive QRS complexes, determine the number of small squares, and divide 1500 by that number. This method is used only when the heart rhythm is regular.
2. Measure the interval between consecutive QRS complexes, determine the number of large squares, and divide 300 by that number. This method is used only when the heart rhythm is regular.
3. Determine the number of RR intervals within 6 seconds and multiply by 10. The ECG paper is conveniently marked at the top with slashes that represent 3-second intervals. This method can be used when the rhythm is irregular. If the rhythm is extremely irregular, an interval of 30 to 60 seconds should be used.

4. Count the number of big blocks between the same point in any two successive QRS complexes (usually R wave to R wave) and divide into 300 because there are 300 big blocks in 1 minute. It is easiest to use a QRS that falls on a dark line. If little blocks are left over when counting big blocks, count each little block as 0.2, add this to the number of big blocks, and then divide by 300.
5. The memory method relies on memorization of the following sequence: 300, 150, 100, 75, 60, 50, 43, 37, 33, 30. Find a QRS complex that falls on the dark line representing 0.2 second or a big block, and count backward to the next QRS complex. Each dark line is a memorized number. This is the method most widely used in hospitals for calculating heart rates for regular rhythms.

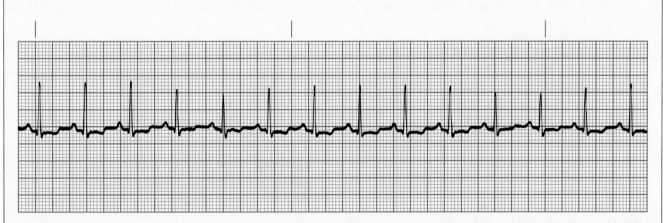

Calculation of heart rate. In this example, the heart rate using the big block method is 300 divided by 4 big blocks (between QRS complexes), or 75 beats/min. The memory method is also demonstrated with a heart rate of 75 beats/min. (Figure from Ignatavicius DD, Workman ML. *Medical-surgical nursing: patient-centered collaborative care*, ed 7, St. Louis, 2013, Saunders.)

(Data from Monahan F, Sands J, Neighbors M, et al: *Phipps' medical-surgical nursing: health and illness perspectives*, ed 8, St. Louis, 2007, Mosby; Ignatavicius DD, Workman ML: *Medical-surgical nursing: patient-centered collaborative care*, ed 7, St. Louis, 2013, Saunders.)

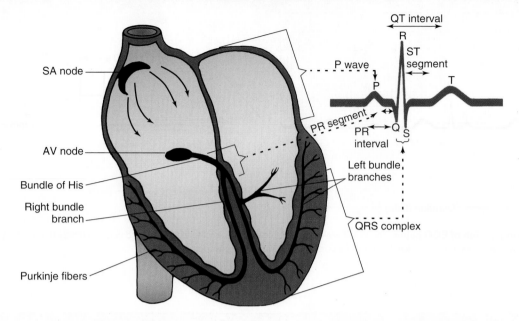

FIGURE 3-7 The cardiac conduction system. (From Ignatavicius DD, Workman ML: *Medical-surgical nursing: patient-centered collaborative care*, ed 7, St. Louis, 2013, Saunders.)

a. It is the easiest means of calculating the heart rate.
b. It cannot be used when the heart rate is irregular.
c. Thirty large squares equal one 6-second time interval.
d. Count the number of RR intervals in the 30 large squares and multiply by 10 to determine the heart rate for 1 minute (the R is the high peak on the strip; Fig. 3-7).

H. Composition of the ECG:
1. P wave: atrial systole
   a. Represents depolarization of the atrial muscle
   b. Should be rounded and without peaking or notching
2. QRS complex: ventricular systole
   a. Represents depolarization of the ventricular muscle
   b. Normally follows the P wave
   c. Is measured from the beginning of the QRS to the end of the QRS (normal <0.12 second)
   d. T wave: ventricular diastole
      (1) Represents repolarization of the ventricular muscle
      (2) Follows the QRS complex
      (3) Usually is slightly rounded, without peaking or notching

HESI Hint • The T wave represents repolarization of the ventricle, so this is a critical time in the heartbeat. This action represents a resting and regrouping stage so that the next heartbeat can occur. If defibrillation occurs during this phase, the heart can be thrust into a life-threatening dysrhythmia.

3. ST segment
   a. Represents early ventricular repolarization
   b. Is measured from the end of the S wave to the beginning of the T wave

4. PR interval
   a. Represents the time required for the impulse to travel from the atria (sinoatrial [SA] node), through the atrioventricular (AV) node, to the Purkinje fibers in the ventricles
   b. Is measured from the beginning of the P wave to the beginning of the QRS complex
   c. Represents AV nodal function (normal 0.12 to 0.20 second)
5. U wave
   a. Is not always present
   b. Is most prominent in the presence of hypokalemia
6. QT interval
   a. Represents the time required to completely depolarize and repolarize the ventricles
   b. Is measured from the beginning of the QRS complex to the end of the T wave
7. RR interval
   a. Reflects the regularity of the heart rhythm
   b. Is measured from one QRS to the next QRS

HESI Hint • Observe the client for tolerance of the current rhythm. This information is the most important data the nurse can collect on a client with an arrhythmia.

HESI Hint • NCLEX-RN questions are likely to relate to early recognition of abnormalities and associated nursing actions. Remember to monitor the client as well as the machine! If the ECG monitor shows a severe dysrhythmia but the client is sitting up quietly watching television without any sign of distress, assess to determine whether the leads are attached properly.

Review of Electrocardiogram (ECG)

1. Identify the waveforms found in a normal ECG.
2. In an ECG reading, which wave represents depolarization of the atrium?
3. In an ECG reading, what complex represents depolarization of the ventricle?
4. What does the PR interval represent?
5. If the U wave is most prominent, what condition might the nurse suspect?
6. Describe the calculation of the heart rate using an ECG rhythm strip.
7. What is the most important assessment data for the nurse to obtain in a client with an arrhythmia?
8. Calculate the rate of this rhythm strip.

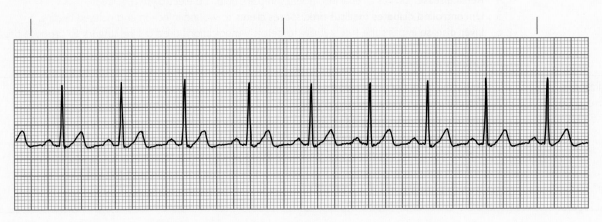

(From Ignatavicius DD, Workman ML. *Medical-surgical nursing: patient-centered collaborative care,* ed 7, St. Louis, 2013, Saunders.)

Answers to Review

1. P wave, QRS complex, T wave, ST segment, PR interval
2. Represented by the P wave
3. QRS complex
4. The time required for the impulse to travel from the atria through the AV node
5. Hypokalemia
6. Count the number of RR intervals in the 30 large squares and multiply by 10 to determine the heart rate for 1 minute.
7. Ability of the client to tolerate the arrhythmia
8. 80 beats per minute (bpm)

Perioperative Care

Description: The perioperative period includes client care before surgery (preoperative), during surgery (intraoperative), and after surgery (postoperative).
A. The nurse's role is to
   1. Educate and advocate
   2. Reduce anxiety
   3. Promote an uncomplicated perioperative period for the client and family
B. Surgery is performed under aseptic conditions in either a hospital or an alternative hospital setting (ambulatory surgical center or health care provider's office).
C. Client safety is a serious concern during the perioperative period. Steps should be implemented to ensure safety. An implementation plan for the reduction and elimination of preventable surgical complications known as the *Surgical Care Improvement Project (SCIP) core measures* is mandatory for patient safety.

Surgical Risk Factors

Refer to Table 3-21.

Preoperative Care

Description: Care provided from the time the client and family make the decision to have surgery until the client is taken to the operative suite

TABLE 3-21 Surgical Risk Factors

Age	The **very young** and **very old** are greater surgical risks than children and adults.
Nutrition	**Obesity** and **malnutrition** increase surgical risk.
Fluid and Electrolyte	**Dehydration** and **hypovolemia** increase surgical risk because of imbalances in **calcium**, **magnesium**, **potassium**, and **phosphorus**.
General Health: Any infection or pathology increases surgical risk.	1. **Cardiac conditions:** Angina, MIs, hypertension, heart failure; well-controlled cardiac problems pose little risk. 2. **Blood coagulation disorders** can lead to severe bleeding, hemorrhage, and shock. 3. **Upper respiratory tract infections** (surgery is usually delayed when the client has an upper respiratory infection) and **COPD** are exacerbated by general anesthesia and adversely affect pulmonary function. 4. **Renal disease,** such as a renal insufficiency, impairs fluid and electrolyte regulation. 5. **Uncontrolled diabetes mellitus** predisposes clients to wound infection and delayed healing. 6. **Liver disease** impairs the liver's ability to detoxify medications used during surgery to produce prothrombin or to metabolize nutrients for wound healing. 7. **Obesity** exacerbates risk.
Medications (prescribed and OTCs)	1. **Anticoagulants** (increase blood coagulation time) 2. **Tranquilizers** (may cause hypotension) 3. **Heroin** (decreases CNS response) 4. **Antibiotics** (may be incompatible with anesthetics) 5. **Diuretics** (may precipitate electrolyte imbalance) 6. **Steroids** 7. Over-the-counter **herbal preparations** 8. **Vitamin E**

Data to Obtain When Taking a Preoperative Nursing History

A. Age
B. Allergies to medications, foods, and topical antiseptics (especially iodine)
C. Current medications: prescriptions, over-the-counter, and herbal preparations
D. History of medical and surgical problems of the patient and immediate family members
E. Previous surgical experiences
F. Previous experience with anesthesia
G. Tobacco, alcohol, and drug abuse
H. Understanding of surgical procedure and risks involved
I. Coping resources
J. Cultural and ethnic factors that may affect surgery

Key Components of Preoperative Teaching Plans

A. Regulations concerning valuables, jewelry, dentures, and hearing aids
B. Food and fluid restrictions such as nothing by mouth (NPO) after midnight per prescription by health care provider; clear liquids may be given up to 6 hours before surgery for the no-risk client per prescription by the health care provider.
C. Invasive procedures such as urinary catheters, IVs, nasogastric (NG) tubes, enemas, douches
D. Preoperative medications
E. Operating room, transportation, skin preparation, postanesthesia

F. Postoperative procedures:
  1. Respiratory care, such as ventilator, incentive spirometer, deep breather, splinting
  2. Activity, such as range of motion (ROM), leg exercises, early ambulation, turning
  3. Pain control, such as IM medications, patient-controlled analgesia (PCA)
  4. Dietary restrictions
  5. ICU or postanesthesia care unit (PACU) orientation (recovery room)

Preoperative Checklist Information

A. Informed consent, surgical consent, signed and witnessed consent to treatment within 24 hours; signature must be obtained before administration of any narcotics or other medications affecting client cognition. Consents are valid for 45 days.
B. Site is marked by the person performing surgery. Before the incision is initiated all team members confirm identity, procedure, site of surgery, and consents.
C. History and physical examination (by health care provider) are noted in chart. History and physical are valid for 30 days.
D. Chest radiograph, ECG, and urinalysis have been performed, when prescribed.
E. Hemoglobin, hematocrit, electrolytes, glucose, and type/crossmatch for blood have been determined, if prescribed.
F. Old chart is on hand.
G. Identification band is on client and allergies are noted.
H. Client identification information is clear (hard-copy charting may use an addressograph card).

I. Contact lenses, glasses, dentures, partial plates, wigs, jewelry, artificial eyes, prostheses, makeup, and nail polish have been removed per institutional policy or as prescribed by health care provider.

J. Client has voided or been catheterized.

K. Client is in hospital gown.

L. Vital signs: BP, temperature, pulse, and respirations have been taken.

M. Premedications, including antibiotics, have been given; types and times have been noted.

N. Skin preparation has been performed (if prescribed by health care provider or physician):
1. Wash skin with soap and water.
2. Do not remove hair unless it will interfere with the operation, and remove it using only electric clippers if possible.
3. Follow shave with scrub or shower with antibacterial solution.

O. Signature of nurse certifies completion.

> **HESI Hint** • Marking the operative site is required for procedures involving right/left distinctions, multiple structures (fingers, toes), and levels (spinal procedures). Site marking should be done with the involvement of the client.

Intraoperative Care

Description: From the time the client is received in the operative suite until admission to the PACU, an OR nurse is in charge of care.

A. Maintain quiet during induction.

B. Maintain safety:
1. Conduct client identification: right client, right procedure, right anatomic site.
2. Ensure that sponge, needle, and instrument counts are accurate. Counts are to be done and verified and documented by two personnel before, during, before closing incision(s), and end of the surgery.
3. Position client during procedure to prevent injury.
4. Strictly adhere to asepsis during all intraoperative procedures.
5. Ensure adequate functioning suction setups are in place.
6. Take responsibility for correct labeling, handling, and deposition of any and all specimens.

C. Monitor physical status:
1. If excessive blood loss occurs, calculate effect on client.
2. Report changes in pulse, temperature, respirations, and BP to surgeon, in conjunction with anesthesiologist/certified registered nurse anesthetist (CRNA).
3. Positioning the patient is a critical part of every procedure and usually follows administration of the anesthetic.

D. Provide psychological support:
1. Provide emotional support to client and family immediately before, during, and after surgery.
2. Arrange with physician to provide information to the family if surgery is prolonged or complications or unexpected findings occur.
3. Communicate emotional state of client to other health care team members.

Postoperative Care

Description: From admission to PACU, until client has recovered

A. Initially, the client goes to the PACU.

B. On arrival, the client is assessed for vital signs (BP, pulse, respirations, temperature), level of consciousness, skin color and condition, dressing location and condition, intravenous fluids, drainage tubes, position, and oxygen saturation levels.

C. When client has been stabilized, and it has been prescribed by the health care provider, the client is then transferred to the general nursing unit or the ICU.

D. Immediate postoperative nursing care should include:
1. Monitoring for signs of shock and hemorrhage: hypotension, narrow pulse pressure, rapid weak pulse, cold moist skin, increased capillary filling time, and decreased urine output (Table 3-22)
2. Positioning client on side (if not contraindicated) to prevent aspiration and to allow client to cough out airway; side rails should be up at all times
3. Providing warmth with heated blanket
4. Managing nausea and vomiting with antiemetic drugs and NG suctioning
5. Managing pain with intravenous analgesics
6. Checking with anesthesiologist about intraoperative medications before administering pain medications
7. Determining intraoperative irrigations and instillations with drains to help evaluate amount of drainage on dressing and in drainage collection devices.
8. Most PACU settings use a scoring system to determine whether the client meets the criteria to be discharged from the PACU.

> **HESI Hint** • NCLEX-RN items may focus on the nurse's role in terms of the entire perioperative process.
>
> Example: A 43-year-old mother of two teenage daughters enters the hospital to have her gallbladder removed in a same-day surgery using an endoscope instead of an incision. What nursing needs will dominate each phase of her short hospital stay?
>
> Preparation phase: education about postoperative care, including NPO, assistance with meeting family needs
>
> Operative phase: assessment, management of the operative suite
>
> Postanesthesia phase: pain management, postanesthesia precautions
>
> Postoperative phase: prevention of complications, assessment for pain management, and teaching about dietary restrictions and activity levels

TABLE 3-22 Common Postoperative Complications

Postoperative Complication	Occurrence	Interventions for Prevention
Urinary retention	8-12 hr postoperatively	• Monitor hydration status and encourage oral intake if allowed. • Offer bedpan or assist to commode.
Pulmonary problems • Atelectasis • Pneumonia • Embolus	1-2 days postoperatively	• Assist client to turn, cough, deep breathe every 2 hr. • Keep client hydrated. • Enable early ambulation. • Provide early incentive spirometer.
Wound-healing problems	5-6 days postoperatively	• Teach splinting of incision when client coughs. • Monitor for signs of infection, malnutrition, dehydration. • Provide high-protein diet.
Urinary tract infections	5-8 days postoperatively	• Oral fluid intake. • Emptying of bladder every 4-6 hr. • Monitor intake and output. • Avoid catheterization if possible.
Thrombophlebitis	6-14 days postoperatively	• Leg exercises every 8 hr while in bed. • Early ambulation. • Apply antiembolus (TED) stockings or sequential compression devices as prescribed; remove TEDs every 8 hr and reapply. • Avoid pressure that may obstruct venous flow; do not raise knee gatch on bed; do not place pillows beneath knees; client should avoid crossing legs at knees. • Low-dose heparin may be used prophylactically.
Decreased gastrointestinal peristalsis • Constipation • Paralytic ileus	2-4 days postoperatively	• NG tubing to decompress GI tract. • Client to limit use of narcotic analgesics, which decrease peristalsis. • Encourage early ambulation.

HESI Hint • Wound dehiscence is separation of the wound edges; it is more likely to occur with vertical incisions. It usually occurs after the early postoperative period, when the client's own granulation tissue is "taking over" the wound, after absorption of the sutures has begun. Evisceration of the wound is protrusion of intestinal contents (in an abdominal wound) and is more likely in clients who are older, diabetic, obese, or malnourished and have prolonged paralytic ileus.

HESI Hint • NCLEX-RN items may focus on delivery of safe effective care.

Time Out, Surgical Care Improvement Project (SCIP) protocol implementation, and Hand-Off communication are all best practices implemented to prevent serious medical error during the perioperative period. **Time Out** occurs before making the incision, and the entire surgical team pauses as the surgical site listed on the consent is read aloud. The entire team confirms that this information is correct. **SCIP** protocols are best prac- tices for safety and quality that are implemented during the preoperative period and followed up on during the postoperative period. The focus of the SCIP protocol is on prevention of infection, prevention of serious cardiac events, and prevention of venous thromboembolism. The **Hand-Off** communication is the transfer of relevant patient information during the perioperative period, which is standardized and must include an opportunity to ask and to respond to questions.

Review of Perioperative Care

1. List five variables that increase surgical risk.
2. Why is a client with liver disease at increased risk for operative complications?
3. Preoperative teaching should include demonstration and explanation of expected postoperative client activities. What activities should be included?
4. What items should the nurse assist the client in removing before surgery?
5. How is the client positioned in the immediate postoperative period, and why?
6. List three nursing actions that prevent postoperative wound dehiscence and evisceration.
7. Identify three nursing interventions that prevent postoperative urinary tract infections.
8. Identify nursing/medical interventions that prevent postoperative paralytic ileus.
9. List four nursing interventions that prevent postoperative thrombophlebitis.
10. During the intraoperative period, what activities should the OR nurse perform to ensure safety during surgery?

Answers to Review

1. Age: very young and very old, obesity and malnutrition, preoperative dehydration/hypovolemia, preoperative infection, use of anticoagulants (aspirin) preoperatively
2. Impairs ability to detoxify medications used during surgery; impairs ability to produce prothrombin to reduce hemorrhage
3. Respiratory activities: coughing, breathing, use of spirometer; exercises: ROM, leg exercises, turning; pain management: medications, splinting; dietary restrictions: NPO evolving to progressive diet; dressings and drains; orientation to recovery room environment
4. Contact lenses, glasses, dentures, partial plates, wigs, jewelry, prostheses, makeup, and nail polish
5. Usually on the side or with head to side to prevent aspiration of any emesis
6. Teaching client to splint incision when coughing; encouraging coughing and deep breathing in early postoperative period when sutures are strong; monitoring for signs of infection, malnutrition, and dehydration; encouraging high-protein diet
7. Avoiding postoperative catheterization; increasing oral fluid intake; emptying bladder every 4 to 6 hours; early ambulation
8. Early ambulation; limiting use of narcotic analgesics; NG tube decompression
9. Teaching performance of in-bed leg exercises; encouraging early ambulation; applying antiembolus stockings; teaching avoidance of positions and pressures that obstruct venous flow
10. Ascertain correct sponge, needle, and instrument count; position client to avoid injury; apply ground during electrocautery use; apply strict use of surgical asepsis

HIV Infection

Description: Infection with human immunodeficiency virus (HIV). The infection is a blood-borne pathogen. Exposure to this blood pathogen is generally acquired through contact of infected blood or blood products, unprotected sex with an infected individual, or fetal exposure from an infected mother through placental transmission or exposure of maternal bodily fluids during birth. In the United States, the Centers for Disease Control and Prevention (CDC) reports over 1.2 million people are infected with the HIV virus and that 1 out of 8 infected individuals are unaware that they are infected (Box 3-5).

A. HIV is caused by a retrovirus, which is attracted to CD4 T cells, lymphocytes, macrophages, and cells of the central nervous system (CNS).
B. The virus enters the cell and begins to replicate. An event, such as cofactors (herpes simplex and cytomegalovirus [CMV]), can stimulate this replication.

BOX 3-5 *Factors Affecting Patterns of Disease*
Age (place in the life cycle, i.e., infant, adult, older adult)
Ethnic group (may be less relevant in multi-ethnic cultures)
Gender
Socioeconomic factors
Lifestyle decisions
Geographic location

Data from Copstead L-E, Banasik J: *Pathophysiology*, ed 5, St. Louis, 2014, Saunders.

C. The destruction of the CD4 T cell causes depletion in the number of CD4 T cells and a loss of the body's ability to fight infection. Individuals with fewer than 200 CD4 T cells are at risk for opportunistic infections. (Normal CD4 T-cell count is 600 to 1200.)

TABLE 3-23 Stages of HIV

Stage	Description and Symptoms
Primary infection (acute HIV infection or acute HIV syndrome) CD4 T-cell counts of at least 800 cells/mm³	• Flulike symptoms, fever, malaise • Mononucleosislike illness, lymphadenopathy, fever, malaise, rash • Symptoms usually occur within 3 weeks of initial exposure to HIV, after which the person becomes asymptomatic
HIV asymptomatic (CDC Category A) CD4 T-cell counts more than 500 cells/mm³	• No clinical problems • Characterized by continuous viral replication • Can last for many years (10 years or longer)
HIV symptomatic (CDC Category B) CD4 T-cell counts between 200 and 499 cells/mm³	• Persistent generalized lymphadenopathy • Persistent fever • Weight loss, diarrhea • Peripheral neuropathy • Herpes zoster • Candidiasis • Cervical dysplasia • Hairy leukoplakia, oral
AIDS (CDC Category C) CD4 T-cell counts less than 200 cells/mm³	• Occurs when a variety of bacteria, parasites, or viruses overwhelm the body's immune system • Once classified as Category C, the patient remains classified as Category C; this has implications for entitlements (e.g., health benefits, housing, food stamps).

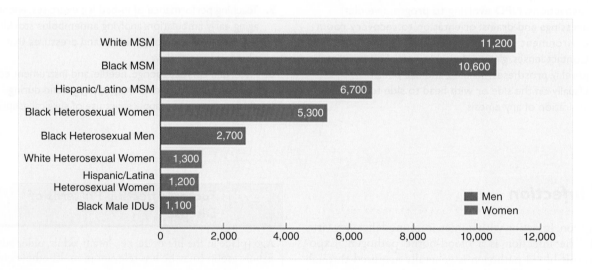

FIGURE 3-8 Estimated new HIV infections in the United States, 2010, for the most affected subpopulations. (From CDC. Estimated HIV incidence among adults and adolescents in the United States, 2007-2010. *HIV Surveillance Supplemental Report* 2012;17(4).) Subpopulations representing 2% or less are not reflected in this chart. *IDU,* Injection of drug user; *MSM,* men who have sex with men.

D. Initially, an individual commonly suffers an acute infection that is quite similar to mononucleosis (Table 3-23).
E. Initial symptoms usually occur within 3 weeks of first exposure to HIV, after which the person becomes asymptomatic. Persons infected with HIV can transmit the virus to others any time after infection has occurred, whether they are symptomatic or asymptomatic. See Figure 3-8 for subpopulations most affected by new HIV infections in the United States.

F. Current CDC definition of AIDS (end-stage infection) includes persons with specific serious opportunistic infections such as *Pneumocystis jiroveci* pneumonia (PCP), disseminated CMV, or Kaposi sarcoma.
G. Risk groups include the following:
1. Homosexual or bisexual males
2. IV drug abusers and those who have had tattoos or acupuncture
3. Heterosexual partners of a risk-group member

① ACUTE INFECTION:	② CLINICAL LATENCY:	③ AIDS:
During this time, large amounts of the virus are being produced in your body. Many, but not all, people develop flu-like symptoms often described as the "worst flu ever."	During this stage of the disease, HIV reproduces at very low levels, although it is still active. During this period, you may not have symptoms. With proper HIV treatment, people may live with clinical latency for several decades. Without treatment, this period lasts an average of 10 years, but some people may progress through this stage faster.	As your CD4 cells fall below 200 cells/mm³, you are considered to have progressed to AIDS. Without treatment, people typically survive 3 years.

FIGURE 3-9 Stages of HIV infection (From CDC)

4. Recipients of blood products before blood product screening (e.g., those with hemophilia who were diagnosed and treated before 1985)
5. Individuals taking medications such as steroids or other agents that cause immunosuppression are an increased risk for acquiring HIV/AIDS once exposed to the HIV virus.
6. Infants born to infected mothers
7. Breastfeeding infants of infected mothers

Nursing Assessment

A. Laboratory testing
   1. Positive ELISA (enzyme-linked immunosorbent assay); false-positive results can occur.
   2. Confirmation by the Western blot test, which uses electrophoresis and evaluates virus-specific bands
   3. Polymerase chain reaction (PCR) test may be used to differentiate between HIV infection in the neonate and antibodies the neonate receives from the mother.
   4. Seroconversion to positive on these tests occurs usually within 6 weeks to 3 months but may take as long as 12 months.
   5. Before seroconversion to antibody-positive status, a P24 antigen assay will be positive. (This test detects the core antigen of the virus.)

HESI Hint • An individual exposed to HIV may remain asymptomatic for many years dependent on various factors and if he or she is actively under a medical regimen of antiretroviral therapy (ART). The stages of HIV infection are presented in Figure 3-9.

Clients usually are not admitted to the hospital for treatment until their HIV status has progressed to an "AIDS" diagnosis.

B. Symptoms
   1. Extreme fatigue
   2. Loss of appetite and unexplained weight loss of more than 10 pounds in 2 months
   3. Swollen glands
   4. Leg weakness or pain
   5. Unexplained fever for more than 1 week
   6. Night sweats
   7. Unexplained diarrhea
   8. Dry cough; may represent PCP
   9. White spots in the mouth and throat; may represent candidiasis
   10. Painful blisters; may represent shingles
   11. Painless purple-blue lesions on the skin
   12. Confusion, disorientation
   13. In women, recurrent vaginal infections that are resistant to treatment
C. Opportunistic infections
   Refer to Table 3-24.

HESI Hint • HIV clients with tuberculosis require respiratory isolation. Tuberculosis is the only real risk to nonpregnant caregivers that is not related to a break in standard precautions (e.g., needle sticks).

Analysis (Nursing Diagnoses)

A. *Risk for infection* related to…
B. *Imbalanced nutrition: less than body requirements* related to…
C. *Impaired urinary elimination* related to…
D. *Ineffective breathing pattern* related to…
E. *Ineffective sexuality patterns* related to…
F. *Fatigue* related to…
G. *Risks for complicated grieving* related to…

Nursing Plans and Interventions

A. Assess respiratory functioning frequently.
B. Avoid known sources of infection.
C. Use strict asepsis for all invasive procedures.
D. Obtain vital signs frequently.
E. Plan activities to allow for rest periods.
F. Elevate HOB.

TABLE 3-24 **Opportunistic Infections**

Pneumocystis carinii Pneumonia	Kaposi Sarcoma	Cryptosporidiosis	Candidiasis of Oral Cavity and Esophagus
• Fever • Dry cough • Dyspnea at rest • Chills	• Purple-blue lesions on skin, often arms and legs • Invasion of gastrointestinal tract, lymphatic system, lungs, and brain	• Severe watery diarrhea (may be 30-40 stools per day) • Abdominal cramps • Nausea • Electrolyte imbalance • Malaise	• Thick white exudate in the mouth • Unusual taste to food • Retrosternal burning • Oral ulcers
Cryptococcal Meningitis	**Cytomegalovirus (CMV) Retinitis**	**CMV Colitis**	**Disseminated CMV**
• Headache • Changes in level of consciousness • Nausea, vomiting • Stiff neck • Blurred vision	• Most common CMV infection in persons with AIDS • Impaired vision in one or both eyes • Can lead to blindness	• Diarrhea • Malabsorption of nutrients • Weight loss	• Malaise • Fever • Pancytopenia • Weight loss • Positive cultures from blood, urine, or throat
Perirectal Muco-cutaneous Herpes Simplex Virus	**Lymphomas of Central Nervous System**	**Tuberculosis (TB)**	**HIV Encephalopathy**
• Severe pain • Bleeding, rectal discharge • Ulceration in the rectal area	• Change in mental status • Apathy • Psychomotor slowing • Seizures	• Pulmonary and extrapulmonary • Lymphatic and hematogenous TB are common • Negative skin testing does not rule out TB	• Memory loss and impaired concentration • Apathy • Depression • Psychomotor slowing (most prominent symptom) • Incontinence • CT scan findings: diffuse atrophy and ventricular enlargement

G. Refer client to nutritionist.

H. Offer small, frequent feedings.

I. Weigh daily.

J. Encourage client to avoid fatty foods.

K. Monitor for skin breakdown, and offer good skin care.

L. Use safety precautions for clients with neurologic symptoms or loss of vision.

M. Orient client who is confused.

> **HESI Hint** • Standard Precautions
> - Wash hands, even if gloves have been worn to give care.
> - Wear examination gloves for touching blood or body fluids or any nonintact body surface.
> - Wear gowns during any procedure that might generate splashes (e.g., changing clients with diarrhea).
> - Use masks and eye protection during activity that might disperse droplets (e.g., suctioning).

> - Do not recap needles; dispose of in puncture-resistant containers.
> - Use mouthpiece for resuscitation efforts.

N. Provide emotional, cultural, and spiritual support for the grieving client who is losing all relationships and skills.

O. Provide emotional support for significant others: family, family of choice, partners, and friends.

P. Administer IV fluids for hydration, as prescribed.

Q. Administer total parenteral nutrition (TPN) as prescribed.

R. Administer agents that treat specific opportunistic infections and medications for HIV (Table 3-25).

S. Assist with pain management; administer prescribed narcotics or analgesics.

> **HESI Hint** • It is recommended that caregivers who are pregnant not provide care for a client with cytomegalovirus (CMV) because fetal exposure to CMV can be detrimental to a developing fetus.

TABLE 3-25 HIV Drugs

Drugs	Indications	Adverse Reactions	Nursing Implications
NRTI (nucleotide) inhibitors • Tenofovir	• HIV infection • Classifications used in various combinations to reduce viral load and slow development of resistance	• Headache • Renal insufficiency • Fever, rash, N/V, abdominal cramps	• Monitor for lactic acidosis.
Non-NRT inhibitors • Efavirenz • Delavirdine • Nevirapine • Etravirine		• CNS changes • Nausea • Rash • Triglycerides • Hepatotoxicity	• Many drug-drug interactions. • Monitor liver function tests. • Reduces contraceptive effects. • Do not confuse Viramune with Viracept.
Protease inhibitors • Indinavir • Amprenavir • Saquinavir • Ritonavir • Nelfinavir • Lopinavir + ritonavir • Fosamprenavir • Atazanavir		• Depression • Ketoacidosis • Seizures • Angioedema • Stevens-Johnson syndrome	• Many drug-drug interactions. • High-fat, high-protein foods reduce absorption. • Give most of these *with* food. • Reduces contraceptive effects. • Do not confuse ritonavir with trade name zidovudine.
Combination products • Lamivudine + zidovudine • Zidovudine + lamivudine + abacavir • Emtricitabine + tenofovir • Tenofovir + emtricitabine + efavirenz		• Monitor for side effects associated with the individual drugs	• Note implications of the individual drugs in the combination product.
CCR5 inhibitors • Maraviroc		• Hepatotoxicity • Cough, fever, rash, hypotension • Increased risk of infection	• Use cautiously in patients with underlying liver, renal, and cardiac disease.
Fusion inhibitor • Enfuvirtide		• Infection risk and lipodystrophy if injection site is not rotated	• Monitor skin reactions at injection site.
Antiprotozoals • Atovaquone • Trimethoprim/sulfamethoxazole • Pentamidine isethionate	• (Valtrex) used for PCP in those unable to tolerate trimethoprim/sulfamethoxazole prophylaxis • Prophylaxis for PCP • Treatment of PCP	• CNS disturbances • Agranulocytosis • Phlebitis if IV • Renal calculi with Bactrim • Leukopenia • ECG abnormalities	• Enhances effects of oral hypoglycemic. • Increases thrombocytopenia risk if given with thiazide diuretics. • Check for allergy to sulfonamide. • IV or aerosol; not oral. • Use careful precautions against potential spread of TB.

TABLE 3-25 HIV Drugs—cont'd

Drugs	Indications	Adverse Reactions	Nursing Implications
Antivirals • Acyclovir sodium (Valacyclovir) • Famciclovir (Famvir) • Ganciclovir • Valganciclovir	• Herpes simplex CMV retinitis	• Granulocytopenia • Thrombocytopenia	• Give with or without food. • Many incompatibilities IV PO, IV, topical. • Monitor liver function tests.
Antifungals • Amphotericin B • Caspofungin • Fluconazole • Flucytosine • Anidulafungin • Posaconazole • Itraconazole • Micafungin • Voriconazole	• IV: Cryptococcal meningitis • PO: Oral candidiasis	• Nephrotoxicity • Hypotension • Hypokalemia • Febrile reaction • Muscle cramps • Circulatory problems	• Many drug-drug interactions. • Vesicant: Monitor IV site closely; premedicate with antipyretic; give slowly. • Swish as long as possible before swallowing PO form.

Note: Client should have regular blood counts to track CD4 levels and viral load.

Pediatric HIV Infection

Description: Infection with HIV in infants and children
A. Sources of infection in pediatric clients
   1. Perinatal transmission. Up to 35% of children born to HIV-positive mothers who are not treated with antiretroviral will become infected. If the mother is treated with zidovudine during pregnancy and the neonate is delivered by cesarean section and the neonate is treated with zidovudine 2 mg/kg/dose four times a day for period of 6 weeks after birth, the rate decreases to below 5%.
   2. HIV-infected blood products
   3. Breast milk
   4. Sexual abuse
B. At birth, the mother's antibodies for the HIV infection may passively pass onto the infant. It usually takes approximately 18 months for these maternal antibodies to clear from the infant's system; if the infant is not HIV-positive the test results will be negative.

Nursing Assessment

A. Risk groups
   1. Infants born to mothers who are HIV-positive
   2. Hemophiliacs
   3. Infants and children who have received blood transfusions
B. Symptoms
   1. Failure to thrive
   2. Lymphadenopathy
   3. Organomegaly
   4. Neuropathy
   5. Cardiomyopathy
   6. Chronic recurrent infections such as thrush
   7. Unexplained fevers

HESI Hint • Pediatric HIV is often evidenced by lymphoid interstitial pneumonitis, pulmonary lymphoid hyperplasia, and opportunistic infections.

HESI Hint • The focus of NCLEX-RN questions is likely to be assessment of early signs of the disease and management of complications associated with HIV.

Analysis (Nursing Diagnoses)

A. All diagnoses for adults may be experienced by children, depending on the age of the child.
B. *Interrupted family processes* related to…
C. *Delayed growth and development* related to…

Nursing Plans and Interventions

A. Avoid exposure to persons with infections, especially chickenpox.
B. Administer *no* live virus vaccines.
C. Teach the family to:
   1. Use gloves when diapering the child.
   2. Clean any soiled surfaces (wearing gloves) with a 1:10 bleach-to-water solution.
   3. Identify signs of opportunistic infections.
D. Monitor growth parameters.
E. Administer gamma globulin as prescribed, usually each month.
F. Support use of social services.
G. Support child's attending school as much as child is able.
H. Assist in community and school education programs.

Review of HIV Infection

1. Identify the ways HIV is transmitted.
2. Vertical transmission (from mother to fetus) occurs how often if the mother is not treated during pregnancy?
3. Describe universal precautions.
4. What are the side effects of amphotericin B?

5. What does the CD4 T-cell count describe?
6. Why does the CD4 T-cell count drop in HIV infections?
7. Describe the ways a pediatric client might acquire HIV infection.

Answers to Review

1. HIV is transmitted through blood and body fluids—for example, unprotected sexual contact with an infected person, sharing needles with drug-abusing persons, infected blood products (rare), breast milk (mother-to-fetus transmission), and breaks in universal precautions (needle sticks or similar occurrences).
2. Vertical transmission occurs 30% to 50% of the time.
3. Protection from blood and body fluids is the goal of standard precautions. Standard precautions initiate barrier protection between caregiver and client through handwashing; using gloves; using gowns and masks; using eye protection as indicated, depending on activity of

care and the likelihood of exposure; preventing needle sticks by not recapping needles.
4. Side effects of amphotericin B can be quite severe; they include anorexia, chills, cramping, muscle and joint pain, and circulatory problems.
5. CD4 T-cell count describes the number of infection-fighting lymphocytes the person has.
6. CD4 T-cell count drops because the virus destroys CD4 T cells as it invades them and replicates.
7. Pediatric acquisition may occur through infected blood products, through sexual abuse, and through breast milk.

Pain: Fifth Vital Sign

Description: An individual's subjective experience of something that is an unpleasant sensation or emotion.
A. Clients' pain often goes unrecognized and untreated.
   1. Health care professionals are poorly educated about identifying, assessing, and managing pain.
   2. Health care professionals often cling to outdated beliefs and biases, including fear of addiction.
B. An individual's response to pain is influenced by several factors:
   1. Anxiety: Reduction of anxiety can help to control pain.
   2. Past experience with pain: The more pain experienced in childhood, the greater the perception of pain in adulthood.
   3. Culture and religion: Cultural and religious practices learned from one's family play an important role in determining how a person experiences and expresses pain.
   4. Gender affects the expression of pain.
   5. Communication, whether it is a language barrier and/or a client who is unable to speak.
   6. Altered level of consciousness.
C. Pain is classified as either acute or chronic.
   1. Acute pain:
      a. Is temporary (30 days in relationship to injury; no longer than 6 months)
      b. Occurs after an injury to the body
      c. Includes postoperative pain, labor pain, and renal calculus pain

   2. Chronic pain (usually lasting beyond 6 months after initial injury)
      a. Nonmalignant (e.g., low back pain, rheumatoid arthritis)
      b. Intermittent (e.g., migraine headaches)
      c. Malignant, associated with neoplastic diseases

Theory of Pain

A. Gate control theory: Pain impulses travel from the periphery to the gray matter in the dorsal horn of the spinal cord along small nerve fibers.
   1. A "gating" mechanism called the *substantia gelatinosa* either opens to or closes off the transmission of pain impulses to the brain.
   2. It is thought that the stimulation of large, fast-conducting sensory fibers opposes the input from small pain fibers, thus blocking pain transmission.
   3. Modalities used: Stimulation of large fibers by massage, heat, cold, acupuncture, transcutaneous electrical nerve stimulation (TENS)
B. Endorphin/enkephalin theory:
   1. Endorphins: Naturally occurring compounds that have morphinelike qualities; they modulate pain by preventing the conduction of pain impulses in the CNS.
   2. Enkephalins: Specific neurotransmitters that bind with opiate receptors in the dorsal horn of the spinal cord; they modulate pain by closing the gate and stopping the pain impulse.
   3. Modalities used: Stimulation of endogenous opiate release through acupuncture, placebos, TENS

Nursing Assessment

A. Location: Pain may be localized, radiating, or referred.
B. Intensity: Ask client to rate pain before and after an intervention such as medication (use scale such as 0 to 10, with 0 being no pain).
C. Comfort: Often clients can describe what relieves pain better than they can describe the pain itself.
D. Quality: Pain may be sharp, dull, aching, sore, etc.
E. Chronology: Ask client when pain started, what time of day it occurs, how often it appears, how long it lasts, whether it is constant or intermittent, whether the intensity changes.
F. Subjective experience: Determine what decreases or aggravates pain, what other symptoms are associated with pain, what interventions provide relief, what limitations the pain inflicts.

HESI Hint • The alphabet mnemonic "PQRST" is an easy tool to use when assessing and documenting a client's experience of pain.

P	Provocative and Palliative or Aggravating Factors	What provokes the painful sensation? What makes it worse or better?
Q	Quality	Type of sensation → dull, aching, sharp, stabbing, burning
R	Region or Location, Radiation	Where is the pain located and does it radiate anywhere?
S	Severity	Ask the client to rate pain on a scale.
T	Timing	How long has it been hurting? How often does it occur? When did it occur?
U	Understanding	Ask the client what he or she thinks may be the cause or the problem causing the pain.

(From Ignatavicius, D, Workman, L: *Medical-surgical nursing: patient-centered collaborative care*, 7 ed.)

Analysis (Nursing Diagnoses)

A. *Acute or chronic pain* related to…
B. *Ineffective coping* related to…
C. *Disturbed sleep pattern* related to…
D. *Activity intolerance* related to…
E. *Self-care deficit (specify)* related to…

Nursing Plans and Interventions for Pain Management

A. Pharmacologic interventions (Table 3-26)
1. Nonnarcotics, nonsteroidal antiinflammatory drugs (NSAIDs; see Table 4-28)
   a. Act by means of a peripheral mechanism at level of damaged tissue by inhibiting prostaglandin and other chemical mediator syntheses involved in pain
   b. Show antipyretic activity through action on the hypothalamic heat-regulating center to reduce fever
   c. Examples: salicylate—aspirin nonsalicylates, acetaminophen ibuprofen
2. Narcotic mixed agonists/antagonists
   a. Bind to both a receptor that produces pain relief, which is the agonist portion, and to another receptor that does not produce a physiologic effect, which is the antagonist portion. Patients are less likely to have respiratory depression.
   b. May cause withdrawal symptoms if administered after client has been receiving narcotics.
   c. Produce side effects, including drowsiness, occasionally, nausea, and psychomimetic effects, such as hallucinations and euphoria.
   d. Examples: butorphanol nalbuphine

TABLE 3-26 Routes of Administration for Analgesics

Route	Administration
Oral	• Preferred method of administration • Drug level peak: 1-2 hr
Intramuscular	• Acceptable method of managing acute short-term pain • Onset 30 min; peak effect 1-3 hr; duration of action: 4 hr
Rectal	• Useful for clients with nausea and inability to take analgesics by mouth • Useful for home care and for elderly clients as an alternative to PO and IV administration • Reduced effectiveness with constipation
IV bolus (IV push)	• Provides the most rapid onset (5 min) but has the shortest duration (1 hr) • Useful for acute pain, such as a client in labor
Patient-controlled analgesia (PCA)	• Ideal method of pain control; client is able to prevent pain by self-administering smaller doses of the narcotic (usually morphine) as soon as the first sign of discomfort arises • Usually administered IV • A predetermined dose and a set lockout interval (5-20 min) are prescribed by physician; pump is calibrated to deliver the specified dose whenever client hits the button. • Lock-out mechanism prevents overdose. • Pump can record number of times the client uses the pump and the cumulative dose delivered.

Continued

TABLE 3-26 **Routes of Administration for Analgesics—cont'd**

Route	Administration
Continuous subcutaneous narcotic infusion (CSI)	• Useful for clients who are NPO but require prolonged administration of parenteral narcotics • Provides a constant level of analgesia by continuous infusion of a narcotic • Site should be inspected every 8 hr and changed at least every 7 days • Risk for respiratory depression
Continuous epidural analgesia	• Catheter threaded into epidural space with continuous infusion of fentanyl citrate, morphine, or other narcotic analgesics • Risk for respiratory depression
Transdermal patches	• Applied to skin (self-adhesive or with overlay to secure patch) • Also used to deliver hormonal therapy, nitroglycerin, and nicotine • Sites for application and frequency of application are specific to each medication • Document removal of old patch, site, and application date and time of new patch

TABLE 3-27 **Onset of Commonly Administrated Narcotics**

Medication	Mode	Onset	Comments
Codeine	PO IM or SC	30-45 min 10-30 min	• Do *not* administer discolored injection solutions. • May also be prescribed as an antitussive or antidiarrheal
Hydromorphone	PO IM IV	30 min 15 min 10-15 min	• Fast-acting, potent narcotic • More likely to cause appetite loss than other narcotics
Morphine sulfate	PO IM IV	60-90 min 10-30 min 10 min	• Drug of choice in relieving pain associated with myocardial infarction • May cause transient decrease in blood pressure • Drug of choice for use with chronic cancer pain
Fentanyl citrate	IM IV Intradermal Intrabuccal Intrathecal	7-15 min Within 5 min Within 12 hr 5-15 min Immediate	• Synthetic narcotic • Acts quicker; less duration

3. Narcotics
   a. Act as opioids, binding with specific opiate receptors throughout the CNS to reduce pain perception.
   b. Cause such side effects as nausea and vomiting, constipation, respiratory depression, and CNS depression.
   c. Examples: hydromorphone morphine sulfate (Table 3-27)

HESI Hint • For narcotic-induced respiratory depression, naloxone may be administered as prescribed by the health care provider.

B. Adjuvants to analgesics
   1. Are given in combination with an analgesic to potentiate or enhance the analgesic's effectiveness
   2. Are helpful in controlling discomfort associated with pain, such as nausea, anxiety, and depression (e.g., promethazine)

HESI Hint • Use noninvasive methods for pain management when possible:
Relaxation exercises
Distraction
Imagery
Biofeedback
Interpersonal skills
Physical care: altering positions, touch, hot and cold applications

Nursing Assessment of Pain Relief Techniques

A. Pain (Table 3-28)
B. Response to pharmacologic intervention: Tolerance to pharmacologic interventions may occur—that is, the client physiologically requires increasingly larger doses to provide the same effect.
   1. The first sign of tolerance is a decreased duration of a drug's effectiveness.

2. The need for increased doses can be the result of increased pain rather than tolerance (e.g., clients with advanced cancer).

> **HESI Hint** • Narcotic analgesics are preferred for pain relief because they bind to the various opiate receptor sites in the CNS. Morphine is often the

preferred narcotic (*remember*, it causes respiratory depression).

Another agonist is methadone. Narcotic antagonists block the attachment of narcotics such as naloxone to the receptors. Once naloxone has been given, additional narcotics cannot be given until the naloxone effects have passed.

TABLE 3-28 **Pain Relief Techniques**

Noninvasive
Cutaneous stimulation that is useful alone or in combination with other pain management techniques
• Heat and cold applications decrease pain and muscle spasm.
• Transcutaneous electrical nerve stimulation (TENS) provides continuous mild electrical current to the skin via electrodes.
• Massage provides a simple, inexpensive, and effective method of pain relief.
• Distraction diverts client's attention from the pain, useful during short periods of pain or during painful procedures such as intravenous venipunctures.
• Relaxation can be used as a distraction and to facilitate sedation or sleep; it rarely decreases pain sensation.
• Biofeedback techniques enable control of autonomic responses (tachycardia, muscle tension) to pain through electrical feedback.
Invasive
Any procedure that invades the body and is used to relieve pain
• Nerve blocks involve injection of anesthetic into or near a nerve to decrease pain pathways (e.g., deadening area for dental work, regional anesthesia used in obstetrics).
• Neurosurgical procedures include surgical or chemical (alcohol) interruption of nerve pathways; it is commonly used in clients with cancer who have severe pain.
• Acupuncture is the insertion of needles at various points in the body to relieve pain.

Review of Pain

1. What modalities are associated with the gate control pain theory?
2. How does past experience with pain influence current pain experience?
3. What modalities are thought to increase the production of endogenous opiates?
4. What six factors should the nurse include when assessing the pain experience?
5. What mechanism is involved in the reduction of pain through the administration of NSAIDs?
6. If narcotic agonist/antagonist drugs are administered to a client already taking narcotic drugs, what may be the result?
7. List four side effects of narcotic medications.
8. What is the antidote for narcotic-induced respiratory depression?
9. What is the first sign of tolerance to pain analgesics?
10. Which route of administration for pain medications has the quickest onset and the shortest duration?
11. List the six modalities that are considered noninvasive, nonpharmacologic pain relief measures.

Answers to Review

1. Massage, heat and cold, acupuncture, TENS
2. The more pain experienced in childhood, the greater is the perception of pain in adulthood or with the current pain experience.
3. Acupuncture, administration of placebos, TENS
4. Location, intensity, comfort measures, quality, chronology, and subjective view of pain
5. NSAIDs act via a peripheral mechanism at the level of damaged tissue by inhibiting prostaglandin synthesis and other chemical mediators involved in pain transmission.
6. Initiation of withdrawal symptoms
7. Nausea/vomiting; constipation; CNS depression; respiratory depression
8. Narcan
9. Decreased duration of drug effectiveness
10. Intravenous push, or bolus
11. Heat and cold applications; TENS; massage; distraction; relaxation techniques; biofeedback techniques

Death and Grief

Description: Death is the last developmental task for an individual. It completes the life cycle. Grief is the process an individual goes through to deal with loss. How each person deals with these situations is dependent on the individual. An individual's past experience and coping skills and what other stresses he or she may have going on in his or her life can largely affect how the person responds and reacts to these situations.

Nursing Assessment

A. Types of death
   1. Natural/expected
   2. Sudden/unexpected
   3. Suicide
B. Stages of preparing for an expected death may not be sequential. An individual may fluctuate between the stages. An individual may not experience every stage.
   1. Denial
      a. Coping style used to protect self/ego
      b. Noncompliance, refusal to seek treatment, ignoring of symptoms
      c. Changing the subject when speaking about illness
      d. Stating, "Not me, it must be a mistake."
   2. Anger
      a. Often directing it at family or health care team members
      b. Stating, "Why me? It's not fair."
   3. Bargaining
      a. Making a deal with God to prolong life
      b. Usually not sharing this with anyone, keeping it a very private experience
   4. Depression
      a. Results from the losses experienced because of health status and hospitalization
      b. Anticipating the loss of life
   5. Acceptance
      a. Accepting of the inevitable
      b. Beginning to separate emotionally

C. Stages of dealing with loss (grief)
   1. Shock, disbelief, rejection, or denial
      a. Anger and crying
      b. Conflicting emotions
      c. Anger toward the deceased
      d. Guilt
      e. Preoccupation with loss
   2. Resolution
      a. Process taking up to 1 year or more
      b. Renewed interest in activities
D. Complicated grief
   1. Unresolved grief
      a. Determine level of dysfunction
   2. Physical symptoms similar to those of the deceased
   3. Clinical depression
   4. Social isolation
   5. Failure to acknowledge loss

Analysis (Nursing Diagnoses)

A. *Complicated grief* related to…
B. *Powerlessness* related to…

Nursing Plans and Interventions

A. Encourage client to express anger in a supportive, non-threatening environment.
B. Discourage rumination.
C. Assist client in giving up idealized perception of deceased; point out misrepresentations.
D. Encourage interaction with others.
E. Assist client with identification of support systems.
F. Consult spiritual leader as indicated by client need and preference.
G. Assist client toward a comfortable, peaceful death.

> **HESI Hint** • Do not take away the coping style used in a crisis state.
>   Denial is a very useful and needed tool for some at the initial stage. Support, do not challenge, unless it hinders or blocks treatment, endangering the patient.

Review of Death and Grief

1. Identify the five stages of grief associated with dying.
2. A client has been told of a positive breast biopsy report. She asks no questions and leaves the health care provider's office. She is overheard telling her husband, "The doctor didn't find a thing." What coping style is operating at this stage of grief?
3. Your client, an incest survivor, is speaking of her deceased father, the perpetrator. "He was a wonderful man, so good and kind. Everyone thought so." What would be the most useful intervention at this time?
4. Your client feels responsible for his sister's death because he took her to the hospital where she died. "If I hadn't taken her there, they couldn't have killed her." It has been 1 month since her death. Is this response indicative of a normal or a complicated grief reaction?
5. Mrs. Green lost her husband 3 years ago. She has not disturbed any of his belongings and continues to set a place at the table for him nightly. Is this response indicative of a normal or a complicated grief reaction?

Answers to Review

1. Denial, anger, bargaining, depression, acceptance
2. Denial
3. Gently point out both the positive and negative aspects of her relationship with her father. Try to minimize the idealization of the deceased.
4. This is a normal expression of the anger and guilt that occur. Try to minimize rumination on these thoughts.
5. This is a dysfunctional grief reaction. Mrs. Green has never moved out of the denial stage of her grief work. For more review, go to http://evolve.elsevier.com/HESI/RN for HESI's online study examinations.

4 MEDICAL-SURGICAL NURSING

HESI Hint • Safety is a priority with all clients. Ascertain the use of complementary therapies by addressing contraindications and side effects. Safety includes safe handoff, interprofessional communication, fall prevention, assessing, and reporting changes in condition, as well as responses to treatments and medications.

Communication

HESI Hint • Therapeutic communication is necessary to elicit important information from clients and their families in all nursing interventions and settings. It is important in crisis intervention to ascertain cultural awareness/cultural influences on health; to note and address religious and spiritual influences on health; to assess family dynamics; and to detect sensory alterations, such as hearing loss or speech deficits.

Nurses coordinate client care through communication. Excellent communication allows nurses to not only relay empathy and knowledge to clients, but also to prevent adverse effects clients may experience and promote quality outcomes. As the nurse communicates with the client, a partnership develops to promote client health and well-being.

Characteristics of Communication

Professional communication is the assimilation of nursing skills and knowledge integrated with dignity and respect for all human beings, incorporating the assumptions and values of the profession while maintaining accountability and self-awareness.
A. Collegial
B. Collaborative
C. Interdisciplinary/interprofessional

HESI Hint • The SBAR format is used in many institutions during communication processes with other nurses, physicians, physician assistants, physical therapists, social workers, pharmacists, laboratory technicians, etc. SBAR stands for Situation, Background, Assessment, and Recommendations.

D. Confidential
　　1. Health Insurance Portability and Accountability Act (HIPAA)
　　2. Ethical

HESI Hint • Nonverbal communication may be more important than verbal communication. Body language, use of personal space, and verbal/oral messages should be congruent. Tone of voice and facial expression are part of body language. An example of positive body language is leaning in toward a client while talking. Recognition of cultural differences regarding personal space is an important component of communication. Most Americans maintain half a meter (1.7 or 1½ feet) distance between people when talking. Body language and verbal/oral communication should be congruent; state messages in a positive manner even when providing negative feedback.

Types of Communication

A. Oral/verbal communication
B. Body language communication
　　1. Eye contact
　　2. Shifting away from nurse
　　3. Grimacing
　　4. Angry or fearful expression
C. Written communication
D. Technology
　　1. Electronic medical records
　　2. Bar coding

HESI Hint • Clear verbal communication and accurate written records are critical during care transitions. Care transitions include such times as changes of shift, when the client moves from unit to unit, or when the client moves to a new care setting.

E. Basic communication standards can be applied to all clients:
　　1. Establish trust.
　　2. Offer self; be empathetic.
　　3. Demonstrate a nonjudgmental attitude (examine your bias in order to remain nonjudgmental).
　　4. Use active listening.

5. Identify the client's communication deficits and make adjustments to meet the client's abilities.
6. Accept and support the client's feelings.
7. Clarify and validate the client's statements.
8. Provide a matter-of-fact approach.

Multiple factors affect client responses to nurses, including pain, anxiety, life-altering changes, physiologic needs, temperature changes (from room to operating room or postanesthesia care unit [PACU]), new nurses, difficulty tracking time, and various and different stimuli encountered in a hospital or setting that is unusual to the client.

> **HESI Hint** • Therapeutic communication is necessary in eliciting important information from clients and their families in all nursing interventions and settings, including crisis intervention, cultural awareness/cultural influences on health, religious and spiritual influences on health, family dynamics, and sensory alterations.

Communication Strategies

A. Assess client for hearing deficits or hearing loss
B. Determine whether client understands questions
C. Take time to ask yes/no questions if the client is having difficulty communicating
D. Observe client's nonverbal communication cues (grimacing indicating pain, fear in a child)
E. When possible, provide continuity of care by assigning the same nurse
F. Encourage presence of family members to reassure client

Health Promotion and Disease Prevention

Health

A frequently used definition for health is "the state of complete physical, mental, and social well-being; not merely the absence of disease or infirmity."[1] Health promotion actions work toward the goal of developing client attitudes and behaviors that maintain health or enhance well-being. Disease prevention actions work toward the goal of safeguarding clients from real or potential health risks. There are three levels of prevention.

A. Primary prevention is intended to reduce health risks and increase healthy behaviors. Examples: providing immunizations, teaching nutrition classes, and requiring smoke-free zones.
B. Secondary prevention is intended to detect disease (through screening) and treat the disease as early as possible. Examples: a colonoscopy allows colon cancer to be detected so that an intervention can be initiated as early as possible.
C. Tertiary prevention is intended to prevent disability and complications and to provide for a peaceful death. Tertiary prevention includes rehabilitation. Examples: rehabilitation after a stroke or hip replacement surgery, hospice care.

Healthy Behaviors

Healthy behaviors are associated with longer, more productive lives. Lifestyle choices affect health. Unhealthy behaviors are risk factors for developing disease. It is difficult to change health behavior, especially when the behavior is ingrained in a person's lifestyle patterns. The nurse's role in helping the client to make positive changes includes:

A. Identifying unhealthy behaviors as an initial step in health promotion/disease prevention.
B. Asking questions that uncover and define the client's motivation.
C. Delineating behaviors and health status indicators that are outcomes of behavior change.

> **HESI Hint** • Changing unhealthy behaviors can modify or even prevent some chronic illnesses. Nurses play a major role in helping clients manage their chronic illnesses and disabilities through behavioral changes. Health teaching and counseling often are the role of the nurse in helping the client focus on improving health habits.
> Areas of behavioral change include:
> 1. Physical activity
> 2. Nutrition
> 3. Stress
> 4. Use of tobacco or marijuana
> 5. Use of alcohol
> 6. Spiritual perspective
> 7. Coping skills
> 8. Support systems

> **HESI Hint** • According to the American Lung Association smoke is harmful to lung health. Burning wood, tobacco, or marijuana releases toxins and carcinogens.

Teaching/Learning

Nurses possess specific professional knowledge, skills, and values that make them well suited to teach clients and families how to care for their health. Teaching is a deliberate process whereby the nurse implements a series of actions to bring about learning in the client.

Learning is the act of acquiring new, reinforced, or modified knowledge, behaviors, skills, or values. Learning can be achieved only by the learner. The teaching–learning process is an interactive, individualized interaction between the nurse and the client.

> **HESI Hint** • To develop a collaborative learning environment between the nurse and the client, nurses must be acutely aware of their own beliefs and values about the teaching–learning process, including client empowerment.

The teaching–learning process has four steps: assessment, planning, implementation, and evaluation. The process is iterative, where reassessment continually follows evaluation.

A. Assessment: Systematically assess the client's learning needs that relate to the health behaviors and health problems
   1. Assess learning needs from three domains
      a. Knowledge
      b. Skills
      c. Values
   2. Identify the client characteristics
      a. Nonmodifiable—for example: age, cultural background, cognitive abilities
      b. Modifiable—for example: knowledge base, and use of community resources
   3. Examine the client's readiness to learn
      a. Motivation to learn
      b. Attitudes and beliefs
   4. Recognize potential barriers to client learning
      a. Involve family members/significant others
      b. Home environment
      c. Community environment
B. Planning: Shows plan to measure client's achievement toward improving knowledge or health behaviors
   1. Collaborate with client about learning needs
   2. Determine client's priorities regarding learning needs
   3. Write behavioral goals/objectives that reflect changes in the client's behavior that are observable or measurable.
C. Implementation: Carry out the teaching strategies with the client
   1. Identify teaching strategies to use—for example: group or videos.
   2. Actively involve the client in the learning activities
   3. Include family members/significant others
D. Review outcomes after implementing a plan.
   1. Determine the effectiveness of teaching strategies.
   2. Determine whether goals/objectives were met
   3. Alter strategies if goals are not met.

Spiritual Assessment

During times of illness, religious or spiritual practices may be a source of comfort for the client. While obtaining a spiritual assessment, you can discover information about the client's preference for a personal clergy member or the hospital chaplain. A spiritual assessment tool may assist the nurse to integrate a spiritual assessment into the client's plan of care. FICA is an acronym for Faith and Belief: Importance, Community, and address in Care.[2]

Sometimes a simple question can be used to obtain a spiritual history. Ask the client, "Do you have any spiritual needs or concerns related to your health?"[3]

FICA: Taking a Spiritual History

Faith, Belief, Meaning: Do you consider yourself spiritual or religious? Do you have spiritual beliefs that help you cope with stress? Or if the client says no, ask, "What gives your life meaning?"

Importance: Have your beliefs influenced how you take care of yourself? What importance does your faith or beliefs have in your life? Have your beliefs influenced how you take care of yourself in this illness/situation?

Community: Are you part of a spiritual or religious community? Is this of support to you, and if so, how? Is there a group of people (communities such as friends, church, temple, synagogue, mosque, or support group)?

Address in care: How would you like me, your nurse, to address these issues in your health care?

When nurses empathize with clients, they recognize the concept of humanity in each of us. A client may or may not be open to praying with a nurse. A nurse should be honest in letting a client know that the nurse is not comfortable praying with the client. If comfortable, the nurse can tell the client, "I'll stay with you while you pray but I would rather not join in praying." Remember that prayer may help the client with feelings of loneliness or isolation. Prayer traditions vary for clients.

Cultural Diversity

Nurses frequently provide care for clients of different cultural backgrounds. Nurses need to be cognizant of their own cultural biases because everyone has biases. How nurses communicate with clients may be influenced by bias and may create a barrier between client and nurse. Therefore nurses must learn to accept that differences exist and to accept those cultural differences. Whenever possible if cultural traditions do not pose a harm to clients, they should be incorporated into client treatment if the client and health care provider include these requests in the treatment plan.

> **HESI Hint** • Obtain a cultural and spiritual assessment and include cultural and spiritual preferences in the plan of care when appropriate and feasible. Nurses are expected to provide care for all clients. It is important to note that clients are

culturally diverse, regardless of their ethnicity, race, or socioeconomic status and to note that in every culture subgroups may form. However, culturally diverse clients may be distinguished from mainstream culture by ethnicity, social class, and/or language. Since the 2000 census there has been a notable change in the cultural, ethnic, and racial alignment of the United States.

Culture influences how clients seek medical attention or treat themselves.

Complementary and Alternative Interventions

> **HESI Hint** • Reasons why clients use herbal medications:
> - Cultural influence
> - Perception that supplements are safer and "healthier" than conventional drugs
> - Sense of control over one's care
> - Emotional comfort from taking action
> - Limited access to professional care
> - Lack of health insurance
> - Convenience
> - Media hype and aggressive marketing
> - Recommendation from family and friends

The Institute of Medicine (IOM) is actively involved in studying "innovative" treatments such as acupuncture, yoga, and the therapeutic use of animals.[4] Acupuncture and massage have also been successfully implemented to decrease pain or decrease the need for pain medication. In the treatment for posttraumatic stress disorder (PTSD), for example, the use of eye movement desensitization reprocessing (EMDR) emphasizes the focus on mental images and muscle tension, creating positive images and thoughts while following particular eye movements that create different scenarios for the reality of the traumatic event.

For example, conventional medicine treats premenstrual syndrome (PMS) with selective serotonin reuptake inhibitors (SSRIs) such as fluoxetine, paroxetine, sertraline, and citalopram or a tricyclic antidepressant related to SSRI such as clomipramine.[5] A simpler but almost as effective method can be a large block of chocolate! Chocolate has been found to increase serotonin and has been dubbed "the Prozac of plants" by *Forbes* magazine.[6,7]

Acupressure and herbal medicines are among the traditional medical practices used by Asian clients to reestablish the balance between yin and yang. In some Asian countries, healers use a process of "coining," in which a coin is heated and vigorously rubbed on the body to draw illness out of the body. The resulting welts can mistakenly be attributed to child abuse if this practice is not understood. Traditional healers, such as Buddhist monks, acupuncturists, and herbalists, also may be consulted when someone is ill.[8]

A Japanese technique used to promote healing, reduce stress, and induce relaxation is called reiki. The process for administering reiki is by "laying on hands," and it is based on the idea that an unseen "life force energy" flows through us and is what causes us to be alive. It is believed that when a person's "life force energy" is low, then the person is more apt to become ill or feel stress. When the life force energy is high, an individual is believed to be more prone to being happy and healthy.

Smell connects to the part of the brain that controls the autonomic nervous system. Aromatherapy is the introduction of essential oils, such as sweet orange to grapefruit scents, that are effective in managing the odor of dressing changes in some hospice settings. It is believed that essential oils stimulate the release of neurotransmitters in the brain. The type of essential oil may induce pain reduction, induce sedation, or stimulate clients to a sense of well-being. Many clients also use herbal medications that they used in their country of origin or that they learned about from family traditions. To maintain client safety, nurses need to be aware of those herbal medications, their mechanisms of action, side effects, and food or drug interactions. See Figure 4-1 and Table 4-1.[7,9]

Respiratory System

Pneumonia

Description: Inflammation of the lower respiratory tract
A. Pneumonia can be caused by infectious agents.
B. Organisms that cause pneumonia reach the lungs by three methods.
   1. Aspiration
   2. Inhalation
   3. Hematogenous spread

Essential Oil	Disorder Treated
True lavender	Anxiety
True lavender	Breast tenderness
Juniper	Fluid retention
Juniper	Breast tenderness
Clary sage	Low-back pain
Geranium	Mood swings
Geranium	Nervous tension

FIGURE 4-1 Examples of essential oils. (From Buckle J: *Clinical aromatherapy: essential oils in practice* (revised), ed 2. St. Louis, Elsevier, 2003. Page 299.

TABLE 4-1 Herbal Medications, Uses, Mechanisms of Action, Side Effects, and Interactions

Herbal Medication	Application	Mechanism of Action	Side Effects	Drug Interaction	Efficacy
Bitter orange	Weight reduction	CNS stimulant catecholaminergic	High BP and tachycardia in healthy adults with a normal BP	It can interact with many drugs	Unproven
Black cohosh	Alleviate hot flashes of menopause	Acts on neurotransmitter systems; binds with serotonin receptor subtypes	No evidence of severe side effects		
Echinacea	Reduction in duration of common cold	Stimulation of immune cell function and cytokine production	Allergic reactions	Potential inhibition of CYP450 isoforms	Proven
Ephedra	Reduction of fatigue	CNS stimulation	Excessive adrenergic stimulation	Numerous	Proven
	Weight reduction	CNS stimulant catecholaminergic	Hypertension, MI, stroke Extensive CNS stimulation Agitation, sleep disturbances, psychosis	Synergistic interaction with methylxanthines Synergistic interaction with monoamine oxidase inhibitors (MAOIs) Inhibition of antihypertensive effects	Proven
Garlic	Reduction of hyperlipidemia	HMG-CoA reductase inhibitor	Odor, diaphoresis, bleeding	Potentiation of anticoagulant and antiplatelet medications Decreased plasma levels of protease inhibitor drug saquinavir	
Ginger	Treatment of nausea in motion sickness and pregnancy	Serotonin antagonist	No major adverse effects	Potential potentiation of anticoagulant antiplatelet drugs (controversial)	Proven
Ginkgo	Enhancement of mental performance	Vasodilator	No major adverse effects	Synergistic interaction with other stimulants (e.g., caffeine)	Unproven
Ginseng	Treatment of erectile dysfunction	Antiandrogen	No major adverse effects	No consistent reports	Supportive
	Reduction of fatigue	unknown			Unproven
	Enhancement of mental performance	Unknown			Unproven

Continued

TABLE 4-1 **Herbal Medications, Uses, Mechanisms of Action, Side Effects, and Interactions—cont'd**

Herbal Medication	Application	Mechanism of Action	Side Effects	Drug Interaction	Efficacy
Hoodia gordonii Also known as Hoodia, Veldkos, Slimming cactus, *Trichocaulon gordonii*, *Stapelia gordonii*	Weight reduction	P57, the main ingredient cannot actively reach the brain to suppress the appetite. (not proven effective)	May be mildly toxic (confirmed in mice but not humans) increased heart rate. Possible hepatotoxic as evidenced by increase in alkaline phosphatase (ALP) in health women.		Unproven
Kava	Treatment of anxiety	Modulatory effect at GABA receptors	Hepatotoxicity	Inhibition of CYP4502EI Potentiation of other sedatives (benzodiazepines) Inhibition of effects of levodopa in Parkinson disease clients	Proven
Red yeast rice	Reduction of hyperlipidemia	Precise mechanism of action unknown Lovastin is principal active ingredient 7 other HMG-CoA reductase inhibitors (statins)	Unknown adverse effects	Unknown	Partly understood
Saw palmetto	Relief of benign prostate hypertrophy	Antiandrogen	None	No major interactions reported	Unproven
Soy	Therapeutic for menopausal vasomotor symptoms Prevention of breast cancer Prevention of osteoporosis	Phytoestrogens help balance wildly fluctuating hormone levels Structurally similar to estradiol (major endogenous estrogen)	Can provoke asthma Gastrointestinal disturbance	Dangerous interaction with MAOI inhibitors leading to serotonin syndrome Inhibition of actions of tamoxifen	Proven
Soy protein	Reduction of hyperlipidemia	Unknown			Proven
St. John's wort	Depression	Inhibition of norepinephrine, dopamine, and serotonin reuptake	Mania in bipolar clients Photosensitivity	Many Serotonin syndrome when combined with selective serotonin reuptake inhibitors or tricyclic antidepressants Reduced plasma concentrations of many drugs such as oral contraceptives, statins, warfarin	Proven

From Buckle J. *Clinical Aromatherapy: Essential Oils in Practice.* 2nd ed. St Louis: Elsevier; 2003.

C. Pneumonia is generally classified according to causative agent.
   1. Bacterial (gram-positive and gram-negative)
   2. Viral
   3. Fungal (rare)
   4. Chemical

> **HESI Hint** • Pneumonia affects people of all ages, especially those 65 or older or infants under age 2 (because their immune systems are still developing).

D. Pneumonia may be community-acquired or medical care–associated pneumonia that encompasses hospital-associated, ventilator-associated, and health care–associated pneumonia.
E. High-risk groups include individuals who are:
   1. Debilitated by accumulated lung secretions (e.g., asthma, chronic obstructive pulmonary disease [COPD], sickle cell anemia)
   2. Cigarette smokers
   3. Immobile
   4. Immunosuppressed
   5. Experiencing a depressed gag and/or cough reflex
   6. Sedated
   7. Experiencing neuromuscular disorders
   8. Nasogastric/orogastric intubation
   9. Hospitalized client

Nursing Assessment

A. Tachypnea: shallow respirations, often with use of accessory muscles
B. Abrupt onset of fever with shaking and chills (not reliable in older adults)
C. Productive cough with pleuritic pain
D. Rapid, bounding pulse
E. In older adults, symptoms include:
   1. Confusion
   2. Lethargy/malaise
   3. Anorexia
   4. Rapid respiratory rate
   5. Tachycardia
F. Pain and dullness to percussion over the affected lung area
G. Bronchial breath sounds, crackles
   1. Bronchial breath sounds "E" to "A" changes in lungs (egophony); client says letter while nurse listens to the chest. Pneumonia may cause "E" to sound like letter "A" when heard via stethoscope.
   2. Tactile fremitus: nurse can feel the chest vibrations when client says "99." Increased fremitus is heard because solid tissue conducts sound in the pneumonia client.
H. Chest radiograph indication of infiltrates with consolidation or pleural effusion
I. Elevated white blood cell (WBC) count

J. Arterial blood gas (ABG) indication of hypoxemia
K. On pulse oximetry, a drop in O_2 saturation (should be >90%, ideally >95%)

> **HESI Hint** • Increased temperature also increases metabolism and the demand for O_2. Fever can also cause dehydration because of excessive fluid loss due to diaphoresis.

> **HESI Hint** • *Clients at High Risk for Pneumonia*
> - Altered level of consciousness
> - Brain injury
> - Depressed or absent gag and cough reflexes
> - Susceptible to aspirating oropharyngeal secretions, including alcoholics, anesthetized individuals
> - Drug overdose
> - Stroke victims
> - Immunocompromised

Analysis (Nursing Diagnoses)

A. *Impaired gas exchange* related to …
B. *Ineffective airway clearance* related to …
C. *Activity intolerance* related to …
D. *Risk for deficient fluid volume* related to …
E. *Ineffective breathing pattern* related to …
F. *Risk for imbalanced body temperature*

Nursing Plans and Interventions

A. Assess sputum for volume, color, consistency, clarity, and distinct odors like *Pseudomonas*.
B. Assist client to cough productively by:
   1. Deep breathing every 2 hours (may use incentive spirometer)
   2. Using humidity to loosen secretions (may be oxygenated)
   3. Suctioning the airway, if necessary
   4. Chest physiotherapy
C. Provide fluids up to 3 L/day unless contraindicated (helps liquefy lung secretions).
D. Assess lung sounds before and after coughing.
E. Assess rate, depth, and pattern of respirations regularly (normal adult rate is 16 to 20 breaths/min; assess for accessory muscle).
F. Monitor ABGs (Po_2 >80 mm Hg; Pco_2 <45 mm Hg).
G. Monitor O_2 saturation with pulse oximetry (ideally >95%).
H. Assess skin color (nail beds, mucous membranes, color for appropriate ethnic population).
I. Assess mental status, restlessness, and irritability.
J. Administer humidified O_2 as prescribed.
K. Monitor temperature regularly.
L. Provide adequate rest periods throughout the day, including uninterrupted sleep.
M. Administer antibiotics as prescribed (Table 4-2).

TABLE 4-2 Antiinfectives

Drugs	Indications	Adverse Reactions	Nursing Implications
Penicillins			
• Procaine penicillin G • Benzathine penicillin • Penicillin V	• Antiinfectives • Used primarily for gram-positive infections	• Allergic reactions • Anaphylaxis • Phlebitis at IV site • Diarrhea • GI distress • Superinfection	• Use with caution in clients allergic to cephalosporins. • Monitor for allergic reactions. • Observe all clients for at least 30 minutes after parenteral administration. • Oral penicillin G should be taken on an empty stomach. • Probenecid decreases renal excretion, thereby resulting in an increased blood level of the drug. • Alters contraceptive effectiveness
Semisynthetic			
• Oxacillin sodium • Nafcillin sodium • Cloxacillin sodium • Dicloxacillin sodium	• Antiinfectives • Used primarily for gram-positive infections	• Allergic reactions • Anaphylaxis • Superinfection • See Penicillins	• Cannot be used in clients allergic to penicillin • Caution in clients allergic to cephalosporins • Monitor for superinfection (sore mouth, vaginal discharge, diarrhea, cough). • See Penicillins.
Antipseudomonal Penicillins and Combinations			
• Ampicillin • Ticarcillin + clavulanate • Piperacillin + tazobactam • Ampicillin + sulbactam	• Antiinfectives • Broad spectrums	• Similar to penicillin • Ampicillin rash	• Contraindicated in clients allergic to penicillin • See Penicillins.
Tetracyclines			
• Tetracycline HCl • Doxycycline hyclate • Minocycline	• Antiinfectives	• Hypersensitivity reactions • Photosensitivity	• Decrease the effectiveness of oral contraceptives • Avoid concurrent use of antacids, milk products • Inspect IV site frequently. • Monitor for superinfections. • Avoid exposure to sunlight during use. • Avoid use in pregnant clients and children under 8 years; can cause yellow-brown discoloration of teeth and growth retardation.
Aminoglycosides			
• Gentamicin sulfate • Tobramycin sulfate • Amikacin sulfate	• Antiinfectives • Used with gram-negative bacteria	• Neuromuscular blockade • Nephrotoxicity • Ototoxicity	• Monitor renal function, BUN, creatinine, and I&O. • Monitor for ototoxicity: headache, dizziness, hearing loss, tinnitus. • Monitor for superinfection. • Peak and trough levels required

Drugs	Indications	Adverse Reactions	Nursing Implications
Miscellaneous Agents • Vancomycin hydrochloride • Metronidazole			• Monitor vancomycin serum drug concentrations. • Peak and trough levels required
Cephalosporins			
First Generation • Cefazolin • Cephalexin *Second Generation* • Cefaclor • Cefamandole • Cefuroxime • Cefoxitin • Cefotetan • Cefprozil *Third Generation* • Cefotaxime • Ceftriaxone • Ceftazidime • Cefdinir • Cefixime • Cefpodoxime • Ceftibuten (Cedax) *Fourth Generation* • Cefepime	• Antiinfectives	• Allergic reactions • Thrombophlebitis • GI distress • Superinfection	• Use with caution in clients allergic to penicillin and cephalo-sporins. • See Penicillins.
Carbapenems			
• Imipenem • Meropenem • Ertapenem			
Monobactam			
• Aztreonam	• *Pseudomonas aeruginosa* + many otherwise resistant organisms • Most effective against gram-nega-tives	• Phlebitis • Pseudomembranous colitis • CNS changes • EEG changes • Headache, diplopia • Hypotension	• Monitor renal and hepatic function, especially in older adults. • Carefully monitor for diarrhea. • Assess motor sensory function and cardiac rhythm.

Continued

TABLE 4-2 Antiinfectives—cont'd

Drugs	Indications	Adverse Reactions	Nursing Implications
Macrolides			
• Clarithromycin • Azithromycin • Erythromycin	• Clarithromycin (PO): URI, including streptococci; as adjunct treatment for *Helicobacter pylori* • Clarithromycin (IV): gram-negative and gram-positive organisms	• Pseudomembranous colitis • Phlebitis: a vesicant • Superinfections • Dizziness • Dyspnea	• Give clarithromycin XL with food. • Space monoamine oxidase inhibitors (MAOI) 14 days before start and after end of clarithromycin • Report diarrhea, abdominal cramping (all macrolides). • Monitor liver and renal labs. • PO clarithromycin give on empty stomach.
Fluoroquinolones			
• Ciprofloxacin • Levofloxacin • Moxifloxacin	• Used to treat respiratory infections, UTIs, skin, bone, and joint infections • Has been used as conjunctive treatment for TB and AIDS	• Superinfections • CNS disturbances • Arroyos and cataracts possible with ciprofloxacin • Ciprofloxacin: a vesicant	• Prompt onset • Crosses placenta and in breast milk • Can lower seizure threshold • Monitor liver, renal, and blood counts. • Safety for children not known • Many drug-drug interactions
Lincosamides			
• Clindamycin	• Soft tissue infections caused by streptococci, staphylococci, and anaerobes • Infections resistant to penicillins and cephalosporins • Used in penicillin- and erythromycin-sensitive clients	• Agranulocytosis • Pseudomembranous colitis • Superinfections	• Periodic liver, renal, and blood count monitoring • Report diarrhea immediately.
Streptogramin			
• Quinupristin/dalfopristin	• Life-threatening VRE	• Arthralgia, myalgia • Severe vesicant • Pseudomembranous colitis • Nausea/vomiting, diarrhea • Rash, pruritus	• Incompatible with any saline solutions or heparin • Functionally related to both macrolides and lincosamides • Monitor total bilirubin. • Many drug-drug interactions
Oxazolidinone			
• Linezolid	• Life-threatening VRE and MRSA	• GI disturbances • Headache • Pancytopenia • Pseudomembranous colitis • Superinfections	• Monitor renal and liver labs and blood count. • May exacerbate HTN, especially if patient ingests foods with tyramine (MAOI-like properties) • Report diarrhea immediately.

HTN, Hypertension; *MRSA*, methicillin-resistant *Staphylococcus aureus*; *PCP*, *Pneumocystic pneumonia*; *VRE*, vancomycin-resistant enterococcus.

N. Teach high-risk clients and their families about risk factors and include preventive measures.
O. Encourage at-risk groups to get pneumonia and annual influenza ("flu") vaccinations. Healthy adults develop protection within 2 to 3 weeks after receiving the vaccine.[10]
P. Promote rest and conserve energy.

> **HESI Hint** • Bronchial breath sounds are heard over areas of density or consolidation. Sound waves are easily transmitted over consolidated tissue.

> **HESI HINT** • *Hydration*
> • Thins out the mucus trapped in the bronchioles and alveoli, facilitating expectoration
> • Is essential for client experiencing fever
> • Is important because 300 to 400 mL of fluid is lost daily by the lungs through evaporation

> **HESI Hint** • Irritability and restlessness are early signs of cerebral hypoxia; the client's brain is not receiving enough O_2.

> **HESI Hint** • *Pneumonia Preventives*
> • Older adults: Annual flu vaccinations; pneumococcal vaccination at age 65 or older and younger clients who are at high risk. (Repeat vaccinations may be recommended. See Centers for Disease Control and Prevention [CDC] guidelines);[11] avoiding sources of infection and indoor pollutants (dust, smoke, and aerosols); no smoking
> • Immunosuppressed and debilitated persons: Annual flu vaccinations, pneumonia vaccination, avoid infections, sensible nutrition, adequate fluid intake, appropriate balance of rest and activity
> • Comatose and immobile persons: Elevation of head of bed at least 30 degrees for feeding and for 1 hour after feeding; turn frequently
> • Patients with functional or anatomic asplenia: Flu and pneumonia vaccinations

Chronic Airflow Limitation (CAL)

Description: Chronic lung disease includes chronic bronchitis, pulmonary emphysema, and asthma (Table 4-3).
A. Emphysema and chronic bronchitis, termed *chronic obstructive pulmonary disease* (COPD), are characterized by bronchospasm and dyspnea. The damage to the lung is not reversible and increases in severity.

> **HESI Hint** • Exposure to tobacco smoke is the primary cause of COPD in the United States.

B. Asthma, unlike COPD, is an intermittent disease with reversible airflow obstruction and wheezing.

> **HESI Hint**
> 1. Compensation occurs over time in clients with chronic lung disease, and ABGs are altered.
> 2. As COPD worsens, the amount of O_2 in the blood decreases (hypoxemia) and the amount of carbon dioxide (CO_2) in the blood increases (hypercapnia), causing chronic respiratory acidosis (increased arterial carbon dioxide [$PaCO_2$]), which results in kidneys retaining bicarbonate as compensation.
> 3. Not all clients with COPD are CO_2 retainers, even when hypoxemia is present, because CO_2 diffuses more easily across lung membranes than O_2.
> 4. In advanced emphysema, due to the alveoli being affected, hypercarbia is a problem, rather than in bronchitis, where the airways are affected.
> 5. It is imperative that baseline data be obtained for the client.

Nursing Assessment
A. Changes in breathing pattern (e.g., an increase in rate with a decrease in depth)
B. Overinflation of the lungs causes the rib cage to remain partially expanded (barrel chest)
C. Generalized cyanosis of lips, mucous membranes, face, nail beds ("blue bloater")
D. Cough (dry or productive)
E. Higher CO_2 than average
F. Low O_2, as determined by pulse oximetry (<90% to 92%)
G. Decreased breath sounds
H. Coarse crackles in lung fields that tend to disappear after coughing, wheezing
I. Dyspnea, orthopnea
J. Poor nutrition, weight loss
K. Activity intolerance
L. Anxiety concerning breathing; manifested by:
  1. Anger
  2. Fear of being alone
  3. Fear of not being able to catch breath

> **HESI Hint** • Productive cough and comfort can be facilitated by semi-Fowler or high-Fowler position, which lessens pressure on the diaphragm by abdominal organs. Gastric distention becomes a problem in these clients because it elevates the diaphragm and inhibits full lung expansion.

> **HESI Hint** • *Normal ABG Values*
>
> | Blood Gas | Adult | Child |
> | --- | --- | --- |
> | Blood gas | 7.35-7.45 | 7.36-7.44 |
> | P_{CO_2} | 35-45 mm Hg | Same as adult |
> | P_{O_2} | 80-100 mm Hg | Same as adult |
> | HCO_3^- | 21-28 mEq/L | Same as adult |

TABLE 4-3 Chronic Airflow Limitation

Chronic Bronchitis	Emphysema	Asthma
Pathophysiology		
• Chronic sputum with cough production on a daily basis for a minimum of 3 onths in each of 2 consecutive years • Chronic hypoxemia, cor pulmonale • Increase in mucus, cilia production • Increase in bronchial wall thickness (obstructs air flow) • Reduced responsiveness of respiratory center to hypoxemic stimuli	• Reduced gas exchange surface area • Increased air trapping (increased AP diameter) • Decreased capillary network • Increased work, increased O_2 consumption	• Narrowing or closure of the airway due to a variety of stimulants
Precipitating Factors		
• Higher incidence in smokers	• Cigarette smoking • Environmental and/or occupational exposure • Genetic	• Mucosal edema • $\dot{V}/\dot{Q}$ abnormalities • Increased work of breathing • Beta blockers • Respiratory infection • Allergic reaction • Emotional stress • Exercise • Environmental or occupational exposure • Reflux esophagitis
Assessment		
• Generalized cyanosis • "Blue bloaters" • Right-sided heart failure • Distended neck veins • Crackles • Expiratory wheezes	• "Pink puffers" • Barrel chest • Pursed-lip breathers • Distant, quiet breath sounds • Wheezes • Pulmonary blebs on radiograph	• Dyspnea, wheezing, chest tightness • Assess precipitating factors. • Medication history
Nursing Plans and Interventions		
• Lowest F_{IO_2} possible to prevent CO_2 retention • Monitor for signs and symptoms of fluid overload • Maintain Pa_{O_2} between 55 and 60 • Baseline ABGs • Teach pursed-lip breathing and diaphragmatic breathing. • Teach tripod position. • Administer bronchodilators and antiinflammatory agents.	• Lowest F_{IO_2} possible to prevent CO_2 retention • Monitor for signs and symptoms of fluid overload. • Maintain Pa_{O_2} between 55 and 60. • Baseline ABGs • Teach pursed-lip breathing and diaphragmatic breathing. • Teach tripod position. • Administer bronchodilators and antiinflammatory agents	• Administer bronchodilators. • Administer fluids and humidification. • Education (causes, medication regimen) • ABGs • Ventilatory patterns • C-PAP and Bi-PAP

HESI Hint • Overinflation of the lungs causes the rib cage to remain partially expanded, giving the characteristic appearance of a barrel chest. The person works harder to breathe, but the amount of O_2 taken in is not adequate to oxygenate the tissues.

Insufficient oxygenation occurs with chronic bronchitis and leads to generalized cyanosis and often right-sided heart failure (cor pulmonale).

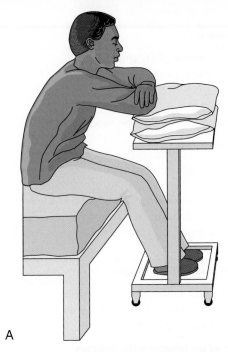

A

Sitting on the edge of a bed with the arms folded and placed on two or three pillows positioned over a nightstand.

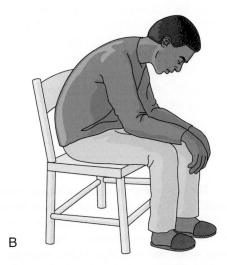

B

Sitting in a chair with the feet spread shoulder-width apart and leaning forward with the elbows on the knees. Arms and hands are relaxed.

FIGURE 4-2 Forward-leaning position. *A,* The patient sits on the edge of the bed with arms folded on a pillow placed on the elevated bedside table. *B,* Patient in three-point position. The patient sits in a chair with the feet approximately 1 foot apart and leans forward with elbows on knees. (From Ignatavicius DD, Workman ML: *Medical-surgical nursing: Patient-centered collaborative care,* ed 7, St. Louis, 2013, Saunders.)

Analysis (Nursing Diagnoses)

A. *Ineffective airway clearance* related to …
B. *Ineffective breathing pattern* related to …
C. *Impaired gas exchange* related to …
D. *Anxiety related activity intolerance* related to…

> **HESI Hint** • Cells of the body depend on O_2 to carry out their functions. Inadequate arterial oxygenation is manifested by cyanosis and slow capillary refill (<3 seconds). A chronic sign is clubbing of the fingernails, and a late sign is clubbing of the fingers.

Nursing Plans and Interventions

A. Teach client to sit upright and bend slightly forward to promote breathing.
  1. In bed: Teach client to sit with arms resting on over-bed table (tripod position).
  2. In chair: Teach client to lean forward with elbows resting on knees (tripod position; Fig. 4-2).
B. Teach diaphragmatic and pursed-lip breathing. Teach prolonged expiratory phase to prevent bronchiolar collapse and prevent air trapping.
C. Administer O_2 at 1 to 2 L per nasal cannula (Table 4-4).
D. Pace activities to conserve energy.
E. Maintain adequate dietary intake.
  1. Small, frequent meals
  2. Increase calories and protein, but do not overfeed
  3. Favorite foods
  4. Dietary supplements
    a. For people continuing to smoke tobacco, additional vitamin C may be necessary.
    b. Magnesium and calcium, because of their role in muscle contraction and relaxation, may be important for people with COPD.
    c. Routine monitoring of magnesium and phosphorus levels is important because of their role related to bone mineral density (osteoporosis).
F. Provide an adequate fluid intake (minimum 3 L/day) unless contraindicated.
G. Fluids should be taken between meals (rather than with them) to prevent excess stomach distention and to decrease pressure on the diaphragm.
H. Instruct client in relaxation techniques (teach when not in distress).
I. Teach prevention of secondary infections.
J. Teach about medication regimen (Table 4-5).
K. Smoking cessation is imperative.
L. Encourage health-promoting activities.

> **HESI Hint** • *Health Promotion*
> - Eating consumes energy needed for breathing. Offer mechanically soft diets, which do not require as much chewing and digestion. Assist with feeding if needed.
> - Prevent secondary infections; avoid crowds, contact with persons who have infectious diseases, and respiratory irritants (tobacco smoke).

TABLE 4-4 Nursing Skills: Respiratory Client

Suctioning (Tracheal)

- Suction when adventitious breath sounds are heard, when secretions are present at endotracheal tube, and when gurgling sounds are noted.
- Use aseptic/sterile technique throughout procedure.
- Wear mask and goggles.
- Advance catheter until resistance is felt.
- Apply suction only when withdrawing catheter (gently rotate catheter when withdrawing).
- Never suction for more than 10 to 15 seconds, and pass the catheter only three or fewer times.
- Oxygenate with 100% O_2 for 1 to 2 minutes before and after suctioning to prevent hypoxia.

Ventilator Setting Maintenance

- Verify that alarms are on.
- Maintain settings and check often to ensure that they are specifically set as prescribed by health care provider.
- Verify functioning of ventilator at least every 4 hours.

Oxygen Administration

- Nasal cannula: low O_2 flow for low O_2 concentrations (good for COPD)
- Simple face mask: low flow, but effectively delivers high O_2 concentrations; cannot deliver <40% O_2
- Nonrebreather mask: low flow, but delivers high O_2 concentrations (60% to 90%)
- Partial rebreather mask: low-flow O_2 reservoir bag attached; can deliver high O_2 concentrations
- Venturi mask: high-flow system; can deliver exact O_2 concentration
- C-PAP and Bi-PAP

Pulse Oximetry

- Easy measurement of O_2 saturation
- Should be >90%, ideally above 95%
- Noninvasive, fastens to finger, toe, or earlobe
- No nail polish
- Must have good peripheral perfusion to be accurate

Tracheostomy Care

- Aseptic technique (remove inner cannula only from stoma)
- Clean nondisposable inner cannula with H_2O_2; rinse with sterile saline in accordance with hospital policy
- 4 × 4 gauze dressing is butterfly folded after inner cannula is inserted.

Respiratory Isolation Technique

- Mask is required for anyone entering room.
- Private room is required with negative air pressure.
- Client must wear mask if leaving room.

Proper Use of an Inhaler with Spacers

- Have client exhale completely.
- Grip mouthpiece (in mouth) only if client has a spacer; otherwise, keep the mouth open to bring in volume of air with misted medication. While inhaling slowly, push down firmly on the inhaler to release the medication.
- Use bronchodilator inhaler before steroid inhaler.
- Wait at least 1 minute between puffs (inhaled doses).
- After steroid inhaler use, patient must perform oral care to prevent fungal infections.

- Teach client to report any change in characteristics of sputum.
- Encourage client to hydrate well (3 L/day) and decrease caffeine due to diuretic effect.
- Obtain immunizations when needed (flu and pneumonia).

HESI Hint • When asked to prioritize nursing actions, use the ABC rule:
- Airway first
- Then breathing
- Then circulation

In cardiopulmonary resuscitation (CPR) circumstances, follow the CAB guidelines.

HESI Hint • Look and listen! If breath sounds are clear but the client is cyanotic and lethargic, adequate oxygenation is not occurring.

HESI Hint • The key to respiratory status is assessment of breath sounds, as well as visualization of the client. Breath sounds are better described, not named; for example, sounds should be described as crackles, wheezes, or high-pitched whistling sounds rather than rales, rhonchi, etc., which may not mean the same thing to each clinical professional.

HESI Hint • Watch for NCLEX-RN® questions that deal with O_2 delivery. In adults, O_2 must bubble through some type of water solution so it can be humidified if given at >4 L/min or delivered directly to the trachea. If given at 1 to 4 L/min or by mask or nasal prongs, the oropharynx and nasal pharynx provide adequate humidification.

Cancer of the Larynx

Description: Neoplasm occurring in the larynx, most commonly squamous cell in origin

A. Prolonged use of combined effects of alcohol and tobacco is directly related to development.

TABLE 4-5 **Bronchodilators and Corticosteroids**

Drugs	Indications	Adverse Reactions	Nursing Implications
Adrenergics and Sympathomimetics			
• Epinephrine • Isoproterenol HCl • Albuterol • Isoetharine • Terbutaline • Salmeterol • Metaproterenol (inhaled) • Levalbuterol	• Bronchodilator	• Anxiety • Increased heart rate • Nausea, vomiting • Urinary retention	• Check heart rate. • Monitor for urinary retention, especially in men over 40. • Instruct in proper use of inhaler. • Use bronchodilator inhaler before steroid inhaler. • May cause sleep disturbance.
Methylxanthine			
• Aminophylline (IV) • Theophylline (PO)	• Bronchodilator	• GI distress • Sleeplessness • Cardiac dysrhythmias • Hyperactivity • Tachycardia	• Administer oral forms with food. • Avoid foods containing caffeine. • Check heart rate. • Instruct in proper use of inhaler. • Monitor therapeutic range. • Crosses placenta.
Corticosteroids			
• Prednisone (PO) • Solu-Medrol (IV) • Beclomethasone dipropionate (inhaled) • Budesonide (inhaled) Fluticasone (inhaled) • Triamcinolone (inhaled) • Flunisolide (inhaled) • Mometasone (inhaled)	• Antiinflammatory	• Cardiac dysrhythmias occur with long-term steroid use	• See Endocrine System • Instruct in proper use of inhaler. • Encourage oral care after use.
Anticholinergics			
• Ipratropium • Tiotropium	• Bronchodilator • Control of rhinorrhea	• Dry mouth • Blurred vision • Cough	• Do not exceed 12 doses in 24 hours (ipratropium).
Combination Products			
• Fluticasone + salmeterol • Ipratropium + albuterol • Budesonide + formoterol	• See individual drugs.	• See individual drugs.	• See individual drugs.
Phosphodiesterase 4 Inhibitors			
• Roflumilast	• Reduced lung inflammation in severe COPD	• Insomnia • Weight loss • Depression	• Many drug-drug interactions

B. Other contributing factors include:
  1. Vocal straining
  2. Chronic laryngitis
  3. Family predisposition
  4. Industrial exposure to carcinogens
  5. Nutritional deficiencies: riboflavin
C. Men are affected eight times more often than are women.
D. Diagnosis usually occurs between the ages of 55 and 70.

E. The earliest sign is hoarseness or a change in vocal quality that lasts more than 2 weeks.
F. Medical management includes radiation therapy, often with adjuvant chemotherapy or surgical removal of the larynx (laryngectomy).

Nursing Assessment

A. Magnetic resonance imaging (MRI)
B. Direct laryngoscopy

C. Assessing for hoarseness of longer than 2 weeks (early changes)
D. Assessing for color changes in mouth or tongue

> **HESI Hint** • With cancer of the larynx, the tongue and mouth often appear white, gray, dark brown, or black and may appear patchy.

E. Assessing for dysphagia, dyspnea, cough, hemoptysis, weight loss, neck pain radiating to the ear, enlarged cervical nodes, and halitosis (later changes)
F. Radiographs of head, neck, and chest
G. Computed tomography (CT) scan of neck and biopsy

Analysis (Nursing Diagnoses)

Client undergoing a laryngectomy:
A. *Risk for aspiration* related to …
B. *Anxiety* related to …
C. *Ineffective airway clearance* related to …
D. *Impaired verbal communication* related to …
E. *Ineffective breathing pattern* related to …
F. *Imbalanced nutrition: less than body requirements* related to…

Nursing Plans and Interventions

A. Provide preoperative teaching.
   1. Allow client and family to observe and handle tracheostomy tubes and suctioning equipment.
   2. Explain how and why suctioning will take place after surgery.
   3. Plan for acceptable communication methods after surgery.
   4. Consider literacy level.
   5. Refer client to speech pathologist.
   6. Discuss the planned rehabilitation program.
B. Provide postoperative care.
   1. Simplify communications.
   2. Use planned alternative communication methods.
   3. Keep call bell/light within reach at all times.
   4. Ask client yes/no questions whenever possible.
C. Promote respiratory functioning.
   1. Assess respiratory rate and characteristics every 1 to 2 hours.
   2. Keep bed in semi-Fowler position at all times.
   3. Keep laryngeal airway humidified at all times.
   4. Auscultate lung sounds every 2 to 4 hours.
      a. Clients retain secretions
      b. Suction excess secretions from mouth and tracheostomy as needed immediately after surgery
   5. Provide tracheostomy care every 2 to 4 hours and as needed (PRN).

> **HESI Hint** • Tracheostomy care involves cleaning the inner cannula, suctioning, and applying clean dressings.

6. Administer tube feedings as prescribed.
7. Encourage ambulation as early as possible.
8. Refer for speech rehabilitation with artificial larynx or to learn esophageal speech.
9. Humidification of environment.

> **HESI Hint** • Air entering the lungs is humidified along the nasobronchial tree. This natural humidifying pathway is gone for the client who has had a laryngectomy. If the air is not humidified before entering the lungs, secretions tend to thicken and become crusty.

> **HESI Hint** • A laryngectomy tube has a larger lumen and is shorter than the tracheostomy tube. Observe the client for any signs of bleeding or occlusion, which are the greatest immediate postoperative risks (first 24 hours).

> **HESI Hint** • Always have suction equipment available at the bedside for new and chronic tracheostomy clients.

> **HESI Hint** • Fear of choking is very real for laryngectomy clients. They cannot cough as they could earlier because the glottis is gone. Teach the glottal stop technique to remove secretions (take a deep breath, momentarily occlude the tracheostomy tube, cough, and simultaneously remove the finger from the tube).

Pulmonary Tuberculosis

Description: Communicable lung disease caused by an infection by *Mycobacterium tuberculosis* bacteria
A. Transmission is by airborne droplets.
B. After initial exposure, the bacteria encapsulate (form a Ghon lesion).
C. Bacteria remain dormant until a later time, when clinical symptoms appear.

Nursing Assessment

A. It is often asymptomatic.
B. Symptoms include:
   1. Fever with night sweats
   2. Anorexia, weight loss
   3. Malaise, fatigue
   4. Cough, hemoptysis
   5. Dyspnea, pleuritic chest pain with inspiration
   6. Cavitation or calcification as evidenced on chest radiograph
   7. Positive sputum culture is positive for *M. tuberculosis*
   8. Repeated upper respiratory infections (URIs)

Tuberculosis Skin Test (TST) (Mantoux); A positive TB skin test in a healthy client is exhibited by an induration 10 mm or greater in diameter 48 to 72 hours after the skin test. Anyone who has received a bacillus Calmette-Guérin (BCG) vaccine will have a positive skin test and must be evaluated with an initial chest radiograph. A health history with signs and symptoms form may be filled out annually until signs and symptoms arise; then another radiograph is required. Chest x-rays are required on new employment; employer may require an x-ray every 5 years depending on exposure risk.

CDC guidelines indicate that the QuantiFeron-TB Gold test, a new blood test, is more reliable for TB skin testing. Nucleic acid amplification (NAA) testing may be recommended when a client has signs and symptoms of TB.

Analysis (Nursing Diagnoses)

A. *Ineffective breathing pattern…*
B. *Ineffective air clearance…*
C. *Noncompliance…*
D. *Ineffective self-health management related to lack of knowledge…*

Nursing Plans and Interventions

A. Provide client teaching.
   1. Cough into tissues and dispose of immediately into biohazardous waste bags.
   2. Take all medications as prescribed daily for 9 to 12 months.
   3. Wash hands using proper handwashing technique.
   4. Report symptoms of deteriorating condition, especially hemorrhage.
B. Collect sputum cultures as needed; client may return to work after three negative cultures.
C. Place client in respiratory isolation while hospitalized.
D. Administer anti-TB medications as prescribed (Table 4-6).
E. Refer client and high-risk persons to local or state health department for testing and prophylactic treatment.
F. Promote adequate nutrition.

Lung Cancer

Description: Neoplasm occurring in the lung
A. Lung cancer is the leading cause of cancer-related death in the United States.
B. Cigarette smoking is responsible for 80% to 90% of all lung cancers.
C. Exposure to occupational hazards such as asbestos and radioactive dust poses significant risk.
D. Lung cancer tends to appear years after exposure; it is most commonly seen in persons after ages 50 or 60.
E. Lung cancer has a poor prognosis.

Nursing Assessment

A. Persistent dry, hacking cough early, with cough turning productive as disease progresses
B. Hoarseness
C. Dyspnea
D. Hemoptysis; rust-colored or purulent sputum

TABLE 4-6 Drug Therapy for Tuberculosis (TB)

Drug	Mechanisms of Action	Side Effects	Comments
First-Line Drugs			
• Isoniazid (INH)	• Interferes with DNA metabolism of tubercle bacillus	• Nausea, vomiting, abdominal pain • Rare: neurotoxicity, optic neuritis, and hepatotoxicity • Peripheral neuritis	• Metabolism primarily by liver and excretion by kidneys; pyridoxine (vitamin B_6) administration during high-dose therapy as prophylactic measure; use as single prophylactic agent for active TB in individuals whose PPD converts to positive; ability to cross blood–brain barrier • Drug interaction with alcohol, Antabuse, and phenytoin
• Rifampin	• Has broad-spectrum effects, inhibits RNA polymerase of tubercle bacillus	• Hepatitis, febrile reaction, GI disturbance, peripheral neuropathy, hypersensitivity • Orange body secretions	• Used in conjunction with at least one other antitubercular agent; low incidence of side effects; suppression of effect of birth control pills; possible orange urine • Increases metabolism of digoxin and oral hypoglycemics

Continued

TABLE 4-6 Drug Therapy for Tuberculosis (TB)—cont'd

Drug	Mechanisms of Action	Side Effects	Comments
• Ethambutol	• Inhibits RNA synthesis and is bacteriostatic for the tubercle bacillus	• Skin rash, GI disturbance, malaise, peripheral neuritis, optic neuritis	• Side effects uncommon and reversible with discontinuation of drug; most common use as substitute drug when toxicity occurs with isoniazid or rifampin
• Pyrazinamide	• Bactericidal effect (exact mechanism is unknown)	• Fever, skin rash, hyperuricemia, jaundice (rare) • Hepatotoxicity, arthralgias, GI distress	• High rate of effectiveness when used with streptomycin or capreomycin
• Rifapentine	• Inhibits DNA-dependent RNA polymerase	• Red discoloration of body fluids and tissues	• Many drug interactions • Always use in conjunction with at least one other antituberculosis drug.
Second-Line Drugs			
• Ethionamide	• Inhibits protein synthesis	• GI disturbance, hepatotoxicity, hypersensitivity • Peripheral neuritis	• Valuable for treatment of resistant organisms; contraindicated in pregnancy. • Give with meals; avoid alcohol. • If neuropathy exists, give pyridoxine.
• Capreomycin	• Inhibits protein synthesis and is bactericidal	• Ototoxicity, nephrotoxicity	• Cautious use in older adults. • Undergo periodic hearing evaluation.
• Kanamycin and amikacin	• Interferes with protein synthesis	• Ototoxicity, nephrotoxicity	• Use in select cases for treatment of resistant strains. • Evaluate hearing after starting medication.
• Paraaminosalicylic acid (PAS)	• Interferes with metabolism of tubercle bacillus	• GI disturbance (common), hypersensitivity, hepatotoxicity	• Interferes with absorption of rifampin; used uncommonly. • Give with meals.
• Streptomycin	• Inhibits protein synthesis and is bactericidal	• Ototoxicity (eighth cranial nerve), nephrotoxicity, hypersensitivity	• Cautious use in older adults, those with renal disease, and pregnant women; must be given parenterally.
• Levofloxacin and moxifloxacin	• Inhibits DNA gyrase	• Increased risk of tendinitis	• Many drug-drug interactions.
Second-Line Drugs			
• Cycloserine	• Inhibits cell wall synthesis	• Personality changes, psychosis, rash	• Contraindicated in individuals with histories of psychosis; used in treatment of resistant strains.

HESI Hint • Teaching is very important with the client with TB. Drug therapy is usually long term (6 months or longer). It is essential that the client take the medications as prescribed for the entire time. Skipping doses or prematurely terminating the drug therapy can result in a public health hazard.

HESI Hint • *Teaching Points*
Rifampin: Reduces effectiveness of oral contraceptives; client should use other birth control methods during treatment; gives body fluids orange tinge; stains soft contact lenses
Isoniazid (INH): Increased phenytoin levels
Ethambutol: Vision check before starting therapy and monthly thereafter; may have to take for 1 to 2 years
Teach rationale for combination drug therapy to increase compliance. Resistance develops more slowly if several anti-TB drugs given, instead of just one drug at a time.

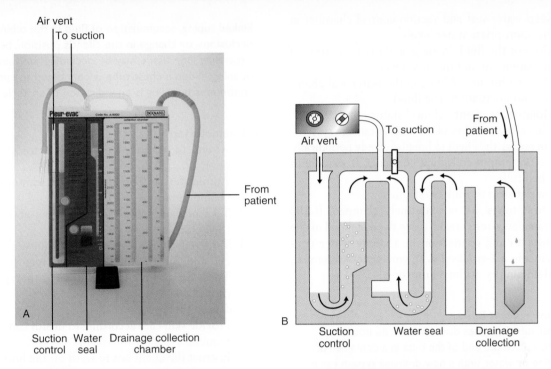

FIGURE 4-3 Chest tubes. Chest tubes are used to remove or drain blood or air from the intrapleural space, to expand the lung after surgery, or to restore subatmospheric pressure to the thoracic cavity. Many brands of commercial chest drainage systems are available; all are based upon the traditional three-bottle water seal system. *A,* The Pleur-evac drainage system, a commercial three-chamber chest drainage device. *B,* Schematic of the drainage device. (From Ignatavicius DD, Workman ML: *Medical-surgical nursing: Patient-centered collaborative care,* ed 8, St. Louis, 2016, Saunders.)

E. Pain in the chest area
F. Diminished breath sounds, occasional wheezing
G. Abnormal chest radiograph
H. Positive sputum for cytology and for pleural fluid

Analysis (Nursing Diagnoses)

A. *Chronic pain* related to …
B. *Ineffective breathing pattern* related to …
C. *Impaired gas exchange* related to …
D. *Imbalanced nutrition: less than body requirements* related to …
E. *Anxiety* related to …

Nursing Plans and Interventions

A. Nursing interventions are similar to those implemented for the client with COPD.
B. Place client in semi-Fowler position.
C. Teach pursed-lip breathing to improve gas exchange.
D. Teach relaxation techniques; client often becomes anxious about breathing difficulty.
E. Administer O_2 as indicated by pulse oximetry or ABGs.
F. Take measures to allay anxiety.
   1. Keep client and family informed of impending tests and procedures.
   2. Give client as much control as possible over personal care.
   3. Encourage client and family to verbalize concerns.

G. Decrease pain to manageable level by administering analgesics as needed (within safety range for respiratory difficulty).
H. Surgery
   1. Thoracotomy for clients who have a resectable tumor. (Unfortunately, detection commonly occurs so late that the tumor is no longer localized and is not amenable to resection.)
   2. Pneumonectomy (removal of entire lung)
      a. Position client on operative side or back.
      b. Chest tubes are not usually used.
   3. Lobectomy and segmental resection
      a. Position client on back.
      b. Chest tubes are usually inserted (Fig. 4-3).
      c. Check to ensure tubing is not kinked or obstructed.

HESI Hint • Some tumors are so large that they fill entire lobes of the lung. When removed, large spaces are left. Chest tubes are not usually used with these clients because it is helpful if the mediastinal cavity, where the lung used to be, fills up with fluid. This fluid helps to prevent the shift of the remaining chest organs to fill the empty space.

   4. Chest tubes
      a. Keep all tubing coiled loosely below chest level, with connections tight and taped.

b. Keep water seal and suction control chamber at the appropriate water levels.

c. Monitor the fluid drainage, and mark the time of measurement and the fluid level.

d. Observe for air bubbling in the water seal chamber and fluctuations (tidaling).

e. Monitor the client's clinical status.

f. Check the position of the chest drainage system.

g. Encourage the client to breathe deeply periodically.

h. Do not empty collection container. Replace unit when full.

i. Do not strip or milk chest tubes.

j. Chest tubes are not routinely clamped. If the drainage system breaks, place the distal end of the chest tubing connection in a sterile water container at a 2-cm level as an emergency water seal.

k. Maintain dry occlusive dressing.

HESI Hint • Chest Tubes

If the chest tube becomes disconnected, do not clamp! Immediately place the end of the tube in a container of sterile saline or water until a new drainage system can be connected.

If the chest tube is accidentally dislodged from the client, the nurse should cover with a dry sterile dressing taped on three sides. If an air leak is noted, tape the dressing on three sides only; this allows air to escape and prevents the formation of a tension pneumothorax. Notify the health care provider.

HESI Hint • NCLEX-RN Content on Chest Tubes

Fluctuations (tidaling) in the fluid will occur if there is no external suction. These fluctuating movements are a good indicator that the system is intact; they should move upward with each inspiration and downward with each expiration. If fluctuations cease, check for kinked tubing, accumulation of fluid in the tubing, occlusions, or change in the client's position, because expanding lung tissue may be occluding the tube opening. When a chest tube is connected to suction, continuous bubbling is an indication of an air leak.

I. Chemotherapy
  1. Attend to immunosuppression factor. (See Oncology)
  2. Administer antiemetics before administration of chemotherapy.
  3. Take precautions in administrating antineoplastics. (See Oncology)
  4. Targeted therapy is used for nonsmall cell cancer and for treatment of late-stage lung cancer. These drugs are not used alone as therapy for lung cancer.

J. Radiation therapy
  1. Provide skin care according to health care provider's request.
  2. Instruct the client not to wash off the lines drawn by the radiologist.
  3. Instruct client to wear soft cotton garments only.
  4. Avoid use of powders and creams on radiation site unless specified by the radiologist.

HESI Hint • Various pathophysiologic conditions can be related to the nursing diagnosis
Ineffective breathing patterns:

1. Inability of air sacs to fill and empty properly (emphysema, cystic fibrosis)
2. Obstruction of the air passages (carcinoma, asthma, chronic bronchitis)
3. Accumulation of fluid in the air sacs (pneumonia)
4. Respiratory muscle fatigue (COPD, pneumonia)

Review of Respiratory System

1. List four common symptoms of pneumonia the nurse might note on physical examination.
2. State four nursing interventions for assisting the client to cough productively.
3. What symptoms of pneumonia might the nurse expect to see in an older client?
4. How does the nurse prevent hypoxia during suctioning?
5. During mechanical ventilation, what are three major nursing interventions?
6. When examining a client with emphysema, what physical findings is the nurse likely to see?
7. What is the most common risk factor associated with lung cancer?
8. Describe the preoperative nursing care for a client undergoing a laryngectomy.
9. List five nursing interventions after chest tube insertion.
10. What immediate action should the nurse take when a chest tube becomes disconnected from a bottle or suction apparatus? What should the nurse do if a chest tube is accidentally removed from the client?
11. What instructions should be given to a client after radiation therapy?
12. What precautions are required for clients with TB when placed on respiratory isolation?
13. List four components of teaching for the client with tuberculosis.

Answers to Review

1. Tachypnea, fever with chills, productive cough, bronchial breath sounds
2. Encourage deep breathing; increase fluid intake to 3 L/day; use humidity to loosen secretions; suction airway to stimulate coughing.
3. Confusion, lethargy, anorexia, rapid respiratory rate
4. Deliver 100% O_2 (hyperinflating) before and after each endotracheal suctioning.
5. Monitor client's respiratory status and secure connections; establish a communication mechanism with the client; keep airway clear by coughing and suctioning.
6. Barrel chest, dry or productive cough, decreased breath sounds, dyspnea, crackles in lung fields
7. Smoking (cigarettes or marijuana)
8. Involve family and client in manipulation of tracheostomy equipment before surgery; plan acceptable communication methods; refer to speech pathologist; discuss rehabilitation program.
9. Maintain a dry occlusive dressing on chest tube. Keep all tubing connections tight and taped. Monitor client's clinical status. Encourage the client to breathe deeply periodically. Monitor the fluid drainage, and mark the time of measurement and the fluid level.
10. Place the end of the tube in a sterile water container at a 2-cm level. Apply an occlusive dressing, and notify health care provider stat.
11. Do not wash off lines; wear soft cotton garments; avoid use of powders and creams on radiation site.
12. A mask for anyone entering room; private room; client must wear mask if leaving room.
13. Cough into tissues and dispose of immediately in special bags. Long-term need for daily medication. Good handwashing technique. Report symptoms of deterioration, for example, blood in secretions.

Renal System

Acute Kidney Injury

Description: A potentially reversible disorder, it is a rapid loss of kidney function accompanied by a rise in serum creatinine and/or a reduction in urine output.

> **HESI Hint** • Normally, kidneys excrete approximately 1 mL of urine per kg of body weight per hour.
>
> For adults, total daily urine output ranges between 1500 and 2000 mL depending on the amount and type of fluid intake, amount of perspiration, environmental or ambient temperature, and the presence of vomiting or diarrhea.

A. Acute kidney failure (AKI) occurs when metabolites accumulate in the body and urinary output changes.
B. There are three major types of AKI (Table 4-7).
C. There are three phases of AKI.
  1. Oliguric phase
  2. Diuretic phase
  3. Recovery phase

Nursing Assessment

A. History of taking nephrotoxic drugs (salicylates, antibiotics, nonsteroidal antiinflammatory drugs [NSAIDs], angiotensin-converting enzyme [ACE] inhibitors, angiotensin receptor blocker [ARBs])
B. Alterations in urinary output
C. Edema, weight gain (ask if waistbands have suddenly become too tight)

TABLE 4-7 Acute Renal Failure

Types	Description	Causative Factors
• Prerenal	• Interference with renal perfusion	• Hemorrhage • Hypovolemia • Decreased cardiac output • Decreased renal perfusion
• Intrarenal	• Damage to renal parenchyma	• Prolonged prerenal state • Nephrotoxins • Intratubular obstruction • Infections (glomerulonephritis) • Renal injury • Vascular lesions • Acute pyelonephritis
• Postrenal	• Obstruction in the urinary tract anywhere from the tubules to the urethral meatus	• Calculi • Prostatic hypertrophy • Tumors

D. Change in mental status
E. Hematuria
F. Dry mucous membranes
G. Drowsiness, headache (HA), muscle twitching, seizures

HESI Hint • Electrolytes are profoundly affected by kidney problems (a favorite NCLEX-RN topic). There must be a balance between extracellular fluid and intracellular fluid to maintain homeostasis. A change in the number of ions or in the amount of fluid will cause a shift in one direction or the other. Sodium and chloride are the primary extracellular ions. Potassium and phosphate are the primary intracellular ions.

H. Diagnostic findings in the oliguric phase
   1. Increased blood urea nitrogen (BUN) and creatinine
   2. Increased potassium (hyperkalemia)
   3. Decreased sodium (hyponatremia)
   4. Decreased pH (acidosis)
   5. Fluid overload (hypervolemic)
   6. High urine specific gravity (>1.020 g/mL)
I. Diagnostic findings in the diuretic phase
   1. Decreased fluid volume (hypovolemia)
   2. Decreased potassium (hypokalemia)
   3. Further decrease in sodium (hyponatremia)
   4. Low urine specific gravity (<1.020 g/mL)
J. Diagnostic laboratory work returns to normal range in recovery phase.

HESI Hint • In some cases, persons in AKI may not experience the oliguric phase but may progress directly to the diuretic phase, during which the urine output may be as much as 10 L per day.

Analysis (Nursing Diagnoses)

A. *Excess fluid volume* related to …
B. *Deficient fluid volume* related to …
C. *Anxiety* related to …
D. *Risk for electrolyte imbalance* related to …

HESI Hint • Clients at risk for developing AKI in the acute care setting are those with chronic kidney disease (CKD), older age, massive trauma, major surgical procedures, extensive burns, cardiac failure, sepsis, or obstetric complications.

Nursing Plans and Interventions

A. Monitor intake and output (I&O) accurately: Fluid restriction during the oliguric phase (600 mL plus previous 24-hr fluid loss)
B. Weigh daily: in oliguric phase, client may gain up to 1 lb/day.
C. Document and report any change in fluid volume status.
D. Nutritional therapy
E. Adequate protein intake (0.6 to 2 g/kg/day) depending on degree of catabolism
F. Monitor laboratory values of both serum and urine to assess electrolyte status, especially hyperkalemia

indicated by serum potassium levels over 5 mEq/L and electrocardiogram (ECG) changes.

G. Potassium restriction and measures to lower potassium (if elevated). Sodium polystyrene (Kayexalate) may be prescribed if K⁺ is too elevated.
H. Restrict sodium restriction.
I. Assess level of consciousness for subtle changes.
J. Prevent cross-infection.

HESI Hint • Body weight is a good indicator of fluid retention and renal status. Obtain accurate weights of all clients with renal failure; obtain weight on the same scale at the same time every day.

HESI Hint • *Fluid Volume Alterations*

Excess Fluid	Fluid-Deficient Symptoms
• Dyspnea	• Decreased urine output
• Weight gain	
• Tachycardia	• Reduction in body weight
• Jugular vein distention	
• Peripheral edema	• Decreased skin turgor
• Elevated blood pressure	
• Dyspnea	• Dry mucous membranes
• Signs and symptoms of pulmonary edema	• Hypotension
• Weight gain	• Tachycardia
	• Weight loss

HESI Hint • Watch for signs of hyperkalemia: dizziness, weakness, cardiac irregularities, muscle cramps, diarrhea, and nausea.

HESI Hint • Potassium has a critical safe range (3.5 to 5.0 mEq/L) because it affects the heart, and any imbalance must be corrected by medications or dietary modification. Limit high-potassium foods (bananas, orange juice, cantaloupe, strawberries, avocados, spinach, fish) and salt substitutes, which are high in potassium.

HESI Hint • Clients with renal failure retain sodium. With water retention, the sodium becomes diluted and serum levels may appear near normal. With excessive water retention, the sodium levels appear decreased (dilution). Limit fluid and sodium intake in AKI clients.

K. Monitor cardiac rate and rhythm (acute cardiac dysrhythmias are usually related to hyperkalemia).
L. Monitor drug levels and interactions.

HESI Hint • During oliguric phase, minimize protein breakdown and prevent rise in BUN by limiting protein intake. When the BUN and creatinine return to normal, acute renal failure (ARF) is determined to be resolved.

Chronic Renal Failure (CRF): End-Stage Renal Disease (ESRD)

Description: Progressive, irreversible damage to the nephrons and glomeruli, resulting in uremia
A. Causes of chronic renal failure are multitudinous.
B. As renal function diminishes, dialysis becomes necessary.
C. Transplantation is an alternative to dialysis for some clients.

Nursing Assessment

A. History of high medication usage
B. Family history of renal disease
C. Increased blood pressure (BP) and/or chronic hypertension (HTN)

D. Diabetes
E. Edema, pulmonary edema
F. Decreasing urinary function
 1. Hematuria
 2. Proteinuria
 3. Cloudy urine
 4. Oliguric (100 to 400 mL/day)
 5. Anuric (<100 mL/day)

HESI Hint • Accumulation of waste products from protein metabolism is the primary cause of uremia. Protein must be restricted in CRF clients. However, if protein intake is inadequate, a negative nitrogen balance occurs, causing muscle wasting. The glomerular filtration rate (GFR) is most often used as an indicator of the level of protein consumption.

H. Dialysis (Table 4-8)

TABLE 4-8 **Renal Dialysis**

Types of Dialysis	Description	Nursing Implications
• Hemodialysis	• Requires venous access (AV shunt, fistula, or graft) • Treatment is 3-8 hours in length, 3 times per week • Correction of fluid and electrolyte imbalance is rapid • Potential blood loss • Does not result in protein loss	• Heparinization is required. • Requires expensive equipment. • Rapid shifts of fluid and electrolytes can lead to disequilibrium syndrome (an unpleasant sensation and a potentially dangerous situation). • Potential hepatitis B and C • Do *not* take blood pressure or perform venipunctures on the arm with the AV shunt, fistula, or graft. • Assess access site for thrill and bruit.
• Continuous arteriovenous hemofiltration (CAVH)	• Requires vascular access: usually femoral or subclavian catheters • Slow process • Correction of fluid and electrolyte imbalance is slow • Does not cause blood loss • Does not result in protein loss	• Requires heparinization of filter tubing. • Filters are costly. • Equipment is simple to use but requires specialized training to monitor. • Limited to special care units; not for home use. • Filter may rupture, causing blood loss.

• Peritoneal	• Surgical placement of abdominal catheter is required (Tenckhoff, Gore-Tex, column-disk)
	• Slow process; up to 8-10 hours for repeated cycles
	• Correction of fluid and electrolyte imbalance is slow
	• Does not cause blood loss
	• Protein is lost in dialysate.
		• Heparinization is not required.
		• Fairly expensive.
		• Simple to perform.
		• Easy to use at home.
		• Dialysate is similar to IV fluid and is prescribed for the individual client's electrolyte needs.
		• Potential complications:
		  • Bowel or bladder perforation
		  • Exit-site and tunnel infection
		  • Peritonitis

HESI Hint • The major difference between dialysate for hemodialysis and peritoneal dialysis is the amount of glucose. Peritoneal dialysis dialysate is much higher in glucose. For this reason, if the dialysate is left in the peritoneal cavity too long, hyperglycemia may occur.

HESI Hint • *Dialysis Covered by Medicare*
- All persons in the United States are eligible for Medicare as of their first day of dialysis under special ESRD funding.
- Medicare card will indicate ESRD.
- Transplantation is covered by Medicare procedure; coverage terminates 6 months postoperative if dialysis is no longer required.

I. Previous kidney transplant
J. Laboratory information
  1. Azotemia
  2. Increased creatinine and BUN
  3. Decreased calcium
  4. Elevated phosphorus, magnesium, potassium, and sodium
  5. Anemia

Analysis (Nursing Diagnoses)

A. *Risk for electrolyte imbalance…*
B. *Excess fluid volume* related to …
C. *Imbalanced nutrition: less than body requirements* related to …
D. *Decreased cardiac output* related to …

Nursing Plans and Interventions

A. Monitor serum electrolyte levels.
B. Weigh daily.
C. Monitor strict I&O.
D. Check for jugular vein distention (JVD) and other signs of fluid overload.
E. Monitor for peripheral edema and pulmonary edema.
F. Provide low-protein, low-sodium, low-potassium, low-phosphate diet.
G. Provide low-protein, low-sodium, low-potassium, low-phosphate diet

HESI Hint • Protein intake is restricted until blood chemistry shows ability to handle the protein catabolites, urea and creatinine. Ensure high caloric intake so protein is spared for its own work; give hard candy, jelly beans, or flavored carbohydrate powders.

HESI Hint • Frequent monitoring of laboratory parameters, especially serum albumin, prealbumin (may be a better indicator of recent or current nutritional status than albumin), and ferritin are necessary to evaluate nutritional status. All patients with CKD should be referred to a dietitian for nutritional education and guidance.

H. Administer phosphate binders with food because client is unable to excrete phosphates (no magnesium-based antacids). Timing is important!
I. Encourage client's protein intake to be of high biologic value (eggs, milk, meat) because the client is on a low-protein diet.
J. Teach client fluid allowance is 500 to 600 mL greater than the previous day's 24-hour output.
K. Alternate periods of rest with periods of activity.
L. Encourage strict adherence to medication regimen; teach client to obtain health care provider's permission before taking any over-the-counter medications.
M. Administer prescribed sodium polystyrene sulfonate (Kayexalate) for acute hyperkalemia.
N. Observe for complications.
  1. Anemia (administer antianemic drug; Table 4-9)
  2. Renal osteodystrophy (abnormal calcium metabolism causes bone pathology)

TABLE 4-9 Antianemic: Biologic Response Modifier (BRM)

Drugs	Indications	Adverse Reactions	Nursing Interventions
• Erythropoietin	• Anemia due to decreased production of erythropoietin in end stage renal disease • Stimulates RBC production, increases Hgb, reticulocyte count, and Hct	• Use with caution in older adults because of increased risk for thrombosis. • HTN, seizures, depletion of body iron stores	• Monitor Hct weekly; report levels over 30%-33% and increases of more than 4 points in less than 2 weeks. • Monitor serum iron and ferritin levels. • Monitor blood pressure and potassium levels. • Explain that pelvic and limb pain should dissipate after 12 hours. • Do not shake vial; shaking may inactivate the glycoprotein. • Discard unused contents; does not contain preservatives.

HESI Hint • As kidneys fail, medications must often be adjusted. Of particular importance is digoxin toxicity because digitalis preparations are excreted by the kidneys. Signs of toxicity in adults include nausea, vomiting, anorexia, visual disturbances, restlessness, headache, cardiac dysrhythmias, and pulse <60 bpm.

3. Severe, resistant HTN
4. Infection
5. Metabolic acidosis
O. Living related or cadaver renal transplant (Table 4-10)
   1. Monitor for rejection.
   2. Monitor for infection.
   3. Teach client to maintain immunosuppressive drug therapy meticulously.

Urinary Tract Infections (UTIs)

Description: Infection or inflammation at any site in the urinary tract (kidney, pyelonephritis; urethra, urethritis; bladder, cystitis; prostate, prostatitis)
A. Normally, the entire urinary tract is sterile.
B. The most common infectious agent is *Escherichia coli*.
C. Persons at highest risk for acquiring UTIs:
   1. Clients diagnosed with diabetes
   2. Pregnant women
   3. Men with prostatic hypertrophy
   4. Immunosuppressed persons
   5. Catheterized clients
   6. Anyone with urinary retention, either short term or long term
   7. Older women (bladder prolapse)
D. Diagnosis
   1. Clean-catch midstream urine collection for culture to identify specific causative organism
   2. Intravenous pyelogram (IVP) to determine kidney functioning
   3. Cystogram to determine bladder functioning
   4. Cystoscopy to determine bladder or urethral abnormalities

Nursing Assessment
A. Signs of infection, including fever and chills
B. Urinary frequency, urgency, or dysuria
C. Hematuria
D. Pain at the costovertebral angle
E. Elevated serum WBCs (>10,000)
F. Disorientation or confusion in older adults may be a sign of UTI.

Analysis (Nursing Diagnoses)
A. *Acute pain* related to …
B. *Impaired urinary elimination* related to …
C. *Deficient knowledge* (specify) related to …
D. *Risk for infection* related to…

Nursing Plans and Interventions
A. Administer antibiotics specific to infectious agent.
B. Instruct client in the appropriate medication regimen.
C. Encourage fluid intake of 3000 mL of fluid/day.
D. Maintain I&O.
E. Administer mild analgesics (phenazopyridine [Pyridium], acetaminophen, or aspirin).
F. Encourage client to void every 2 to 3 hours to prevent residual urine from stagnating in bladder.
G. Avoid unnecessary catheterization.
H. Remove indwelling catheters within 24 to 48 of insertion during hospitalizations.

TABLE 4-10 Postoperative Care: Kidney Surgery

Assessment	Nursing Interventions	Rationale
• Respiratory status	• Auscultate lung sounds to detect "wet" sounds indicating infection. • Demonstrate method of splinting incision for comfort when coughing and deep breathing.	• Flank incision causes pain with both inspiration and expiration. Therefore client avoids deep breathing and coughing; this can lead to respiratory difficulties, including pneumonia.
• Circulatory status	• Check vital signs to detect early signs of bleeding, shock. • Monitor skin color and temperature (pallor and cold skin are signs of shock). • Monitor urinary output (decreases with circulatory collapse). • Monitor surgical site for frank bleeding.	• The kidney is very vascular. • Bleeding is a constant threat. • Circulatory collapse will occur with hemorrhage and can occur very quickly.
• Pain relief status	• Administer narcotic analgesics as needed to relieve pain.	• Relief of pain will improve the client's cooperation with deep-breathing exercises. • Relief of pain will improve client's cooperation with early ambulation.
• Urinary status	• Check urinary output and drainage from all tubes inserted during the surgery. • Maintain accurate intake and output.	• Mechanical drainage of bladder will be implemented after surgery.

I. Routine perineal hygiene especially with use of bedpan or if fecal incontinence is present.

> **HESI Hint** • The key to resolving UTIs with most antibiotics is to keep the blood level of the antibiotic constant. It is important to tell the client to take the antibiotics around the clock and not to skip doses so that a consistent blood level can be maintained for optimal effectiveness.

J. Develop and implement a teaching plan:
 1. Take entire prescription as directed.
 2. Consume oral fluids up to 3 L/day (water, juices); should not consume *citrus* juices.
 3. Shower rather than bathe as a preventive measure. If bathing is necessary, never take a bubble or oil bath and avoid feminine hygiene sprays.
 4. Cleanse from front to back after toileting (women and girls).
 5. Avoid urinary tract irritants: alcohol, sodas, citrus juices, spices.
 6. Void immediately after intercourse (women).
 7. Void every 2 to 3 hours during the day.
 8. Wear cotton undergarments and loose clothing to help decrease perineal moisture.
 9. Practice good handwashing technique.
 10. Obtain follow-up care.

Urinary Tract Obstruction

Description: Partial or complete blockage of the flow of urine at any point in the urinary system
A. Urinary tract obstruction may be caused by:
 1. Foreign body (calculi)
 2. Tumors
 3. Strictures
 4. Functional (e.g., neurogenic bladder)
B. When urinary tract obstruction occurs, urine is retained above the point of obstruction.
 1. Hydrostatic pressure builds, causing dilation of the organs above the obstruction.
 2. If hydrostatic pressure continues to build, hydronephrosis develops, and it can lead to renal failure.

Nursing Assessment

A. Pain
 1. May experience renal colic
 2. Radiating down the thigh and to the genitalia
B. Symptoms of obstruction
 1. Fever, chills
 2. Nausea, vomiting, diarrhea
 3. Abdominal distention

> **HESI Hint** • Location of the pain can help to determine the location of the stone.
> • Flank pain usually means the stone is in the kidney or upper ureter. If the pain radiates to the abdomen or scrotum, the stone is likely to be in the ureter or bladder.

> • Excruciating spastic-type pain is called *colic.*
> • During kidney stone attacks, it is preferable to administer pain medications at regularly scheduled intervals rather than PRN to prevent spasm and optimize comfort.

C. Change in voiding pattern
 1. Dysuria, hematuria
 2. Urgency, frequency, hesitancy, nocturia, dribbling
 3. Difficulty in starting a stream
 4. Incontinence
D. Clients with the following conditions are at risk for developing calculi:
 1. Strictures
 2. Prostatic hypertrophy
 3. Neoplasms
 4. Congenital malformations
 5. History of calculi
 6. Family history of calculi

Analysis (Nursing Diagnoses)

A. *Acute pain* related to …
B. *Impaired urinary elimination* related to…
C. *Urinary retention* related to…
D. *Risk for infection* related to …
E. *Risk for injury* related to …

Nursing Plans and Interventions

A. Administer narcotic analgesics to control pain and alpha-adrenergic blockers to relax smooth muscle in the ureter to facilitate stone passage.
B. Apply moist heat to the painful area unless prescribed otherwise.
C. Encourage high oral fluid intake to help dislodge the stone.
D. Administer intravenous (IV) antibiotics if infection is present.
E. Strain all urine!
F. Send any stones found when straining to the laboratory for analysis.
G. Accurately document I&O.
H. Endourologic procedures
 1. Cystoscopy
 2. Cystolitholapaxy
 3. Ureteroscopy
 4. Percutaneous nephrolithotomy
I. Lithotripsy
 1. Ultrasonic
 2. Electrohydraulic
 3. Laser
 4. Extracorporeal shockwave
J. Surgical therapy
 1. Nephrolithotomy
 2. Pyelolithotomy
 3. Ureterolithotomy
 4. Cystotomy

> **HESI Hint** • Percutaneous nephrostomy: A needle or catheter is inserted through the skin into the calyx of the kidney. The stone may be dissolved by percutaneous irrigation with a liquid that dissolves the stone or by ultrasonic sound waves (lithotripsy) that can be directed through the needle or catheter to break up the stone, which then can be eliminated through the urinary tract.

K. Develop and implement a teaching plan to include:
1. Pursue follow-up care, because stones tend to recur.
2. Maintain a high fluid intake of 3 to 4 L/day.
3. Follow prescribed diet (based on composition of stone).
4. Avoid long periods of remaining in supine position.

Benign Prostatic Hyperplasia (BPH)

Description: Enlargement or hypertrophy of the prostate (sometimes called *hypertrophy of the prostate*)
A. BPH tends to occur in men over 40 years of age.
B. Intervention is required when symptoms of obstruction occur.
C. There are three treatment approaches: active surveillance (watchful waiting), drug therapy with 5-alpha-reductase inhibitors such as finasteride (Proscar) and alpha-adrenergic receptor blockers (tamsulosin), or surgery.
D. The most common treatment is transurethral resection of the prostate gland (TURP). The prostate is removed by endoscopy (no surgical incision is made), allowing for a shorter hospital stay.

Nursing Assessment

A. Increased frequency of voiding, with a decrease in amount of each voiding
B. Nocturia
C. Hesitancy
D. Terminal dribbling
E. Decrease in size and force of stream
F. Acute urinary retention
G. Bladder distention
H. Recurrent UTIs

Analysis (Nursing Diagnoses)

A. *Acute or chronic pain* related to …
B. *Risk for injury: hemorrhage* related to …
C. *Risk for injury: infection* related to …
D. *Risk for urinary retention* related to …

Nursing Plans and Interventions

A. Preoperative teaching: include information concerning pain from bladder spasms that occurs postoperatively.
B. Maintain patent urinary drainage system (large three-way indwelling catheter with a 30-mL balloon) to decrease the spasms.

C. Provide pain relief as prescribed: analgesics, narcotics, and antispasmodics.
D. Minimize catheter manipulation by taping catheter to abdomen or leg, or use a leg strap.
E. Maintain gentle traction on urinary catheter.
F. Check the urinary drainage system for clots.
G. Irrigate bladder as prescribed (may be continuous or rarely intermittent). If continuous, keep Foley bag emptied to avoid retrograde pressure.

> **HESI Hint** • Bladder spasms frequently occur after TURP. The catheter may cause a continuous sensation of bladder fullness. The client should not try to void around the catheter because bladder spasms may occur. Client can request medication to reduce or prevent spasms.

> **HESI Hint** • Instillation of hypertonic or hypotonic solution into a body cavity will cause a shift in cellular fluid. Use only sterile saline for bladder irrigation after TURP because the irrigation must be isotonic to prevent fluid and electrolyte imbalance.
>
> Clients with Foley catheters require perineal care *and* Foley care twice per day.

H. Observe the color and content of urinary output.
1. Normal drainage after prostate surgery is reddish pink, clearing to light pink within 24 hours after surgery. Some small to medium-sized blood clots may be present.
2. Monitor for bright-red bleeding with large clots and increased viscosity.
I. Monitor vital signs frequently for indication of hemorrhagic or hypovolemic shock (circulatory collapse).
J. Monitor hemoglobin (Hgb) and hematocrit (Hct) for pattern of decreasing values that indicates bleeding.
K. After catheter is removed:
1. Monitor amount and number of times client voids.
2. Encourage fluids.
3. Have the client use urine cups to provide a specimen with each voiding.
4. Observe for hematuria after each voiding (urine should progress to clear yellow color by the fourth day).
5. Inform client that burning on urination and urinary frequency are usually experienced during the first postoperative week.
6. Generally the client is not impotent after surgery, but sterility may occur.
7. Instruct client to report any frank bleeding to physician immediately.
8. Monitor for signs of urethral stricture: straining, dysuria, weak urinary stream.
9. Administer antispasmodics as ordered.
10. Ambulate first postop day, if possible.

L. Instruct client to increase fluid intake to 3000 mL/day.
M. Prepare client for discharge with instructions to:
  1. Continue to drink 12 to 14 glasses of water a day.
  2. Avoid constipation, straining.
  3. Avoid strenuous activity, lifting, intercourse, and engaging in sports during the first 3 to 4 weeks after surgery.
  4. Schedule a follow-up appointment.

> **HESI Hint** • Inform the client before discharge that some bleeding is expected after TURP. Large amounts of blood or frank bright bleeding should be reported. However, it is normal for the client to pass small amounts of blood, as well as small clots, during the healing process. He should rest quietly and continue drinking large amounts of fluid.

Review of Renal System

1. Differentiate between acute renal failure and chronic renal failure.
2. During the oliguric phase of renal failure, protein should be severely restricted. What is the rationale for this restriction?
3. Identify two nursing interventions for the client on hemodialysis.
4. What is the highest priority nursing diagnosis for clients in any type of renal failure?
5. A client in renal failure asks why antacids are being given. How should the nurse reply?
6. List four essential elements of a teaching plan for clients with frequent urinary tract infections.
7. What are the most important nursing interventions for clients with possible renal calculi?
8. What discharge instructions should be given to a client who has had urinary calculi?
9. After transurethral resection of the prostate gland (TURP), hematuria should subside by what postoperative day?
10. After the urinary catheter is removed in the TURP client, what are three priority nursing actions?
11. After kidney surgery, what are the primary assessments the nurse should make?

Answers to Review

1. Acute renal failure: often reversible, abrupt deterioration of kidney function. Chronic renal failure: irreversible, slow deterioration of kidney function characterized by increasing BUN and creatinine. Eventually dialysis is required.
2. Toxic metabolites that accumulate in the blood (urea, creatinine) are derived mainly from protein catabolism.
3. Do not take BP or perform venipuncture on the arm with the atrioventricular (AV) shunt, fistula, or graft. Assess access site for thrill and bruit.
4. Risk for imbalanced fluid volume
5. Calcium and aluminum antacids bind phosphates and help keep phosphates from being absorbed into bloodstream, thereby preventing rising phosphate levels; must be taken with meals.
6. Fluid intake 3 L/day; good handwashing; void every 2 to 3 hours during waking hours; take all prescribed medications; wear cotton undergarments.
7. Straining all urine is the most important intervention. Other interventions include accurate I&O documentation and administering analgesics as needed.
8. Maintain high fluid intake of 3 to 4 L/day. Pursue follow-up care (stones tend to recur). Follow prescribed diet based on calculi content. Avoid supine position.
9. The fourth day
10. Continued strict I&O. Continued observations for hematuria. Inform client burning and frequency may last for a week.
11. Respiratory status (breathing is guarded because of pain); circulatory status (the kidney is very vascular and excessive bleeding can occur); pain assessment; urinary assessment (most important, assessment of urinary output).

Cardiovascular System

> **HESI Hint** • What is the relationship of the kidneys to the cardiovascular system?
> • The kidneys filter about 1 L of blood per minute.
> • If cardiac output is decreased, the amount of blood going through the kidneys is decreased; urinary output is decreased. Therefore a decreased urinary output may be a sign of cardiac problems.
> • When the kidneys produce and excrete 0.5 mL of urine/kg of body weight or average 30 mL/hr output, the blood supply is considered to be minimally adequate to perfuse the vital organs.

Angina

Description: Chest discomfort or pain that occurs when myocardial O_2 demands exceed supply

Common Causes

A. Atherosclerotic heart disease
B. HTN
C. Coronary artery spasm
D. Hypertrophic cardiomyopathy
E. Any activity that increases the heart's oxygen demand; physical exertion, cold temperatures

Nursing Assessment

A. Pain
   1. Mild to severe intensity, described as heavy, squeezing, pressing, burning, choking, aching, and feeling of apprehension
   2. Substernal, radiating to left arm and/or shoulder, jaw, right shoulder
   3. Transient or prolonged, with gradual or sudden onset; typically of short duration
   4. Often precipitated by exercise, exposure to cold, a heavy meal, mental tension, sexual intercourse
   5. Relieved by rest and/or nitroglycerin
B. Dyspnea, tachycardia, palpitations
C. Nausea, vomiting
D. Fatigue
E. Diaphoresis, pallor, weakness
F. Syncope
G. Dysrhythmias
H. Diagnostic information
   1. ECG: Is generally at client baseline unless taken during anginal attack, when ST-segment depression and T-wave inversion may occur
   2. Exercise stress test: Shows ST-segment depression and hypotension
   3. Stress echocardiogram: Looks for changes in wall motion (indicated in women)
   4. Coronary angiogram: Detects coronary artery spasms
   5. Cardiac catheterization: Detects arterial blockage
I. Risk factors
   1. Nonmodifiable
      a. Heredity
      b. Gender: male > female until menopause, then equal risk
      c. Ethnic background: African Americans
      d. Age
   2. Modifiable
      a. Hyperlipidemia
      b. Total serum cholesterol above 300 mg/dL: Four times greater risk for developing coronary artery disease (CAD) than those with levels less than 200 mg/dL (desirable level)
      c. Low-density lipoprotein (LDL), "bad cholesterol": A molecule of LDL is approximately 50% cholesterol by weight (<100 mg/dL desirable).
      d. High-density lipoprotein (HDL), "good cholesterol": HDL is inversely related to the risk for developing CAD (>60 mg/dL is desirable). In fact, HDL may serve to remove cholesterol from tissues.
      e. HTN
      f. Cigarette smoking
      g. Obesity
      h. Physical inactivity
      i. Metabolic syndrome
      j. Stress
      k. Elevated homocysteine level
      l. Substance abuse

Analysis (Nursing Diagnoses)

A. *Decreased cardiac output* related to …
B. *Acute pain* related to …
C. *Anxiety* related to …

Nursing Plans and Interventions

A. Monitor medications, and instruct client in proper administration.
B. Determine factors precipitating pain, and assist client and family in adjusting lifestyle to decrease these factors.
C. Teach risk factors, and identify client's own risk factors.
D. During an attack
   1. Provide immediate rest.
   2. Take vital signs.
   3. Record an ECG.
   4. Administer no more than three nitroglycerin tablets, 5 minutes apart (Table 4-11).
   5. Seek emergency treatment if no relief has occurred after taking nitroglycerin.
E. Physical activity
   1. Teach avoidance of isometric activity.
   2. Implement an exercise program.
   3. Teach that sexual activity may be resumed after exercise is tolerated, usually when able to climb two flights of stairs without exertion. Nitroglycerin can be taken prophylactically before intercourse.
F. Provide nutritional information about modifying fats (saturated) and sodium. Antilipemic medications may be prescribed to lower cholesterol levels (Table 4-12).
G. Medical interventions include:
   1. Percutaneous transluminal coronary angioplasty (PTCA), also known as *percutaneous coronary intervention (PCI)*. A balloon catheter is repeatedly inflated to split or fracture plaque, and the arterial wall is stretched, enlarging the diameter of the vessel. A rotoblade is used to pulverize plaque.
   2. Arthrectomy. A catheter with a collection chamber is used to remove plaque from a coronary artery by shaving, cutting, or grinding.
   3. Coronary artery bypass graft (CABG)

TABLE 4-11 Antianginals

Drugs	Indications/Actions	Adverse Reactions	Nursing Implications
Nitrates			
• Nitroglycerin (NTG) • Isosorbide dinitrate • Isosorbide mononitrate	• Anginal prophylaxis • Acute attack • Reduces vascular resistance	• Headache • Flushing • Dizziness • Weakness • Hypotension • Nausea	• Monitor relief. • Have client rest. • Monitor vital signs. • Store medication in original container. • Protect from light.
Beta Blockers			
• Propranolol HCl Atenolol • Nadolol • Metoprolol	• Anginal prophylaxis • Reduces O_2 demand	• Fatigue • Lethargy • Hallucinations • Impotence • Bradycardia • Hypotension • HF • Wheezing	• Monitor apical heart rate. • Assess for decreased BP. • Do not stop medication abruptly. • Clients with HF, bronchitis, asthma, COPD, or renal or hepatic insufficiency have increased likelihood of incurring adverse reactions.
Calcium Channel Blockers			
• Verapamil • Nifedipine HCl Diltiazem HCl	• Anginal prophylaxis • Inhibits influx of calcium ions • Decreases sinoatrial node automaticity and atrioventricular node conduction	• Dizziness • Hypotension • Fatigue • Headache • Syncope • Peripheral edema • Hypokalemia • Dysrhythmia • HF • Gastric distress	• Clients with HF and older adults have an increased likelihood of incurring adverse reactions. • Assess for decreased BP. • Monitor serum potassium. • Swallow pills whole. • Store at room temperature. • Do not stop abruptly. • Take 1 hour before meals or 2 hours after meals.
Other			
• Ranolazine	• Anginal prophylaxis • Inhibits influx of sodium ions	• Dysrhythmia • Constipation	• Many drug-drug interactions. • Contraindication in all levels of hepatic cirrhosis.

4. Coronary laser therapy
5. Coronary artery stent or drug-eluding stents

Myocardial Infarction (MI)

Description: Disruption in or deficiency of coronary artery blood supply, resulting in necrosis of myocardial tissue

Causes of MI

A. Thrombus or clotting
B. Shock or hemorrhage

Nursing Assessment

A. Sudden onset of pain in the lower sternal region (substernal)
  1. Severity increases until it becomes nearly unbearable.
  2. Heavy and viselike pain often radiates to the shoulders and down the arms and/or to the neck, jaw, and back. Common locations for pain are substernal, retrosternal, or epigastric areas. Pain of MI differs from angina pain in its sudden onset.
    a. Women may also present with shortness of breath or fatigue.
    b. Pain differs from anginal pain in its onset.
  3. Pain is not relieved by rest.
  4. Nausea and vomiting
  5. Anxiety, feeling of impending doom/death
  6. Pain is not relieved by nitroglycerin.
  7. Pain may persist for hours or days.
  8. Client may not have pain (silent MI), especially those with diabetic neuropathy.
B. Rapid, irregular, and thready pulse
C. Decreased level of consciousness indicating decreased cerebral perfusion
D. Left heart shift sometimes occurring after MI
E. Cardiac dysrhythmias, occurring in about 90% of MI clients
F. Cardiogenic shock or fluid retention

TABLE 4-12 Antilipemics

Drugs	Indications	Adverse Reactions	Nursing Implications
Bile Sequestrants			
• Colestipol HCl Colesevelam • Cholestyramine	• Treat type IIA hyperlipidemia (hypercholesterolemia) when dietary changes fail	• Abdominal pain, nausea and vomiting, distention, flatulence, belching, constipation • Reduced absorption of lipid-soluble vitamins: A, D, E, and K • Alteration in absorption of other oral medications	• Teach client to mix powder forms with adequate amounts of liquid or fruits high in moisture content such as applesauce to prevent accidental inhalation or esophageal distress. • Monitor prothrombin times. • Assess for visual changes and rickets • Administer other oral medications 1 hour before or 6 hours after giving bile sequestrants.
HMG-CoA Reductase Inhibitors (Statins)			
• Atorvastatin • Fluvastatin • Pravastatin • Simvastatin • Lovastatin • Pitavastatin • Rosuvastatin		• Side effects similar to bile sequestrants • May elevate liver enzymes • Hepatitis or pancreatitis • Rhabdomyolysis	• Obtain liver enzymes baseline and monitor every 6 months. • Monitor CPK levels. • Review specific drug–food interactions; avoid grapefruit juice. • Timing with or without food varies with drug. • Instruct client to report any muscle tenderness. • Monitor dose limits when interacting medications prescribed.
Fibric Acid Derivatives			

• Gemfibrate
• Fenofibrate
• Fenofibric acid
• Clofibrate
	• Used with diet changes to lower elevated cholesterol and triglycerides	• Abdominal and epigastric pain; diarrhea—most common
		• Flatulence, nausea, and vomiting
		• Heartburn
		• Dyspepsia
		• Gallstones
		• Tricor: weakness, fatigue, headache
		• Myopathy
			• Obtain baseline labs: liver function, CBC, and electrolytes; monitor every 3-6 months.
			• Administer:
			  • Lopid: 30 minutes before breakfast and dinner
			  • Tricor: with meals

Water-Soluble Vitamins			
• Niacin • Nicotinic acid	• Large doses decrease lipoprotein and triglyceride synthesis and increase HDL	• Flushing of face and neck • Pruritus • Headache • Orthostatic hypotension • (ER form): Hepatotoxicity • Hyperglycemia • Hyperuricemia • Upper GI distress	• Give with milk or food to avoid GI irritation. • Client to change positions slowly. • Instruct client taking extended-release (ER) form to report darkened urine, light-colored stools, anorexia, yellowing of eyes or skin, severe stomach pain.

HESI Hint • Angina is caused by myocardial ischemia. Which cardiac medications would be appropriate for acute angina?
Digoxin: *not appropriate*; increases the strength and contractility of the heart muscle; the problem in angina is that the muscle is not receiving enough O_2. Digoxin will not help.
Nitroglycerin: *appropriate*; causes dilatation of the coronary arteries, allowing more O_2 to get to the heart muscle.
Atropine: *not appropriate*; increases heart rate by blocking vagal stimulation, which suppresses the heart rate; does not address the lack of O_2 to the heart muscle.
Propranolol (Inderal): *not appropriate* for acute angina attack; however, is *appropriate* for long-term management of stable angina because it acts as a beta blocker to control vasoconstriction.

G. Serum cardiac markers
   1. Cardiac-specific troponin is a myocardial muscle protein released into circulation after MI or injury with greater sensitivity and specificity for myocardial injury than CK-MB.
   2. Creatine kinase (CK), intracellular enzymes that are released into circulation after an MI, can also be elevated after other intracoronary procedures.
      a. Rise 3 to 12 hours after an MI
      b. Peak within up to 24 hours
      c. Return to normal within 2 to 3 days
   3. CK-MB band is specific to myocardial cells and can help quantify myocardial damage.
      a. Cardiac-specific troponin T (cTnT) and cardiac-specific troponin I (cTnI)
      b. Increase 3 to 12 hours after the onset of MI
      c. Peak at 10 to 24 hours
      d. Return to baseline over 5 to 14 days
H. Narrowed pulse pressure, for example, 90/80 mm Hg
 I. Bowel sounds are absent or high pitched, indicating possibility of mesenteric artery thrombosis, which acts as an intestinal obstruction. (See Gastrointestinal System, p. 120.)
 J. Heart failure indicated by crackles in the lungs sounds
K. ECG changes occur as early as 2 hours after MI or as late as 72 hours after MI (Table 4-13)
L. Nausea, vomiting, gastric discomfort, indigestion
M. Anxiety, restlessness, feeling of impending doom or death
N. Cool, pale, diaphoretic skin
O. Dizziness, fatigue, syncope
 P. Women more commonly experience dyspnea, unusual fatigue, and sleep disturbances.

Analysis (Nursing Diagnoses)

A. *Risk for decreased cardiac tissue perfusion* related to …
 B. *Decreased cardiac output* related to …
C. *Activity intolerance* related to …
D. *Acute pain* related to …

Nursing Plans and Interventions

A. Administer medications as prescribed.
   1. For pain and to increase O_2 perfusion, IV morphine sulfate (acts as a peripheral vasodilator and decreases venous return)
   2. Other medications often prescribed include (see Table 4-11):
      a. Nitrates (e.g., nitroglycerin)
      b. ACE inhibitors
      c. Beta blockers
      d. Calcium channel blockers (when beta blockers are contraindicated)
      e. Aspirin
      f. Antiplatelet aggregates
B. Obtain vital signs, including ECG rhythm strip regularly, per agency policy.
C. Administer O_2 at 2 to 6 L per nasal cannula.
D. Obtain cardiac enzymes as prescribed.
E. Provide a quiet, restful environment.
F. Assess breath sounds for rales (indicating pulmonary edema).
G. Maintain patent IV line for administration of emergency medications.
H. Monitor fluid balance.
 I. Keep in semi-Fowler position to assist with breathing.
 J. Maintain bed rest for 12 hours.
K. Encourage client to resume activity gradually.
L. Encourage verbalization of fears.
M. Provide information about the disease process and cardiac rehabilitation.
N. Consider medical interventions (see HESI Hint regarding Angina, p. 101):
   1. Thrombolytic agents, within 1 to 4 hours of MI, but not more than 12 hours of MI (Table 4-14)
   2. Intraaortic balloon pump (IABP) to improve myocardial perfusion
   3. Surgical reperfusion with CABG
   4. PCI with stenting.

> **HESI Hint** • Remember MONA when administering medications and treatments in the patient with myocardial infarction. MONA: morphine, oxygen, nitroglycerin, aspirin.

Hypertension

Description: Persistent seated BP levels equal to or greater than 140/90 mm Hg
A. Essential (primary) HTN has no known cause (idiopathic).
B. Secondary HTN develops in response to an identifiable mechanism or another disease.

TABLE 4-13 Postmyocardial Infarction Cardiac Enzyme Elevations

Enzyme/Marker	Onset	Peak	Return to Normal
CK-MB (recognized indicator of MI by most clinicians)	4-8 hr	12-24 hr	48-72 hr
Myoglobin	1-4 hr (elevate before CK-MB)	12 hr	24 hr
Cardiac troponins	As early as 1 hr post injury	10-24 hr	5-14 days

HESI Hint • Blood pressure is created by the difference in the pressure of the blood as it leaves the heart and the resistance it meets flowing out to the tissues. Diet and exercise, smoking cessation, weight control, and stress management can control many factors that influence the resistance blood meets as it flows from the heart.

Nursing Assessment

A. BP equal to or greater than 140/90 mm Hg on two separate occasions

1. Obtain BP while client is lying down, sitting, and standing.
2. Compare readings taken lying down, sitting, and standing. A difference of more than 10 mm Hg of

TABLE 4-14 Fibrinolytic Agents

Drugs	Indications	Adverse Reactions	Nursing Implications
• Streptokinase	• Deep vein thrombosis • Pulmonary embolism • Arterial thrombosis and embolism • Coronary thrombosis • Dissolving clots in arteriovenous cannula	• Anaphylactic response ranging from breathing difficulties to bronchospasm, periorbital swelling, or angioneurotic edema • Increased risk for bleeding • Hemorrhagic infarction at site of myocardial damage • Reperfusion dysrhythmias	• Assess for bleeding at puncture site; apply pressure to control bleeding. • Assess for allergic reactions and dysrhythmias during intracoronary perfusion. • Immobilize client's leg for 24 hours after femoral coronary cannulation and perfusion; assess pedal pulses for adequate circulation. • Monitor client's thrombin time after therapy. Do *not* administer heparin or oral anticoagulants until thrombin time is less than twice that of control. • Do *not* shake vial when reconstituting; roll and tilt vial gently to mix.
• Tenecteplase • Reteplase	• Acute management of coronary thrombosis	• Do not give if history of uncontrolled HTN. • Can cause hypotension.	• Obtain baseline studies before administration: PT, PTT, CBC, fibrinogen level, renal studies, cardiac enzymes. • Check for abnormal pulse, neurologic vital signs, and presence of skin lesions, which may indicate coagulation defects. • Avoid needle punctures because of the possibility of bleeding; apply pressure for 10 minutes to venous puncture sites and for 30 minutes to arterial puncture sites; follow with pressure dressing. • Be prepared to treat reperfusion dysrhythmias.
• Urokinase	• Pulmonary embolism • Coronary thrombosis • IV catheter clearance	• Is nonantigenic and does not cause allergic reactions; otherwise has the same adverse reactions as those cited for streptokinase.	• Infuse heparin and an oral anticoagulant after urokinase therapy to prevent rethrombosis. • Is much more expensive than streptokinase, but does not cause allergic reactions found with streptokinase therapy. • Reconstitute immediately before use.
• Alteplase • Anistreplase	• Deep vein thrombosis • Pulmonary embolism • Coronary thrombosis	• Interacts with heparin, oral anticoagulants, and antiplatelet drugs to increase the risk for bleeding.	• Alters coagulation only at the thrombus, *not* systemically (bleeding complications associated with streptokinase and urokinase are reduced with t-PA therapy). • Because t-PA is a human protein, allergic response is unlikely to occur. • Half-life is 3-7 minutes; use immediately.

either systolic or diastolic indicates postural hypotension. Take pressure in both arms.

B. Genetic risk factors (nonmodifiable)
1. Positive family history for HTN
2. Gender (men have a greater risk for being hypertensive at an earlier age than women).
3. Age (risk increases with increasing age).
4. Ethnicity (African Americans are at greater risk than whites).

C. Lifestyle and habits that increase risk for becoming hypertensive (modifiable)
1. Use of alcohol, tobacco, and caffeine
2. Sedentary lifestyle, obesity
3. Nutrition history of high salt and fat intake
4. Use of oral contraceptives or estrogens
5. Stress

D. Associated physical problems
1. Renal failure
2. Impaired renal function
3. Respiratory problems, especially COPD
4. Cardiac problems, especially valvular disorders
5. Dyslipidemia
6. Diabetes

E. Pharmacologic history
1. Steroids (increase BP)
2. Estrogens (increase BP)

F. Assess for headache, edema, nocturia, nosebleeds, and vision changes (may be asymptomatic).

G. Assess level of stress and source of stress (related to job, economics, family).

H. Assess personality type (i.e., determine whether client exhibits perfectionist behavior).

> **HESI Hint** • Remember the risk factors for HTN: heredity, race, age, alcohol abuse, increased salt intake, obesity, and use of oral contraceptives.

Analysis (Nursing Diagnoses)

A. *Deficient knowledge* related to …
B. *Noncompliance* related to …
C. *Ineffective tissue perfusion (peripheral)* related to …

Nursing Plans and Interventions

A. Develop a teaching plan to include:
1. Information about disease process
   a. Risk factors
   b. Causes
   c. Long-term complications
   d. Lifestyle modifications
   e. Relationship of treatment to prevention of complications
2. Information about treatment plan
   a. How to take own BP
   b. Reasons for each medication (Tables 4-15 and 4-16)
   c. How and when to take each medication
   d. Necessity of consistency in medication regimen

e. Need for ongoing assessment while taking antihypertensives

> **HESI Hint** • The number-one cause of a stroke in hypertensive clients is noncompliance with medication regimen. HTN is often symptomless, and antihypertensive medications are expensive and have side effects. Studies have shown that the more clients know about their antihypertensive medications, the more likely they are to take them; teaching is important!

f. Need to monitor serum electrolytes every 90 to 120 days for duration of treatment
g. Need to monitor renal functioning (BUN and creatinine) every 90 to 120 days for duration of treatment
h. Need to monitor BP and pulse rate, usually weekly

B. Encourage client to implement nonpharmacologic measures to assist with BP control, such as:
1. Stress reduction
2. Weight loss
3. Tobacco cessation
4. Exercise

C. Determine medication side effects experienced by client (see Table 4-16).
1. Impotence
2. Insomnia

D. Provide nutrition guidance, including a sample meal plan and how to dine out (low-salt, low-fat, low-cholesterol diet).

Peripheral Vascular Disease (PVD)

Description: Circulatory problems that can be due to arterial or venous pathology

Nursing Assessment

A. The signs, symptoms, and treatment of PVD can vary widely, depending on the source of pathology. Therefore careful assessment is very important.

B. Predisposing factors
1. Arterial
   a. Arteriosclerosis (95% of all cases are caused by atherosclerosis)
   b. Advanced age
2. Venous
   a. History of deep vein thrombosis (DVT)
   b. Valvular incompetence

C. Associated diseases
1. Arterial
   a. Raynaud disease (nonatherosclerotic, triggered by extreme heat or cold, spasms of the arteries)
   b. Buerger disease (occlusive inflammatory disease, strongly associated with smoking)

TABLE 4-15 Diuretics

Drugs	Indications	Adverse Reactions	Nursing Implications
Thiazides			

• Chlorthalidone
• Hydrochlorothiazide
• Indapamide
• Metolazone
	• To decrease fluid volume
	• To increase excretion of water, sodium, potassium, and chloride
	• Inexpensive
	• Effective
	• Useful in severe HTN
	• Effective orally
	• Enhances other antihypertensives
		• Hypokalemia symptoms include:
		  • Dry mouth
		  • Thirst
		  • Weakness
		  • Drowsiness
		  • Lethargy
		  • Muscle aches
		  • Tachycardia
		• Hyperuricemia
		• Glucose intolerance
		• Hypercholesterolemia
		• Sexual dysfunction
			• Observe for postural hypotension; can be potentiated by:
			  • Alcohol
			  • Barbiturates
			  • Narcotics
			• Caution with:
			  • Renal failure
			  • Gout
			  • Client taking lithium
			• Hypokalemia increases risk for digitalis toxicity.
			• Administer potassium supplements.
			• Encourage intake of potassium-rich foods.

Loop			
• Furosemide • Torsemide • Bumetanide	• Rapid action • Potent for use when thiazides fail • Cause volume depletion	• Hypokalemia • Hyperuricemia • Glucose intolerance • Hypercholesterolemia • Hypertriglyceridemia • Sexual dysfunction • Weakness	• Volume depletion and electrolyte depletion are rapid. • All nursing implications cited for thiazides.
Potassium-Sparing			
• Spironolactone • Amiloride • Triamterene • Eplerenone	• Volume depletion without significant potassium loss	• Hyperkalemia • Gynecomastia • Sexual dysfunction	• Watch for hyperkalemia and renal failure in those treated with ACE inhibitors or NSAIDs. • Watch for increase in serum lithium levels. • Give after meals to decrease GI distress.
Combination Thiazide and Potassium-Sparing			
• HCTZ and Triamterene • HCTZ + Amiloride HCTZ + Spironolactone	• Decreases fluid volume while minimizing K$^+$ loss	• Side effects of individual drug offset or minimized by its partner	• Caution client previously on a loop or thiazide alone not to overdo K$^+$ foods now because of K$^+$-sparing component in new drug. • Follow scheduling doses to avoid sleep disruption.

    c. Diabetes
    d. Acute occlusion (emboli/thrombi)
  2. Venous
    a. Varicose veins
    b. Thrombophlebitis
    c. Venous stasis ulcers
D. Skin
  1. Arterial
    a. Smooth skin
    b. Shiny skin
    c. Loss of hair
    d. Thickened nails
    e. Dry, thin skin

  2. Venous
    a. Brown pigment around ankles
E. Color
  1. Arterial
    a. Pallor on elevation
    b. Rubor when dependent
  2. Venous—cyanotic when dependent
F. Temperature
  1. Arterial
    a. Cool
  2. Venous
    a. Warm
G. Pulses

TABLE 4-16 Antihypertensives

Drugs	Indications	Adverse Reactions	Nursing Implications
Alpha-Adrenergic Blockers			

• Prazosin HCl
• Terazosin
• Phentolamine mesylate
• Doxazosin
	• Used as peripheral vaso-dilator that acts directly on the blood vessels
	• Used in extreme HTN of pheochromocytoma
		• Orthostatic hypotension
		• Weakness
		• Palpitations
			• Use cautiously in older clients.
			• Occasional vomiting and diarrhea
			• Warn clients of possible:
			  • Drowsiness
			  • Lack of energy
			  • Weakness

Combined Alpha/Beta Blockers			

• Labetalol
• Carvedilol
	• Produces decrease in BP without reflex tachycardia or bradycardia	• HF
		• Ventricular dysrhythmias
		• Blood dyscrasias
		• Bronchospasm
		• Orthostatic hypotension
			• Contraindicated with:
			  • HF
			  • Heart block
			  • COPD
			  • Asthma

Beta Blockers			
• Metoprolol tartrate • Nadolol • Propranolol HCl • Timolol maleate • Atenolol • Bisoprolol • Metoprolol	• Blocks the sympathetic nervous system, especially to the heart • Produces a slower heart rate • Lowers blood pressure • Reduces O_2 consumption during myocardial contraction	• Bradycardia • Fatigue • Insomnia • Bizarre dreams • Sexual dysfunction • Hypertriglyceridemia • Decreased HDL • Depression	• Check apical or radial pulse daily. • Monitor for GI distress. • Do not discontinue abruptly. • Watch for shortness of breath; give cautiously with bronchospasm. • Do not vary how taken (with or without food). • Do not vary time taken. • May mask symptoms of hypoglycemia or may prolong a hypoglycemic reaction • Contraindicated in asthma
Central-Acting Inhibitors			
• Clonidine • Guanabenz acetate • Guanfacine • Methyldopa	• Decreases BP by stimulating central alpha receptors, resulting in decreased sympathetic outflow from the brain	• Drowsiness • Dry mouth • Fatigue • Sexual dysfunction	• Watch for rebound HTN if abruptly discontinued. • Use caution to make position changes slowly, avoid standing still and taking hot baths and showers.
Vasodilators			
• Hydralazine HCl • Minoxidil	• Decreases BP by decreasing peripheral resistance	• Headache • Tachycardia • Fluid retention (HF, pulmonary edema) • Postural hypotension	• Monitor BP, pulse routinely. • Observe for peripheral edema. • Monitor I&O. • Weigh daily.
Angiotensin II Receptor Antagonists			
• Losartan • Valsartan • Irbesartan • Azilsartan • Candesartan • Eprosartan • Olmesartan • Telmisartan	• Blocks the vasoconstrictor and aldosterone-producing effects of angiotensin II at various sites (vascular smooth muscle and adrenal glands)	• Hypotension • Fatigue • Hepatitis • Renal failure • Hyperkalemia (rare)	• Monitor liver enzymes, electrolytes. • Monitor for angioedema in those with history of it when on ACE inhibitors previously.

TABLE 4-16 Antihypertensives—cont'd

Drugs	Indications	Adverse Reactions	Nursing Implications
Angiotensin-Converting Enzyme (ACE) Inhibitors			
• Captopril • Enalapril maleate • Lisinopril • Ramipril • Benazepril • Quinapril • Fosinopril • Moexipril • Trandolapril	• Decreases BP by suppressing renin-angiotensin aldosterone system and inhibiting conversion of angiotensin I into angiotensin II • Useful with clients diagnosed with diabetes	• Proteinuria • Neutropenia • Skin rash • Cough	• Observe for acute renal failure (reversible). • Routine renal function tests. • Remain in bed 3 hours after first dose.
Calcium Channel Blockers			
• Diltiazem • Nifedipine • Verapamil HCl • Nisoldipine • Felodipine • Nicardipine • Amlodipine	• Inhibits calcium ion influx during cardiac depolarization • Decreases SA/AV node conduction	• Headache • Hypotension • Dizziness • Edema • Nausea • Constipation • Tachycardia • HF • Dry cough	• Check BP and pulse routinely. • Limit caffeine consumption. • Take medications before meals. • Avoid grapefruit juice with these drugs; it increases serum levels, causing hypotension. • High-fat meals elevate serum levels.

1. Arterial
   a. Decreased or absent
2. Venous
   a. Normal

H. Pain
1. Arterial
   a. Sharp
   b. Increases with walking and elevation
   c. Intermittent claudication: Classic presenting symptom; occurs in skeletal muscles during exercise; is relieved by rest
   d. Rest pain: Occurs when the extremities are horizontal; may be relieved by dependent position; often appears when collateral circulation fails to develop
2. Venous
   a. Persistent, aching, full feeling, dull sensation
   b. Relieved when horizontal (elevate and use compression stockings)
   c. Nocturnal cramps

I. Ulcers
1. Arterial
   a. Usually very painful; however, occasionally may not be painful
   b. Occur on lateral lower legs, toes, heels
   c. Demarcated edges
   d. Small, but deep
   e. Circular in shape
   f. Necrotic
   g. Not edematous
2. Venous

   a. Slightly painful (dull ache or heaviness)
   b. Occur on medial legs, ankles
   c. Uneven edges
   d. Superficial, but large
   e. Marked edema
   f. Highly exudative

Analysis (Nursing Diagnoses)

A. *Ineffective tissue perfusion (peripheral)* related to …
B. *Activity intolerance* related to …
C. *Impaired skin integrity* related to …
D. *Risk for infection* related to …
E. *Acute pain* related to …

Treatment

A. Noninvasive treatment
1. Arterial
   a. Elimination of smoking
   b. Topical antibiotic
   c. Saline dressing
   d. Bed rest, immobilization
   e. Fibrinolytic agents if clots are the problem (not used for Raynaud or Buerger disease; see Table 4-14)
2. Venous
   a. Systemic antibiotics
   b. Compression dressing (snug) or alginate dressing if ulcerated
   c. Limb elevation
   d. For thrombosis: fibrinolytic agents (see Table 4-14) and anticoagulants (Table 4-17)

TABLE 4-17 Anticoagulants

Drugs	Indications	Adverse Reactions	Nursing Implications
• Heparin sodium	• Administered parenterally (SQ or IV) as an antagonist to thrombin and to prevent the conversion of fibrinogen to fibrin	• Hemorrhage • Agranulocytosis • Leukopenia • Hepatitis • Heparin-induced thrombocytopenia	• Assess PTT, Hgb, Hct, platelets. • Assess stools for occult blood. • Avoid IM injection. • Notify anyone performing diagnostic testing of medication. • *Antagonist:* protamine sulfate
• Warfarin sodium	• Blocks the formation of prothrombin from vitamin K	• Hemorrhage • Agranulocytosis • Leukopenia • Hepatitis	• See Heparin. • Given orally. • Assess PT. • Avoid sudden change in intake of foods high in vitamin K. • *Antagonist:* vitamin K.
Antiplatelet Agents • Ticlopidine • Dipyridamole • Clopidogrel • Prasugrel • Ticagrelor	• Short-term use after cardiac interventions • Reduce risk for thrombolytic stroke for those intolerant to aspirin • Prevention of thrombolytic disorders	• Neutropenia • Thrombocytopenia • Agranulocytosis • Leukopenia • Hemorrhage • GI irritation, bleeding • Pancytopenia	• Give PO or with food to decrease gastric irritation with ticlopidine (Ticlid). • Advise not to take antacids within 2 hours of taking ticlopidine. • Monitor CBC every 2 weeks for 3 months, and thereafter if signs of infection develop. • Monitor for signs of bleeding. • Give 1 hour AC (Persantine); (Plavix) no regard for meals
Low-Molecular–Weight Heparins • Enoxaparin • Tinzaparin • Dalteparin	• Prevention of thrombolytic formation (deep vein)	• Hemorrhage • GI irritation, bleeding • Thrombocytopenia	• Monitor for signs of bleeding. • Give subcutaneously. • Monitor CBC. • Use soft toothbrush; avoid cuts.
Factor Xa Inhibitor • Fondaparinux	• Prevention of thrombolytic formation (deep vein)	• Hemorrhage • GI irritation, bleeding	• Monitor for signs of bleeding. • Give subcutaneously. • Monitor CBC. • Use soft toothbrush; avoid cuts.

Drugs	Indications	Adverse Reactions	Nursing Implications
Group IIa-IIIb Inhibitor (Platelet Antiaggregant) • Eptifibatide • Tirofiban • Abciximab	• Acute coronary syndrome (unstable angina or non–Q wave MI) • Used in combination with heparin, aspirin, and, in selected situations, Ticlid and Plavix	• Bleeding, most frequent • Hypotension • Thrombocytopenia • Acute toxicity: decreased muscle tone, dyspnea, loss of righting reflex	• Check drug–drug interactions before giving other medications. • Obtain baseline PT/aPTT, Hgb, Hct, and platelet count, and monitor. • Dose adjusted by weight for older adults • Same client teaching as with heparin; review activities to avoid. • Watch for bleeding. • Quickly reversible, so emergency procedures may still be performed shortly after discontinuing infusion.

New Oral Anticoagulants (NOAC)
• Dabigatran
• Rivaroxaban
• Apixaban
	For all three:
	• Prevention of VTE in orthopedic surgery
	• Prevention of stroke and systemic embolism in patients with atrial fibrillation
		• >to 50% in anticoagulant plasma when used with ketoconazole
		  Quinidine
		  Verapamil
		• < 50% in anticoagulant plasma concentrations when used with carbamazepine, rifampin, St John's wort
		• >Risk of bleeding with ASA, NSAID, platelet aggregation inhibitors, anticoagulants, thrombolytics
		• >to 50% in anticoagulant plasma when used with clarithromycin, ketoconazole, ritonavir
		• < 50% in anticoagulant plasma concentrations when used with carbamazepine, phenytoin, phenobarbital, rifampin, St John's wort
		• >Risk of bleeding with ASA, NSAID, platelet aggregation inhibitors, anticoagulants, thrombolytics
		• >to 50% in anticoagulant plasma when used with ketoconazole, itraconazole, ritonavir
		• < 50% in anticoagulant plasma concentrations when used with carbamazepine, phenobarbital, phenytoin rifampin, St John's wort
		• >Risk of bleeding with ASA, NSAID, platelet aggregation inhibitors, anticoagulants, thrombolytics
			• For all three: Maintain prescribed length of administration can be 28 or > for hip surgery
			• And 10 days or > for knee surgery
			• Presence of conditions predisposing to bleeding risks
			• Avoid concomitant use with other anticoagulants
			• Renal impairment
			• Use with care >age 80; <60 kg; serum creatinine > 133 umol/L

Continued

TABLE 4-17 Anticoagulants—cont'd

Drugs	Indications	Adverse Reactions	Nursing Implications
• Rivaroxaban	• Oral anticoagulant	• Increases the risk of bleeding and can cause serious or fatal bleeding. • Cease use at once if there is easy bruising, unusual bleeding (nose, mouth, vagina, or rectum); bleeding from wounds or injection; any bleeding that will not stop; heavy menstrual periods. • Clients with atrial fibrillation are at increased risk of forming blood clots in the heart. Do not stop taking without contacting the health care provider. • Increased risk of bleeding when taken in conjunction with aspirin or aspirin-containing products, NSAIDS, warfarin sodium, any medicine that contains heparin, clopidogrel, or other medications used to prevent or treat blood clots.	• Give orally. Does not require monitoring like warfarin
• Dabigatran	• Oral anticoagulant	• Contraindicated in concomitant use with dronedarone. • Make have an effect on some pathology tests. • There is an increased risk of bleeding especially for clients 75 years old or older, having moderate kidney impairment (creatinine 3050 mL/min); use with clients with congenital or acquired coagulation disorders, thrombocytopenia or functional platelet defects, active ulcerative GI disease, recent biopsy or major trauma, recent intracranial hemorrhage, brain, spinal, or ophthalmic surgery, or bacterial endocarditis. Must not be used with clients with prosthetic heart valves. • Medication must be stored and dispensed in the original packaging (blister pack or bottle) because of the increased risk of exposure to moisture or humidity causing breakdown and loss of potency.	• Give orally. Does not require monitoring like warfarin.

B. Surgery
1. Arterial
   a. Embolectomy: removal of clot
   b. Endarterectomy: removal of clot and stripping of plaque
   c. Arterial bypass: Teflon or Dacron graft or autograft
   d. Percutaneous transluminal angioplasty (PTA): compression of plaque
   e. Amputation: removal of extremity
2. Venous
   a. Vein ligation
   b. Thrombectomy
   c. Débridement

Nursing Plans and Interventions

A. Monitor extremities at designated intervals.
   1. Color
   2. Temperature
   3. Sensation and pulse quality in extremities
B. Schedule activities within client's tolerance level.
C. Encourage rest at the first sign of pain.
D. Encourage client to keep extremities elevated (if venous) when sitting and to change position often.
E. Encourage client to avoid crossing legs and to wear nonrestrictive clothing.
F. Encourage client to keep the extremities warm by wearing extra clothing, such as socks and slippers, and not to use external heat sources such as electric heating pads.
G. Teach methods of preventing further injury.
   1. Change position frequently.
   2. Wear nonrestrictive clothing (no knee-high hose).
   3. Avoid crossing legs or keeping legs in a dependent position.
   4. Wear support hose or antiembolism stockings.
   5. Wear shoes when ambulating.
   6. Obtain proper foot and nail care.

> **HESI Hint** • Decreased blood flow results in diminished sensation in the lower extremities. Any heat source can cause severe burns before the client realizes damage is being done.

H. Discourage cigarette smoking (causes vasoconstriction and spasm of arteries).
I. Provide preoperative and postoperative care if surgery is required.
   1. Preoperative: Maintain affected extremity in a level position (if venous) or in a slightly dependent position (if arterial; 15 degrees), at room temperature, and protect from trauma.
   2. Postoperative: Assess surgical site frequently for hemorrhage, and check distal peripheral pulses.
   3. Anticoagulants may be continued after surgery to prevent thrombosis of affected artery and to diminish development of thrombi at the initiating site.

Abdominal Aortic Aneurysm (AAA)

Description: Dilatation of the abdominal aorta caused by an alteration in the integrity of its wall
A. The most common cause of AAA is atherosclerosis. It is a late manifestation of syphilis.
B. Without treatment, rupture and death will occur.
C. AAA is often asymptomatic.
D. The most common symptom is abdominal pain or low back pain, with the complaint that the client can feel his or her heart beating.
E. Those taking antihypertensive drugs are at risk for developing AAA.

> **HESI Hint** • A client is admitted with severe chest pain and states that he feels a terrible tearing sensation in his chest. He is diagnosed with a dissecting aortic aneurysm. What assessments should the nurse obtain in the first few hours?
> • Vital signs every hour
> • Neurologic vital signs
> • Respiratory status
> • Urinary output
> • Peripheral pulses

Nursing Assessment

A. Bruit (swooshing sound heard over a constricted artery when auscultated) heard over abdominal aorta, pulsation in upper abdomen
B. Abdominal or lower back pain
C. May feel heartbeat in abdomen, or feel an abdominal mass
D. Abdominal radiograph (aortogram, angiogram, abdominal ultrasound) to confirm diagnosis if aneurysm is calcified
E. Symptoms of rupture: hypovolemic or cardiogenic shock with sudden, severe abdominal pain

Analysis (Nursing Diagnoses)

A. *Activity intolerance* related to …
B. *Risk for vascular trauma* related to …
C. *Anxiety* related to …
D. *Acute pain* related to …

Nursing Plans and Interventions

A. Assess all peripheral pulses and vital signs regularly.
   1. Radial
   2. Femoral
   3. Popliteal
   4. Posterior tibial
   5. Dorsalis pedis
B. Observe for signs of occlusion after graft.
   1. Change in pulses
   2. Severe pain
   3. Cool to cold extremities below graft
   4. White or blue extremities

C. Observe renal functioning for signs of kidney damage (artery clamped during surgery may result in kidney damage).
 1. Output of less than 30 mL/hr
 2. Amber urine
 3. Elevated BUN and creatinine (early signs of renal failure)

> **HESI Hint** • During aortic aneurysm repair, the large arteries are clamped for a certain period, and kidney damage can result. Monitor daily BUN and creatinine levels. Normal BUN is 10 to 20 mg/dL, and normal creatinine is 0.6 to 1.2 mg/dL. The ratio of BUN to creatinine is 20:1. When this ratio increases or decreases, suspect renal problems.

D. Observe for postoperative ileus.
 1. Nasogastric (NG) tube to low continuous suction for 1 to 2 days postoperative (may help to prevent ileus)
 2. Bowel sounds checked every shift

Thrombophlebitis

Description: Inflammation of the venous walls with the formation of a clot; also known as *venous thrombosis, phlebothrombosis*, or *DVT*

Nursing Assessment

A. Calf tenderness, redness or pain, calf pain with dorsiflexion of the foot
B. Functional impairment of extremity
C. Edema and warmth in extremity
D. Asymmetry
 1. Inspect legs from groin to feet
 2. Measure diameters of calves
E. Tender areas on affected extremity with very gentle palpation
F. Occlusion with diagnostic testing
 1. Venogram
 2. Doppler ultrasound
 3. Fibrinogen scanning
G. Risk factors
 1. Prolonged, strict bed rest
 2. General surgery
 3. Leg trauma
 4. Previous venous insufficiency
 5. Obesity
 6. Oral contraceptives
 7. Pregnancy
 8. Malignancy

Analysis (Nursing Diagnoses)

A. *Acute pain* related to ...
B. *Ineffective peripheral tissue perfusion* related to ...

> **HESI Hint** • Heparin prevents conversion of fibrinogen to fibrin and prothrombin to thrombin, thereby inhibiting clot formation. Because the clotting mechanism is prolonged, do not cause tissue trauma, which may lead to bleeding when giving heparin subcutaneously. Do not massage area or aspirate; give in the abdomen between the pelvic bones, 2 inches from umbilicus; rotate sites.

Nursing Plans and Interventions

A. Administer anticoagulant therapy as prescribed (see Table 4-17).

> **HESI Hint** • *Anticoagulants*
>
> **Heparin**
>   Antagonist: protamine sulfate
>   Laboratory: PTT or aPTT determines efficacy
>   Keep 1.5 to 2.5 times normal control
>
> **Warfarin (Coumadin)**
>   Antagonist: vitamin K
>   Laboratory: PT determines efficacy
>   Keep 1.5 to 2.5 times normal control
>   INR (international normalized ratio): desirable therapeutic level usually 2:3 (reflects how long it takes a blood sample to clot)

1. Observe for side effects, especially bleeding.
2. Teach client side effects of medications included in treatment regimen.
3. Monitor laboratory data to determine the efficacy of medications included in treatment regimen.
4. Note on all laboratory requests that client is receiving anticoagulants.
5. Partial thromboplastin time (PTT) determines efficacy of heparin.
6. Prothrombin time (PT) or INR determines efficacy of Coumadin.
7. Maintain pressure on venipuncture sites to minimize hematoma formation.
8. Notify physician of any unusual bleeding.
 a. Abnormal vaginal bleeding
 b. Nosebleeds
 c. Melena
 d. Hematuria
 e. Gums
 f. Hemoptysis
9. Advise client to use soft toothbrush, floss with waxed floss.
10. Advise client to wear medical alert symbol.
11. Advise client to avoid alcoholic beverages.
12. Advise client to avoid safety razors if taking warfarin (Coumadin).

13. Advise client to avoid aspirin and aspirin products and NSAIDs.
B. Advise client to wear antiembolic stockings and to elevate extremity and use shock blocks at foot of bed.
C. Advise bed rest; strict, if prescribed, means no bathroom privileges! Advise client to avoid straining.
D. Monitor for decreasing symptomatology.
  1. Pain
  2. Edema
E. Monitor for pulmonary embolus (chest pain, shortness of breath).
F. Teach client that there is increased risk for DVT formation in the future.
G. Dietary precautions if taking warfarin (Coumadin).

> **HESI Hint** • Clients may ingest foods high in Vitamin K to maintain therapeutic blood levels based on their dietary intake.

Dysrhythmias

Description: Disturbance in heart rate or heart rhythm
A. Dysrhythmias are caused by a disturbance in the electrical conduction of the heart, not by abnormal heart structure.
B. Client is often asymptomatic until cardiac output is altered.
C. Common causes of dysrhythmias
  1. Drugs (e.g., digoxin, quinidine, caffeine, nicotine, alcohol), illicit drugs
  2. Acid–base and electrolyte imbalances (potassium, calcium, and magnesium)
  3. Marked thermal changes
  4. Disease and trauma
  5. Stress

Nursing Assessment

A. Change in pulse rate or rhythm
  1. Tachycardia: fast rates (>100 bpm)
  2. Bradycardia: slow rates (<60 bpm)
  3. Irregular rhythm
  4. Pulselessness
B. ECG changes
C. Complaints of:
  1. Palpitations
  2. Syncope
  3. Pain
  4. Dyspnea
D. Diaphoresis
E. Hypotension
F. Electrolyte imbalances

Analysis (Nursing Diagnoses)

A. *Risk for decreased tissue perfusion* related to …
B. *Activity intolerance* related to …
C. *Decreased cardiac output* related to…

Selected Dysrhythmias

A. Atrial fibrillation (Fig. 4-4, *A*)
  1. Description
    a. Chaotic activity in the AV node
    b. No true P waves visible
    c. Irregular ventricular rhythm
  2. Assessment and treatment
    a. Anticoagulant therapy due to risk for stroke
    b. Antidysrhythmic drugs
    c. Cardioversion to treat atrial dysrhythmias.
    d. Cardiac catheter ablation
B. Atrial flutter (see Fig. 4-4, *A*)
  1. Description
    a. Saw-toothed waveform
    b. Fluttering in chest
    c. Ventricular rhythm stays regular
  2. Assessment and treatment
    a. Cardioversion to treat atrial dysrhythmia
    b. Antidysrhythmic drugs
    c. Radiofrequency catheter ablation
C. Ventricular tachycardia
  1. Description
    a. Wide, bizarre QRS
  2. Assessment and treatment
    a. Pulse
    b. Impaired cardiac output
    c. Synchronized cardioversion if pulse present (if no pulse, treat as ventricular fibrillation)
    d. Antidysrhythmic drugs
D. Ventricular fibrillation
  1. Description
    a. Cardiac emergency
    b. Irregular undulations of varying amplitudes, from coarse to fine
    c. No cardiac output (no pulse or BP)

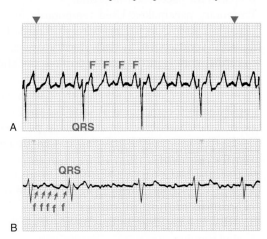

FIGURE 4-4 *A,* Atrial flutter with a 4:1 conduction (four flutter *[F]* waves to each QRS complex). *B,* Atrial fibrillation. Note the chaotic fibrillatory *(f)* waves between the QRS complexes. Note: Recorded from lead V₁. (*A* from Urden L, Stacy K, Lough M: *Priorities in critical care nursing,* ed 6, 2013, St. Louis, Elsevier/Mosby; *B,* from Sole M, Klein D, Moseley M: *Introduction to critical care nursing,* ed 6, St. Louis, 2013, Elsevier/Saunders.)

2. Assessment and treatment
   a. CPR
   b. Defibrillation as quickly as possible
   c. Antidysrhythmic drugs

Nursing Plans and Interventions

A. Determine medications client is currently taking.
B. Determine serum drug levels, especially digitalis.
C. Determine serum electrolyte levels, especially K^+ and Mg^{++}.
D. Obtain ECG reading on admission, and monitor continuously.
E. Holter monitoring, either event monitor or loop recorder.

> **HESI Hint** • A Holter monitor offers continuous observation of the client's heart rate. To make assessment of the rhythm strips most meaningful, teach the client to keep a record of:
> • Medication times and doses
> • Chest pain episodes: type and duration
> • Valsalva maneuver (straining at stool, sneezing, coughing)
> • Sexual activity
> • Exercise and other activities

F. Approach client in a calm, reassuring manner.
G. Monitor client's activity, and observe for any symptoms occurring during activity.
H. Ensure proper administration of medications, and monitor for side effects (Table 4-18).
I. Be prepared for emergency measures, such as cardioversion or defibrillation.

> **HESI Hint** • Cardioversion is the delivery of synchronized electrical shocks to the myocardium.

J. Be prepared for pacemaker insertion.
   1. Temporary pacemaker: Used temporarily in emergency situations. A pacing wire is threaded into the right ventricle via the superior vena cava, or an epicardial wire is put in place (through the client's chest incision) during cardiac surgery.
   2. Permanent internal pacemaker with pulse generator implanted in the abdomen or shoulder: may be single or dual chambered. Programmable pacemakers can be reprogrammed by placing a magnetic device over the generator.
   3. Instruct the client to:
      a. Report pulse rate lower than the set rate of the pacemaker.
      b. Avoid leaning over an automobile with the engine running.
      c. Stand 4 to 5 feet away from high-output generators and electromagnetic sources, such as operating radar detectors.
      d. Avoid MRI diagnostic testing.
      e. For airport travel, notify Transportation Security Administration (TSA) of the presence of a pacemaker. Handheld screening rod should not be placed directly over the pacemaker.

> **HESI Hint** • Difference in synchronous and asynchronous pacemakers:
> • Synchronous, or demand: Pacemaker fires only when the client's heart rate falls below a rate set on the generator.
> • Asynchronous, or fixed: Pacemaker fires at a constant rate.
> • Implantable cardioverter defibrillator (ICD); device defibrillates to detect life-threatening ventricular arrhythmias. May have dual function as a pacemaker.

K. Recognize and treat symptomatic premature ventricular contractions (PVCs) as prescribed (Fig. 4-5). A PVC is a contraction originating in an ectopic focus in the ventricles. It is the premature occurrence of a QRS complex that is wide and distorted in shape (report and treat PVCs):
   1. If they occur more often than once in 10 beats.
   2. If they occur in groups of two or three; three consecutive PVCs is ventricular tachycardia.
   3. If they occur near the T wave (R-on-T phenomenon).
   4. If they take on multiple configurations.

Heart Failure (HF)

Description: Inability of the heart to pump enough blood to meet the tissue's O_2 demands
A. Primary underlying conditions causing HF:
   1. Ischemic heart disease
   2. MI
   3. Cardiomyopathy
   4. Valvular heart disease
   5. HTN

Nursing Assessment

A. Observe for symptoms associated with left-sided or right-sided failure.
   1. Left-sided heart failure: pulmonary edema (left ventricular failure)
      a. Description: Results in pulmonary congestion due to the inability of the left ventricle to pump blood to the periphery
      b. Symptoms
         (1) Dyspnea
         (2) Orthopnea
         (3) Crackles
         (4) Cough
         (5) Fatigue
         (6) Tachycardia
         (7) Anxiety
         (8) Restlessness
         (9) Confusion
         (10) Paroxysmal nocturnal dyspnea (PND)

TABLE 4-18 Antidysrhythmics

Drugs	Indications	Adverse Reactions	Nursing Implications
Class I (A, B, C)			
• Quinidine • Disopyramide phosphate • Procainamide • Moricizine • Lidocaine HCl • Mexiletine • Tocainide HCl • Phenytoin sodium • Propafenone • Flecainide acetate	• Premature beats • Atrial flutter, fibrillation • Contraindicated in heart block • Ventricular dysrhythmias • Unlabeled use: digitalis for induced dysrhythmias • Ventricular dysrhythmias	• Diarrhea • Hypotension • ECG changes • Cinchonism • Interacts with many common drugs • Hypotension • CNS effects • Seizures • GI distress • Bradycardia • Dizziness • Slurred speech • Ventricular dysrhythmias	• Instruct client to monitor pulse rate and rhythm. • Monitor ECG. • Monitor for tinnitus and visual disturbances. • Lidocaine administered IV bolus and by infusion. • Monitor for confusion, drowsiness, slurred speech, seizures with lidocaine. • Administer oral drugs with food. • May cause digoxin toxicity.
Class II			
• Propranolol HCl • Metoprolol • Atenolol	• Supraventricular and ventricular tachydysrhythmias	• Hypotension • Bradycardia • Bronchospasm	• Monitor vital signs. • Contraindicated in asthma.
Class III (Inotropics)			
• Amiodarone HCl • Sotalol • Dofetilide • Dronedarone • Ibutilide	• Ventricular dysrhythmias	• Dysrhythmias • HTN or hypotension • Muscle weakness, tremors • Photophobia	• Amiodarone is now one of the first-choice drugs. • Monitor vital signs, ECG. • Instruct client taking amiodarone to wear sunglasses and sunscreens when outside.
Class IV			
• Verapamil HCl • Diltiazem	• Supraventricular dysrhythmias	• Hypotension • Bradycardia • Constipation	• Monitor BP and pulse. • Instruct client to change positions slowly.
Miscellaneous Agents			
• Atropine sulfate	• Bradycardia	• Chest pain • Urinary retention • Dry mouth	• Monitor heart rate and rhythm. • Assess for chest pain. • Assess for urinary retention. • Avoid use with glaucoma.
• Digoxin	• Supraventricular dysrhythmias • Atrial fibrillation	• Bradycardia • Dysrhythmias • Anorexia, nausea, vomiting, diarrhea, visual disturbances	• Monitor pulse rate and rhythm. • Check apical pulse for one full minute before administering; hold if blood pressure is less than 60 bpm and notify health care provider. • Instruct client to report signs of toxicity. • Hypokalemia increases the risk for toxicity. • Causes hypercalcemia.
• Epinephrine	• Cardiac arrest	• Tachycardia • HTN	• Impaired renal function can cause toxicity; monitor BUN and creatinine. • Monitor pulse return in asystole. • Monitor vital signs.

Continued

TABLE 4-18 Antidysrhythmics—cont'd

Additional Drugs that Promote Cardiovascular Perfusion in the Failing Heart			
Drugs	**Indications**	**Adverse Reactions**	**Nursing Implications**
Vasopressors			
• Norepinephrine bitartrate	• Dilated coronary arteries and causes peripheral vasoconstriction for emergency hypotensive states not caused by blood loss, vascular thrombosis, or anesthesia using cyclopropane or halothane	• Can cause *severe* tissue necrosis, sloughing, and gangrene if infiltrates (blanching along vein pathway is preliminary sign of extravasation)	• Rapidly inactivated by various body enzymes; need to ensure IV patency. • Use cautiously in previously hypertensive clients. • Check BP every 2-5 minutes. • Use large veins to avoid complications of prolonged vasoconstriction. • Pressor effects potentiated by many drugs; check drug–drug interactions. • Have phentolamine (Regitine) diluted per protocol for local injection if infiltrates.
Cardiotonic/Vasodilator (Human B-type Natriuretic Peptide: HBNP)			
• Nesiritide	• Treatment of acutely decompensated HF in clients who have dyspnea at rest or with minimal activity • Reduces PCWP and reduces dyspnea	• Hypotension is primary side effect and can be dose limiting • Dysrhythmias • Headache, dizziness, insomnia, tremors, paresthesias • Abdominal pain, nausea and vomiting	• Many drug–drug interactions. • Monitor BP and telemetry. • As diuresis occurs, monitor electrolytes, especially K⁺. • Watch for overresponse to treatment in older adults.

PCWP, Pulmonary capillary wedge pressure.

2. Right-sided heart failure: Peripheral edema (right ventricular failure)
   a. Description: Results in peripheral congestion due to the inability of the right ventricle to pump blood out to the lungs; often results from left-sided failure or pulmonary disease
   b. Symptoms
      (1) Peripheral edema
      (2) Weight gain
      (3) Distended neck veins
      (4) Anorexia, nausea
      (5) Nocturia
      (6) Weakness
      (7) Hepatomegaly
      (8) Ascites
B. Enlargement of ventricles as indicated by chest radiograph
C. Brain natriuretic peptide test (BPN) measures levels of protein in heart and blood vessels. High BPN levels occur with heart failure.
D. N-terminal probrain natriuretic peptide (NT-proBNP) is used for diagnosis of impaired left ventricular ejection fraction (LVEF) after myocardial infarction.

HESI Hint • Restricting sodium reduces salt and water retention, thereby reducing vascular volume and preload.

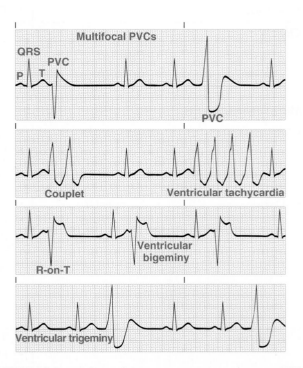

FIGURE 4-5 Various forms of premature ventricular contractions (PVCs). Note: Recorded from lead II. (From Sole M, Klein D, Moseley M: *Introduction to critical care nursing*, ed 6, St. Louis, 2013, Elsevier/Saunders.)

TABLE 4-19 Digitalis Preparations

Drugs	Indications	Adverse Reactions	Nursing Implications
• Digoxin	• HF • Increases the contractility of cardiac muscle • Slows heart rate and conduction	• Severe: AV block • Headache • Dysrhythmias • Nausea • Vomiting • Blurred vision • Yellow-green halos • Hypotension • Fatigue	• Monitor serum electrolytes; hypokalemia increases risk for digoxin toxicity. • Monitor serum digitalis levels if any side effects are present. • Check apical pulse before administration; call health care provider if rate is <60 bpm. • Teach client to take radial pulse before administration and call health care provider if <60 bpm in adults. • Therapeutic range: 0.5-2 mg.
• Digoxin-immune Fab	• Antidote for digitalis toxicity • Binds with digoxin to prevent binding at the site of action	• Decreased cardiac output • Atrial tachydysrhythmias • Use with caution in children and older adults.	• Use with 0.22-mcm filter. • Place client on continuous cardiac monitor. • Have resuscitation equipment at bedside before giving first dose.

HESI Hint • *Digitalis*
- Side effects of digitalis are increased when the client is hypokalemic.
- Digitalis has a negative chronotropic effect (i.e., it slows the heart rate). Hold the digitalis if the pulse rate is <60 or >120 bpm (<90 bpm in an infant) or has markedly changed rhythm.
- Bradycardia, tachycardia, and dysrhythmias may be signs of digitalis toxicity; these signs include nausea, vomiting, and headache in adults.
- If withheld, consult with physician.

Analysis (Nursing Diagnoses)

A. *Decreased cardiac output* related to ...
B. *Impaired urinary elimination* related to ...
C. *Activity intolerance* related to ...
D. *Anxiety* related to ...
E. *Ineffective tissue perfusion* related to ...

Nursing Plans and Interventions

A. Monitor vital signs at least every 4 hours for changes.
B. Monitor apical heart rate with vital signs to detect dysrhythmias, or abnormal heart sounds such as S3 or S4.
C. Assess for hypoxia.
   1. Restlessness
   2. Tachycardia
   3. Angina
D. Auscultate lungs for indication of pulmonary edema (wet sounds or crackles).
E. Administer O$_2$ as needed.
F. Elevate head of bed to assist with breathing.
G. Observe for signs of edema.
   1. Weigh daily.
   2. Monitor I&O.
   3. Measure abdominal girth; observe ankles and fingers.
H. Limit sodium intake.
I. Elevate lower extremities while sitting.
J. Check apical heart rate before administration of digitalis; withhold medication and call physician if rate is <60 bpm (Table 4-19).
K. Administer diuretics in the morning if possible (see Table 4-15).
L. Provide periods of rest after periods of activity.

Inflammatory and Infectious Heart Disease

Description: Inflammatory and infectious process involving the endocardium and pericardium

A. Endocarditis is an inflammatory disease involving the inner surface of the heart, including the valves. Organisms travel through the blood to the heart, where vegetations adhere to the valve surface or endocardium and can break off and become emboli.
B. Causes of endocarditis
   1. Rheumatic heart disease
   2. Congenital heart disease
   3. IV drug abuse
   4. Cardiac surgery
   5. Immunosuppression
   6. Dental procedures
   7. Invasive procedures
C. Pericarditis is an inflammation of the outer lining of the heart.

D. Causes of pericarditis
1. MI
2. Trauma
3. Neoplasm
4. Connective-tissue disease
5. Heart surgery
6. Idiopathic
7. Infections

Nursing Assessment

A. Endocarditis
1. Fever
2. Chills, malaise, night sweats, fatigue
3. Murmurs
4. Symptoms of heart failure
5. Atrial embolization
B. Pericarditis
1. Pain: sudden, sharp, severe:
a. Substernal, radiating to the back or arm
b. Aggravated by coughing, inhalation, deep breathing
c. Relieved by leaning forward
2. Pericardial friction rub heard best at left lower sternal border
3. Fever

HESI Hint • Infective endocarditis damage to heart valves occurs with the growth of vegetative lesions on valve leaflets. These lesions pose a risk for embolization, erosion, or perforation of the valve leaflets or abscesses within adjacent myocardial tissue. Valvular stenosis or regurgitation (insufficiency), most commonly of the mitral valve, can occur, depending on the type of damage inflicted by the lesions, and can lead to symptoms of left- or right-sided heart failure (see Valvular Heart Disease on this page and Heart Failure, p. 114).

HESI Hint • *Pericarditis*
The presence of a friction rub is an indication of pericarditis (inflammation of the lining of the heart). ST-segment elevation and T-wave inversion are also signs of pericarditis.

HESI Hint • *Acute and Subacute Infective Endocarditis*
There are two types of infective endocarditis: acute, which often affects individuals with previously normal hearts and healthy valves and carries a high mortality rate, and subacute, which typically affects individuals with preexisting conditions, such as rheumatic heart disease, mitral valve prolapse, or immunosuppression. Intravenous drug abusers are at risk for both acute and subacute bacterial endocarditis. When this population develops subacute infective endocarditis, the valves on the right side of the heart (tricuspid and pulmonic) are typically affected because of the introduction of common pathogens that colonize the skin (*Staphylococcus epidermis* or *Candida* spp.) into the venous system.

Analysis (Nursing Diagnoses)

A. *Decreased cardiac output* related to …
B. *Risk for injury: emboli* related to …

Nursing Plans and Interventions

A. Endocarditis
1. Monitor hemodynamic status (vital signs, level of consciousness, urinary output).
2. Administer antibiotics IV for 4 to 6 weeks. The American Heart Association recommends administration of antibiotics before dental or genitourinary procedures in high-risk patients.
3. Clients may be instructed in IV therapy for home health care.
4. Teach clients about anticoagulant therapy if prescribed.
5. Encourage client to maintain good hygiene.
6. Instruct client to inform dentist and other health care providers of history.
B. Pericarditis
1. Provide rest and maintain position of comfort.
2. Administer analgesics and antiinflammatory drugs.

Valvular Heart Disease

Description: Heart valves that are unable to open fully (stenosis) or close fully (insufficiency or regurgitation)
A. Valve dysfunction most commonly occurs on the left side of the heart; the mitral valve is most commonly involved, followed by the aortic valve.

HESI Hint • In mitral valve stenosis, blood is regurgitated back into the left atrium from the left ventricle. In the early period, there may be no symptoms, but as the disease progresses, the client will exhibit excessive fatigue, dyspnea on exertion, orthopnea, dry cough, hemoptysis, or pulmonary edema. There will be a rumbling apical diastolic murmur, and atrial fibrillation is common.

B. Common causes of valvular disease
1. Rheumatic fever
2. Congenital heart diseases
3. Syphilis
4. Endocarditis
5. HTN
C. Prevention of rheumatic heart disease would reduce the incidence of valvular heart disease.

Nursing Assessment

A. Pericardial effusion with possible tamponade that requires pericardiocentesis
B. Fatigue
C. Dyspnea, orthopnea
D. Hemoptysis and pulmonary edema
E. Murmurs
F. Irregular cardiac rhythm
G. Angina

Analysis (Nursing Diagnoses)

A. *Decreased cardiac output* related to …
B. *Impaired gas exchange* related to …
C. *Excess fluid volume* related to fluid retention secondary to valvular-induced heart failure related to…
D. *Activity intolerance* related to …

Nursing Plans and Interventions

A. See Heart Failure, p. 114.
B. Monitor client for atrial fibrillation with thrombus formation.
C. Teach the necessity for prophylactic antibiotic therapy before any invasive procedure, such as dental procedures, that is likely to produce gingival or mucosal bleeding: bronchoscopy, esophageal dilation, upper endoscopy, colonoscopy, sigmoidoscopy, or cystoscopy.
D. Prepare the client for surgical repair or replacement of heart valves.
E. Instruct clients receiving mechanical valve replacement of the need for lifelong anticoagulant therapy to prevent thrombus formation. Tissue (biologic) valves and autografts do not require lifelong anticoagulant therapy.

Review of Cardiovascular System

1. How do clients experiencing angina describe that pain?
2. Develop a teaching plan for a client taking nitroglycerin.
3. List the parameters of BP for diagnosing HTN.
4. Differentiate between essential and secondary HTN.
5. Develop a teaching plan for a client taking antihypertensive medications.
6. Describe intermittent claudication.
7. Describe the nurse's discharge instructions to a client with venous PVD.
8. What is often the underlying cause of an abdominal aortic aneurysm?
9. What laboratory values should be monitored daily in a client with thrombophlebitis who is undergoing anticoagulant therapy?
10. When do PVCs present a grave danger?
11. Differentiate between the symptoms of left-sided cardiac failure and right-sided cardiac failure.
12. List three symptoms of digitalis toxicity.
13. What condition increases the likelihood that digitalis toxicity will occur?
14. What lifestyle changes can the client who is at risk for HTN initiate to reduce the likelihood of becoming hypertensive?
15. What immediate actions should the nurse implement when a client is having a myocardial infarction?
16. What symptoms should the nurse expect to find in a client with hypokalemia?
17. Bradycardia is defined as a heart rate below _____ bpm. Tachycardia is defined as a heart rate above _____ bpm.
18. What precautions should clients with valve disease take before invasive procedures or dental work?

Answers to Review

1. Described as squeezing, heavy, burning, radiates to left arm or shoulder, transient or prolonged
2. Take at first sign of anginal pain. Take no more than three, 5 minutes apart. Call for emergency attention if no relief in 10 minutes.
3. >140/90
4. Essential HTN has no known cause; secondary HTN develops in response to an identifiable mechanism.
5. Explain how and when to take medication, reason for medication, necessity of compliance, need for follow-up visits while on medication, need for certain laboratory tests, and vital sign parameters while initiating therapy.
6. Pain related to PVD; the pain occurs with exercise and disappears with rest.
7. Keep extremities elevated when sitting, rest at first sign of pain, keep extremities warm (but do not use heating pad), change position often, avoid crossing legs, wear unrestrictive clothing.
8. Atherosclerosis
9. PTT, PT, Hgb, Hct, platelets
10. When they begin to occur more often than once in 10 beats, occur in twos or threes, land near the T wave, or take on multiple configurations
11. Left-sided failure results in pulmonary congestion due to backup of circulation in the left ventricle. Right-sided failure results in peripheral congestion due to backup of circulation in the right ventricle.
12. Dysrhythmias, headache, nausea, and vomiting

13. Hypokalemia (which is more common when diuretics and digitalis preparations are given together)
14. Cease cigarette smoking, if applicable; control weight; exercise regularly; and maintain a low-fat, low-cholesterol diet.
15. Administer O_2 by nasal cannula at 2 to 5 L/min; ensure patent IV or start an IV to deliver emergency medication; take measures to alleviate pain and anxiety (administer PRN pain medications and antianxiety medications); place the client on immediate strict bed rest to lower O_2 demands on heart.
16. Dry mouth and thirst, drowsiness and lethargy, muscle weakness and aches, and tachycardia
17. 60 bpm; 100 bpm
18. Take prophylactic antibiotics.

Gastrointestinal System

Hiatal Hernia and Gastroesophageal Reflux Disease

A. Hiatal hernia is a herniation of the esophagogastric junction and a portion of the stomach into the chest through the esophageal hiatus of the diaphragm.
   1. Sliding hernia is the most common type, accounting for 75% to 90% of adult hiatal hernias.
B. Gastroesophageal reflux disease (GERD) is the result of an incompetent lower esophageal sphincter that allows regurgitation of acidic gastric contents into the esophagus.
   1. Multiple factors determine whether GERD is present.
      a. Efficiency of antireflux mechanism
      b. Volume of gastric contents
      c. Potency of refluxed material
      d. Efficiency of esophageal clearance
      e. Resistance of the esophageal tissue to injury and the ability to repair tissue
   2. The client must have several episodes of reflux for GERD to be present.

Nursing Assessment

A. Heartburn after eating that radiates to arms and shoulders
B. Feeling of fullness and discomfort after eating
C. Positive diagnosis determined by fluoroscopy, barium swallow, or gastroscopy

Analysis (Nursing Diagnoses)

A. *Acute pain* related to …
B. *Deficient knowledge* (specify) related to …
C. *Anxiety* related to …
D. Imbalanced nutrition: less than body requirements due to…

Nursing Plans and Interventions

A. Determine an eating pattern that alleviates symptoms.
   1. Encourage small, frequent meals.
   2. Encourage elimination of foods that are determined to aggravate symptoms (these foods are client specific but can include caffeine, catsup, strawberries, and chocolate).
   3. Encourage client to sit up while eating and remain in an upright position for at least 1 hour after eating.
   4. Encourage client to stop eating 3 hours before bedtime.
   5. Elevate the head of the bed on 6- to 8-inch blocks.
   6. Teach about commonly prescribed medications (H2 antagonists, antacids).

> **HESI Hint** • A Fowler or semi-Fowler position is beneficial in reducing the amount of regurgitation, as well as in preventing the encroachment of the stomach tissue upward through the opening in the diaphragm.

B. Teaching plan for client and family should include the following:
   1. Differentiate between the symptoms of hiatal hernia and those of MI.
   2. Be alert to the possibility of aspiration.
   3. Give information about drugs used for treatment (Table 4-20).

Peptic Ulcer Disease (PUD)

Description: Ulceration that penetrates the mucosal wall of the gastrointestinal (GI) tract
A. Gastric ulcers tend to occur in the lesser curvature of the stomach.
B. Duodenal ulcers occur in the duodenum, which is the most common location of PUD.
C. Esophageal ulcers occur in the esophagus.
D. The cause of some PUD is unknown. A significant number of gastric ulcers are caused by a bacterium, *Helicobacter pylori*, and can be successfully treated by drug therapy. Risk factors for the development of peptic ulcers include:
   1. Drugs (NSAIDs, corticosteroids)
   2. Alcohol
   3. Cigarette smoking
   4. Acute medical crisis or trauma
   5. Familial tendency
   6. Blood type O
E. Symptoms common to all types of ulcers include the following:
   1. Belching
   2. Bloating
   3. Epigastric pain radiating to the back (not associated with the type of food eaten) and relieved by antacids

TABLE 4-20 Antiulcer Drugs

Drugs	Indications	Adverse Reactions	Nursing Implications
Antacids			
• Aluminum hydroxide/ magnesium hydroxide	• Treatment of peptic ulcers • Work by neutralizing or reducing acidity of stomach contents • Differences in absorption rate	• Constipation • Diarrhea • Drug interactions	• Need to take several times a day. • Administer after meals. • Assess for history of renal diseases when client is taking magnesium products; electrolyte readjustment occurs and can result in renal insufficiency and calcinosis.
Histamine-2 Antagonists			
• Ranitidine HCl • Cimetidine • Famotidine • Nizatidine	• Treatment of peptic ulcers • Prophylactic treatment for clients at risk for developing ulcers (those on steroids or highly stressed)	• Multiple drug interactions	• Cigarette smoking interferes with drug action. • Expensive.
Mucosal Healing Agents			

• Sucralfate	• Treatment of peptic ulcers	• Constipation
		• Drug interaction with:
		  • Tetracycline
		  • Phenytoin sodium
		  • Digoxin
		  • Cimetidine
			• Medication to be taken at least 1 hour before meals.
			• Antacids interfere with absorption.

Proton Pump Inhibitors			

• Lansoprazole
• Pantoprazole (available PO and IV)
• Esomeprazole
• Omeprazole
• Rabeprazole
• Dexlansoprazole
	• Treatment of erosive esophagitis associated with GERD	• Constipation
		• Heartburn
		• Anxiety
		• Diarrhea
		• Abdominal pain, hepatocellular damage, pancreatitis, gastroenteritis
		• Tinnitus, vertigo, confusion, headache
		• Blurred vision, hypokinesia
		• Chest pain, dyspnea
			• Taken before meals.
			• Do not crush or chew pantoprazole IV:
			  • Resume oral therapy as soon as feasible.
			  • Long-lasting effects of drug may inhibit absorption of other drugs.
			  • Not removed by hemodialysis.
			  • Monitor for indications of adverse reactions.

Additional Drugs			
• Prokinetic agents • Antiemetics • Cough suppressants • Stool softeners	• Treatment of slow peristalsis and increased intraabdominal pressure in clients with GERD	• Diarrhea	• Monitor for indications of adverse reactions.

Nursing Assessment

A. Determine how food intake affects pain.
B. Take history of antacid, histamine antagonist, or proton pump inhibitor use.
C. Determine presence of melena (black tarry stools).
D. Determine presence and location of peptic ulcer as determined by:
   1. Esophagogastroduodenoscopy (EGD)
   2. Barium swallow
   3. Gastric analysis indicating increased levels of stomach acid
E. Potential complications
   1. Hemorrhage
   2. Perforation (which always requires surgery)
   3. Obstruction

Analysis (Nursing Diagnoses)

A. *Acute pain* related to …
B. *Imbalanced nutrition: less than body requirements* related to …
C. *Deficient knowledge* related to …
D. *Risk for injury* related to …

Nursing Plans and Interventions

A. Determine symptom onset and how symptoms are relieved.
B. Monitor color, quantity, consistency of stools and emesis, and test for occult blood.
C. Administer medications as prescribed, usually 1 to 2 hours after meals and at bedtime (see Table 4-20).
D. Administer mucosal healing agents at least 1 hour before meals, as prescribed (see Table 4-20).
E. Encourage small, frequent meals; no bedtime snacks; and avoidance of beverages containing caffeine.
F. Prepare client for surgery if uncontrolled bleeding, obstruction, or perforation occurs.
   1. Gastric resection
   2. Vagotomy
   3. Pyloroplasty
G. Teach client that dumping syndrome may occur postoperatively.
   1. Secondary to rapid entry of hypertonic food into jejunum (pulls water out of bloodstream)
   2. Occurs 5 to 30 minutes after eating
   3. Characterized by vertigo, syncope, sweating, pallor, tachycardia, and/or hypotension
   4. Minimized by small, frequent meals: high-protein, high-fat, low-carbohydrate diet
   5. Exacerbated by consuming liquids with meals; helped by lying down after eating
   6. Can also be observed in clients on hypertonic tube feeding
H. Teach client to avoid medications that increase the risk for developing peptic ulcers.
   1. Salicylates
   2. NSAIDs such as ibuprofen
   3. Corticosteroids in high doses
   4. Anticoagulants
I. Teach client the importance of informing all health care personnel of ulcer history.
J. Teach client symptoms of GI bleeding.
   1. Dark, tarry stools
   2. Coffee-ground emesis
   3. Bright-red rectal bleeding
   4. Fatigue
   5. Pallor
   6. Severe abdominal pain, which should be reported immediately (could denote perforation)
K. Teach client importance of smoking cessation and stress management.

> **HESI Hint** • Stress can cause or exacerbate ulcers. Teach stress-reduction methods, and encourage those with a family history of ulcers to obtain medical surveillance for ulcer formation.

> **HESI Hint** • Clinical manifestations of GI bleeding:
> • Pallor: conjunctival, mucous membranes, nail beds
> • Dark, tarry stools
> • Bright-red or coffee-ground emesis
> • Abdominal mass or bruit
> • Decreased BP, rapid pulse, cool extremities (shock), increased respirations

Inflammatory Bowel Diseases

Description: Consists of Crohn's disease and ulcerative colitis

Crohn's Disease (Regional Enteritis)

Description: Subacute, chronic inflammation extending throughout all layers of intestinal mucosa (most commonly found in terminal ileum), which has a cobblestone appearance of the GI mucosa, with periods of remission interspersed with periods of exacerbation. Crohn's disease occurs during the teenage years and early adulthood, but has a second peak in the sixth decade. Capsule endoscopy has shown greater sensitivity than radiography when diagnosing Crohn's disease. There is speculation that Crohn's disease could be caused by a combination of environmental factors and genetic predisposition, but as of now, there is no cure, so treatment relies on medications to treat the acute inflammation and maintain a remission. Surgery is reserved for patients who are unresponsive to medications or who develop life-threatening complications. In a total proctocolectomy (the colon and rectum are removed and the anus is closed), the terminal ileum is brought through the abdominal wall, and a permanent ileostomy is formed.

Nursing Assessment

A. Abdominal pain (unrelieved by defecation), right lower quadrant
B. Diarrhea, steatorrhea (fatty diarrheal stools), and weight loss, with client becoming emaciated
C. Constant fluid loss
D. Low-grade fever
E. Perforation of the intestine occurring due to severe inflammation; constitutes a medical emergency
F. Anorexia related to pain after eating
G. Weight loss, anemia, malnutrition

Analysis (Nursing Diagnoses)

A. *Risk for bleeding* related to…
B. *Risk for deficient fluid volume* related to …
C. *Chronic pain* related to …
D. *Imbalanced nutrition: less than body requirements* related to …

Nursing Plans and Interventions

A. Determine bowel elimination pattern, and control diarrhea with diet and medication as indicated.
B. Provide a nutritious, well-balanced, low-residue, low-fat, high-protein, high-calorie diet, with no dairy products.
C. Administer vitamin supplements and iron.
D. Advise client to avoid foods that are known to cause diarrhea, such as milk products and spicy foods.
E. Advise client to avoid smoking, caffeinated beverages, pepper, and alcohol.
F. Provide complete bowel rest with IV total parenteral nutrition (TPN) if necessary.
G. Administer medications as prescribed: aminosalicylates, antimicrobials, corticosteroids, immunosuppressants, and biologic therapy as necessary for acute symptoms and chronic treatment.
H. Monitor I&O and serum electrolytes.
I. Weigh at least twice a week.
J. Provide emotional support, and encourage use of support groups such as the Crohn's and Colitis Foundation of America.
K. Encourage client to talk with the enterostomal therapists before surgery.
L. If ileostomy is performed, teach stoma care (see Stoma Care, p. 126).

> **HESI Hint** • The GI tract usually accounts for only 100 to 200 mL of fluid loss per day, although it filters up to 8 L per day. Large fluid losses can occur if vomiting or diarrhea exists.

Ulcerative Colitis

Description: Disease that affects the superficial mucosa of the large intestines and rectum, causing the bowel to eventually narrow, shorten, and thicken due to muscular hypertrophy. Sigmoidoscopy and colonoscopy allow direct examination of the large intestinal mucosa and are used for diagnosis of ulcerative colitis.

Nursing Assessment

A. Diarrhea
B. Abdominal pain and cramping
C. Intermittent tenesmus (anal contractions) and rectal bleeding
D. Liquid stools containing blood, mucus, and pus (may pass 10 to 20 liquid stools per day)
E. Weakness and fatigue
F. Anemia

Analysis (Nursing Diagnoses)

A. *Risk for deficient fluid volume* related to …
B. *Acute pain* related to …
C. *Imbalanced nutrition: less than body requirements* related to …

Nursing Plans and Interventions

A. Determine bowel elimination pattern, and control diarrhea with diet and medication as indicated.
B. Provide a nutritious, well-balanced, low-residue, low-fat, high-protein, high-calorie diet, with no dairy products.
C. Administer vitamin supplements and iron.
D. Advise client to avoid foods that are known to cause diarrhea, such as milk products and spicy foods.
E. Advise client to avoid smoking, caffeinated beverages, pepper, and alcohol.
F. Provide complete bowel rest with IV hyperalimentation if necessary.
G. Administer medications as prescribed, often corticosteroids, antidiarrheals, sulfasalazine (Azulfidine), mesalamine (various brands), and infliximab (Remicade) or other biologic treatments, if there is no response to previous medications.
H. Monitor I&O and serum electrolytes.
I. Weigh at least twice a week.
J. Provide emotional support, and encourage use of support groups such as the local Ileitis and Colitis Foundation.
K. Encourage client to talk with the enterostomal therapists before surgery.
L. If ileostomy is performed, teach stoma care (see Stoma Care, p. 126).

> **HESI Hint** • Opiate drugs tend to depress gastric motility. However, they should be given with caution. The nurse should assess for abdominal distention, abdominal pain, abdominal rigidity, signs and symptoms of shock-increased HR, and decreased BP, indicating possible perforation/GI bleed.

Diverticular Diseases

Description: Manifested in two clinical forms: diverticulosis and diverticulitis

A. Diverticulosis: bulging pouches in the GI wall (diverticula), which push the mucosa lining through the surrounding muscle
B. Diverticulitis: inflamed diverticula, which may cause obstruction, infection, and hemorrhage

> **HESI Hint** • Diverticulosis is the presence of pouches in the wall of the intestine. There is usually no discomfort, and the problem goes unnoticed unless seen on radiologic examination (usually prompted by some other condition). Diverticulitis is an inflammation of the diverticula (pouches), which can lead to perforation of the bowel.

Nursing Assessment

A. Left lower quadrant pain
B. Increased flatus
C. Rectal bleeding
D. Signs of intestinal obstruction:
   1. Constipation alternating with diarrhea
   2. Abdominal distention
   3. Anorexia
   4. Low-grade fever
E. Barium enema or colonoscopy positive for diverticular disease: obstruction, ileus, or perforation confirmed by abdominal radiograph (barium not used during acute phase of illness)

Analysis (Nursing Diagnoses)

A. *Risk for bleeding* due to…
B. *Ineffective tissue perfusion* related to …
C. *Acute pain* related to …
D. *Imbalanced nutrition: less than body requirements* related to …

Nursing Plans and Interventions

A. Provide a well-balanced, high-fiber diet unless inflammation is present, in which case client is NPO, followed by low-residue bland foods.

> **HESI Hint** • A client admitted with complaints of severe lower abdominal pain, cramping, and diarrhea is diagnosed as having diverticulitis. What are the nutritional needs of this client throughout recovery?
> • Acute phase: NPO, graduating to liquids
> • Recovery phase: no fiber or foods that irritate the bowel
> • Maintenance phase: high-fiber diet with bulk-forming laxatives to prevent pooling of foods in the pouches where they can become inflamed; avoidance of small, poorly digested foods such as popcorn, nuts, seeds, etc.

B. Include bulk-forming laxatives such as Metamucil in daily regimen.
C. Increase fluid intake to 3 L/day.

D. Monitor I&O and bowel elimination; avoid constipation (administer stool softener or bulk laxatives).
E. Observe for complications.
   1. Obstruction
   2. Peritonitis or other infections
   3. Hemorrhage (treatment for ruptured diverticula is a temporary colostomy and is maintained for approximately 3 months to allow the bowel to rest)
   4. Infection

Intestinal Obstruction

Description: Partial or complete blockage of intestinal flow (fluids, feces, gas) that occurs mostly in the small intestines
A. Mechanical causes of intestinal obstruction
   1. Adhesions (most common cause)
   2. Hernia (strangulates the gut)
   3. Volvulus (twisting of the gut)
   4. Intussusception (telescoping of the gut within itself)
   5. Tumors; develop slowly; usually a mass of feces becomes lodged against the tumor
B. Neurogenic causes of intestinal obstruction
   1. Paralytic ileus (usually occurs in postoperative clients)
   2. Spinal cord lesion
C. Vascular cause of intestinal obstruction
   1. Mesenteric artery occlusion (leads to gut infarct)

> **HESI Hint** • *Bowel Obstructions*
> • Mechanical: Due to disorders outside the bowel (hernia, adhesions) caused by disorders within the bowel (tumors, diverticulitis) or by blockage of the lumen in the intestine (intussusception, gallstone)
> • Nonmechanical: Due to paralytic ileus, which does not involve any actual physical obstruction but results from inability of the bowel itself to function

Nursing Assessment

A. Sudden onset of abdominal pain, tenderness, or guarding
B. History of abdominal surgeries
C. History of obstruction
D. Distention
E. Increased peristalsis when obstruction first occurs, then peristalsis becoming absent when paralytic ileus occurs
F. Bowel sounds that are high pitched with early mechanical obstruction and diminish to absent with neurogenic or late mechanical obstruction

Analysis (Nursing Diagnoses)

A. *Risk for dysfunctional GI motility* related to …
B. *Deficient volume* related to …
C. *Acute pain* related to …

Nursing Plans and Interventions

A. Maintain client NPO, with IV fluids and electrolyte therapy.

B. Monitor I&O; a Foley catheter maintains strict output.
C. Implement nasogastric (NG) intubation.
  1. Attach to low suction (intermittent; 80 mm Hg).
  2. Document output every 8 hours.
  3. Irrigate with normal saline if policy dictates.
D. NG tube (passed through the nose into the stomach; Miller-Abbott tube is used for decompression; it is passed through the nose and the stomach into the small intestines then connected to suction; placement is usually performed by the health care provider.
  1. Nasogastric tube
    a. Measure correct length of tubing to be inserted by measuring from the tip of the client's nose to the client's earlobe to the xiphoid process.
  2. Advance decompression tube every 1 to 2 hours.
  3. Do not secure to nose until tube reaches specified position.
  4. Reposition client every 2 hours to assist with placement of the tube.
  5. Connect tube to suction.
  6. Irrigate NG tube with normal saline; irrigate Miller-Abbott tube with air only.
  7. Note amount, color, consistency, and any unusual odor of drainage.
  8. Assess for signs of dehydration (skin turgor, amount and color of urine).
  9. Monitor electrolyte values.

HESI Hint • A client admitted with complaints of constipation, thready stools, and rectal bleeding over the past few months is diagnosed with a rectal mass. What are the nursing priorities for this client?
- NPO
- NG tube (possibly an intestinal tube such as a Miller-Abbott)
- IV fluids
- Surgical preparations of bowel (if obstruction is complete)
- Foods and fluids are restricted for 8 to 10 hours before surgery if possible.
- If the patient has a bowel obstruction or perforation, bowel cleansing is contraindicated.
- Oral erythromycin and neomycin are given to further decrease the amount of colonic and rectal bacteria.
- If possible, all clients who require surgery for obstruction undergo NG intubation and suction before surgery. However, in cases of complete obstruction, surgery should proceed without delay
- Teaching (preoperative nutrition, etc.)

E. Document pain; medicate as prescribed.
F. Assess abdomen regularly for distention, rigidity, change in status of bowel sounds.
G. If conservative medical interventions fail, surgery will be required to remove obstruction.

Colorectal Cancer

Description: Tumors occurring in the colon
A. Cancer of the colon is the fourth most common cancer in the United States.
B. This is the second-leading cause of cancer-related deaths in the United States.
C. Approximately 45% of cancerous tumors of the colon occur in the rectal or sigmoid area, 25% in the cecum and ascending colon, and 30% in the remainder of colon.
D. The highest incidence occurs in persons older than 50 years of age.
E. A diet of high-fiber, low-fat foods, including cruciferous vegetables, may be a factor in the prevention of colon cancer.

HESI Hint • Diet recommended by the American Cancer Society to prevent bowel cancer:
- Eat more cruciferous vegetables (those from the cabbage family, such as broccoli, cauliflower, Brussels sprouts, cabbage, and kale).
- Increase fiber intake.
- Maintain average body weight.
- Eat less animal fat.

F. Early detection is important.

HESI Hint • American Cancer Society recommendations for early detection of colon cancer:
- A digital rectal examination (DRE) every year after 40.
- A stool blood test every year after 50.
- A colonoscopy or sigmoidoscopy examination every 10 years after the age of 50 in average-risk clients, or more often based on the advice of a physician.

G. Usual treatment is surgical removal of the tumor, with adjuvant radiation or antineoplastic chemotherapy.
H. Diagnosis is made by digital examination, flexible fiber-optic sigmoidoscopy with biopsy, colonoscopy, and barium enema.
I. Carcinoembryonic antigen (CEA) serum level is used to evaluate effectiveness of chemotherapy.

Nursing Assessment

A. Rectal bleeding
B. Change in bowel habits
C. Sense of incomplete evacuation, tenesmus
D. Abdominal pain, nausea, vomiting
E. Weight loss, cachexia
F. Abdominal distention or ascites
G. Family history of cancer, particularly cancer of the colon
H. History of polyps

Analysis (Nursing Diagnoses)

A. *Deficient knowledge* related to ...
B. *Ineffective coping* (specify) related to ...
C. *Disturbed body image* related to ...

Nursing Plans and Interventions

A. Prepare client for surgery
B. Prepare client for bowel preparation, which may include laxatives and gut lavage with polyethylene glycol (GoLYTELY).
C. If colostomy has been performed, teach stoma care (see Stoma Care below
D. Provide high-calorie, high-protein diet.
E. Promote prevention of constipation with high-fiber diet.

> **HESI Hint** • An early sign of colon cancer is rectal bleeding. Encourage patients 50 years of age or older and those with increased risk factors to be screened yearly with fecal occult blood testing. Routine colonoscopy at 50 is also recommended.

Stoma Care

A. General information
   1. The more distal the stoma is, the greater chance for continence. Greatest chance for continence is with a stoma created from the sigmoid colon on the left side of the abdomen.
   2. An ileostomy drains liquid material; peristomal skin is prone to breakdown by enzymes.
   3. The lower the stoma's location is in the GI tract, the more solid, or formed, is the effluence (stoma drainage).
   4. The greatest chance for continence is with a stoma created from the sigmoid colon on the left side of the abdomen.
   5. Consultation with an enterostomal therapist is essential.
B. Preoperative care
   1. Client and family must be informed about what to expect postoperatively:
      a. Proposed location of the stoma
      b. Approximate size
      c. What it will look like (provide picture, if indicated)
   2. The family should be included in teaching, but it should be emphasized that the client is ultimately responsible for his or her own care.
C. Pouch care
   1. Ostomates often wear pouches.
   2. The adhesive-backed opening, designed to cover the stoma, should provide about ⅛-inch clearance from the stoma.
   3. A rubber band or clip is used to secure the bottom of the pouch and prevent leakage.
   4. A simple squirt bottle is used to remove effluence from the sides of the bag. Pouch system is changed every 3 to 7 days.
   5. Clients should maintain an extra supply of pouches so that they never run out and should change the pouch when bowel is inactive.
   6. Pouch should be emptied when one third to one half full.
D. Irrigation
   1. Those with descending-colon colostomies can irrigate to provide control over effluence.
      a. Clients should irrigate at approximately the same time daily.
      b. Clients should use warm water (cold or hot water causes cramping).
      c. Clients should wash around stoma with lukewarm water and a mild soap.
      d. Commercial skin barriers may be purchased for home use.
   2. Odor control
      a. Commercial preparations are available.
      b. Foods in diet that cause offensive odors can be eliminated.
E. Diet
   1. Ileostomy
      a. Clients should chew food thoroughly.
      b. High-fiber foods (popcorn, peanuts, unpeeled vegetables) can cause severe diarrhea and may have to be eliminated.
   2. Colostomy
      a. Client should resume the regular diet gradually. Foods that were a problem preoperatively should be tried cautiously.

Cirrhosis

Description: Degeneration of liver tissue, causing enlargement, fibrosis, and scarring
A. Causes of cirrhosis include the following:
   1. Chronic alcohol ingestion (Laënnec cirrhosis)
   2. Viral hepatitis
   3. Exposure to hepatotoxins (including medications)
   4. Infections
   5. Congenital abnormalities
   6. Chronic biliary tree obstruction
   7. Chronic severe right-sided HF
   8. Idiopathy
B. Initially, hepatomegaly occurs; later, the liver becomes hard and nodular.

Nursing Assessment

A. History of alcohol, prescriptive and street drug use
B. Work history of exposure to toxic chemicals (pesticides, fumes, etc.)
C. Medication history of long-term use of hepatotoxic drugs
D. Family health history of liver abnormalities
E. Physical findings
   1. Weakness, malaise
   2. Anorexia, weight loss
   3. Palpable liver (early); abdominal girth increases as liver enlarges
   4. Jaundice

5. Fetor hepaticus (fruity or musty breath)

> **HESI Hint • *Clinical Manifestations of Jaundice***
> - Yellow skin, sclera, or mucous membranes (bilirubin in skin)
> - Dark-colored urine (bilirubin in urine)
> - Chalky or clay-colored stools (absence of bilirubin in stools)

> **HESI Hint •** Fetor hepaticus is a distinctive breath odor of chronic liver disease. It is characterized by a fruity or musty odor that results from the damaged liver's inability to metabolize and detoxify mercaptan, which is produced by the bacterial degradation of methionine, a sulfurous amino acid.

6. Asterixis (hand-flapping tremor that often accompanies metabolic disorders)
7. Mental and behavioral changes
8. Bruising, erythema
9. Dry skin, spider angiomas
10. Gynecomastia (breast development), testicular atrophy
11. Ascites, peripheral neuropathy
12. Hematemesis
13. Palmar erythema (redness in palms of the hands)

> **HESI Hint •** For treatment of ascites, paracentesis and peritoneovenous shunts (LeVeen and Denver shunts) may be indicated.

> **HESI Hint •** Esophageal varices may rupture and cause hemorrhage. Immediate management includes insertion of an esophagogastric balloon tamponade (a Blakemore-Sengstaken or Minnesota tube). Other therapies include vasopressors, vitamin K, coagulation factors, and blood transfusions.

F. Clotting defects noted in laboratory findings include:
   1. Elevated bilirubin, AST, ALT, alkaline phosphatase, PT, and ammonia
   2. Decreased Hgb, Hct, electrolytes, K, Na, and albumin

> **HESI Hint •** Ammonia is not broken down as usual in the damaged liver; therefore the serum ammonia level rises.
>   The metabolism of drugs is slowed down so they remain in the system longer.

G. Complications include:
   1. Ascites, edema
   2. Portal HTN
   3. Esophageal varices

4. Encephalopathy
5. Respiratory distress
6. Coagulation defects

Analysis (Nursing Diagnoses)

A. *Excess fluid volume* related to …
B. *Risk for bleeding* related to …
C. *Pain* related to …
D. *Ineffective breathing pattern* related to …
E. *Imbalanced nutrition: less than body requirements* related to …
F. *Risk for infection* related to …
G. *Impaired skin integrity* related to…

Nursing Plans and Interventions

A. Eliminate causative agent (alcohol, hepatotoxin).
B. Administer vitamin supplements (A, B complex, C, K), and teach client and family the need for continuing these supplements.
C. Observe mental status frequently (at least every 2 hours); note any subtle changes.
D. Avoid initiating bleeding, and observe for bleeding tendencies.
   1. Avoid injections whenever possible.
   2. Use small-bore needles for IV insertion.
   3. Maintain pressure to venipuncture sites for at least 5 minutes.
   4. Use electric razor.
   5. Provide a soft-bristle toothbrush, and encourage careful mouth care.
   6. Check stools and emesis for frank or occult blood.
   7. Prevent straining at stool.
      a. Administer stood softeners as prescribed.
      b. Provide high-fiber diet.
E. Provide special skin care.
   1. Avoid soap, rubbing alcohol, and perfumed products (these are drying to the skin).
   2. Apply moisturizing lotion or baby oil frequently.
   3. Observe skin for any lesions, including scratch marks.
   4. Turn frequently, and provide lotion to exposed skin.
F. Monitor fluid and electrolyte status daily.
   1. I&O (accurate output measurement may require Foley catheter)
   2. Observe for edema, pulmonary edema.
   3. Measure abdominal girth (determines increase or decrease of ascites).
   4. Weigh daily (determines increase or decrease of edema and ascites).
   5. Restrict fluids to 1500 mL/day (may help to reduce edema and ascites).
G. Monitor dietary intake carefully, especially protein intake. Restrict protein if client has hepatic coma; otherwise, encourage foods with high biologic protein.
H. Explain dietary restrictions: low sodium, low potassium, low fat, high carbohydrate.

I. If encephalopathy is present, lactulose is used to decrease ammonia levels (Table 4-21).

J. If esophageal varices are present, esophagogastric balloon tamponade (Blakemore tube), sclerotherapy, and/or portal systemic shunts may be used for treatment.

Hepatitis

Description: Widespread inflammation of liver cells, usually caused by a virus (Table 4-22)

Nursing Assessment

A. Known exposure to hepatitis

B. Individuals at risk for contracting hepatitis
   1. Homosexual males engaging in unprotected sex
   2. IV drug users (disease transmitted by dirty needles)
   3. Those who received tattoos or body piercing that could have been applied using dirty needles.
   4. Those living in crowded conditions
   5. Health care workers who do not use personal protective equipment (PPE) properly are at high risk

C. Monitor clients with the following symptoms
   1. Fatigue, malaise, weakness
   2. Anorexia, nausea, and vomiting
   3. Jaundice, dark urine, clay-colored stools
   4. Myalgia (muscle aches), joint pain
   5. Dull headaches, irritability, depression
   6. Abdominal tenderness in right upper quadrant
   7. Fever (with hepatitis A)
   8. Elevations of liver enzymes (ALT, AST, alkaline phosphatase), bilirubin

TABLE 4-21 Ammonia Detoxicants/Stimulant Laxative

Drug	Implications	Adverse Reactions	Nursing Implications
• Lactulose • Rifaximin	• Encephalopathy • Used to decrease ammonia levels and bowel pH	• Diarrhea	• Instruct client regarding need for medication. • Observe for diarrhea. • Monitor ammonia levels.

TABLE 4-22 Comparison of Three Types of Hepatitis

Characteristics	Hepatitis A (Infectious Hepatitis)	Hepatitis B (Serum Hepatitis)	Hepatitis C (Non-A, Non-B Hepatitis)
• Source of infection	• Contaminated food • Contaminated water or shellfish	• Contaminated blood products • Contaminated needles or surgical instruments • Mother to child at birth	• Contaminated blood products • Contaminated needles; IV drug use • Dialysis
• Route of infection	• Oral • Fecal • Parenteral • Person to person	• Parenteral • Oral • Fecal • Direct contact • Breast milk • Sexual contact	• Parenteral • Sexual contact
• Incubation period	• 15-50 days	• 14-180 days	• Average: 14-180 days
• Onset	• Abrupt	• Insidious	• Insidious
• Seasonal variation	• Autumn • Winter	• All year	• All year
• Age group affected	• Children • Young adults	• Any age	• Any age
• Vaccine	• Yes	• Yes	• No
• Inoculation	• Yes	• Yes	• Yes
• Potential for chronic liver disease	• No	• Yes	• Yes
• Immunity	• Yes	• Yes	• No

Analysis (Nursing Diagnoses)

A. *Risk for impaired liver function* related to ...
B. *Imbalanced nutrition: less than body requirements* related to ...
C. *Risk for infection* related to ...
D. *Activity intolerance* related to...

Nursing Plans and Interventions

A. Assess client's response to activity, and plan periods of rest after periods of activity.
B. Assist client with care as needed; encourage client to get help with daily activities at home (caring for children, preparing meals, etc.)
C. Provide high-calorie, high-carbohydrate diet with moderate fats and proteins.
   1. Serve small, frequent meals.
   2. Provide vitamin supplements.
   3. Provide foods the client prefers.
D. Administer medications, interferon, nucleoside and nucleotide analogs, protease inhibitors, and antiemetics as prescribed.

> **HESI Hint • *Provide an Environment Conducive to Eating***
> For clients who are anorexic or nauseated:
> - Remove strong odors immediately; they can be offensive and increase nausea.
> - Encourage client to sit up for meals; this can decrease the propensity to vomit.
> - Serve small, frequent meals.
> - Give antiemetic before eating.

E. Teach client importance of adhering to personal hygiene, using individual drinking and eating utensils, toothbrushes, and razors. Prevention of spread to others must be emphasized.
F. Teach client to avoid hepatotoxic substances such as alcohol, aspirin, acetaminophen, and sedatives.

> **HESI Hint** • Liver tissue is destroyed by hepatitis. Rest and adequate nutrition are necessary for regeneration of the liver tissue being destroyed by the disease. Many drugs are metabolized in the liver, so drug therapy must be scrutinized carefully. Caution the client that recovery takes many months, and previously taken medications and/or over-the-counter drugs should not be resumed without the health care provider's directions.

Pancreatitis

Description: Nonbacterial inflammation of the pancreas
A. Acute pancreatitis occurs when there is digestion of the pancreas by its own enzymes, primarily trypsin.
B. Alcohol ingestion and biliary tract disease are major causes of acute pancreatitis.
C. Chronic pancreatitis is a progressive, destructive disease that causes permanent dysfunction.
D. Long-term alcohol use is the major factor in chronic pancreatitis.
E. Alcohol consumption should be stopped when acute pancreatitis is suspected and consumption completely avoided in chronic pancreatitis.

Nursing Assessment

A. Acute pancreatitis
   1. Severe midepigastric pain radiating to back; usually related to excess alcohol ingestion or a fatty meal
   2. Abdominal guarding; rigid, boardlike abdomen, and abdominal pain
   3. Nausea and vomiting
   4. Elevated temperature, tachycardia, decreased BP
   5. Bluish discoloration of flanks (Grey Turner sign) or periumbilical area (Cullen sign)
   6. Elevated amylase, lipase, triglycerides, and glucose levels
   7. Low serum calcium levels
B. Chronic pancreatitis
   1. Continuous burning or gnawing abdominal pain
   2. Recurring attacks of severe upper abdominal and back pain
   3. Ascites
   4. Steatorrhea, diarrhea
   5. Weight loss
   6. Jaundice, dark urine
   7. Signs and symptoms of diabetes mellitus

Analysis (Nursing Diagnoses)

A. *Acute pain* related to ...
B. *Chronic pain* related to ...
C. *Imbalanced nutrition: less than body requirements* related to ...
D. *Deficient fluid volume* related to ...
E. *Risk for electrolyte imbalance*

Nursing Plans and Interventions

A. Acute pancreatitis
   1. Maintain NPO status.
   2. Maintain NG tube to suction; TPN may be prescribed.
   3. Administer hydromorphone (Dilaudid) or fentanyl (Sublimaze) as needed.
   4. Administer antacids, histamine H2 receptor-blocking drugs, anticholinergics, proton pump inhibitors.
   5. Assist client to assume position of comfort on side with legs drawn up to chest.
   6. Teach client to avoid alcohol, caffeine, and fatty and spicy foods.
   7. If severe, blood sugar monitoring and regular insulin coverage may be needed temporarily.
   8. Monitor for neuromuscular manifestations of hypocalcemia (e.g., tetany, muscle twitching, cramping, grimacing, seizure, altered deep tendon reflexes, and spasm).

9. Place in semi-Fowler position to decrease pressure on the diaphragm.
10. Encourage client to cough and deep breathe and/or use incentive spirometry.
11. Monitor ECG for dysrhythmias related to electrolyte imbalances.

> **HESI Hint** • Acute pancreatic pain is located retroperitoneally. Any enlargement of the pancreas causes the peritoneum to stretch tightly. Therefore sitting up or leaning forward reduces the pain.

B. Chronic pancreatitis
   1. Administer analgesics such as hydromorphone (Dilaudid), fentanyl (Sublimaze), and morphine (narcotic tolerance and dependency may be a problem).
   2. Administer pancreatic enzymes such as pancreatin (Creon) or pancrelipase (Viokase) with meals or snacks. Powdered forms should be mixed with fruit juice or applesauce (mixing with proteins should be avoided).
   3. Monitor client's stools for number and consistency to determine effectiveness of enzyme replacement.
   4. Teach client about consuming a bland, low-fat diet and to avoid rich foods, alcohol, and caffeine.
   5. Monitor for signs and symptoms of diabetes mellitus.

Cholecystitis and Cholelithiasis

Description: Cholecystitis: acute inflammation of the gallbladder; cholelithiasis: formation or presence of stones in the gallbladder
A. Incidence of these diseases is greater in females who are multiparous and overweight.
B. Treatment for cholecystitis consists of IV hydration, administration of antibiotics, and pain control with morphine or NSAIDs; anticholinergics are administered to decrease smooth muscle spasms.
C. Treatment for cholelithiasis consists of nonsurgical removal of stones.
   1. Dissolution therapy (administration of bile salts; used rarely)
   2. Endoscopic retrograde cholangiopancreatography (ERCP)
   3. Lithotripsy (not covered by many insurance carriers, thereby limiting its use)
D. Cholecystectomy is performed if stones are not removed nonsurgically and inflammation is absent. It may be done through laparoscope.

> **HESI Hint** • After an ERCP, the client may feel sick. The scope is placed in the gallbladder, and the stones are crushed and left to pass on their own. These clients may be prone to pancreatitis.

Nursing Assessment
A. Pain, anorexia, vomiting, or flatulence precipitated by ingestion of fried, spicy, or fatty foods
B. Fever, elevated WBCs, and other signs of infection (cholecystitis)
C. Abdominal tenderness
D. Jaundice and clay-colored stools (blockage)
E. Elevated liver enzymes, bilirubin, and WBCs

Analysis (Nursing Diagnoses)
A. *Acute pain* related to …
B. *Deficient knowledge* (specify) related to …
C. *Deficient fluid volume* related to…

Nursing Plans and Interventions
A. Administer analgesic for pain as needed.
B. Maintain NPO status.
C. Maintain NG tube to suction if indicated.
D. Administer IV antibiotics for cholecystitis, and administer antibiotics prophylactically for cholelithiasis.
E. Monitor I&O.
F. Monitor electrolyte status regularly.
G. Teach client to avoid fried, spicy, and fatty foods and to reduce caloric intake if indicated.

> **HESI Hint** • Nonsurgical management of a client with cholecystitis includes:
> - Low-fat diet
> - Decompression of the stomach via NG tube
> - Medications for pain and clotting if required

H. Provide preoperative and postoperative care if surgery is indicated
I. Monitor T-tube drainage.

Review of Gastrointestinal System

1. List four nursing interventions for the client with a hiatal hernia.
2. List three categories of medications used in the treatment of PUD.
3. List the symptoms of upper and lower GI bleeding.
4. What bowel sound disruptions occur with an intestinal obstruction?
5. List four nursing interventions for postoperative care of a client with a colostomy.
6. List the common clinical manifestations of jaundice.
7. What are the common food intolerances for clients with cholelithiasis?
8. List five symptoms indicative of colon cancer.

9. In a client with cirrhosis, it is imperative to prevent further bleeding and observe for bleeding tendencies. List six relevant nursing interventions.
10. What is the main side effect of lactulose, which is used to reduce ammonia levels in clients with cirrhosis?
11. List four groups who have a high risk for contracting hepatitis.
12. How should the nurse administer pancreatic enzymes?

Answers to Review

1. Sit up while eating and for 1 hour after eating. Eat frequent, small meals. Eliminate foods that are problematic.
2. Antacids, H2 receptor blockers, mucosal healing agents, proton pump inhibitors
3. Upper GI: melena, hematemesis, tarry stools; lower GI: bloody stools, tarry stools; common to both: tarry stools
4. Early mechanical obstruction: high-pitched sounds; late mechanical obstruction: diminished or absent bowel sounds
5. Irrigate daily at same time; use warm water for irrigations; wash around stoma with mild soap and water after each ostomy bag change; ensure that pouch opening extends at least ⅛ inch around the stoma.
6. Scleral icterus (yellow sclera), dark urine, chalky or clay-colored stools
7. Fried, spicy, and fatty foods
8. Rectal bleeding, change in bowel habits, sense of incomplete evacuation, abdominal pain with nausea, weight loss
9. Avoid injections; use small-bore needles for IV insertion; maintain pressure for 5 minutes on all venipuncture sites; use electric razor; use soft-bristle toothbrush for mouth care; check stools and emesis for occult blood.
10. Diarrhea
11. Homosexual males, IV drug users, those who have had recent ear piercing or tattooing, and health care workers
12. Give with meals or snacks. Powder forms should be mixed with fruit juices.

Endocrine System

. . . .

Hyperthyroidism (Graves Disease, Goiter)

Description: Excessive activity of thyroid gland, resulting in an elevated level of circulating thyroid hormones. Possibly long-term or lifelong treatment.
A. Hyperthyroidism can result from a primary disease state; from the use of replacement hormone therapy; or from excess thyroid-stimulating hormone (TSH) being produced by an anterior pituitary tumor.
B. Graves disease is thought to be an autoimmune process and accounts for most cases.
C. Diagnosis is made on the basis of serum hormone levels
D. Common treatment for hyperthyroidism—goal is to create a euthyroid state
  1. Thyroid ablation by medication
  2. Radioactive iodine therapy
  3. Thyroidectomy
  4. Adenectomy of portion of anterior pituitary where TSH-producing tumor is located
E. All treatments make the client hypothyroid, requiring hormone replacement.

Nursing Assessment

A. Enlarged thyroid gland
B. Acceleration of body processes
  1. Weight loss
  2. Increased appetite

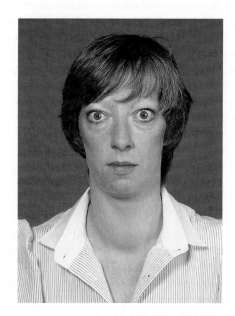

FIGURE 4-6 Graves disease. This woman has a diffuse goiter and exophthalmos. (From Forbes CD, Jackson WF: *Colour atlas and text of clinical medicine,* ed 3, London, 2003, Mosby.)

  3. Diarrhea
  4. Heat intolerance
  5. Tachycardia, palpitations, increased systolic BP
  6. Diaphoresis, wet or moist skin
  7. Nervousness, insomnia
C. Exophthalmos (Fig. 4-6)

D. T_3 elevated above 220 ng/dL

E. T_4 elevated above 12 mcg/dL

F. Low level of TSH indicates primary disease; elevated T_4 level suppresses thyroid-releasing hormone (TRH), which suppresses TSH secretion. If source is anterior pituitary, both will be elevated.

G. Radioactive iodine uptake (^{131}I) (indicates presence of goiter)

H. Thyroid scan (indicating presence of goiter)

Analysis (Nursing Diagnoses)

A. *Activity intolerance* related to …

B. *Deficient knowledge* (specify) related to …

C. *Imbalanced nutrition: less than body requirements* related to …

D. *Risk for injury* related to …

Nursing Plans and Interventions

A. Provide a calm, restful atmosphere.

B. Observe for signs of thyroid storm (sudden oversecretion of thyroid hormone; is life threatening).

> **HESI Hint** • Thyroid storm is a life-threatening event that occurs with uncontrolled hyperthyroidism due to Graves disease. Other causes include childbirth, congestive heart failure (CHF), diabetic ketoacidosis, infection, pulmonary embolism, emotional distress, trauma, and surgery. Symptoms include fever, tachycardia, agitation, anxiety, and HTN. Primary nursing interventions include maintaining an airway and adequate aeration.
>
> Propylthiouracil (PTU) and methimazole (Tapazole) are antithyroid drugs used to treat thyroid storm. Propranolol (Inderal) may be given to decrease excessive sympathetic stimulation.

C. Teach the following:
1. After treatment, resulting hypothyroidism will require daily hormone replacement.
2. Client should wear MedicAlert jewelry in case of emergency.
3. Signs of hormone replacement overdosage are the signs for hyperthyroidism (see Nursing Assessment, Hyperthyroidism, p. 131).
4. Signs of hormone replacement underdosage are the signs for hypothyroidism (see Nursing Assessment, Hypothyroidism, p. 133).

D. Explain to client the recommended diet: high-calorie, high-protein, low-caffeine, low-fiber diet (if diarrhea is present).

E. Perform eye care for exophthalmos.
1. Artificial tears to maintain moisture
2. Sunglasses when in bright light
3. Annual eye examinations

F. Prepare client for treatment of hyperthyroidism.
1. Thyroid ablation

a. Propylthiouracil (PTU) and methimazole (Tapazole) act by blocking synthesis of T_3 and T_4.

b. Dosage is calculated based on body weight and is given over several months.

c. Client should take medication exactly as prescribed so that the desired effect can be achieved.

d. The expected effect is to make the client euthyroid, often given to prepare the client for thyroidectomy.

2. Radiation
a. ^{131}I is given to destroy thyroid cells.
b. ^{131}I is very irritating to the GI tract.
c. Clients commonly vomit (vomitus is radioactive).
d. Place client on radiation precautions. Use time, distance, and shielding as means of protection against radiation (see Reproductive System, p. 177).

3. Thyroidectomy

> **HESI Hint** • After a thyroidectomy, be prepared for the possibility of laryngeal edema. Put a tracheostomy set at the bedside along with O_2 and a suction machine; calcium gluconate should be easily accessible if parathyroid glands have been accidently removed.

a. Check frequently for bleeding (on the anterior or posterior of the dressing), irregular breathing, neck swelling, frequent swallowing, and sensations of fullness at the incision site.

b. Support the neck when moving client (do not hyperextend).

c. Check for laryngeal edema, laryngeal nerve damage leads to vocal cord paralysis; therefore observe for hoarseness or inability to speak clearly.

d. Monitor Trousseau and Chvostek signs, because removal of the parathyroid(s) may lead to tetany.

e. Keep drainage devices, like Jackson-Pratt (JP) drains, compressed and empty.

4. Hypophysectomy (pituitary adenectomy)
a. Is employed if the client's condition is the result of increased pituitary secretion of adrenocorticotropic hormone (ACTH).

b. TSH-secreting pituitary tumors are resected using a transnasal approach (transsphenoidal hypophysectomy) via endoscopic transnasal approach.

c. Monitor for nasal discharge or postnasal drip that may be indicative of cerebrospinal leakage (assess drainage for glucose).

> **HESI Hint** • Normal serum calcium is 9.0 to 10.5 mEq/L. The best indicator of parathyroid problems is a decrease in the client's calcium compared with the preoperative value.

HESI Hint • If two or more parathyroid glands have been removed, the chance of tetany increases dramatically:
- Monitor serum calcium levels (9.0 to 10.5 mg/dL is normal range).
- Check for tingling of toes and fingers and around the mouth.
- Check Chvostek sign (twitching of lip after a tap over the facial nerve at the angle of the jaw means it is positive; Fig. 4-7).
- Check Trousseau sign (carpopedal spasm after BP cuff is inflated above systolic pressure and held for 3 minutes means it is positive; see Fig. 4-7).

Hypothyroidism (Hashimoto Disease, Myxedema)

Description: Hypofunction of the thyroid gland, with resulting insufficiency of thyroid hormone
A. Early symptoms of hypothyroidism are nonspecific but gradually intensify.
B. Hypothyroidism is treated by hormone replacement.
C. Endemic goiters occur in individuals living in areas where there is a deficit of iodine. Iodized salt has helped to prevent this problem.

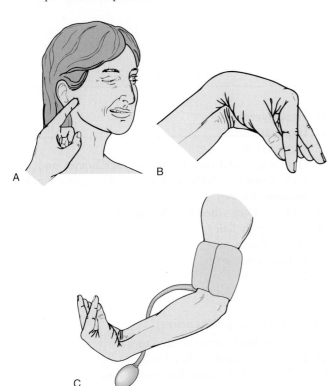

FIGURE 4-7 Tests for hypocalcemia. *A,* Chvostek sign is contraction of facial muscles in response to a light tap over the facial nerve in front of the ear. *B,* Trousseau sign is a carpal spasm induced by *C,* inflating a blood pressure cuff above the systolic pressure for a few minutes. (From Lewis SM, Heitkemper MM, Dirksen SR: *Medical-surgical nursing: assessment and management of clinical problems,* ed 9, St. Louis, 2013, Mosby.)

HESI Hint • Myxedema coma can be precipitated by acute illness, withdrawal of thyroid medication, anesthesia, use of sedatives, or hypoventilation (with the potential for respiratory acidosis and CO_2 narcosis). The airway must be kept patent and ventilator support used as indicated.

Nursing Assessment

A. Fatigue
B. Thin, dry hair; dry skin
C. Thick, brittle nails
D. Constipation
E. Bradycardia, hypotension
F. Goiter
G. Periorbital edema, facial puffiness
H. Cold intolerance
I. Weight gain
J. Dull emotions and mental processes
K. Diagnosis
   1. Low T_3 (below 70)
   2. Low T_4 (below 5)
   3. Presence of T_4 antibody (indicating that T_4 is being destroyed by the body)
L. Husky voice
M. Slow speech

Analysis (Nursing Diagnoses)

A. *Imbalanced nutrition: more than body requirements; constipation* related to…
B. *Deficient knowledge* related to …
C. *Noncompliance* related to …
D. *Activity intolerance* related to …

Nursing Plans and Interventions

A. Teach the following:
   1. Medication regimen: daily dose of prescribed hormone
   2. Medication effects and side effects (Table 4-23)
   3. Ongoing follow-up to determine serum hormone levels
   4. Signs and symptoms of myxedema coma (hypoventilation, hypotension, hypothermia, hyponatremia, hypoglycemia, lactic acidosis, and respiratory failure)
B. Develop a bowel elimination plan to prevent constipation:
   1. Fluid intake to be 3 L/day
   2. High-fiber diet, including fresh fruits and vegetables
   3. Increased activity
   4. Little or no use of enemas and laxatives
C. Avoid sedating client; it can lead to respiratory difficulties.

Addison Disease (Primary Adrenocortical Deficiency)

Description: Autoimmune process commonly found in conjunction with other endocrine diseases of an autoimmune nature; a primary disorder; hypofunction of the adrenal cortex

TABLE 4-23 Thyroid Preparations

Drugs	Indications	Adverse Reactions	Nursing Implications
• Levothyroxine • Liothyronine sodium • Desiccated thyroid	• Action is to increase metabolic rates • Synthetic T$_4$	• Anxiety • Insomnia • Tremors • Tachycardia • Palpitations • Angina • Dysrhythmias	• Give in early am before meals. • Check serum hormone levels routinely. • Check BP and pulse regularly. • Weigh daily. • Report side effects to health care provider. • Avoid foods and products containing iodine. • Initiate cautiously in clients with cardiovascular disease.

TABLE 4-24 Corticosteroids

Drugs	Indications	Adverse Reactions	Nursing Implications
• Hydrocortisone • Prednisone • Dexamethasone • Methylprednisolone	• Hormone replacement • Severe rheumatoid arthritis • Autoimmune disorders	• Emotional lability • Impaired wound healing • Skin fragility • Abnormal fat deposition • Hyperglycemia • Hirsutism • Moon face • Osteoporosis • All symptoms of Cushing syndrome if overdosage occurs	• Wean slowly (administer a high dose, then taper off); careful monitoring is required during withdrawal. • Monitor serum potassium, glucose (can become diabetic), and sodium. • Weigh daily; report weight gain of more than 5 lb per week. • Administer with antiulcer drugs or food. • Use care to prevent injuries. • Teach symptoms of Cushing syndrome. • Monitor BP and pulse closely.

A. Sudden withdrawal from corticosteroids may precipitate symptoms of Addison disease (Table 4-24).

B. Addison disease is characterized by lack of cortisol, aldosterone, and androgens.

C. Definitive diagnosis is made using an ACTH stimulation test.

D. If ACTH production by the anterior pituitary has failed, it is considered secondary Addison disease.

> **HESI Hint** • Many people take steroids for a variety of conditions. NCLEX-RN questions often focus on the need to teach clients the importance of following the prescribed regimen precisely. They should be cautioned against stopping the medications suddenly and should be informed that it is necessary to taper off the dosage when taking steroids.

Nursing Assessment

A. Fatigue, weakness

B. Weight loss, anorexia, nausea, vomiting

C. Postural hypotension

D. Hypoglycemia

E. Hyponatremia

F. Hyperkalemia

G. Hyperpigmentation of mucous membranes and skin (only if primary Addison disease; not seen in secondary Addison disease)

H. Signs of shock when in Addison crises

I. Loss of body hair

J. Hypovolemia
  1. Hypotension
  2. Tachycardia
  3. Fever

Analysis (Nursing Diagnoses)

A. *Deficient fluid volume* related to …

B. *Deficient knowledge* related to …

C. *Risk for electrolyte imbalance* related to…

Nursing Plans and Interventions

A. Take vital signs frequently (every 15 minutes if in crisis).

B. Monitor I&O and weigh daily.

C. Instruct client to rise slowly because of the possibility of postural hypotension.

D. During Addison crises, administer IV glucose with parenteral hydrocortisone, a steroid with both mineralocorticoid and glucocorticoid properties; requires large fluid volume replacement.

E. Monitor serum electrolyte levels.

F. Maintain low-stress environment (protect patient from noise, light, and temperature extremes because patient cannot physiologically cope with stress).

G. Teach
   1. Need for lifelong hormone replacement
   2. Need for close medical supervision
   3. Need for MedicAlert jewelry
   4. Signs and symptoms of overdosage and underdosage of medication
   5. Diet requirements: high sodium, low potassium, and high carbohydrate (complex carbohydrates)
   6. Fluid requirements: intake of at least 3 L of fluid per day

H. Provide ulcer prophylaxis.

HESI Hint • *Addison crisis is a medical emergency.* It is brought on by sudden withdrawal of steroids or a stressful event (trauma, severe infection) or exposure to cold, overexertion, or decrease in salt intake.
- Vascular collapse: Hypotension and tachycardia occur; administer IV fluids at a rapid rate until stabilized.
- Hypoglycemia: Administer IV glucose.
- Essential to reversing the crisis: Administer parenteral hydrocortisone.
- Aldosterone replacement: Administer fludrocortisone acetate (Florinef) PO (available only as oral preparation) with simultaneous administration of salt (sodium chloride) if client has a sodium deficit.

Cushing Syndrome

Description: Excess adrenocorticoid activity

A. Cause is usually chronic administration of corticosteroids.

B. Cushing syndrome can also be caused by adrenal, pituitary, or hypothalamus tumors.

Nursing Assessment

A. Physical symptoms include:
   1. Moon face
   2. Truncal obesity
   3. Buffalo hump
   4. Abdominal striae
   5. Muscle atrophy
   6. Thinning of the skin
   7. Hirsutism in females
   8. Hyperpigmentation
   9. Amenorrhea
   10. Edema, poor wound healing
   11. Impotence
   12. Bruises easily

B. HTN

C. Susceptibility to multiple infections

D. Osteoporosis

E. Peptic ulcer formation

F. Many false positives and false negatives in laboratory testing

G. Laboratory data often include the following findings:
   1. Hyperglycemia
   2. Hypernatremia
   3. Hypokalemia
   4. Decreased eosinophils and lymphocytes
   5. Increased plasma cortisol
   6. Increased urinary 17-hydroxycorticoids

Analysis (Nursing Diagnoses)

A. *Excess fluid volume* related to …

B. *Risk for infection* related to …

C. *Disturbed body image* related to …

D. *Imbalanced nutrition: more than body requirements* related to …

E. *Impaired skin integrity* related to …

Nursing Plans and Interventions

A. Encourage the client to protect himself or herself from exposure to infection.

B. Wash hands; use good handwashing technique.

C. Monitor client for signs of infection:
   1. Fever
   2. Oral infection by *Candida* spp.
   3. Vaginal yeast infections
   4. Adventitious lungs sounds
   5. Skin lesions
   6. Elevated WBCs

D. Teach safety measures.
   1. Position bed close to floor, with call light within easy reach.
   2. Encourage use of side rails.
   3. Be sure walkways are unobstructed.
   4. Encourage wearing shoes when ambulating.

E. Provide low-sodium diet; encourage consumption of foods that contain vitamin D and calcium.

F. Provide good skin and perineal care.

G. Discuss possibility of weaning from steroids after surgery. (If weaning is done too quickly, symptoms of Addison disease will occur.)

H. Encourage selection of clothing that minimizes visible aberrations; encourage maintenance of normal physical appearance.

I. Monitor I&O and weigh daily.

J. Provide ulcer prophylaxis.

HESI Hint • Teach clients to take steroids with meals to prevent gastric irritation. They should never skip doses. If they have nausea or vomiting for more than 12 to 24 hours, they should contact the physician.

Diabetes Mellitus (DM)

Description: A metabolic disorder characterized by high levels of glucose resulting from defects in insulin secretion, insulin action, or both

A. Diabetes mellitus is characterized by hyperglycemia.

B. Diabetes mellitus affects the metabolism of protein, carbohydrate, and fat.

C. Four ways to diagnose DM:
1. Fasting plasma glucose (FPG) greater than or equal to 126 mg/dL
2. Glycosylated Hgb (HbA$_{1c}$) greater than or equal to 6.5%
3. Random blood glucose greater than or equal to 200 mg/dL in a client with classic symptoms of hyperglycemia
4. Oral glucose tolerance test (OGTT) greater than 200
   a. Use plasma glucose, not fingersticks, to diagnose diabetes.
   b. Results should be confirmed on a subsequent visit.

D. The major classifications of diabetes are:
1. Type 1: results from B-cell destruction
2. Type 2: results from progressive secretory insulin deficit and or defect in insulin uptake
3. Other: transplant-related diabetes, cystic fibrosis–related diabetes, iatrogenic-induced (stress, hospital) diabetes, steroid-induced diabetes
4. Gestational diabetes
5. Prediabetes: Blood glucose levels when fasting are 100 to 125 mg/dL or HbA$_{1C}$ of 5.7% to 6.4%.

E. Many clients diagnosed with type 2 DM use insulin but retain some degree of pancreatic function.

F. Obesity is a major risk factor in type 2 DM (Table 4-25).

Clinical Characteristics and Treatment of Diabetes Mellitus

A. Type 1
1. Description: Results from the progressive autoimmune-based destruction of beta cells
   a. Can become hyperglycemic and ketosis-prone relatively easily
   b. Precipitating factors for diabetic ketoacidosis (DKA) include infection and inadequate or undermanagement of glucose.
2. Clinical characteristics of DKA
   a. Serum glucose of 250 and above
   b. Ketonuria in large amounts
   c. Arterial pH of <7.30 and HCO$_3$ <15 mEq/L
   d. Nausea, vomiting, dehydration, abdominal pain, Kussmaul's respirations, acetone odor to breath
3. Treatment
   a. Usually with isotonic IV fluids, 0.9% NaCl solution until BP stabilized and urine output 30 to 60 mL/hr
   b. Slow infusion by IV pump of regular insulin, too

TABLE 4-25 Comparison of Type 1 and Type 2 Diabetes Mellitus

Variable	Type 1 DM	Type 2 DM
Prevalence	5% of U.S. population with DM	90%-95% of U.S. population with DM
Pathology	Beta-cell destruction leading to absolute insulin deficiency	Basic defect is insulin resistance and usually have relative rather than absolute insulin deficiency
Onset	Sudden	Gradual, insidious
Signs and symptoms	Polyuria, polydipsia, polyphagia, weight loss	Polydipsia, polyuria, polyphagia, weight loss, fatigue, frequent infections, blurred vision, impotence
Age at onset	Any age but mostly young, under 21	Any age but mostly in adults
Weight	Thin, slender	Overweight, obese
Ketosis	Common	Rare
Pathology	Autoimmune and viral component	Obesity, cardiovascular disease (CVD) an equal comorbidity Genetic predisposition
Lifestyle management	Medical nutrition therapy: carbohydrate counting Physical activity	Medical nutrition therapy: Heart-healthy, portion-controlled diet Physical activity
Pharmacologic management	Intensive insulin therapy	Typically a stepwise approach Diet, exercise Oral agents Oral agents and insulin Insulin

rapid infusion of insulin to lower serum glucose can lead to cerebral edema

c. Careful replacement of potassium based on laboratory data

B. Type 2

1. Description: Results from either the inadequate production of insulin by the body or lack of sensitivity to the insulin being produced
   a. Rare development of ketoacidosis
   b. With extreme hyperglycemia, hyperosmolar hyperglycemia nonketotic syndrome (HHNKS) develops.
2. Clinical characteristics of HHNKS
   a. Hyperglycemia >600 mg/dL
   b. Plasma hyperosmolality
   c. Dehydration
   d. Changed mental status
   e. Absent ketone bodies
3. Treatment
   a. Usually with isotonic IV fluid replacement and careful monitoring of potassium and glucose levels
   b. Intravenous insulin given until blood glucose stable at 250 mg/dL

Nursing Assessment

Complications of diabetes

A. Integument
   1. Skin infections
   2. Wounds that do not heal
   3. Acanthosis

> **HESI Hint** • Why do clients with diabetes have trouble with wound healing? High blood glucose contributes to damage of the smallest vessels, the capillaries. This damage causes permanent capillary scarring, which inhibits the normal activity of the capillary. This phenomenon causes disruption of capillary elasticity and promotes problems such as diabetic retinopathy, poor healing of breaks in the skin, and cardiovascular abnormalities.

B. Oral cavity
   1. Periodontal disease
   2. Candidiasis (raised, white patchy areas on mucous membranes)
C. Eyes
   1. Cataracts
   2. Retinopathy
D. Cardiopulmonary system
   1. Angina
   2. Dyspnea
   3. HTN
E. Periphery
   1. Hair loss on extremities, indicating poor perfusion
   2. Other signs of poor peripheral circulation:
      a. Coolness

   b. Skin shininess and thinness
   c. Weak or absent peripheral pulses
   d. Ulcerations on extremities
   e. Pallor
   f. Thick nails with ridges
F. Kidneys
   1. Edema of face, hands, and feet
   2. Symptoms of urinary tract infection (UTI)
   3. Symptoms of renal failure: Edema, anorexia, nausea, fatigue, difficulty in concentrating
   4. Diabetic nephropathy is the primary cause of end-stage renal failure in the United States
G. Neuromusculature
   1. Neuropathies
   2. Symptoms of neuropathies: numbness, tingling, pain, burning
H. Gastrointestinal disturbances
   1. Nighttime diarrhea
   2. Gastroparesis (faulty absorption)
I. Reproductive
   1. Male: impotence
   2. Female: vaginal dryness, frequent vaginal infections
   3. Menstrual irregularities
J. Psychosocial issues
   1. Depression: Persons with DM have a high rate of depression. Depression contributes to poor DM regimen adherence, feelings of helplessness, and poor health outcomes.
   2. Increased risk of developing anorexia nervosa and bulimia nervosa in women with type 1 DM.

> **HESI Hint** • *Glycosylated Hgb (HbA$_{1c}$)*
> • Indicates glucose control over previous 90 to 120 days (life of red blood cells [RBCs])
> • Is a valuable measurement of diabetes control
> • Informs diagnosis of diabetes and prediabetes

Analysis (Nursing Diagnoses)

A. *Readiness for enhanced knowledge* related to …
B. *Risk for injury* related to …
C. *Readiness for enhanced coping* related to …
D. *Deficit fluid volume* related to …
E. *Readiness for enhanced self-health management* related to …

Nursing Plans and Interventions

A. Determine baseline laboratory data.
   1. Serum glucose
   2. Electrolytes
   3. Creatinine
   4. BUN
   5. Cholesterol, both LDL and HDL
   6. Triglycerides
   7. ABGs as indicated

B. Teach injection technique and/or oral medication(s).
1. Identify the prescribed dose and type of insulin (Tables 4-26 and 4-27).
2. For insulin:
   a. Lift skin; use 90-degree angle. If client is very thin or using 5/16-inch needle, the nurse may need to use a 45-degree angle.
   b. Do not reuse syringes or needles.
3. Rotate injection sites.
4. Usually insulins are premixed; if insulin is not pre-mixed draw regular insulin into syringe first when mixing insulins.
C. Teach about medical nutrition therapy (MNT).
1. Work with dietitian to reinforce specific meal plan.
2. Overall goal is to make healthy nutritional choices and eat a varied diet.
3. Encourage carbohydrate counting for those on complex insulin regimens.
4. Teach that meals should be timed according to medication (insulin) peak times.
5. Teach diet regimen.
   a. 45% to 50% carbohydrates
   b. 15% to 20% protein
   c. 30% or less fat
   d. Foods high in complex carbohydrates, high in fiber, and low in fat, whenever possible

e. Alcoholic beverages can be included in diet with proper planning
6. Teach about managing sick days (illness raises blood glucose).
   a. Teach client to keep taking insulin.
   b. Monitor glucose more frequently.
   c. Watch for signs of hyperglycemia.

> **HESI Hint** • The body's response to illness and stress is to produce glucose. Therefore any illness results in hyperglycemia.

D. Teach exercise regimen because exercise decreases blood sugar levels.
1. Exercise after mealtime; either exercise with someone or let someone know where exercise will take place to ensure safety.
2. A snack may be needed before or during exercise.
3. Monitor blood glucose before, during, and after exercise when beginning a new regimen.
E. Teach signs and symptoms of hyperglycemia and hypoglycemia (Table 4-28).

> **HESI Hint** • If in doubt whether a client is hyperglycemic or hypoglycemic, treat for hypoglycemia.

TABLE 4-26 Oral Hypoglycemics

Drugs	Indications	Adverse Reactions	Nursing Implications
Sulfonylureas			
First Generation • Tolbutamide • Chlorpropamide *Second Generation* • Glyburide • Glipizide • Glimepiride	• Lowers blood sugar by stimulating the release of insulin by the beta cells of the pancreas and causes tissues to take up and store glucose more easily • First generation is low potency and short acting • Second generation is high potency and longer acting	*First Generation* • Hypoglycemia • Nausea, heartburn, constipation, anorexia • Agranulocytosis • Allergic skin reactions *Second Generation* • Weight gain • Hypoglycemia, particularly in older adults	*First Generation* • Responsiveness may decline over time. • Given once daily with first meal. • Monitor blood sugar. • Hard to detect hypoglycemia if older adult or also on beta blockers. *Second Generation* • Less likely to interact with other medications.
Biguanides			
• Metformin	• Lowers serum glucose levels by inhibiting hepatic glucose production and increasing sensitivity of peripheral tissue to insulin	• Abdominal discomfort • Diarrhea • Lactic acidosis	• Many drug–drug interactions. • Extended-release tablets should be taken with the evening meal. • Use cautiously with preexisting renal or liver disease or HF. • Discontinue 48 hours before and wait 48 hours to restart dosage after diagnostic studies requiring IV iodine contrast media. • Can lead to vitamin B_{12} deficiency.

TABLE 4-26 Oral Hypoglycemics—cont'd

Drugs	Indications	Adverse Reactions	Nursing Implications
Alpha-Glucosidase Inhibitors			
• Acarbose • Miglitol	• Lowers blood glucose by blunting sugar levels after meals	• Hypoglycemia	• Optimally, must be taken with the *first* bite of each meal. • May be taken with other classes of oral hypoglycemics. • Monitor blood sugar. • Use is controversial in IBD client.
Thiazolidinediones			
• Rosiglitazone • Pioglitazone	• Lowers blood sugar by decreasing the insulin resistance of the tissues	• Hypoglycemia • Increased total cholesterol, weight gain • Edema, anemia	• Many drug–drug interactions. • Skip dose if meal skipped. • Monitor liver function. • Caution with use in CAD; may precipitate HF.
Meglitinides			
• Repaglinide • Nateglinide	• Lowers blood sugar by stimulating beta cells in pancreas to release insulin; does this by closing K^+ channels and opening Ca^{2+} channels	• Hypoglycemia • Angina, chest pain • Arthralgia, back pain • Nausea and vomiting, dyspepsia, constipation, or diarrhea	• May be used with metformin. • Give before meals; if a meal is skipped, skip the dose. • Monitor blood sugar.
Incretin Enhancer			
• Linagliptin • Saxagliptin • Sitagliptin	• Lowers blood glucose by inhibiting degradation of incretins, which increases insulin secretion	• Hypoglycemia	• Not considered a first-line agent.
Combinations			
• Glyburide + metformin • Pioglitazone + metformin • Rosiglitazone + glimepiride • Rosiglitazone + metformin • Glipizide + metformin	• Lowers blood sugar by combining the advantages of two classes of hypoglycemics	• Note possible adverse reactions to both classes • Hypoglycemia (severe)	• Note implications of both classes of drugs.

TABLE 4-27 Types of Insulin and Other Injectable Therapies

Type	Name	Onset	Peak Action	Duration	Nursing Implications
• Rapid-acting	• Human insulin lispro Aspart • Glulisine	• 15-30 min • 15-30 min • 15-30 min	• 30-90 min • 30-90 min • 30-90 min	• 3-5 hr • 3-5 hr • 3-5 hr	• Give within 15 min of a meal.
• Short-acting	• Regular insulin (human)	• 30-60 min	• 2-3 hr	• 5-7 hr	• Regular insulin may be given IV.
• Intermediate-acting	• Isophane insulin (human)	• 1-2 hr	• 4-6 hr	• 14-24 hr	• Not to be given IV. • Mixtures combine rapid-acting regular insulin with intermediate-acting NPH insulin in a 30% regular with 70% NPH proportion or at 50/50 combination.

Continued

TABLE 4-27 Types of Insulin and Other Injectable Therapies—cont'd

Type	Name	Onset	Peak Action	Duration	Nursing Implications
• Long-acting	• Glargine • Detemir	• 1 hr • 1.1 hr	• 14-20 hr • 5 hr peak-less (source: niddk.nih.gov)	• 24 hr	• Not to be given IV. • Recommended: give once daily (subcutaneous) at bedtime. • In some cases, given two times a day. • Acts as basal insulin. • Caution: Solution is clear, but bottle is distinctly different shape from regular insulin. • Do not confuse insulins. • Do not shake solution. • Do not mix other insulins with Lantus. • Use cautiously if patient is NPO.
• Premix	• Humalog 75/25 • Human 70/30 • NovoLog 70/30 • Humalog 50/50	• 10-30 min • 5-10 min	• Varies 1-4 hr	• 10-16 hr	• For all premixes: Offer when food readily available • 25% Lispro/75% Humulin N (NPH) • 30% Regular/70% NPH • 30% Aspart/70% NPH

Other Injectable Therapies

Drugs	Action/Indications	Adverse Reaction	Implications and Precautions
• Exenatide	• Stimulates release of insulin; ↓ glucagon secretion; ↑ satiety; ↓ gastric emptying; may facilitate weight loss (≈3-5 kg) • Indicated for clients with type 2 DM who are not adequately controlled with oral therapy. It is not indicated for clients with type 1 DM.	• Nausea, vomiting, hypoglycemia, diarrhea, headache	• Not a substitute for insulin • Not recommended for ESRD, pancreatitis, severe renal impairment, or severe gastrointestinal disease • May slow absorption of other drugs
• Pramlintide	• Slows gastric emptying time, suppresses the release of glucagon, and appears to suppress appetite. • Indicated as adjunct treatment in type 1 DM for clients who have not obtained adequate glycemic control with insulin therapy and for clients with type 2 DM who have not obtained adequate glycemic control with insulin with or without oral therapy	• Nausea, vomiting, • Hypoglycemia, diarrhea, headache	• Contraindicated for clients with diabetic gastroparesis. It is also avoided in clients who have exhibited significant hypoglycemic reactions or who are not able to recognize and manage hypoglycemic reactions.

HESI Hint • Insulin is prescribed in basal/bolus and correction factor therapy. The goal of insulin therapy is to mimic the body's normal basal/bolus secretion of insulin. Basal insulin (long-acting and intermediate-acting insulin) suppresses glucose production between meals and overnight. Bolus insulin or mealtime limits hyperglycemia after meals. Correction factor is the amount of insulin needed to correct hyperglycemia, usually given before a meal.

TABLE 4-28 Comparison of Hyperglycemia and Hypoglycemia

Hyperglycemia		Hypoglycemia	
Signs and Symptoms	**Nursing Action**	**Signs and Symptoms**	**Nursing Action**

• Polydipsia
• Polyuria
• Polyphagia
• Blurred vision
• Weakness
• Weight loss
• Syncope
	• Encourage water intake.
	• Check blood glucose frequently.
	• Assess for ketoacidosis:
	  • Urine ketones
	  • Urine glucose
	  • Administer insulin as directed
		• Headache
		• Nausea
		• Sweating
		• Tremors
		• Lethargy
		• Hunger
		• Confusion
		• Slurred speech
		• Tingling around mouth
		• Anxiety, nightmares
			• Usually occurs rapidly and is potentially life threatening; treat immediately with complex carbohydrates (CHO).
			  • Example: fast-acting carbohydrates.
			  • One tube glucose gel, 120-180 mL fruit juice or cola 10-16 jelly beans, 10 gum drops, 3 pieces of hard candy (Jolly Rancher), 5-7 pieces Life Savers–type candy
			• Check blood glucose (may seize if <40).

> **HESI Hint** • *Self-monitoring of blood glucose (SMBG)*
> - Uses techniques that are specific to each meter
> - Frequency of monitoring based on treatment regimen, change in meals, illness, and exercise regimen
> - Requires recording results and reporting results to health care provider at time of visit
> - Results of monitoring used to assess the efficacy of therapy and to guide adjustments in medical nutrition therapy, exercise, and medications to achieve the best possible blood glucose control

F. Teach about foot care.
  1. Feet should be checked daily for changes; signs of injury and breaks in skin should be reported to health care provider.
  2. Feet should be washed daily with mild soap and warm water; soaking is to be avoided; feet should be dried well, especially between toes.
  3. Feet may be moisturized with a lanolin product, but not between the toes.
  4. Well-fitting leather shoes should be worn; going barefoot and wearing sandals are to be avoided.
  5. Clean socks should be worn daily.
  6. Garters and tight elastic-topped socks should never be worn.
  7. Corns and calluses should be removed by a professional.
  8. Nails should be cut or filed straight across.
  9. Warm socks should be worn if feet are cold.
G. Encourage regular health care follow-ups.
  1. Ophthalmologist
  2. Podiatrist
  3. Annual physical examination
H. Teach that immediate attention should be sought if any sign of infection occurs.
I. Refer client to the American Diabetes Association for additional information.

Review of Endocrine System

1. What diagnostic test is used to determine thyroid activity?
2. What condition results from all treatments for hyperthyroidism?
3. State three symptoms of hyperthyroidism and three symptoms of hypothyroidism.
4. List five important teaching aspects for clients who are beginning corticosteroid therapy.
5. Describe the physical appearance of clients who have Cushing syndrome.
6. Which type of diabetes always requires insulin replacement?
7. Which type of diabetes sometimes requires no medication?
8. List five symptoms of hyperglycemia.
9. List five symptoms of hypoglycemia.
10. Name the necessary elements to include in teaching a client newly diagnosed with diabetes.
11. The nurse is in a situation where there is no premixed insulin. In fewer than 10 steps, describe the method of drawing up a mixed dose of insulin (regular with NPH).
12. Identify the peak action time of the following types of insulin: rapid-acting regular insulin, intermediate-acting insulin, and long-acting insulin.
13. When preparing a client with diabetes for discharge, the nurse teaches the client the relationship between stress, exercise, bedtime snacking, and glucose balance. State the relationships among each of these.

14. When making rounds at night, the nurse notes that a client prescribed insulin is complaining of a headache, slight nausea, and minimal trembling. The client's hand is cool and moist. What is the client most likely experiencing?

15. Identify five foot-care interventions that should be taught to a client with diabetes.

Answers to Review

1. T₃, T₄
2. Hypothyroidism, requiring thyroid replacement
3. Hyperthyroidism: weight loss, heat intolerance, diarrhea; hypothyroidism: fatigue, cold intolerance, weight gain
4. Continue medication until weaning plan is begun by physician; monitor serum potassium, glucose, and sodium frequently; weigh daily, and report gain of >5 lb/wk; monitor BP and pulse closely; teach symptoms of Cushing syndrome.
5. Moon face, obesity in trunk, buffalo hump in back, muscle atrophy, and thin skin
6. Type 1
7. Type 2
8. Polydipsia, polyuria, polyphagia, weakness, weight loss
9. Hunger, lethargy, confusion, tremors or shakes, sweating
10. The underlying pathophysiology of the disease; its management and treatment regimen; meal planning; exercise program; insulin administration; sick-day management; symptoms of hyperglycemia (not enough insulin); symptoms of hypoglycemia (too much insulin, too much exercise, not enough food); foot care
11. Identify the prescribed dose and type of insulin per physician order; store unopened insulin in refrigerator. Opened insulin vials may be kept at room temperature. Draw up regular insulin first; rotate injection sites; may reuse syringe by recapping and storing in refrigerator.
12. Rapid-acting regular insulin: 2 to 4 hours; immediate-acting insulin: 6 to 12 hours; long-acting insulin: 14 to 20 hours
13. Stress and stress hormones usually increase glucose production and increase insulin need. Conversely, exercise may increase the chance of a hypoglycemic reaction; therefore the client should always carry a fast-acting source of carbohydrate, such as glucose tablets or hard candies, when exercising.
14. Hypoglycemia/insulin reaction
15. Check feet daily, and report any breaks, sores, or blisters to health care provider; wear well-fitting shoes; never go barefoot or wear sandals; never personally remove corns or calluses; cut or file nails straight across; wash feet daily with mild soap and warm water.

Musculoskeletal System

Rheumatoid Arthritis

Description: Chronic, systematic, progressive deterioration of the connective tissue (synovium) of the joints; characterized by inflammation
A. The exact cause is unknown, but it is classified as an immune complex disorder.
B. Joint involvement is bilateral and symmetrical.
C. Severe cases may require joint replacement (see Joint Replacement, p. 148).

Nursing Assessment

A. Fatigue
B. Generalized weakness
C. Weight loss

> **HESI Hint** • A client comes to the clinic complaining of morning stiffness, weight loss, and swelling of both hands and wrists. Rheumatoid arthritis is suspected. Which methods of assessment might the nurse use, and which methods would the nurse not use? Use inspection, palpation, and strength testing. Do not assess range of motion (ROM); this activity promotes pain because ROM is limited.

D. Anorexia
E. Morning stiffness
F. Bilateral inflammation of joints with the following symptoms:
1. Decreased ROM
2. Joint pain
3. Warmth
4. Edema
5. Erythema
G. Joint deformity

> **HESI Hint** • In the joint, the normal cartilage becomes soft, fissures and pitting occur, and the cartilage thins. Spurs form and inflammation sets in. The result is deformity marked by immobility, pain, and muscle spasm. The prescribed treatment regimen is corticosteroids for the inflammation; splinting, immobilization, and rest for the joint deformity; and NSAIDs for the pain.

H. Diagnosis confirmed by the following:
1. Elevated erythrocyte sedimentation rate (ESR)
2. Positive rheumatoid factor (RF)
3. Presence of antinuclear antibody (ANA)
4. Joint-space narrowing indicated by arthroscopic examination (provides joint visualization)

5. Abnormal synovial fluid (fluid in joint) indicated by arthrocentesis
6. C-reactive protein (CRP) indicated by active inflammation

> **HESI Hint** • Synovial tissues line the bones of the joints. Inflammation of this lining causes destruction of tissue and bone. Early detection of rheumatoid arthritis can decrease the amount of bone and joint destruction. Often the disease goes into remission. Decreasing the amount of bone and joint destruction reduces the amount of disability.

Analysis (Nursing Diagnoses)

A. *Chronic pain* related to …
B. *Impaired physical mobility* related to …
C. *Self-care deficit* (specify) related to …
D. *Ineffective coping* related to …

Nursing Plans and Interventions

A. Implement pain relief measures.
   1. Use moist heat.
      a. Warm, moist compresses
      b. Whirlpool baths
      c. Hot shower in the morning
   2. Use diversionary activities.
      a. Imaging
      b. Distraction
      c. Self-hypnosis
      d. Biofeedback
   3. Administer medications, and teach client about medications (Table 4-29; see Table 4-24).
B. Provide periods of rest after periods of activity.
   1. Encourage self-care to maximal level.
   2. Allow adequate time for the client to perform activities.

3. Perform activities during time of day when client feels most energetic.
C. Encourage the client to avoid overexertion and to maintain proper posture and joint position.

> **HESI Hint** • What activity recommendations should the nurse provide a client with rheumatoid arthritis?
> • Do not exercise painful, swollen joints.
> • Do not exercise any joint to the point of pain.
> • Perform exercises slowly and smoothly; avoid jerky movements.

D. Encourage use of assistive devices.
   1. Elevated toilet seat
   2. Shower chair
   3. Cane, walker, and wheelchair
   4. Reachers
   5. Adaptive clothing with Velcro closures
   6. Straight-backed chair with elevated seat
E. Develop a teaching plan to include the following:
   1. Medication regimen
   2. Need for routine follow-up for evaluation of possible side effects
   3. ROM and stretching exercises tailored to specific client needs
   4. Safety tips and precautions about equipment use and environment

Lupus Erythematosus

Description: Systemic inflammatory connective-tissue disorder
A. There are two classifications of lupus erythematosus:
   1. Discoid lupus erythematosus (DLE) affects skin only.
   2. Systemic lupus erythematosus (SLE) can cause major body organs and systems to fail.
B. SLE is more prevalent than DLE.

TABLE 4-29 Nonsteroidal Antiinflammatory Drugs (NSAIDs)

Drugs	Indications	Adverse Reactions	Nursing Implications
• Aspirin • Ibuprofen • Indomethacin • Ketorolac tromethamine • Celecoxib • Etodolac • Diclofenac • Naproxen • Piroxicam	• Used as antiinflammatory • Antipyretic • Analgesic • Can be used with other agents; only NSAID available for IV administration.	• GI irritation, bleeding • Nausea, vomiting, constipation • Elevated liver enzymes • Prolonged coagulation time • Tinnitus • Thrombocytopenia • Fluid retention • Nephrotoxicity • Blood dyscrasias	• Teach to take with food or milk to reduce GI symptoms. • Teach to watch for signs of bleeding. • Teach to avoid alcohol. • Teach to observe for tinnitus. • Administer corticosteroids for severe rheumatoid arthritis (see Table 4-24). • NSAIDs reduce the effect of ACE inhibitors in hypertensive clients. • Note name similarity of Celebrex with other drugs having one-letter difference in spelling. • Encourage routine appointments to check liver/renal labs and CBC.

C. Lupus is an autoimmune disorder.

D. Kidney involvement is the leading cause of death in clients with lupus; it is followed by cardiac involvement as a leading cause of death.

> **HESI Hint** • NCLEX-RN questions often focus on the fact that avoiding sunlight is key in the management of lupus erythematosus; this is what differentiates it from other connective-tissue diseases.

E. Factors that trigger lupus:
1. Sunlight
2. Stress
3. Pregnancy
4. Drugs

Nursing Assessment

A. DLE
1. Dry, scaly rash on face or upper body (butterfly rash)

B. SLE
1. Joint pain and decreased mobility
2. Fever
3. Nephritis
4. Pleural effusion
5. Pericarditis
6. Abdominal pain
7. Photosensitivity
8. HTN

Analysis (Nursing Diagnoses)

A. *Chronic pain* related to …

B. *Disturbed body image* related to …

C. *Activity intolerance* related to…

D. *Impaired physical mobility* related to…

Nursing Plans and Interventions

A. Instruct client to avoid prolonged exposure to sunlight.

B. Instruct client to clean the skin with mild soap.

C. Monitor and instruct client in administration of steroids.

Osteoarthritis (OA) (Formerly Known as Degenerative Joint Disease [DJD])

Description: Noninflammatory arthritis

A. OA is characterized by a degeneration of cartilage, a wear-and-tear process.

B. It usually affects one or two joints.

C. It occurs asymmetrically.

D. Obesity and overuse are predisposing factors.

Nursing Assessment

A. Joint pain that increases with activity and improves with rest

B. Morning stiffness

C. Asymmetry of affected joints

D. Crepitus (grating sound in the joint)

E. Limited movement

F. Visible joint abnormalities indicated on radiographs

G. Joint enlargement and bony nodules

Analysis (Nursing Diagnoses)

A. *Chronic pain* related to …

B. *Impaired physical mobility* related to …

C. *Deficient self-care* related to …

D. *Deficient knowledge* (specify) related to …

Nursing Plans and Interventions

(See Rheumatoid Arthritis, p. 142.)

A. Instruct in weight-reduction diet.

B. Remind client that excessive use of the involved joint aggravates pain and may accelerate degeneration.

C. Teach the client to:
1. Use correct posture and body mechanics
2. Sleep with rolled terry cloth towel under cervical spine if neck pain is a problem
3. Relieve pain in fingers and hands by wearing stretch gloves at night
4. Keep joints in functional position

Osteoporosis

Description: Metabolic disease in which bone demineralization results in decreased density and subsequent fractures

A. Many fractures in older adults occur as a result of osteoporosis and often occur before the client's falling rather than as the result of a fall.

B. The cause of osteoporosis is unknown.

C. Postmenopausal women are at highest risk.

Nursing Assessment

A. Classic dowager's hump, or kyphosis of the dorsal spine (Fig. 4-8)

B. Loss of height, often 2 to 3 inches

C. Back pain, often radiating around the trunk

D. Pathologic fractures, often occurring in the distal end of the radius and the upper third of the femur

E. Compression fracture of spine: assess ability to void and defecate.

> **HESI Hint** • Postmenopausal, thin, white women are at highest risk for development of osteoporosis. Encourage exercise, a diet high in calcium, and supplemental calcium. Tums are an excellent source of calcium, but they are also high in sodium, so hypertensive or edematous individuals should seek another source of supplemental calcium.

Analysis (Nursing Diagnoses)

A. *Risk for injury* related to …

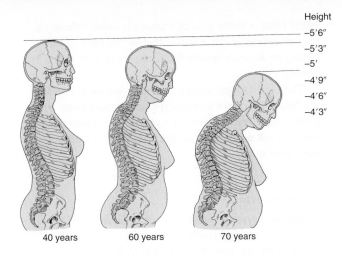

Height
−5′6″
−5′3″
−5′
−4′9″
−4′6″
−4′3″

40 years   60 years   70 years

FIGURE 4-8 Osteoporotic changes: A normal spine at 40 years of age, and osteoporotic changes at ages 60 and 70 years. These changes can cause a loss of height and may result in dorsal kyphosis. (From Black JM, Hawks JH: *Medical-surgical nursing: clinical management for positive outcomes*, ed 8, St. Louis, 2009, Saunders.)

B. *Impaired physical mobility* related to …
C. *Deficient knowledge* related to …

Nursing Plans and Interventions

A. Create a hazard-free environment.
B. Keep bed in low position.
C. Encourage client to wear shoes or nonskid slippers when out of bed.
D. Encourage environmental safety.
   1. Provide adequate lighting.
   2. Keep floor clear.
   3. Discourage use of throw rugs.
   4. Clean spills promptly.
   5. Keep side rails up at all times.

> **HESI Hint** • The main cause of fractures in older adults, especially in women, is osteoporosis. The main fracture sites seem to be hip, vertebral bodies, and Colles fracture of the forearm.

E. Provide assistance with ambulation.
   1. Client may need walker or cane.
   2. Client may need standby assistance when initially getting out of bed or chair.
F. Teach regular exercise program.
   1. ROM exercise several times a day
   2. Ambulation several times a day
   3. Use of proper body mechanics
   4. Regular weight-bearing exercises promote bone formation
G. Provide diet that is high in protein, calcium, and vitamin D; discourage use of alcohol and caffeine.
H. Encourage preventive measures for females.
   1. Hormone replacement therapy (HRT) has been used as a primary prevention strategy for reducing bone loss in the postmenopausal woman. However, recent studies demonstrated that HRT may increase a woman's risk of breast cancer, cardiovascular disease, and stroke. If using HRT, the benefits should outweigh the risks.

2. Take prescribed medications to prevent further loss of bone mineral density (BMD).
   a. Bisphosphonates: inhibit osteoclast-mediated bone resorption, thereby increasing BMD. Common side effects are anorexia, weight loss, and gastritis. Instruct the client to take with full glass of water, take 30 minutes before food or other medications, and remain upright for at least 30 minutes after taking.
      (1) Alendronate (Fosamax)
      (2) Etidronate (Didronel)
      (3) Ibandronate (Boniva)
      (4) Pamidronate (Aredia)
      (5) Risedronate (Actonel)
      (6) Tiludronate (Skelid)
   b. Selective estrogen receptor modulator: to mimic the effect of estrogen on bone by reducing bone resorption without stimulating the tissues of the breast or uterus. The most common side effects are leg cramps and hot flashes.
      (1) Raloxifene (Evista)
      (2) Teriparatide (Forteo)
3. High calcium and vitamin D intake beginning in early adulthood
4. Calcium supplementation after menopause (Tums are an excellent source of calcium).
5. Weight-bearing exercise
I. Dual-energy x-ray absorptiometry (DEXA), which measures bone density in the spine, hips, and forearm, as a baseline after menopause, with frequency as recommended by health care provider
J. Osteopenia is defined as bone loss that is more than normal and has a T-score less than or equal to a range of −1 to −2.5 but is not yet at the level for a diagnosis of osteoporosis. Bone mineral density (BMD) is commonly reported as a "T-score," which is the difference between the client's BMD and the BMD of "young normal adults" of the same gender. The difference between the client's score and the young adult norm is expressed as standard deviation (SD) below or above the average.

Fracture

Description: Any break in the continuity of the bone

A. Fractures are described by the type and extent of the break.
B. Fractures are caused by a direct blow, crushing force, a sudden twisting motion, or a disease such as cancer or osteoporosis.
   1. Complete fracture: A break across the entire cross section of the bone
   2. Incomplete fracture: A break across only part of the bone
   3. Closed fracture: No break in the skin
   4. Open fracture: Broken bone protrudes through skin or mucous membranes (much more prone to infection)
C. Five types of fractures
   1. Greenstick: One side of a bone is broken; the other side is bent.
   2. Transverse: Break occurs straight across the bone shaft.
   3. Oblique: Break occurs at an angle across the bone.
   4. Spiral: Break twists around the bone.
   5. Comminuted: Break has more than three fragments (Table 4-30).

HESI Hint • What type of fracture is more difficult to heal: an extracapsular fracture (below the neck of the femur) or an intracapsular fracture (in the neck of the femur)?

The blood supply enters the femur below the neck of the femur. Therefore an intracapsular fracture heals with greater difficulty, and there is a greater likelihood that necrosis will occur because the fracture is cut off from the blood supply.

Nursing Assessment

A. Signs and symptoms of fracture include:
   1. Pain, swelling, tenderness
   2. Deformity, loss of functional ability
   3. Discoloration, bleeding at the site through an open wound
   4. Crepitus: crackling sound between two broken bones
B. Fracture is evident on radiograph.
C. Therapeutic management is based on:
   1. Reduction of the fracture
   2. Maintenance of realignment by immobilization
   3. Restoration of function

TABLE 4-30 Common Types of Fractures

Description	Illustration	Description	Illustration
Burst: Characterized by multiple pieces of bone; often occurs at bone ends or in vertebrae		Longitudinal: Fracture line extends in the direction of the bone's longitudinal axis	
Comminuted: More than one fracture line; more than two bone fragments; fragments may be splintered or crushed		Nondisplaced: Fragments aligned at fracture site	
Complete: Break across the entire section of bone, dividing it into distinct fragments; often displaced		Oblique: Fracture line occurs at approximately 45-degree angle across the longitudinal axis of the bone	

TABLE 4-30 Common Types of Fractures—cont'd

Description	Illustration	Description	Illustration
Displaced: Fragments out of normal position at fracture site	Torsion	Spiral: Fracture line results from twisting force; forms a spiral encircling the bone	
Incomplete: Fracture occurs through only one cortex of the bone; usually nondisplaced		Stellate: Fracture lines radiate from one central point	
Linear: Fracture line is intact; fracture is caused by minor to moderate force applied directly to the bone		Traverse: Fracture line occurs at 90-degree angle to longitudinal axis of bone	
Avulsion: Bone fragments are torn away from the body of the bone at the site of attachment of a ligament or tendon		Colles: Fracture within the last inch of the distal radius; distal fragment is displaced in a position of dorsal and medial deviation	
Compression: Bone buckles and eventually cracks as the result of unusual loading force applied to its longitudinal axis		Pott: Fracture of the distal fibula, seriously disrupting the tibiofibular articulation; a piece of the medial malleolus may be chipped off as a result of rupture of the internal lateral ligament	
Greenstick: Incomplete fracture in which one side of the cortex is broken and the other side is flexed but intact		Impacted: Telescoped fracture, with one fragment driven into another	

HESI Hint • NCLEX-RN questions focus on safety precautions. Improper use of assistive devices can be very risky. When using a nonwheeled walker, the client should lift and move the walker forward and then take a step into it. The client should avoid scooting the walker or shuffling forward into it; these movements take more energy and provide less stability than does a single movement.

D. Observe client's use of assistive devices.
  1. Crutches
    a. There should be two to three finger widths between the axilla and the top of the crutch.
    b. A three-point gait is most common. The client advances both crutches and the impaired leg at the same time. The client then swings the uninvolved leg ahead to the crutches.

2. Cane
   a. It is placed on the unaffected side.
   b. The top of the cane should be at the level of the greater trochanter.
3. Walker
   a. Strength of upper extremity and unaffected leg is assessed and improved with exercises, if necessary, so that upper body is strong enough to use walker.
   b. Client lifts and advances the walker and steps forward.
E. See, Chapter 5, Pediatric Nursing for cast care and care of a client in traction.

> **HESI Hint** • The risk for the development of a fat embolism, a syndrome in which fat globules migrate into the bloodstream and combine with platelets to form emboli, is greatest in the first 36 hours after a fracture. It is more common in clients with multiple fractures, fractures of long bones, and fractures of the pelvis. The initial symptom of a fat embolism is confusion due to hypoxemia (check blood gases for Po_2). Assess for respiratory distress, restlessness, irritability, fever, and petechiae. If an embolus is suspected, notify physician stat, draw blood gases, administer O_2, and assist with endotracheal intubation.

> **HESI Hint** • In clients with hip fractures, thromboembolism is the most common complication. Prevention includes passive ROM exercises, use of elastic stockings, elevation of the foot of the bed 25 degrees to increase venous return, and low-dose heparin therapy.

> **HESI Hint** • Clients with fractures, edema, or casts on the extremities need frequent neurovascular assessment distal to the injury. Skin color, temperature, sensation, capillary refill, mobility, pain, and pulses should be assessed.

> **HESI Hint** • Assess the 5 Ps of neurovascular functioning: pain, paresthesia, pulse, pallor, and paralysis.

Joint Replacement

Description: Surgical procedure in which a mechanical device, designed to act as a joint, is used to replace a diseased joint
A. The most commonly replaced joints:
   1. Hip
   2. Knee
   3. Shoulder
   4. Finger
B. Prostheses may be ingrown or cemented.
C. Accurate fitting is essential.
D. Client must have healthy bone stock for adequate healing.
E. Joint replacement provides excellent pain relief in 85% to 90% of the clients who have the surgery.
F. Infection is the concern postoperatively.

Nursing Assessment

A. Joint pathology
   1. OA
   2. Rheumatoid arthritis
   3. Fracture
B. Pain not relieved by medication
C. Poor ROM in the affected joint

Analysis (Nursing Diagnoses)

A. *Risk for infection* related to …
B. *Acute pain* related to …
C. *Chronic pain* related to …
D. *Risk for injury to affected limb* related to …
E. *Activity intolerance* related to…
F. *Impaired physical mobility* related to …

Nursing Plans and Interventions

A. Provide postoperative care for wound and joint.
   1. Monitor incision site.
      a. Assess for bleeding and drainage.

> **HESI Hint** • Orthopedic wounds have a tendency to ooze more than other wounds. A suction drainage device usually accompanies the client to the postoperative floor. Check drainage often.

      b. Assess suture line for erythema and edema.
      c. Assess suction drainage apparatus for proper functioning.
      d. Assess for signs of infection.

> **HESI Hint** • NCLEX-RN questions about joint replacement focus on complications. A big problem after joint replacement is infection.

   2. Monitor functioning of extremity.
      a. Check circulation, sensation, and movement of extremity distal to replacement.
      b. Provide proper alignment of affected extremity. (Client will return from the operating room with alignment for the initial postoperative period.)
      c. Provide abductor appliance (hip replacement) or continuous passive motion (CPM) device if indicated.
B. Monitor I&O every shift, including suction drainage.

HESI Hint • Fractures of bone predispose the client to anemia, especially if long bones are involved. Check hematocrit every 3 to 4 days to monitor erythropoiesis.

C. Encourage fluid intake of 3 L per day.
D. Encourage client to perform self-care activities at maximal level.
E. Coordinate rehabilitation: work closely with health care team to increase client's mobility gradually.
   1. Get client out of bed as soon as possible.
   2. Keep client out of bed as much as possible.
   3. Keep abductor pillow in place while client is in bed (hip replacement).
   4. Use elevated toilet seat and chairs with high seats for those who have had hip or knee replacements (prevents dislocation).
   5. Do not flex hip more than 90 degrees (hip replacement).

HESI Hint • After hip replacement, instruct the client not to lift the leg upward from a lying position or to elevate the knee when sitting. This upward motion can pop the prosthesis out of the socket.

F. Provide discharge planning that includes rehabilitation on an outpatient basis as prescribed.

HESI Hint • Immobile clients are prone to complications: skin integrity problems, formation of urinary calculi (client's milk intake may be limited), and venous thrombosis (client may be on prophylactic anticoagulants).

Amputation

Description: Surgical removal of a diseased part or organ
A. Causes for amputation include the following:
   1. Peripheral vascular disease, 80% (75% of these are clients with diabetes)
   2. Trauma
   3. Congenital deformities
   4. Malignant tumors
   5. Infection
B. Amputation necessitates major lifestyle and body-image adjustments.

Nursing Assessment
A. Before amputation, symptoms of PVD include:
   1. Cool extremity
   2. Absent peripheral pulses
   3. Hair loss on affected extremity
   4. Necrotic tissue or wounds

      a. Blue or blue-gray, turning black
      b. Drainage possible, with or without odor
   5. Leathery skin on affected extremity
   6. Decrease of pain sensation in affected extremity
B. Inadequate circulation as determined by:
   1. Arteriogram
   2. Doppler flow studies

Analysis (Nursing Diagnoses)
A. *Risk for ineffective peripheral tissue perfusion* related to…
B. *Acute pain* related to …
C. *Impaired physical mobility* related to …
D. *Disturbed body image* related to …

Nursing Plans and Interventions
A. Provide wound care.
   1. Monitor surgical dressing for drainage.
      a. Mark dressing for bleeding, and check marking at least every 8 hours.
      b. Measure suction drainage every shift.
   2. Change dressing as needed (physician usually performs initial dressing change).
      a. Maintain aseptic technique.
      b. Observe wound color, warmth, and approximation of the incision.
      c. Observe for wound healing.
      d. Monitor for signs of infection.
         (1) Fever
         (2) Tachycardia
         (3) Redness of incision area
B. Maintain proper body alignment in and out of bed.
C. Position client to relieve edema and spasms at residual limb (stump) site.
   1. Elevate residual limb (stump) for the first 24 hours postoperatively.

HESI Hint • The residual limb (stump) should be elevated on one pillow. If the residual limb (stump) is elevated too high, the elevation can cause a contracture.

   2. Do not elevate residual limb (stump) after 48 hours postoperatively.
   3. Keep residual limb (stump) in extended position, and turn client to prone position three times a day to prevent hip flexion contracture.
D. Be aware that phantom pain is real; it will eventually disappear, and it responds to pain medication.
E. Handle affected body part gently and with smooth movements.
F. Provide passive ROM until client is able to perform active ROM. Collaborate with rehabilitation team members for mobility improvement.
G. Encourage independence in self-care, allowing sufficient time for client to complete care and to have input into care.

Review of Musculoskeletal System

1. Differentiate between rheumatoid arthritis and OA in terms of joint involvement.
2. Identify the categories of drugs commonly used to treat arthritis.
3. Identify pain relief interventions for clients with arthritis.
4. What measures should the nurse encourage female clients to take to prevent osteoporosis?
5. What are the common side effects of salicylates?
6. What is the priority nursing intervention used with clients taking NSAIDs?
7. List three of the most common joints that are replaced.
8. Describe postoperative residual limb (stump) care (after amputation) for the first 48 hours.
9. Describe nursing care for the client who is experiencing phantom pain after amputation.
10. A nurse discovers that a client who is in traction for a long bone fracture has a slight fever, is short of breath, and is restless. What does the client most likely have?
11. What are the immediate nursing actions if fat embolization is suspected in a client with a fracture or other orthopedic condition?
12. List three problems associated with immobility.
13. List three nursing interventions for the prevention of thromboembolism in immobilized clients with musculoskeletal problems.

Answers to Review

1. Rheumatoid arthritis occurs bilaterally. OA occurs asymmetrically.
2. NSAIDs, of which salicylates are the cornerstone of treatment, and corticosteroids (used when arthritic symptoms are severe)
3. Warm, moist heat (compresses, baths, showers); diversionary activities (imaging, distraction, self-hypnosis, biofeedback); and medications
4. Possible estrogen replacement after menopause, high calcium and vitamin D intake beginning in early adulthood, calcium supplements after menopause, and weight-bearing exercise
5. GI irritation, tinnitus, thrombocytopenia, mild liver enzyme elevation
6. Administer or teach client to take drugs with food or milk.
7. Hip, knee, finger
8. Elevate residual limb (stump) for first 24 hours. Do not elevate residual limb (stump) after 48 hours. Keep residual limb (stump) in extended position, and turn client to prone position three times a day to prevent flexion contracture.
9. Be aware that phantom pain is real and will eventually disappear. Administer pain medication; phantom pain responds to medication.
10. A fat embolism, which is characterized by hypoxemia, respiratory distress, irritability, restlessness, fever, and petechiae
11. Notify physician stat, draw blood gases, administer O_2 according to blood gas results, assist with endotracheal intubation and treatment of respiratory failure.
12. Venous thrombosis, urinary calculi, skin integrity problems
13. Passive ROM exercises, elastic stockings, and elevation of foot of bed 25 degrees to increase venous return

Neurosensory System

Glaucoma

Chronic open-angle glaucoma is also known as simple adult primary glaucoma and as primary open-angle glaucoma.

Description: Condition characterized by increased intraocular pressure (IOP) that involves gradual painless vision loss that can lead to blindness if untreated.
A. Is the second leading cause of blindness in the United States and especially among those over 80 years old.
B. Glaucoma usually occurs bilaterally in those who have a family history of the condition.
C. Aqueous fluid is inadequately drained from the eye.
D. It is generally asymptomatic, especially in early stages.
E. It tends to be diagnosed during routine visual examinations.
F. It cannot be cured but can be treated with success pharmacologically and surgically.

Nursing Assessment
A. Early signs
   1. Increase in IOP >22 mm Hg
   2. Decreased accommodation or ability to focus

HESI Hint • Glaucoma is often painless and symptom free. It is usually detected as part of a regular eye examination.

B. Late signs include:
1. Loss of peripheral vision
2. Seeing halos around lights
3. Decreased visual acuity not correctable with glasses
4. Headache or eye pain that may be so severe as to cause nausea and vomiting (acute closed-angle glaucoma)
C. Diagnostic tests include the following:
1. Tonometer, used to measure IOP
2. Electronic tonometer, used to detect drainage of aqueous humor
3. Gonioscopy, used to obtain a direct visualization of the lens
D. Risk factors include the following:
1. Family history of glaucoma
2. Family history of diabetes
3. History of previous ocular problems
4. Medication use
   a. Glaucoma is a side effect of many medications (e.g., antihistamines, anticholinergics).
   b. Glaucoma can result from the interaction of medications.

Analysis (Nursing Diagnoses)

A. *Anxiety* related to …
B. *Disturbed sensory perception: visual* related to …
C. *Ineffective health maintenance* related to …

Nursing Plans and Interventions

A. Administer eye drops as prescribed (Table 4-31).

> **HESI Hint** • Eye drops are used to cause pupil constriction because movement of the muscles to constrict the pupil also allows aqueous humor to flow out, thereby decreasing the pressure in the eye. Pilocarpine is commonly used. Caution client that vision may be blurred for 1 to 2 hours after administration of pilocarpine and that adaptation to dark environments is difficult because of pupillary constriction (the desired effect of the drug).

B. Orient client to surroundings.
C. Avoid nonverbal communication that requires visual acuity (e.g., facial expressions).
D. Develop a teaching plan that includes the following:
1. Careful adherence to eye-drop regimen can prevent blindness.
2. Vision already lost cannot be restored.
3. Eye drops are needed for the rest of life.
4. Proper eye-drop instillation technique. Obtain a return demonstration.
   a. Wash hands and external eye.
   b. Tilt head back slightly.
   c. Instill drop into lower lid, without touching the lid with the tip of the dropper.
   d. Release the lid, and sponge excess fluid from lid and cheek.
   e. Close eye gently, and leave closed 3 to 5 minutes.
   f. Apply gentle pressure on inner canthus to decrease systemic absorption.
5. Safety measures to prevent injuries:
   a. Remove throw rugs.
   b. Adjust lighting to meet needs.
6. Avoid activities that may increase IOP.
   a. Emotional upsets
   b. Exertion: pushing, heavy lifting, shoveling
   c. Coughing severely or excessive sneezing (get medical attention before upper respiratory infection [URI] worsens)
   d. Wearing constrictive clothing (tight collar or tie, tight belt, or girdle)
   e. Straining at stool and constipation

> **HESI Hint** • There is an increased incidence of glaucoma in older adult populations. Older clients are prone to problems associated with constipation. Therefore the nurse should assess these clients for constipation and postoperative complications associated with constipation and should implement a plan of care directed at prevention of and, if necessary, treatment for constipation.

Nursing Plans and Interventions: The Nonseeing (Blind) Client

A. On entering room, announce your presence clearly and identify yourself; address client by name.
B. Never touch client unless he or she knows you are there.
C. On admission, orient client thoroughly to surroundings.
1. Demonstrate use of the call bell.
2. Walk client around the room and acquaint him or her with all objects: chairs, bed, TV, telephone, etc.
D. Guide client when walking:
1. Walk ahead of client, and place his or her hand in the bend of your elbow.
2. Describe where you are walking. Note whether passageway is narrowing or you are approaching stairs, curb, or an incline.
E. Always raise side rails for newly sightless persons (e.g., clients wearing postoperative eye patches).
F. Assist with meal enjoyment by describing food and its placement in terms of the face of a clock (e.g., "meat at 6 o'clock").
G. When administering medications, inform client of number of pills, and give only a half glass of water (to avoid spills).

Cataract

Description: Condition characterized by opacity of the lens. Cataracts are the leading cause of blindness in the world.
A. Aging accounts for 95% of cataracts (senile).

TABLE 4-31 **Treatment of Glaucoma**

Drugs	Indications	Adverse Reactions	Nursing Implications
Parasympathomimetics			

• Pilocarpine HCl (multiple brands available); 0.5%-6% is the drug of choice	• Enhances papillary constriction (available in drops, gel, and time-release wafer)	• Bronchospasm
		• Nausea, vomiting, diarrhea
		• Blurred vision, twitching eyelids, eye pain with focusing, reduced visual acuity in dim light
			• Use cautiously with:
			  • Pregnancy
			  • Asthma
			  • HTN
			• Teach proper drop instillation technique.
			• Need for ongoing use of the drug at prescribed intervals.
			• Blurred vision tends to decrease with regular use of this drug.

Beta-Adrenergic Receptor–Blocking Agents			

• Timolol maleate optic
• Carteolol
• Levobunolol
• Betaxolol
• Metipranolol
	• Inhibits formation of aqueous humor	• Side effects are insignificant.
		• Hypotension
		• Bradycardia
			• Use cautiously with
			  • Hypersensitivity
			  • Asthma
			  • Second- or third-degree heart block
			  • HF
			  • Congenital glaucoma
			  • Pregnancy
			  • Teach proper drop instillation technique.
			• Need for ongoing use of the drug at prescribed intervals.
			• Blurred vision tends to decrease with regular use of this drug.

Carbonic Anhydrase Inhibitors			
• Acetazolamide • Brinzolamide • Dorzolamide	• Reduces aqueous humor production	• Numbness, tingling of hands and feet • Nausea • Malaise • Postural hypotension if taken orally	• Administer orally or IV. • Produces diuresis. • Assess for metabolic acidosis. • Contraindicated in clients with sulfa allergy.
Alpha Agonists			
• Brimonidine • Iopidine	• Lowers intraocular pressure of glaucoma by decreasing fluid produced		
Prostaglandin Antagonists			
• Latanoprost • Travoprost • Bimatoprost	• Lowers intraocular pressure of glaucoma by increasing outflow of aqueous humor	• Local irritation • Foreign-body sensation • Increased brown pigmentation of iris • Increased eyelash growth	

B. The remaining 5% result from trauma, toxic substances, or systemic diseases or are congenital.
C. Safety precautions may reduce the incidence of traumatic cataracts.
D. Surgical removal is done when vision impairment interferes with daily activities. Intraocular lens implants may be used.
E. Most operations are performed under local anesthesia on an outpatient basis.

> **HESI Hint** • The lens of the eye is responsible for projecting light onto the retina so that images can be discerned. Without the lens, which becomes opaque with cataracts, light cannot be filtered and vision is blurred.

Nursing Assessment

A. Early signs include:
   1. Blurred vision
   2. Decreased color perception
   3. Photophobia
B. Late signs include:
   1. Diplopia
   2. Reduced visual acuity, progressing to blindness
   3. Clouded pupil, progressing to a milky-white appearance
C. Diagnostic tests include use of the following:
   1. Ophthalmoscope
   2. Slit-lamp biomicroscope
   3. Keratometry and A-scan ultrasound

Analysis (Nursing Diagnoses)

A. *Disturbed sensory perception: visual* related to …
B. *Anxiety* related to …

Nursing Plans and Interventions

A. Preoperative: Demonstrate and request a return demonstration of eye medication instillation from client or family member.
B. Develop a postoperative teaching plan that includes:
   1. Warning not to rub or put pressure on eye
   2. Teaching that glasses or shaded lens should be worn during waking hours. An eye shield should be worn during sleeping hours.
   3. Teaching to avoid lifting objects over 5 pounds, bending, straining, coughing, or any other activity that can increase IOP
   4. Teaching to use a stool softener to prevent straining at stool
   5. Teaching to avoid lying on operative side
   6. Teaching the need to keep water from getting into eye while showering or washing hair
   7. Teaching to observe and report signs of increased IOP and infection (e.g., pain, changes in vital signs)

> **HESI Hint** • When the cataract is removed, the lens is gone, making prevention of falls important. When the lens is replaced with an implant, vision is better.

Eye Trauma

Description: Injury to the eye sustained as the result of sharp or blunt trauma, chemicals, or heat
A. Permanent visual impairment can occur.
B. Every eye injury should be considered an emergency.
C. Protective eye shields in hazardous work environments and during athletic sports may prevent injuries.

Nursing Assessment

A. Determine type of injury and symptoms.
B. Diagnostic tests include:
   1. Slit-lamp examination
   2. Instillation of fluorescein to detect corneal injury
   3. Testing of visual acuity for medical documentation and legal protection

Analysis (Nursing Diagnoses)

A. *Acute pain* related to …
B. *Risk for injury* related to…

Nursing Plans and Interventions

A. Position the client according to the type of injury; a sitting position decreases IOP.
B. Remove conjunctival foreign bodies unless embedded.
C. Never attempt to remove a penetrating or embedded object. Do not apply pressure.
D. Apply cold compresses to eye contusion.
E. After chemical injuries, irrigate the eye with copious amounts of water.
F. Administer eye medications as prescribed.
G. Explain that an eye patch may be applied to rest the eye. Reading and watching TV may be restricted for 3 to 5 days.
H. Explain that a sudden increase in eye pain should be reported.

Detached Retina

Description: Hole or tear in, or separation of the sensory retina from, the pigmented epithelium
A. It can be result of increasing age, severe myopia, eye trauma, retinopathy (diabetic), cataract or glaucoma surgery, family or personal history.
B. Resealing is done by surgery.
   1. Cryotherapy (freezing)
   2. Photocoagulation (laser)
   3. Diathermy (heat)
   4. Scleral buckling (most often used)

Nursing Plans and Interventions

A. The client may be on bed rest.
B. Place eye patch over affected eye.
C. Administer medication to inhibit accommodation and constriction; cycloplegics (mydriatics and homatropine) are given to dilate pupil before surgery.
D. Administer medication for postoperative pain.
E. If gas bubble is used (inserted in vitreous), position client so bubble can rise against area to be reattached.
F. Teach the client not to do any heavy lifting or straining with bowel movement, and no vigorous activity for several weeks.

Hearing Loss

Conductive Hearing Loss

Description: Hearing loss in which sound does not travel well to the sound organs of the inner ear. The volume of sound is less, but the sound remains clear. If volume is raised, hearing is normal.

A. Hearing loss is the most common disability in the United States.
B. It usually results from cerumen (wax) impaction or middle ear disorders such as otitis media.

> **HESI Hint** • The ear consists of three parts: the external ear, the middle ear, and the inner ear. Inner ear disorders, or disorders of the sensory fibers going to the central nervous system (CNS), often are neurogenic in nature and may not be helped with a hearing aid. External and middle ear problems (conductive) may result from infection, trauma, or wax buildup. These types of disorders are treated more successfully with hearing aids.

Sensorineural Hearing Loss

Description: Form of hearing loss in which sound passes properly through the outer and middle ear but is distorted by a defect in the inner ear or damage to cranial nerve VIII, or both

A. It involves perceptual loss, usually progressive and bilateral.
B. It involves damage to the eighth cranial nerve.
C. It is detected easily by the use of a tuning fork.
D. Common causes:
   1. Infections
   2. Ototoxic drugs
   3. Trauma
   4. Neuromas
   5. Noise
   6. Aging process

Nursing Assessment

A. Inability to hear a whisper from 1 to 2 feet away
B. Inability to respond if nurse covers mouth when talking, indicating that client is lip reading
C. Inability to hear a watch tick 5 inches from ear
D. Shouting in conversation
E. Straining to hear
F. Turning head to favor one ear
G. Answering questions incorrectly or inappropriately
H. Raising volume of radio or TV

Analysis (Nursing Diagnoses)

A. *Risk for injury* related to …
B. *Impaired verbal communication* related to …

Nursing Plans and Interventions

A. The nurse should do the following to enhance therapeutic communication with the hearing impaired:
   1. Before starting conversation, reduce distraction as much as possible.
   2. Turn the TV or radio down or off, close the door, or move to a quieter location.
   3. Devote full attention to the conversation; do not try to do two things at once.
   4. Look and listen during the conversation.
   5. Begin with casual topics, and progress to more critical issues slowly.
   6. Do not switch topics abruptly.
   7. If you do not understand, let the client know.
   8. If the client is a lip reader, face him or her directly.
   9. Speak slowly and distinctly; determine whether you are being understood.
   10. Allow adequate time for the conversation to take place; try to avoid hurried conversations.
   11. Use active listening techniques.

> **HESI Hint** • NCLEX-RN questions often focus on communicating with older adults who are hearing impaired.
> • Speak in a low-pitched voice, slowly and distinctly.
> • Stand in front of the person, with the light source behind the client.
> • Use visual aids if available.

B. Be sure to inform the health care staff of the client's hearing loss.
C. Helpful aids may include a telephone amplifier, earphone attachments for the radio and TV, and lights or buzzers that indicate the doorbell is ringing located in the most commonly used rooms of the house.
D. Maintain proper care of hearing aids and cochlear implants

Neurologic System

Altered State of Consciousness

Nursing Assessment

A. Use agency's neurologic vital signs assessment tool. It will sometimes contain a scale for scoring, such as the

Glasgow Coma Scale, which objectively documents the client's level of consciousness (Table 4-32).

1. Maximum total is 15; minimum is 3.
2. A score of 7 or less indicates coma.
3. Clients with low scores (i.e., 3 to 4) have high mortality rates and poor prognosis.
4. Clients with scores greater than 8 have a good prognosis for recovery.

HESI Hint • Use of the Glasgow Coma Scale eliminates ambiguous terms to describe neurologic status, such as *lethargic*, *stuporous*, or *obtunded*.

B. Neurologic vital signs sheet will also address pupil size (with sizing scale), limb movement (with scale), and vital signs (BP, temperature, pulse, respirations).
C. Assess skin integrity and corneal integrity.
D. Check bladder for fullness, auscultate lungs, and monitor cardiac status.
E. Family members and significant others should be assessed for knowledge of client status, coping skills, need for extra support, and the ability to assist or provide care on an ongoing basis.

Analysis (Nursing Diagnoses)

HESI Hint • Almost every diagnosis in the NANDA format is applicable because severely neurologically impaired persons require total care.

A. *Ineffective breathing pattern* related to …
B. *Ineffective airway clearance* related to …
C. *Impaired gas exchange* related to …
D. *Decreased cardiac output* related to …
E. *Risk for imbalanced body temperature* (especially if hypothalamus is involved) related to …
F. *Risk for injury* related to …
G. *Impaired physical mobility* related to …
H. *Risk for impaired skin integrity* related to …
I. *Anxiety* related to …
J. *Self-care deficit:* (specify) *eating, toileting, dressing, grooming* related to …

HESI Hint • A client with an altered state of consciousness is fed via enteral routes because the likelihood of aspiration is high with oral feedings. Residual feeding is the amount of previous feeding still in the stomach. The presence of 100 mL of residual in an adult usually indicates poor gastric emptying, and the feeding should be withheld; however, the residual should be returned because it is partially digested.

HESI Hint • Paralytic ileus is common in comatose clients. A gastric tube aids in gastric decompression.

TABLE 4-32 Glasgow Coma Scale

Variable	Response	Score
Eye opening	Spontaneously	4
	To verbal command	3
	To pain	2
	No response	1
Motor response	To verbal command	6
	To painful stimuli	5
	• Localizes pain	4
	• Flexes/withdraws	3
	• Flexor posturing (decorticate)	2
	• Extensor posturing (decerebrate)	1
	• No response	
Verbal response	Oriented and converses	5
	Disoriented, converses	4
	Uses inappropriate words	3
	Incomprehensible sounds	2
	No response	1

HESI Hint • Any client on bed rest or immobilized must have ROM exercises often and very frequent position changes. Do not leave the client in any one position for longer than 2 hours. Any position that decreases venous return, such as sitting with dependent extremities for long periods, is dangerous.

Nursing Plans and Interventions

A. Maintain adequate respirations, airway, oxygenation.
1. Document and report breathing pattern changes.
2. Position client for maximum ventilation: three-quarters prone position or semiprone position to prevent tongue from obstructing airway and slightly to one side with arms away from chest wall.
3. Insert airway if tongue is obstructing or if client is paralyzed.
4. Prepare for insertion of cuffed endotracheal tube.
5. Keep airway free of secretions with suctioning (see Table 4-4).
6. Monitor arterial Po_2 and Pco_2.
7. Prepare for tracheostomy if ventilator support is needed.
8. Provide chest physiotherapy as prescribed by physician.
9. Hyperventilate with 100% O_2 before and after suctioning.

B. Provide nutritional and fluid and electrolyte support.
1. Keep client NPO until responsive, and provide mouth care every 4 hours.

2. Maintain calorie count.
3. Administer feedings as prescribed (Box 4-1).
4. Monitor I&O.
5. Record client's weight (weigh at same time each day).

C. Prevent complications of immobility.
  1. Monitor impairment in skin integrity.
     a. Turn client every 2 hours, and assess bony prominences.
     b. Use egg-crate or alternating-pressure mattress or waterbed.
     c. Use minimal amount of linens and underpads.
  2. Potential for thrombus formation
     a. Perform passive ROM exercises to lower extremities every 4 hours.
     b. Apply sequential compression device (SCD) or elastic hose (remove and reapply every 8 hours).
     c. Avoid positions that decrease venous return.
     d. Avoid pillows under knees and Gatch bed.

BOX 4-1 *Unconscious Client*

Gastric Gavage
- Check bowel sounds, and begin feeding when gastrointestinal peristalsis returns.
- Place client in high-Fowler position.
- Place towel over chest.
- Check gastric tube placement.
- Connect gastrostomy tube to funnel or large syringe.
- Check gastric residual to assess absorption and client tolerance; return residual.
- Pour feeding into tilted funnel, and unclamp tubing to allow feeding to flow by gravity.
- Regulate flow by raising or lowering container. Feeding too quickly causes diarrhea, gastric distention, pain. Feeding too slowly causes possible obstruction of flow.
- After feeding, irrigate tube with (tepid) water and clamp tube.
- Apply small dressing over tube opening; coil tube and attach to dressing. May cover with an abdominal binder.
- Keep head of bed elevated 30 degrees or more during feeding and for at least 1 hour after feeding.

Bowel Management Program
- Get bowel history from reliable source.
- Establish specific time for evacuation. Regularity is essential.
- An unconscious client can evacuate the bowel after the last tube feeding of day, because the gastrocolic and duodenocolic reflexes are active after "meal."
- Stimulate anorectal reflex by insertion of glycerin suppository 15 to 30 minutes before scheduled evacuation time. May need stronger suppository, such as bisacodyl (Dulcolax).
- Ensure adequate fiber in tube feedings and adequate fluid intake of 2 to 4 L/day.
- May apply a rectal pouch to contain fecal material (ostomy bag with seal over anal opening).

---

3. Urinary calculi
   a. Increase fluid intake by mouth (PO) or via gastric tube or intravenously.
   b. Assess urine for high specific gravity (dehydration) and balance between I&O.
4. Contractures and joint immobility
   a. Perform passive ROM every 4 hours.
   b. Sit client up in bed or chair, if possible, or use neuro chair if necessary.
   c. Reposition every 2 hours, maintaining proper body alignment.
   d. Apply splints or other assistive devices to prevent foot drop, wrist drop, or other improper alignment.

D. Monitor and evaluate the vital sign changes indicating changes in condition.
   1. Pulse: a pulse rate change to <60 or >100 bpm can indicate increased intracranial pressure (ICP). A fast rate (>100 bpm) can indicate infection, thrombus formation, or dehydration.
   2. Blood pressure: rising BP or widening pulse pressure can indicate increased ICP.
   3. Temperature: report any abnormalities; temperature elevation can indicate worsening condition, damage to temperature-regulating area of brain, or infection.
   4. Level-of-consciousness changes: they may range from active to somnolent.
   5. Pupillary changes: they may range from prompt to sluggish or may increase in size.

HESI Hint • If temperature elevates, take quick measures to decrease it, because fever increases cerebral metabolism and can increase cerebral edema.

HESI Hint • Safety features for immobilized clients:
- Prevent skin breakdown by frequent turning.
- Maintain adequate nutrition.
- Prevent aspiration with slow, small feedings or NG feedings or enteral feedings.
- Monitor neurologic signs to detect the first signs that ICP may be increasing.
- Provide ROM exercises to prevent deformities.
- Prevent respiratory complications; frequent turning and positioning provide optimal drainage.

E. Prevent injury and promote safety.
   1. Place bed in low position, and keep side rails up at all times.
   2. Pad side rails if client is agitated or if there is a history of seizure activity.
   3. Restrain client if client is trying to remove tubes or attempting to get out of bed.
   4. Touch gently, and talk softly and calmly to the client, remembering that hearing is commonly intact.

> **HESI Hint** • Restlessness may indicate a return to consciousness but can also indicate anoxia, distended bladder, covert bleeding, or increasing cerebral anoxia. Do not oversedate, and report any symptoms of restlessness.

5. Avoid oversedating the client because sedatives and narcotics depress responsiveness and affect pupillary reaction (an important assessment in neurologic vital signs).
6. During all activities, tell the client what you are doing, regardless of the level of consciousness.

F. Maintain hygiene and cleanliness.
1. Provide bathing, grooming, and dressing.
2. Provide oral hygiene.
3. Wash hair weekly.
4. Provide nail care within agency guidelines.

G. Observe for bladder elimination problems.
1. Insert indwelling catheter if prescribed.
2. Remove indwelling catheter as soon as possible; use adult brief or condom catheter.

H. Document and record bowel movements, and report abnormal patterns of constipation or diarrhea.
1. Rapid infusion of tube feedings may cause diarrhea; lack of fiber and inadequate fluids may cause constipation.
2. Initiate bowel program (see Box 4-1).

I. Prevent corneal injury and drying:
1. Remove contact lenses if present.
2. Irrigate eyes with sterile prescribed solution, and instill ophthalmic ointment in each eye every 8 hours to prevent corneal ulceration.
3. Close eyelids if blink reflex is absent.

Head Injury

Description: Any traumatic damage to the head
A. Open traumatic brain injury (TBI) occurs when there is a fracture of the skull or penetration of the skull by an object.
B. Closed traumatic brain injury (TBI) is the result of blunt trauma (more serious because of chance of increased ICP in closed vault).
C. Increased ICP is the main concern in head injury; it is related to edema, hemorrhage, impaired cerebral autoregulation, and hydrocephalus.

> **HESI Hint** • The forces of impact influence the type of traumatic brain injury (TBI). They include acceleration injury, which is caused by the head being in motion, and deceleration injury, which occurs when the head stops suddenly. Helmets are a great preventive measure for motorcyclists and bicyclists (Fig. 4-9).

Nursing Assessment

A. Unconsciousness or disturbances in consciousness
B. Vertigo

C. Confusion, delirium, or disorientation
D. Symptoms of increased ICP
1. Change in level of responsiveness is the most important indicator of increased ICP.

> **HESI Hint** • Even subtle behavior changes, such as restlessness, irritability, or confusion, may indicate increased ICP.

2. Changes in vital signs
   a. Slowing of respirations or respiratory irregularities
   b. Increase or decrease in pulse
   c. Rising BP or widening pulse pressure
   d. Temperature rise
3. Headache
4. Vomiting (projectile)
5. Pupillary changes reflecting pressure on optic or oculomotor nerves
   a. Decrease or increase in size or unequal size of pupils
   b. Lack of conjugate eye movement
   c. Papilledema

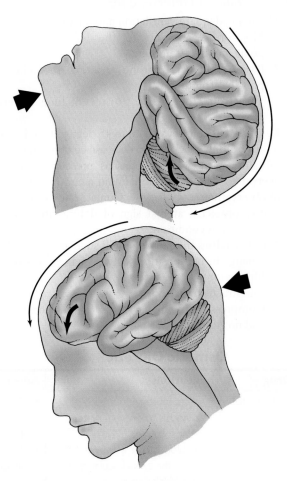

FIGURE 4-9 Head movement during acceleration–deceleration injury, which is typically seen in motor vehicle accidents. (From Ignatavicius DD, Workman ML: *Medical-surgical nursing: patient-centered collaborative care*, ed 7, St. Louis, 2013, Saunders.)

E. Seizures
F. Ataxia
G. Abnormal posturing (decerebrate or decorticate)
H. Cerebrospinal fluid (CSF) leakage through nose (rhinorrhea) or through ear (otorrhea).
I. Hematomas.

> **HESI Hint** • CSF leakage carries the risk for meningitis and indicates a deteriorating condition. Because of CSF leakage, the usual signs of increased ICP may not occur.

J. CT scan or MRI will show a lesion, such as an epidural or subdural hematoma, requiring surgery.
K. Electroencephalograph (EEG) determines presence of seizure activity.

Analysis (Nursing Diagnoses)

A. *Ineffective tissue perfusion* related to …
B. *Risk for injury* related to …
C. *Ineffective family coping* related to …
D. *Risk for infection* related to…

Nursing Plans and Interventions

A. Maintain adequate ventilation and airway.
 1. Monitor Po_2 and Pco_2 for the development of hypoxia and hypercapnia.
 2. Position client semiprone or lateral recumbent to prevent aspiration.
 3. Turn from side to side to prevent lung secretion stasis.
B. Keep head of bed elevated 30 to 45 degrees to aid venous return from the neck and to decrease cerebral volume.
C. Obtain neurologic vital signs as prescribed (at least every 1 to 2 hours), and maintain a continuous record of observations and Glasgow Coma Scale ratings.
D. Notify physician at first sign of deterioration or improvement in condition.
E. Avoid activities that increase ICP such as:
 1. Change in bed position for caregiving and extreme hip flexion
 2. Endotracheal suctioning
 3. Compression of jugular veins (keep head straight and not to one side)

4. Coughing, vomiting, or straining of any type (no Valsalva: increased intrathoracic pressure increases ICP)
F. If temperature increases, take immediate measures to reduce it (aspirin, acetaminophen, cooling blanket) because increased temperature increases cerebral blood flow drastically; avoid shivering.
G. Use intracranial monitoring system when available:
 1. A catheter is inserted into the lateral ventricle, a sensor placed on the dura, or a screw into the subarachnoid space attached to a pressure transducer.
 2. Elevations of ICP over 20 mm Hg should be reported stat.
H. Administer medications prescribed by physician to reduce ICP.
 1. Hyperosmotic agents and diuretics to dehydrate brain and reduce cerebral edema
  a. Mannitol (Table 4-33)
  b. Urea
 2. Steroids
  a. Dexamethasone (Decadron)
  b. Methylprednisolone sodium succinate (Solu-Medrol) to reduce brain edema
 3. Barbiturates
  a. To reduce brain metabolism and systemic BP
I. Insert indwelling Foley catheter to prevent restlessness caused by distended bladder and to monitor balance between restricted fluid I&O, especially if placed on osmotic diuretics.

> **HESI Hint** • Try not to use restraints; they only increase restlessness. Avoid narcotics because they mask the level of responsiveness.

J. Physician may order passive hyperventilation on ventilator: leads to respiratory alkalosis, which causes cerebral vasoconstriction and decreased cerebral blood flow, and therefore decreased ICP.
K. Continue seizure precautions. Health care provider may order prophylactic phenytoin (Dilantin).
L. Prevent complications of immobility (see Nursing Plans and Interventions for Altered State of Consciousness, p. 155).

TABLE 4-33 Osmotic Diuretic

Drug	Indications	Adverse Reactions	Nursing Implications
• Mannitol	• Acts on renal tubules by osmosis to prevent water reabsorption • In bloodstream, draws fluid from the extravascular spaces into the plasma	• Disorientation, confusion, and headache • Nausea and vomiting • Convulsions and anaphylactic reactions	• Use for short-term therapy *only.* • Never give to clients with cerebral hemorrhage. • IV infusion is usually adjusted to urine output; filter and watch for crystals. • Never give to clients with no urine output (anuria); if output is <30 mL/hr, accumulation can cause pulmonary edema and water intoxication.

M. Inform at discharge, if feasible, aftereffects of head injury.
   1. Posttraumatic syndrome: headache, vertigo, emotional instability, inability to concentrate, impaired memory
   2. Posttraumatic epilepsy
   3. Posttraumatic neuroses or psychoses

Spinal Cord Injury

Description: Disruption in nervous system function, which may result in complete or incomplete loss of motor and sensory function. Changes occur in the function of all physiologic systems.

A. Injuries are described by location in the spinal cord. The most common sites are the fifth, sixth, and seventh cervical vertebrae (C5, C6, C7), the twelfth thoracic (T12), and the first lumbar (L1).
B. Damage can range from contusion to complete transection.
C. Permanent impairment cannot be determined until spinal cord edema has subsided, usually by 1 week.

Nursing Assessment

A. Assess breathing pattern, and auscultate lungs.

> **HESI Hint** • Physical assessment should concentrate on respiratory status, especially in clients with injury at C3 to C5, because the cervical plexus innervates the diaphragm.

B. Check neurologic vital signs frequently, especially sensory and motor functions. Assess cardiovascular status.
C. Assess abdomen: girth, bowel sounds; assess lower abdomen for bladder distention.
D. Assess temperature, remembering that hyperthermia occurs commonly.
E. Assess psychosocial status.
F. Hypotension and bradycardia occur with any injury above T6 because sympathetic outflow is affected.

Analysis (Nursing Diagnoses)

A. *Ineffective breathing pattern* related to ...
B. *Ineffective tissue perfusion* related to ...
C. *Impaired skin integrity* related to ...
D. *Self-care deficit* (specify) related to ...
E. *Urinary retention* related to ...
F. *Ineffective coping* related to ...

Nursing Plans and Interventions

A. In acute phase of spinal cord injury:
   1. See Nursing Plans and Interventions for Altered State of Consciousness, p. 156.
   2. Maintain client in an extended position with cervical collar on during any transfer.
   3. Stabilize the client when transferring between the accident scene and the emergency department. The client will be realigned and stabilized in the emergency room.
   4. Maintain a patent airway (most important).
   5. In cervical injuries, skeletal traction is maintained by use of skull tongs or a halo ring (Crutchfield tongs or a Gardner-Wells fixation device).
   6. High-dose corticosteroids are often given to help control edema during the first 8 to 24 hours.
   7. Use a kinetic therapy treatment table (RotoRest bed), which provides continuous side-to-side motion.
   8. Use Stryker frame or very firm mattress with board underneath.
   9. Assess for respiratory failure, especially in clients with high cervical injuries.
   10. Further loss of sensory or motor function below injury can indicate additional damage to cord due to edema and should be reported immediately.
   11. Evaluate for presence of spinal shock (a complete loss of all reflex, motor, sensory, and autonomic activity below the lesion). This is a medical emergency that occurs immediately after the injury.
       a. Hypotension, bradycardia
       b. Complete paralysis and lack of sensation below lesion
       c. Bladder and bowel distention

> **HESI Hint** • It is imperative to reverse spinal shock as quickly as possible. Permanent paralysis can occur if a spinal cord is compressed for 12 to 24 hours.

   12. Evaluate for autonomic dysreflexia (exaggerated autonomic responses to stimuli), which occurs in clients with lesions at or above T6. This is a medical emergency that usually occurs after the period of spinal shock has finished and is usually triggered by a noxious stimulus such as bowel or bladder distention. It may also be triggered by a vaginal examination.
       a. Elevated BP
       b. Pounding headache, sweating, nasal congestion, goose bumps, bradycardia
       c. Bladder and bowel distention
   13. Watch for acute paralytic ileus, lack of gastric activity.
       a. Assess bowel sounds frequently.
       b. Initiate gastric suction to reduce distention, prevent vomiting and aspiration.
       c. Use rectal tube to relieve gaseous distention.
   14. Suction with caution to prevent vagus nerve stimulation, which can cause cardiac arrest.
   15. Administer high-dose corticosteroids intravenously to decrease edema and reduce cord damage.
B. In rehabilitative phase of spinal cord injury:
   1. Encourage deep-breathing exercises.
   2. Administer chest physiotherapy.
   3. Provide kinetic bed to promote blood flow to extremities.
   4. Apply antiembolic stockings or SCDs.
   5. Facilitate ROM exercises.
   6. Mobilize client to chair as soon as possible.

7. Turn client frequently.
8. Keep client clean and dry.
9. Observe for impending skin breakdown.
10. Teach client importance of impeccable skin care.
11. Perform intermittent catheterization every 4 hours.
    a. Begin teaching client catheterization technique.
    b. Teach family member if client is unable.
12. Teach bladder-emptying techniques according to level of injury and bladder muscle response.
    a. UMN (spastic) bladder
    b. LMN (flaccid) bladder
13. Instruct client in monitoring I&O.
14. Encourage the client to drink fluids that promote acidic urine, including cranberry juice, prune juice, bouillon, tomato juice, and water.

> **HESI Hint** • A common cause of death after spinal cord injury is urinary tract infection. Bacteria grow best in alkaline media, so keeping urine dilute and acidic is prophylactic against infection. Also, keeping the bladder emptied assists in avoiding bacterial growth in urine that has stagnated in the bladder.

15. Begin bowel-training program.
16. Talk with client and family about permanence of disability.
17. Encourage rehabilitation facility staff to visit client.
18. Encourage client and family to visit rehabilitation facility.
19. Assist family in finding support group, and refer to community resources after dismissal from rehabilitation facility.

Brain Tumor

Description: Neoplasm occurring in the brain
A. Primary tumors can arise in any tissue of the brain.
B. Secondary tumors are a result of metastasis from other areas (most often from the lungs, followed by breast).
C. Without treatment, benign as well as malignant tumors lead to death.

> **HESI Hint** • Benign tumors continue to grow and take up space in the confined area of the cranium, causing neural and vascular compromise in the brain, increased ICP, and necrosis of brain tissue. Even benign tumors must be treated because they may have malignant effects.

Nursing Assessment

A. Headache that is more severe on awakening
B. Vomiting not associated with nausea
C. Papilledema with visual changes
D. Behavioral and personality changes
E. Seizures

F. Aphasia, hemiplegia, ataxia
G. Cranial nerve dysfunction
H. Abnormal CT scan/MRI or PET scan (looking for metastasis)

Analysis (Nursing Diagnoses)

A. *Ineffective tissue perfusion* related to …
B. *Acute pain* related to …
C. *Risk for injury* related to …
D. *Anxiety* related to …

Nursing Plans and Interventions

A. Institute nursing plans and interventions that are similar to those implemented for the client with a head injury and increased ICP.
B. Elevate the head of the bed 30 to 40 degrees; maintain head in neutral position.
C. Facilitate radiation therapy.
   1. Provide skin care with non–oil-based soap and water. Avoid putting alcohol, powder, or oils on the skin.
   2. Explain that alopecia is temporary.
   3. Instruct client not to wash off the lines drawn by the radiologist.
D. Administer chemotherapy: medications may be injected intraventricularly or intravenously.
E. Facilitate surgical removal of tumor (craniotomy).
   1. Preoperative (shave head)
   2. Postoperative
      a. Perform frequent neurologic and vital sign assessment.
      b. Position client with head of bed elevated for supratentorial lesions and flat for infratentorial lesions.
      c. Position client on side opposite the operative site.
      d. Monitor dressings for signs of drainage (excess amount of CSF).
      e. Monitor respiratory status to prevent hypoventilation.
      f. Avoid activities that cause increased ICP.
      g. Monitor for seizure activity.
      h. Administer medications (see Head Injuries, p. 157).

> **HESI Hint** • Craniotomy preoperative medications:
> • Corticosteroids to reduce swelling
> • Agents and osmotic diuretics to reduce secretions (atropine, glycopyrrolate)
> • Agents to reduce seizures (phenytoin)
> • Prophylactic antibiotics

Multiple Sclerosis (MS)

Description: Demyelinating disease resulting in the destruction of CNS myelin and consequent disruption in the transmission of nerve impulses
A. Onset is insidious, with 50% of clients still ambulatory 25 years after diagnosis.

B. Diagnosis determined by a combination of data:
   1. Presenting symptoms
   2. Increased white matter density seen on CT scan
   3. Presence of plaques seen on MRI
   4. CSF electrophoresis shows presence of oligoclonal (IgG) bands.
C. Current thinking is that MS is autoimmune in origin.

> **HESI Hint** • Symptoms involving motor function usually begin in the upper extremities with weakness progressing to spastic paralysis. Bowel and bladder dysfunction occurs in 90% of cases. MS is more common in women. Progression is not "orderly."

Nursing Assessment

A. Nursing history of client to include:
   1. History of symptoms
   2. Progression of illness
   3. Types of treatment received and the responses
   4. Additional health problems
   5. Current medications
   6. Client's and family's perception of illness
   7. Community resources used by the client
B. Physical assessment to include:
   1. Optic neuritis (loss of vision or blind spots)
   2. Visual or swallowing difficulties
   3. Gait disturbances; intention tremors
   4. Unusual fatigue, weakness, and clumsiness
   5. Numbness, particularly on one side of face
   6. Impaired bladder and bowel control
   7. Speech disturbances
   8. Scotomas (white spots in visual field, diplopia)

Analysis (Nursing Diagnoses)

A. *Impaired physical mobility* related to ...
B. *Fatigue* related to ...
C. *Impaired urinary elimination* related to ...
D. *Impaired home maintenance* related to ...

Nursing Plans and Interventions

A. Allow hospitalized client to keep own routine.
B. Orient client to environment, and teach strategies to maximize vision.
C. Encourage self-care and frequent rest periods.
D. With exercise programs, encourage client to work up to the point just short of fatigue.
E. Teach client that for muscle spasticity, stretch-hold-relax exercises are helpful, as are riding a stationary bicycle and swimming; take precautions against falls.
F. Initially, work with client on a voiding schedule.
G. Teach client that as incontinence worsens, the female may need to learn clean self-catheterization; the male may need a condom catheter.
H. Encourage adequate fluid intake, high-fiber foods, and a bowel regimen for constipation problems.

I. Encourage the client and the family to verbalize their concerns about ongoing care issues.
J. Encourage client to maintain contact with a support group.
K. Refer client for home health care services.
L. Encourage client to contact the local MS Society for emotional support and direct services.
M. Administer steroid therapy and chemotherapeutic drugs in acute exacerbations to shorten length of attack.

> **HESI Hint** • Drug therapy for MS clients: ACTH, cortisone, cyclophosphamide (Cytoxan), and other immunosuppressive drugs. Nursing implications for administration of these drugs should focus on the prevention of infection.

N. Remember that biologic response modifiers such as interferon-beta products (Betaseron, Rebif, and Avonex) have shown recent success for MS relapses.

Myasthenia Gravis

Description: Disorder affecting the neuromuscular transmission of impulses in the voluntary muscles of the body
A. It is considered an autoimmune disease characterized by the presence of acetylcholine receptor (AChR) antibodies, which interfere with neuronal transmission.
B. It usually affects females between ages 10 and 40 and men between ages 50 and 70.

Nursing Assessment

A. Diplopia (double vision), ptosis (eyelid drooping)
B. Masklike affect: sleepy appearance due to facial muscle involvement
C. Weakness of laryngeal and pharyngeal muscles: dysphagia, choking, food aspiration, difficulty speaking
D. Muscle weakness improved by rest, worsened by activity
E. Advanced cases: respiratory failure, bladder and bowel incontinence
F. Myasthenic crisis symptoms (attributed to disease worsening) associated with undermedication. Increase in myasthenic gravis symptoms; more difficulty swallowing, diplopia, ptosis, dyspnea.
G. Cholinergic crisis (attributed to anticholinesterase overdosage): diaphoresis, diarrhea, fasciculations, cramps, marked worsening of symptoms resulting from overmedication

> **HESI Hint** • In clients with myasthenia gravis, be alert for changes in respiratory status; the most severe involvement may result in respiratory failure.

Analysis (Nursing Diagnoses)

A. *Ineffective airway clearance* related to ...
B. *Risk for injury* related to ...

TABLE 4-34 Treatment of Myasthenia Gravis

Drug	Indications	Adverse Reactions	Nursing Implications
• Pyridostigmine bromide	• Inhibits the action of cholinesterase at the cholinergic nerve endings • To promote accumulation of acetylcholine at cholinergic receptor sites	• Cholinergic crisis can occur with overdose	• Atropine is antidote for drug-induced bradycardia • Take drug with milk or food to decrease GI side effects • Dosage regulation required; record keeping, regarding: side effects, drug response • Observe for symptoms of cholinergic crisis • Fasciculations • Abdominal cramps, diarrhea, incontinence of stool or urine • Hypotension, bradycardia, respiratory depression • Lacrimation, blurred vision • Drug therapy is lifelong and requires family teaching and support

C. *Impaired physical mobility* related to …
D. *Risk for imbalanced nutrition: less than body requirements* related to …

Nursing Plans and Interventions

A. If client is hospitalized, have tracheostomy kit available at bedside for possible myasthenic crisis.
B. Teach client the importance of wearing a MedicAlert bracelet.
C. Administer cholinergic drugs as prescribed (Table 4-34).
D. Schedule nursing activities to conserve energy (e.g., complete daily hygiene activities, administration of medications, and treatments all at once), and allow rest periods. Plan activities during high-energy times, often in the early morning.
E. Instruct client to avoid situations that produce fatigue or physical or emotional stress (any type of stress can exacerbate symptoms).

HESI Hint • Bed rest often relieves symptoms. Bladder and respiratory infections are often recurring problems. There is a need for health-promotion teachings.

F. Encourage coughing and deep breathing every 4 to 6 hours. (Muscle weakness limits ability to cough up secretions, promotes URI.)
G. If symptoms worsen, identify type of crisis and report immediately: myasthenic or cholinergic.

HESI Hint • Myasthenic crisis is associated with a positive edrophonium (Tensilon) test, whereas a cholinergic crisis is associated with a negative test.

Parkinson Disease

Description: Chronic, progressive, debilitating neurologic disease of the basal ganglia and substantia nigra, affecting motor ability and characterized by tremor at rest, increased muscle tone (rigidity), slowness in the initiation and execution of movement (bradykinesia), and postural instability (difficulties with gait and balance)

Nursing Assessment

A. Rigidity of extremities
B. Masklike facial expressions with associated difficulty in chewing, swallowing, and speaking
C. Drooling
D. Stooped posture and slow, shuffling gait
E. Tremors at rest, "pill-rolling" movement
F. Emotional lability
G. Increased tremors with stress or anxiety

HESI Hint • NCLEX-RN questions often focus on the features of Parkinson disease: tremors (a coarse tremor of fingers and thumb on one hand that disappears during sleep and purposeful activity; also called "pill rolling"), rigidity, hypertonicity, and stooped posture. Focus: *safety!*

Analysis (Nursing Diagnoses)

A. *Self-care deficit* (specify) related to …
B. *Impaired physical mobility* related to …
C. *Imbalanced nutrition: less than body requirements* related to …
D. *Impaired verbal communication* related to …
E. *Disturbed body image* related to …

Nursing Plans and Interventions

A. Schedule activities later in the day to allow sufficient time for client to perform self-care activities without rushing.
B. Encourage activities and exercise. A cane or walker may be needed.
C. Eliminate environmental noise, and encourage the client to speak slowly and clearly, pausing at intervals.
D. Serve a soft diet, which is easy to swallow.
E. Administer antiparkinsonian drugs as prescribed (Table 4-35).

TABLE 4-35 **Antiparkinsonian Drugs**

Drugs	Indications	Adverse Reactions	Nursing Implications
Anticholinergics (Parasympatholytics [Older Drugs])			
• Atropine sulfate • Benztropine mesylate • Trihexyphenidyl	• Used to treat secondary cholinergic symptoms, such as drooling, sweating, tremors.	• Increased heart rate • Postural hypotension • Dry mouth • Constipation • Urinary retention • Blurred vision	• Review client's history for glaucoma, urinary obstruction. • Warn to avoid rapid position changes. • Avoid extreme heat. • Provide gum, hard candy, and frequent mouth care. • Contraindicated in narrow-angle glaucoma.
Dopamine Replacements			
• Levodopa • Levodopa-carbidopa *Dopamine-Releasing Agents* • Amantadine HCl *Dopamine-Releasing Agonists* • Bromocriptine mesylate • Pramipexole • Ropinirole	• Stimulates dopamine production or increases sensitivity of dopamine receptors • Newer drugs require lower dosage	• Involuntary movements • Nausea • Vomiting	• Explain that drugs may take months to achieve desired effects. • Warn to avoid sudden position changes. • Avoid foods high in vitamin B_6 (meats, liver, i.e., high-protein foods) • If insomnia occurs, suggest taking last dose earlier in day. • May initially cause drowsiness; teach to avoid driving until response is determined.
Monoamine Oxidase Type B Inhibitor			
• Selegiline • Rasagiline	• Used with dopamine agonist when client symptoms do not respond	• Confusion, dizziness • Nausea, dry mouth • Insomnia	• Review drug–drug interactions carefully. • Not an option if client is on antidepressants (selective serotonin reuptake inhibitors or tricyclics). • Can cause hypertensive crisis.
Catechol-O-methyl Transferase (COMT) Inhibitor			
• Entacapone • Tolcapone	• Used with levodopa-carbidopa	• May increase levodopa-carbidopa side effects, including dyskinesias	• Levodopa dose may need to be decreased. • Combination product may decrease pill burden.

HESI Hint • An important aspect of treatment for Parkinson disease is drug therapy. The pathophysiology involves an imbalance between acetylcholine and dopamine, so symptoms can be controlled by administering a dopamine precursor (levodopa).

Guillain-Barré Syndrome

Description: Clinical syndrome of unknown origin involving peripheral and cranial nerves

A. Is usually preceded by a (viral) respiratory or GI infection 1 to 4 weeks before the onset of neurologic deficits

B. Constant monitoring of these clients is required to prevent the life-threatening problem of acute respiratory failure.

C. Full recovery usually occurs within several months to a year after onset of symptoms.

D. About 30% of those diagnosed with Guillain-Barré syndrome are left with a residual disability. Death occurs in 5%.

Nursing Assessment

A. Paresthesia (tingling and numbness)

B. Muscle weakness of legs progressing to the upper extremities, trunk, and face

C. Paralysis of the ocular, facial, and oropharyngeal muscles, causing marked difficulty in talking, chewing, and swallowing. Assess for:
1. Breathlessness while talking
2. Shallow and irregular breathing
3. Use of accessory muscles while breathing
4. Any change in respiratory pattern
5. Paradoxical inward movement of the upper abdominal wall while in a supine position, indicating weakness and impending paralysis of the diaphragm
D. Increasing pulse rate and disturbances in rhythm
E. Transient HTN, orthostatic hypotension
F. Possible pain in the back and in calves of legs
G. Weakness or paralysis of the intercostal and diaphragm muscles; may develop quickly

Analysis (Nursing Diagnoses)

A. *Ineffective breathing pattern* related to …
B. *Impaired verbal communication* related to …
C. *Alteration in bowel or bladder elimination* related to…

Nursing Plans and Interventions

A. Monitor for respiratory distress, and initiate mechanical ventilation if necessary.
B. See Nursing Plans and Interventions for Altered State of Consciousness, p. 155.

Stroke/Brain Attack: Cerebral Vascular Accident (CVA)

Description: Sudden loss of brain function resulting from a disruption in the blood supply to a part of the brain; classified as thrombotic or hemorrhagic

HESI Hint • CNS involvement related to cause of stroke:
• Hemorrhagic: Caused by a slow or fast hemorrhage into the brain tissue; often related to HTN
• Embolic: Caused by a clot that has broken away from a vessel and has lodged in one of the arteries of the brain, blocking the blood supply. It is often related to atherosclerosis (so it may occur again).

A. Risk factors include:
1. HTN
2. Previous transient ischemic attacks (TIAs)
3. Cardiac disease: atherosclerosis, valve disease, history of dysrhythmias (particularly atrial flutter or fibrillation)
4. Advanced age
5. Diabetes
6. Oral contraceptives and HRT
7. Smoking
8. Alcohol more than 2 drinks per day

HESI Hint • Atrial flutter and fibrillation produce a high incidence of thrombus formation after dysrhythmia caused by turbulence of blood flow through all valves and heart.

B. Diagnosis is made by observation of clinical signs and is confirmed by:
1. Cranial CT scan
2. MRI
3. Doppler flow studies
4. Ultrasound imaging
C. Presenting symptoms relate to the specific area of the brain that has been damaged (Table 4-36).

TABLE 4-36 Location of Disruption in the Brain

Feature	Left Hemisphere	Right Hemisphere
• Language	• Aphasia • Agraphia	• May be alert and oriented
• Memory	• No deficit	• Disoriented • Cannot recognize faces
• Vision	• Unable to discriminate words and letters • Reading problems • Deficits in right visual field	• Visual/spatial deficits • Neglect of left visual fields • Loss of depth perception
• Behavior	• Slow • Cautious • Anxious when attempting a new task • Depression or catastrophic response to illness • Sense of guilt • Feeling of worthlessness • Worries over future • Quick anger and frustration	• Impulsive • Unaware of neurologic deficits • Confabulates • Euphoric • Constantly smiles • Denies illness • Poor judgment • Overestimates abilities • Impaired sense of humor
• Hearing	• No deficit	• Loses ability to hear tonal variations

D. Generally there is:
1. Motor loss, usually exhibited as hemiparesis or hemiplegia
2. Communication loss, exhibited as dysarthria, dysphasia, aphasia, or apraxia
3. Perceptual disturbance that can be visual, spatial, and sensory
4. Impaired mental acuity or psychological changes, such as decreased attention span, memory loss, depression, lability, and hostility

E. Bladder dysfunction may be either incontinence or retention.

F. Rehabilitation is begun as soon as the client is stable.

> **HESI Hint** • A woman who had a stroke 2 days earlier has left-sided paralysis. She has begun to regain some movement in her left side. What can the nurse tell the family about the client's recovery period? "The quicker movement is recovered, the better the prognosis is for full or improved recovery. She will need patience and understanding from her family as she tries to cope with the stroke. Mood swings can be expected during the recovery period, and bouts of depression and tearfulness are likely."

Nursing Assessment

A. Change in level of consciousness
B. Paresthesia, paralysis
C. Aphasia, agraphia
D. Memory loss
E. Vision impairment
F. Bladder and bowel dysfunction
G. Behavioral changes
H. Assessment of client's functional abilities, including:
1. Mobility
2. Activities of daily living (ADLs)
3. Elimination
4. Communication
I. Ability to swallow, eat, and drink without aspiration

Analysis (Nursing Diagnoses)

A. *Impaired physical mobility* related to …
B. *Self-care deficit* (specify) related to …
C. *Impaired urinary elimination* related to …
D. *Impaired verbal communication* related to …
E. *Ineffective coping* related to …
F. *Ineffective family coping* related to …
G. *Disturbed body image* related to …

> **HESI Hint** • Words that describe losses in strokes:
> 1. *Apraxia:* inability to perform purposeful movements in the absence of motor problems
> 2. *Dysarthria:* difficulty articulating

> 3. *Dysphasia:* impairment of speech and verbal comprehension
> 4. *Aphasia:* loss of the ability to speak
> 5. *Agraphia:* loss of the ability to write
> 6. *Alexia:* loss of the ability to read
> 7. *Dysphagia:* dysfunctional swallowing

Nursing Plans and Interventions

A. Control HTN to help prevent future stroke.
B. Maintain proper body alignment while client is in bed. Use splints or other assistive devices (including bed rolls and pillows) to maintain functional position.
C. Position client to minimize edema, prevent contractures, and maintain skin integrity.
D. Perform full ROM exercises four times a day. Follow up with program initiated by other team members.
E. Encourage client to participate in or manage own personal care.
F. Set realistic goals; add new tasks daily.
G. Teach client that appropriate self-care activities for the hemiparetic person include:
1. Bathing
2. Brushing teeth
3. Shaving with electric razor
4. Eating
5. Combing hair
H. Encourage client to assist with dressing activities, and modify them as necessary (client will wear street clothes during waking hours).
I. Analyze bladder elimination pattern.
1. Offer bedpan or urinal according to client's particular pattern of elimination.
2. Reassure client that bladder control tends to be regained quickly.
J. Follow-up speech program is initiated by the speech and language therapist.
1. Ensure consistency with this program.
2. Reassure the client that regaining speech is a very slow process.
K. Do not place client in sensory overload; give only one set of instructions at a time.
L. Encourage total family involvement in rehabilitation.
M. Encourage client and family to join a support group.
N. Encourage family members to allow the client to perform self-care activities as outlined by the rehabilitation team.
O. Refer for outpatient follow-up or for home health care.
P. Teach that swallowing modifications may include a soft diet (pureed foods, thickened liquids) and head positioning.

> **HESI Hint** • Steroids are administered after a stroke to decrease cerebral edema and retard permanent disability. H2 inhibitors are administered to prevent peptic ulcers.

Review of Neurologic System

1. What are the classifications of the commonly prescribed eye drops for glaucoma?
2. Identify two types of hearing loss.
3. Write four nursing interventions for the care of the blind person and four nursing interventions for the care of the deaf person.
4. In your own words, describe the Glasgow Coma Scale.
5. List four nursing diagnoses for the comatose client in order of priority. (Remember Maslow's hierarchy of needs to help determine priorities.)
6. State four independent nursing interventions to maintain adequate respiration, airway, and oxygenation in the unconscious client.
7. Who is at risk for stroke?
8. Complications of immobility include the potential for thrombus development. State three nursing interventions to prevent thrombi.
9. List four rationales for the appearance of restlessness in the unconscious client.
10. What nursing interventions prevent corneal drying in a comatose client?
11. When can a comatose client on IV hyperalimentation begin to receive tube feedings instead?
12. What is the most important principle in a bowel management program for a client with neurologic deficits?
13. Define stroke.
14. A client with a diagnosis of stroke presents with symptoms of aphasia and right hemiparesis but no memory or hearing deficit. In what hemisphere has the client suffered a lesion?
15. What are the symptoms of spinal shock?
16. What are the symptoms of autonomic dysreflexia?
17. What is the most important indicator of increased ICP?
18. What vital sign changes are indicative of increased ICP?
19. A neighbor calls the neighborhood nurse stating that he was knocked hard to the floor by his very hyperactive dog. He is wondering what symptoms would indicate the need to visit an emergency department. What should the nurse tell him to do?
20. What activities and situations that increase ICP should be avoided?
21. What is the action of hyperosmotic agents (osmotic diuretics) used to treat ICP?
22. Why should narcotics be avoided in clients with neurologic impairment?
23. Headache and vomiting are symptoms of many disorders. What characteristics of these symptoms would alert the nurse to refer a client to a neurologist?
24. How should the head of the bed be positioned for postcraniotomy clients with infratentorial lesions?
25. Is multiple sclerosis thought to occur because of an autoimmune process?
26. Is paralysis always a consequence of spinal cord injury?
27. What types of drugs are used in the treatment of myasthenia gravis?

Answers to Review

1. Parasympathomimetic for pupillary constriction; beta-adrenergic receptor-blocking agents to inhibit formation of aqueous humor; carbonic anhydrase inhibitors to reduce aqueous humor production; and prostaglandin agonists to increase aqueous humor outflow
2. Conductive (transmission of sound to inner ear is blocked) and sensorineural (damage to eighth cranial nerve)
3. Care of blind: announce presence clearly, call by name, orient carefully to surroundings, guide by walking in front of client with his or her hand in your elbow. Care of deaf: reduce distraction before beginning conversation, look and listen to client, give client full attention if he or she is a lip reader, face client directly.
4. An objective assessment of the level of consciousness based on a score of 3 to 15, with scores of 7 or less indicative of coma
5. Ineffective breathing pattern, ineffective airway clearance, impaired gas exchange, and decreased cardiac output
6. Position for maximum ventilation (prone or semiprone and slightly to one side); insert airway if tongue is obstructing; suction airway efficiently; monitor arterial Po_2 and Pco_2; and hyperventilate with 100% O_2 before suctioning.
7. Persons with histories of HTN, previous TIAs, cardiac disease (atrial flutter or fibrillation), diabetes, or oral contraceptive use; and older adults
8. Frequent ROM exercises, frequent (every 2 hours) position changes, and avoidance of positions that decrease venous return.
9. Anoxia, distended bladder, covert bleeding, or a return to consciousness
10. Irrigation of eyes PRN with sterile prescribed solution, application of ophthalmic ointment every 8 hours, close assessment for corneal ulceration or drying
11. When peristalsis resumes as evidenced by active bowel sounds, passage of flatus or bowel movement
12. Establishment of regularity
13. A disruption of blood supply to a part of the brain, which results in sudden loss of brain function
14. Left

15. Hypotension, bladder and bowel distention, total paralysis, lack of sensation below lesion
16. HTN, bladder and bowel distention, exaggerated autonomic responses, headache, sweating, goose bumps, and bradycardia
17. A change in the level of responsiveness
18. Increased BP, widening pulse pressure, increased or decreased pulse, respiratory irregularities, and temperature increase
19. Call his physician now and inform him or her of the fall. Symptoms needing medical attention would include vertigo, confusion or any subtle behavioral change, headache, vomiting, ataxia (imbalance), or seizure.
20. Change in bed position, extreme hip flexion, endotracheal suctioning, compression of jugular veins, coughing, vomiting, and straining of any kind

21. They dehydrate the brain and reduce cerebral edema by holding water in the renal tubules to prevent reabsorption and by drawing fluid from the extravascular spaces into the plasma.
22. Narcotics mask the level of responsiveness and pupillary responses.
23. Headache that is more severe upon awakening, and vomiting not associated with nausea are symptoms of a brain tumor.
24. Supratentorial: elevated; infratentorial: flat
25. Yes
26. No
27. Anticholinesterase drugs, which inhibit the action of cholinesterase at the nerve endings to promote the accumulation of acetylcholine at receptor sites; this should improve neuronal transmission to muscles.

Hematology and Oncology

Anemia

Description: Deficiency of erythrocytes (RBCs) reflected as decreased Hct, Hgb, and RBCs

Nursing Assessment

A. Pallor, especially of the ears and nail beds; palmar crease; conjunctiva
B. Fatigue, exercise intolerance, lethargy, orthostatic hypotension
C. Tachycardia, heart murmurs, heart failure
D. Signs of bleeding, such as hematuria, melena, menorrhagia
E. Dyspnea
F. Irritability, difficulty concentrating
G. Cool skin, cold intolerance
H. Risk factors
   1. Diet lacking in iron, folate, and/or vitamin B_{12}
   2. Family history of genetic diseases such as sickle cell or congenital hemolytic anemia
   3. Medication history of anemia-producing drugs, such as salicylates, thiazides, and diuretics
   4. Exposure to toxic agents, such as lead or insecticides
I. Diagnostic tests indicate abnormally low results:
   1. Hgb <10 g/dL
   2. Hct <36%
   3. RBCs <4 × 10^{12}
   4. Bone marrow aspiration positive for anemia
J. Blood loss either acute or chronic
K. Medical history of kidney disorders

> **HESI Hint** • Physical symptoms occur as a compensatory mechanism when the body is trying to make up for a deficit somewhere in the system. For instance, cardiac output increases when Hgb levels drop below 7 g/dL.

Analysis (Nursing Diagnoses)

A. *Anxiety* related to …
B. *Ineffective tissue perfusion* related to …
C. *Fatigue* related to…

Nursing Plans and Interventions

A. Administer blood products as prescribed (see Table 3-7)
B. Alternate periods of activity with periods of rest.
C. Teach about diet.
   1. Instruct in food selection and preparation to maximize intake of:
      a. Iron (red meats, organ meats, whole wheat products, spinach, carrots)
      b. Folic acid (green vegetables, liver, citrus fruits)
      c. Vitamin B_{12} (glandular meats, yeast, green leafy vegetables, milk, and cheese)
   2. Instruct in need for prescribed vitamin supplements.
      a. Take iron on an empty stomach to enhance absorption, 1 hour before meals or 2 hours after meals.
      b. Give vitamin C to enhance absorption of iron.
      c. Administer B_{12} and folic acid orally except to clients with pernicious anemia who should receive B_{12} parenterally.
D. If parenteral iron is required, use Z-track method for administration to prevent staining the skin (Table 4-37).
E. Provide genetic information if client has sickle cell or congenital hemolytic anemia.
F. Teach that sickle cell crisis is precipitated by hypoxia (see Chapter 5).
   1. Provide pain relief.
   2. Provide adequate hydration.
   3. Teach client to avoid activities that cause hypoxia.
   4. Teach client when to seek medical attention.
G. Teach client that iron (oral) may turn stools black.
H. Give liquid iron through a straw, with oral care afterward, to prevent discoloring of teeth.

TABLE 4-37 Administration of Iron

Do's	Don'ts
• Use Z-track method of administration. • Use air bubble to avoid withdrawing medication into subcutaneous tissue.	• Do *not* use deltoid muscle. • Do *not* massage injection site.

I. Teach the client to report any unusual bleeding to health care professional.

> **HESI Hint** • Use only normal saline to flush IV tubing or to run with blood. Never add medications to blood products. Two registered nurses should simultaneously check the physician's prescription, the client's identity, and the blood bag label.

Leukemia

Description: Malignant neoplasm of the blood-forming organs

A. Leukemia is characterized by an abnormal overproduction of immature forms of any of the leukocytes. There is an interference with normal blood production that results in decreased numbers of RBCs and platelets.
   1. Anemia results from decreased RBC production and blood loss.
   2. Immunosuppression occurs because of the large number of immature WBCs or profound neutropenia.
   3. Hemorrhage occurs because of thrombocytopenia.
   4. There may be leukemic invasion of other organ systems, such as the liver, spleen, lymph nodes, kidneys, lungs, and brain.
B. The exact cause of leukemia is unknown, but identified precipitating factors include:
   1. Genetic abnormalities
   2. Ionizing radiation (therapeutic or atomic)
   3. Viral infections (human T cells, leukemia virus)
   4. Exposure to certain chemicals or drugs (Box 4-2)
      a. Benzene
      b. Alkylating chemotherapeutic agents
      c. Immunosuppressants
      d. Chloramphenicol
C. Incidence is highest in children 3 to 4 years of age; declines until age 35; then a steady increase occurs.
D. Diagnosis of leukemia is made by biopsy, bone marrow aspiration, lumbar puncture, and frequent blood counts.
E. Leukemia is treated with antineoplastic chemotherapy (Table 4-38).

Types of Leukemia

A. Acute myelogenous leukemia (AML)
   1. It involves the inability of leukocytes to mature; those that do are abnormal.
   2. It can occur at any time during the life cycle.
   3. Onset is insidious.

BOX 4-2 *Administration of Antineoplastic Chemotherapeutic Agents*

• Follow Occupational Safety and Health Administration (OSHA) guidelines for administration as well as for decontamination of nondisposable areas and equipment and of self.
• Obtain complete and detailed instructions about administration (routine knowledge of procedures for IV administration is not sufficient).
• These drugs are toxic to cancer cells and normal cells in both the client and the caregivers who are infusing the drugs.
• Nurses who are pregnant or are considering becoming pregnant should notify supervisor (many agencies discourage or prohibit such caregivers from administering these drugs).
• Wear gloves when handling drugs.
• Check the drug with another nurse against the health care provider's prescription and the client's record to ensure that it is the correct medication.
• If IV catheter line is used for infusion, verify line placement and patency with another nurse and aspirate a blood return.
• If a vesicant (caustic) drug is administered peripherally, stay with the client throughout administration and check IV placement and patency frequently by aspirating a blood return.
• If a peripheral site is used for infusion, use a new site daily.
• Dispose of all IV equipment in the specially provided waste receptacle so that personnel handling trash do not come into contact with vesicant drugs.

> **HESI Hint** • Many health care delivery systems require the nurse to be credentialed in order to administer parental chemotherapy. The practical nurse (PN) should recognize complications of chemotherapy related to administration, safety, side effects, and nursing assessment parameters and should report these to the registered nurse and health care provider.

   4. Prognosis is poor: 5-year survival of 20%; overall, 50% for children.
   5. Cause of death tends to be overwhelming infection.
B. Chronic myelogenous leukemia (CML)
   1. It results from abnormal production of granulocytic cells.
   2. It is a biphasic disease.
   3. The chronic stage lasts approximately 3 years.
   4. The acute phase tends to last 2 to 3 months.

TABLE 4-38 Antineoplastic Chemotherapeutic Agents

Drugs	Indications	Adverse Reactions	Nursing Implications
Alkylating Agents			
• Cyclophosphamide Mechlorethamine HCl • Cisplatin • Busulfan • Procarbazine • Imidazole carboxamide	• Hodgkin disease • Leukemia • Neuroblastoma • Retinoblastoma • Multiple myeloma	• Bone marrow suppression • Nausea and vomiting • Cystitis • Stomatitis • Alopecia • Gonadal suppression • Toxic effects occur slowly with high dosage • Toxic to kidneys and ears • Pleural effusion • Seizures	• Use immediately after reconstitution. • Avoid vapors in eyes. • Vesicant; if comes in contact with skin, flush with water. • Check placement of infusing system. • Hydrate well before and during treatment with IV fluids and mannitol. • Monitor renal functioning and watch for signs of cystitis. • Force fluids. • Monitor hearing and vision.
Antimetabolites			

• Fluorouracil
• Methotrexate sodium; requires leucovorin rescue to prevent toxic effects
• Mercaptopurine/6-MP
• Cytarabine
• Gemcitabine
	• Acute lymphocytic leukemia
	• Acute myelocytic leukemia
	• Brain tumors
	• Ovarian, breast, prostatic, testicular cancers
		• Nausea and vomiting
		• Diarrhea
		• Myelosuppression (bone marrow depression)
		• Proctitis
		• Stomatitis
		• Dermatitis
		• Renal toxicity
		• Hepatotoxicity
		• Anaphylaxis
			• Administer antiemetics as needed.
			• Teach to wear sunscreen when outdoors.
			• Toxic to liver and kidney; avoid:
			  • Aspirin
			  • Sulfonamide
			  • Tetracycline
			  • Vitamins containing folic acid
			• Leucovorin is used with methotrexate as antidote for high doses; called "leucovorin rescue."
			• Give allopurinol concurrently with 6-MP to inhibit uric acid production by cell destruction; it increases drug's potency.
			• Monitor liver function.

Antitumor Antibiotics			
• Dactinomycin • Bleomycin sulfate • Daunorubicin I • Mitomycin • Doxorubicin HCl • Idarubicin	• Sarcoma • Neuroblastoma • Head and neck tumors • Testicular, ovarian, breast cancer • Hodgkin disease • Lymphocytic leukemia • Acute myelocytic leukemia	• Bone marrow suppression • Anorexia • Nausea and vomiting • Alopecia • Cardiac toxicity • Vesicant	• Monitor placement and patency of infusing system. • Monitor for cardiac dysrhythmia. • Inform client that urine turns red. • Administer antiemetics as needed.
Angiogenesis Inhibitors			
• Bevacizumab	• Recombinant humanized monoclonal antibody that prevents neoangiogenesis	• HTN • Bleeding • Thrombosis	• Report abdominal pain. • Monitor for complications. • May inhibit wound healing.

Continued

TABLE 4-38 Antineoplastic Chemotherapeutic Agents—cont'd

Drugs	Indications	Adverse Reactions	Nursing Implications
Endothelial Growth Factor Receptor Inhibitors			
• Cetuximab • Panitumumab	• Inhibits cell growth • Increases programmed cellular death	• Severe infusion reactions with airway obstruction • Hypotension • Acne-like rash • Fatigue • GI disturbances	• Monitor for severe infusion reactions. • Use diphenhydramine before administration.
Miscellaneous Antineoplastics			
• Hydroxyurea • Asparaginase	• Urea-derived antineoplastic agent against solid tumors and CML • Anticancer enzyme against ALL	• Drowsiness • Renal dysfunction • Nausea and vomiting, diarrhea • Hepatitis • Myelosuppression	• Comfort measures for stomatitis, GI discomforts. • Monitor for complications. • Maintain adequate hydration.
Plant Alkaloids			
• Vincristine sulfate • Vinblastine sulfate	• Acute lymphocytic leukemia • Hodgkin disease • Wilms tumor • Sarcoma • Breast cancer • Testicular cancer	• Bone marrow suppression • Neurotoxicity • Weakness • Paresthesia • Jaw pain • Constipation • Stomatitis • Alopecia • Headaches • Minimal nausea and vomiting	• Administer antiemetics as needed. • Monitor for neurotoxicity. • Check placement and patency of infusing system.
Mitotic Inhibitors			
• Paclitaxel • Docetaxel	• Breast cancer • Ovarian cancer • Nonsmall cell lung cancer • Kaposi sarcoma	• Decreased WBCs and RBCs • Alopecia • Nausea and vomiting, diarrhea • Joint, muscle pain	• Monitor for signs and symptoms of infection. • Administer antiemetics and antidiarrheals as needed.
Hormonal Agents (Corticosteroids)			
• Prednisone • Dexamethasone	• Leukemia • Hodgkin disease • Breast cancer • Lymphoma • Multiple myeloma • Cerebral edema (due to brain metastasis)	• See Endocrine.	• See Endocrine.
Male-Specific Hormonal Agents			
• Flutamide • Leuprolide • Goserelin	• Prostate cancers • Testicular cancers	• Headache, paresthesias, cardiac dysrhythmias, nausea and vomiting, hypoglycemia, neuropathies	• Bone pain and voiding problems. • Safety with neuropathies.

TABLE 4-38 **Antineoplastic Chemotherapeutic Agents—cont'd**

Drugs	Indications	Adverse Reactions	Nursing Implications
Female-Specific Hormonal Agents			
• Tamoxifen citrate • Megestrol • Medroxyprogesterone	• Breast cancer	• Hot flashes • Mild nausea	• Administer antiemetics as needed.
Androgens			
• Testosterone • Fluoxymesterone	• Breast cancer (postmenopausal women)	• Fluid retention • Nausea • Masculinization	• Low-salt diet.
Topoisomerase-I Inhibitors			
• Irinotecan • Topotecan	• Used after failure of initial treatment of ovarian, small-cell lung, and colorectal cancers	• Myelosuppression • Moderate nausea and vomiting • Diarrhea	• Camptosar diarrhea treated with atropine due to physiologic cause. • Give antiemetics per protocol.
Monoclonal Antibodies			
• Trastuzumab • Rituximab	• Targets specific malignant cells with less damage to healthy cells in non-Hodgkin lymphoma, breast cancer	• Fever, chills, infection • Nausea and vomiting, diarrhea • Bronchospasm, dyspnea, acute respiratory distress syndrome • Hypotension • Ventricular dysfunction, HF	• Premedicate with antiemetics. • Monitor for identified side effects.
Biologic Response Modifiers			
Antianemic			
• Epoetin	• Anemia due to chronic renal failure, chemotherapy, HIV-related treatments	• Seizures • HTN • Pain at injection site	• Do not shake vial; may cause inactivation of medication. • Monitor Hct levels. • Pain at injection site; give slowly (subcutaneous).
Granulocyte-Stimulating Factor			
• Filgrastim	• Improves immune competence by increasing neutrophils	• Medullary bone pain during initial treatment • Pain at injection site	• Monitor WBC/differential; absolute neutrophil count (ANC). • Give SC slowly due to local pain at site. • Assess bone pain and medicate with analgesics.

Continued

TABLE 4-38 **Antineoplastic Chemotherapeutic Agents—cont'd**

Biologic Response Modifiers			
Thrombotic Growth Factor			
• Oprelvekin	• Stimulates production of megakaryocytes and platelets	• Dizziness, headache, insomnia, blurred vision, nervousness • Pleural effusion • Vasodilation, cardiac dysrhythmias • Bone pain, myalgia • GI upsets • Fluid retention	• Give slowly to reduce pain at injection site. • Assess for complications related to fluid retention. • Start within 6-24 hours of chemotherapy start and continue for 10-21 days. • Monitor CBC: H&H may decrease; monitor platelets.
Interferon-beta Products			
• Interferon beta-1a • Interferon beta-1b	• Relapsing multiple sclerosis • AIDS • Kaposi sarcoma • Malignant melanoma • Hepatitis C	• Seizures, H/A, weakness, insomnia, depression, suicidal ideation • HTN, chest pain, vasodilation, edema, palpitations • Dyspnea • Nausea and vomiting, elevated liver function studies, GI disorders • Myalgia, flulike symptoms	• Anticipate discomfort from side effects and initiate relief measures early. • Notify physician if evidence of depression. • Sunscreen and protective clothing are needed because of photosensitivity. • Do not shake or swirl solution; use soon after reconstitution. • Monitor CBC and blood chemistries.
Interleukins			
• Aldesleukin	• Metastatic renal cell carcinoma	• Respiratory failure; pulmonary edema • HF, MI, dysrhythmias, stroke • Bowel perforation, hepatomegaly, GI disturbances • Serious electrolyte imbalances • Coagulation disorders • Pancytopenia	• Vigilance in monitoring for serious side effects with stat response.
Interferon-Alfa Products			
• Interferon-alfa-2a • Interferon-alfa-2b	• 2a: hairy cell leukemia, Kaposi sarcoma • 2b: chronic hepatitis B and C, Kaposi sarcoma, hairy cell leukemia	• Similar to those of interferon-beta products	• Similar to those of interferon-beta products
Antiemetics			
• Prochlorperazine • Promethazine HCl	• Nausea and vomiting	• Drowsiness • Dizziness • Extrapyramidal symptoms • Orthostatic hypotension • Blurred vision • Dry mouth	• Dilute oral solution with juice, etc. • Determine baseline BP before administration. • Give deep IM. • Monitor BP carefully.

TABLE 4-38 Antineoplastic Chemotherapeutic Agents—cont'd

Antiemetics			
• Metoclopramide HCl • Haloperidol	• Nausea and vomiting	• Drowsiness • Restlessness • Fatigue • Extrapyramidal symptoms	• Caution client of decreased alertness. • Avoid alcohol. • Discontinue if extrapyramidal symptoms occur.
• Diphenhydramine HCl	• Given with Reglan and Haldol to reduce extrapyramidal symptoms	• Sedation • Dizziness • Hypotension • Dry mouth	• Same as above.
Antiemetics			
• Ondansetron HCl	• Prevention of nausea and vomiting associated with cancer • Postoperative nausea and vomiting	• Headache often requiring analgesic for relief	• Administer tablets 30 minutes before chemotherapy and 1-2 hours before radiation therapy. • Dilute IV injection in 50 mL of 5% dextrose or 0.9% NaCl.
• Granisetron	• Nausea and vomiting associated with chemotherapy and abdominal radiation	• HTN • CNS stimulation • Elevated liver enzymes	• Assess for extrapyramidal symptoms. • Monitor liver enzymes. • Give only on day of chemotherapy or radiation treatment and 1 hour before.

ALL, Acute lymphoblastic anemia; *CML,* cell-mediated lympholysis.

5. It occurs in young to middle-aged adults.
6. Known causes include:
   a. Ionizing radiation
   b. Chemical exposure
7. Prognosis is poor: 5-year survival rate of 37%.
8. Treatment is conservative, involving oral antineoplastic agents.
   a. Hydroxyurea (Hydrea, an inhibitor of DNA synthesis)
   b. Interferon (mechanism of action not known)
   c. Imatinib mesylate (Gleevec) targeted therapy if cells are Philadelphia chromosome positive
C. Acute lymphocytic leukemia (ALL)
   1. Abnormal leukocytes are found in blood-forming tissue.
   2. It occurs in children (is the most common childhood cancer).
   3. The prognosis is favorable: 80% of children treated live 5 years or longer.
D. Chronic lymphocytic leukemia (CLL)
   1. It involves increased production of leukocytes and lymphocytes and proliferation of cells within the bone marrow, spleen, and liver.
   2. It occurs after the age of 35, often in older adults.
   3. The 5-year survival rate is 73% overall.
   4. Most clients are asymptomatic and are not treated.

> **HESI Hint** • A 24-year-old is admitted with large areas of ecchymosis on both upper and lower extremities. She is diagnosed with acute myelogenous leukemia. What are the expected laboratory findings for this client, and what is the expected treatment?
> Laboratory: Decreased Hgb, decreased Hct, decreased platelet count, altered WBC (usually quite high)
> Treatment: Prevention of infection; prevention and control of bleeding; high-protein, high-calorie diet; assistance with ADLs; drug therapy

Nursing Assessment

A. Tendency to bleed
   1. Petechiae
   2. Nosebleeds
   3. Bleeding gums
   4. Ecchymoses
   5. Nonhealing skin abrasions
B. Anemia
   1. Fatigue
   2. Pallor
   3. Headache
   4. Bone and joint pain
   5. Hepatosplenomegaly

C. Infection
  1. Fever
  2. Tachycardia
  3. Lymphadenopathy (swollen lymph nodes)
  4. Night sweats
  5. Skin infection, poor healing
D. GI distress
  1. Anorexia
  2. Weight loss
  3. Sore throat
  4. Abdominal pain
  5. Diarrhea
  6. Oral lesions, typically thrush

HESI Hint • Infection in the immunosuppressed person may not be manifested with an elevated temperature. Therefore it is imperative that the nurse perform a total and thorough assessment of the client frequently.

Analysis (Nursing Diagnoses)

A. *Risk for infection* related to …
B. *Risk for bleeding* related to …
C. *Fatigue* related to …
D. *Anxiety* related to …

Nursing Plans and Interventions for Immunosuppressed Clients and Clients with Bone Marrow Suppression

A. Monitor WBC count daily, and inform physician of count.
B. Routinely assess oral cavity and genital area for signs of yeast infection.
C. Monitor vital signs frequently.
  1. Note baseline.
  2. Report fever to physician as requested.
    a. Be aware that parameters for reporting tend to be lower than those in postoperative clients.
    b. Usually report temperature elevations of 38.05°C or above.
D. Administer antibiotics as prescribed, maintaining a strict schedule.
E. Notify physician if delay in administration occurs.
  1. Obtain trough and peak blood levels of antibiotics.
    a. Trough: draw blood sample shortly before administration of antibiotic.
    b. Peak: draw blood sample 30 minutes to 1 hour after administration of drug.
  2. Monitor blood levels of antibiotics for therapeutic dose range.
F. Teach client and family the importance of infection control:
  1. Wash hands using good handwashing technique.
  2. Avoid contact with any infected person.
  3. Avoid crowds.
  4. Maintain daily hygiene to prevent spread of microorganisms.
  5. Avoid eating uncooked foods; they contain bacteria.
  6. Avoid water standing in cups, vases, etc., because they are excellent sources of growth for microorganisms (especially mold spores).
  7. Neutropenic and reverse isolation precautions PRN.
G. Institute an oral hygiene regimen.
  1. Use soft-bristle toothbrush to avoid bleeding.
  2. Use salt and soda mouth rinse.
  3. Perform oral hygiene after each meal and at bedtime.
  4. Lubricate lips with water-soluble gel.
  5. Avoid lemon-glycerin swabs; they dry oral mucosa.
H. Encourage coughing and deep breathing to prevent stasis of secretions in lungs.
I. Avoid rectal thermometers and suppositories to prevent bleeding.
J. Monitor fluid status and balance; febrile clients dehydrate rapidly.
  1. Monitor I&O.
  2. Encourage fluid intake of at least 3 L per day.
K. Encourage mobility to decrease pulmonary stasis.
L. Provide care for invasive catheters and lines (Box 4-3).
  1. Use strict aseptic technique for all invasive procedures.

HESI Hint • Most oncologic drugs cause immunosuppression. Prevention of secondary infections is vital! Advise client to stay away from persons with known infections such as colds. In the hospital, place client in a private room, and maintain an environment as sterile and as clean as possible. These persons should not eat raw vegetables or fruits—only cooked foods—so as to destroy any bacteria.

  2. Change dressings two or three times per week and when soiled.
  3. Use catheter line for piggybacking medication, depending on the purpose of the line and the fluid being infused; no medications can be piggybacked with an infusion of chemotherapeutic agents.
  4. Central lines and implanted ports can often be used for collecting blood samples, bur regular IV sites cannot.
M. Protect the client from bleeding and injury.
  1. Handle the client gently.
  2. Avoid needle sticks. Use smallest gauge needle possible, and apply pressure for 10 minutes after needle sticks.
  3. Encourage use of electric razor only for shaving.
  4. Instruct client to avoid blowing or picking nose.
  5. Assess for signs of bleeding.
  6. Avoid use of salicylates.

Hodgkin Disease

Description: Malignancy of the lymphoid system that initiates in a single lymph node

BOX 4-3 *Care of Intravenous Lines and Catheters*

Types of IV Lines and Catheters	Use and Care of IV Lines and Catheters
• CVC (nontunneled percutaneous central venous catheter) • Hickman (tunneled catheter) • Broviac (tunneled catheter) • CVC, Hickman, and Broviac type catheters • Port-A-Cath (implanted reservoir) • PICC (peripherally inserted central catheter)	• Stays in place for extended periods of time • Used for clients who require immunosuppressive therapy or are receiving long-term IV therapy • Exit sites include: • At the upper chest • Femoral area • Antecubital area • To prevent an air embolus when a central line is open to air, position client in Trendelenburg position or have client perform a Valsalva maneuver if there is no slide clamp on the line. • Maintain a patent IV site by flushing with heparin or saline. (The amount of heparin used depends on size of lumen, length of tubing, whether reservoir exists [e.g., Port-A-Cath].) • Immediately after insertion of a central line, the nurse should auscultate breath sounds. • After insertion of a central line, a chest radiograph must be taken to determine correct placement and detect pneumothorax (observe for unequal expansion of chest wall).

A. Hodgkin disease is characterized by a generalized painless lymphadenopathy.
B. Incidence is higher in males and young adults.
C. Cause is unknown.
D. Prognosis is good: 5-year survival rate of 90%; however, late recurrences after 5 to 10 years are not uncommon.
E. Diagnosis is made by excision of node for biopsy; characteristic cell is called *Reed-Sternberg.*
F. Determination of stage of disease is done by surgical laparotomy.
  1. Stage I: Involvement of single lymph node region or a single extralymphatic organ or site.
  2. Stage II: Involvement of two or more lymph nodes on the same side of the diaphragm or localized involvement of an extralymphatic organ or site.
  3. Stage III: Involvement of lymph node areas on both sides of the diaphragm to localized involvement of one extralymphatic organ, the spleen, or both.
  4. Stage IV: Diffuse involvement of one or more extralymphatic organs, with or without lymph node involvement.
G. Treatment
  1. Radiotherapy
  2. Chemotherapy: ABVD (Adriamycin, Blenoxane, Velban, Dacarbazine)
  3. Splenectomy

Nursing Assessment

A. Enlarged lymph nodes (one or more) usually cervical lymph nodes

B. Anemia, thrombocytopenia, elevated leukocytes, decreased platelets
C. Fever, increased susceptibility to infections
D. Anorexia, weight loss
E. Malaise, bone pain
F. Night sweats
G. Pruritus
H. Pain in affected lymph node after consuming alcohol

Analysis (Nursing Diagnoses)

A. *Risk for infection* related to …
B. *Anxiety* related to …
C. *Imbalanced nutrition: less than body requirements* related to …
D. *Ineffective tissue perfusion* related to …

Nursing Plans and Interventions

A. Protect client from infection; monitor temperature carefully.
B. Observe for signs of anemia.
C. Provide adequate rest.
D. Provide preoperative and postoperative care for laparotomy or splenectomy.
E. Encourage high-nutrient foods.
F. Provide emotional support to client and family.

HESI Hint • Hodgkin disease is one of the most curable of all adult malignancies. Emotional support is vital. Career development is often interrupted for treatment. Chemotherapy renders many male clients sterile. May bank sperm before treatment, if desired.

General Oncology Content

A. Oncology terms
1. Cancer: a disease characterized by uncontrolled growth of abnormal cells
2. Neoplasm: a new formation
3. Carcinoma: a malignant tumor arising from epithelial tissue
4. Sarcoma: a malignant tumor arising from nonepithelial tissue
5. Differentiation: degree to which neoplastic tissue is different from parent tissue
6. Metastasis: spread of cancer from the original site to other parts of the body
7. Adjuvant therapy: therapy supplemental to the primary therapy
8. Palliative procedure: relieves symptoms without curing the cause

B. Tumors identified by tissue of origin
1. Adeno: glandular tissue
2. Angio: blood vessels
3. Basal cell: epithelium (sun-exposed areas)
4. Embryonal: gonads
5. Fibro: fibrous tissue
6. Lympho: lymphoid tissue
7. Melano: pigmented cells of epithelium
8. Myo: muscle tissue
9. Osteo: bone
10. Squamous cell: epithelium

C. Seven warning signs of cancer
1. Change in usual bowel and bladder function
2. A sore that does not heal
3. Unusual bleeding or discharge, hematuria, tarry stools, ecchymosis, bleeding mole
4. Thickening or a lump in the breast or elsewhere
5. Indigestion or dysphagia
6. Obvious changes in a wart or mole
7. Nagging cough or hoarseness

Review of Hematology and Oncology

1. List three potential causes of anemia.
2. Write two nursing diagnoses for the client suffering from anemia.
3. What is the only IV fluid compatible with blood products?
4. What actions should the nurse take if a hemolytic transfusion reaction occurs?
5. List three interventions for clients with a tendency to bleed.
6. Identify two sites that should be assessed for infection in immunosuppressed clients.
7. Name three food sources of vitamin B_{12}.
8. Describe care of invasive catheters and lines.
9. List three safety precautions for the administration of antineoplastic chemotherapy.
10. Describe the use of leucovorin.
11. Describe the method of collecting the trough and peak blood levels of antibiotics.
12. List four nursing interventions for care of the client with Hodgkin disease.
13. List four topics you would cover when teaching an immunosuppressed client about infection control.

Answers to Review

1. Diet lacking in iron, folate, or vitamin B_{12}; use of salicylates, thiazides, diuretics; exposure to toxic agents, such as lead or insecticides
2. Activity intolerance and ineffective tissue perfusion
3. Normal saline
4. Turn off transfusion. Infuse normal saline using a new bag and new tubing. Take temperature. Send blood being transfused to laboratory. Obtain urine sample. Keep vein patent with normal saline.
5. Use a soft toothbrush, avoid salicylates, do not use suppositories.
6. Oral cavity and genital area
7. Glandular meats (liver), milk, green leafy vegetables
8. Use strict aseptic technique. Change dressings two or three times per week or when soiled. Use caution when piggybacking drugs; check purpose of line and drug to be infused. When possible, use lines to obtain blood samples to avoid "sticking" client.
9. Double check order with another nurse. Check for blood return before administration to ensure that medication does not go into tissue. Use a new IV site daily for peripheral chemotherapy. Wear gloves when handling the drugs, and dispose of waste in special containers to avoid contact with toxic substances.
10. Leucovorin is used as an antidote with methotrexate to prevent toxic reactions.
11. Collection of trough: draw blood 30 minutes before administration of antibiotic.
12. Collection of peak: Draw blood 30 minutes after administration of antibiotic.
13. Protect from infection. Observe for anemia. Encourage high-nutrient foods. Provide emotional support to client and family.
14. Handwashing technique. Avoid infected persons. Avoid crowds. Maintain daily hygiene to prevent spread of microorganisms.

Reproductive System

Benign Tumors of the Uterus (Leiomyomas Fibroids, Myomas, Fibromyomas, Fibromas)

Description: Benign tumors arising from the muscle tissue of the uterus

A. Benign tumors are more common in black women than in white women.

B. Benign tumors are more common in women who have never been pregnant.

C. The most common symptom is abnormal uterine bleeding.

D. They tend to disappear after menopause.

E. They rarely become malignant.

F. Treatment for abnormal uterine bleeding (menorrhagia)
   1. Dilation and curettage (D&C)
      a. Used only in extreme cases of bleeding
      b. For older women when endometrial biopsy and ultrasonography have not provided the necessary diagnostic information
   2. Endometrial ablation
      a. Laser or electrosurgical technique
      b. Successful with many clients with menorrhagia

G. Treatment of uterine fibroids with menorrhagia
   1. Myomectomy (removal of fibroids without removal of the uterus) via laparotomy, laparoscopy, or hysteroscopy
   2. Abdominal or vaginal hysterectomy (see Nursing Plans and Interventions for Hysterectomy, p. 178)
   3. Hormonal regimens (e.g., synthetic analog of gonadotropin-releasing hormone [GnRH], nafarelin [Synarel], leuprolide [Lupron] to shrink the tumor)
   4. Uterine artery embolization (UAE) of the blood vessels supplying the fibroid tumor
   5. Cryosurgery

Nursing Assessment

A. Menorrhagia (hypermenorrhea: profuse or prolonged menstrual bleeding)

B. Dysmenorrhea (extremely painful menstrual periods)

C. Uterine enlargement

D. Low back pain and pelvic pain

> **HESI Hint** • Menorrhagia (profuse or prolonged menstrual bleeding) is the most important factor relating to benign uterine tumors. Assess for signs of anemia.

Nursing Plans and Interventions

A. GnRH
   1. Explain regrowth will occur after the treatment is stopped.
   2. A small loss in bone mass and changes in lipid levels can occur.
   3. Amenorrhea may occur.
   4. Adding raloxifene to GnRH administration has been effective in preventing these effects in premenopausal women.
   5. Women who wish to avoid pregnancy should use a nonhormonal or barrier method of contraception.
   6. Discuss administration methods for GnRH agonists (subcutaneous and intramuscular injections, intranasal administration, and subcutaneous implantation).

B. UAE
   1. Preoperative teaching: Do not drink alcohol, smoke, take aspirin or anticoagulant medications 24 hours before the procedure.
   2. During procedure: Expect cramping during injection of the polyvinyl alcohol pellets (PVA) into selected blood vessels.
   3. Postoperatively: Pelvic pain, fever, malaise, and nausea and vomiting may be caused by acute fibroid degeneration.
   4. Pain may be controlled with a patient-controlled analgesia (PCA) pump.
   5. Postoperative nursing assessments: Check for bleeding in the groin and vital signs, assess pain level, check pedal pulse and neurovascular condition of affected leg.
   6. Discharge teaching
      a. Take prescribed medications as ordered.
      b. Call your physician if you have any of the following symptoms: bleeding, pain, swelling or hematoma at the puncture site, fever of 101° F (38.3° C), urinary retention, or abnormal vaginal drainage (foul odor, brown color, tissue).
      c. Eat a normal diet including fluids and fiber.
      d. Do not use tampons or douche or have vaginal intercourse for at least 4 weeks.
      e. Avoid straining during bowel movements.
      f. Keep your follow-up appointment.
   7. An ultrasound or MRI examination may be done after the UAE to determine the effectiveness of the procedure.

Uterine Prolapse, Cystocele, and Rectocele

Description: Uterine prolapse is downward displacement of the uterus. Cystocele is the relaxation of the anterior vaginal wall with prolapse of the bladder. Rectocele is the relaxation of the posterior vaginal wall with prolapse of the rectum.

A. Preventive measures
   1. Postpartum perineal exercises
   2. Spaced pregnancies
   3. Weight control

B. Surgical intervention
   1. Hysterectomy
   2. Anterior and posterior vaginal repair (A&P repair)

C. Nonsurgical intervention (for uterine prolapse)
1. Kegel exercises
2. Knee-chest position
3. Pessary use

> **HESI Hint** • What is the anatomic significance of a prolapsed uterus? When the uterus is displaced, it impinges on other structures in the lower abdomen. The bladder, rectum, and small intestine can protrude through the vaginal wall.

Nursing Assessment

A. Predisposing conditions
1. Multiparity
2. Pelvic tearing during childbirth
3. Vaginal muscle weakness associated with aging
4. Obesity
B. Symptoms associated with uterine prolapse
1. Dysmenorrhea
2. Pulling and dragging sensations in pelvis and back
3. Dyspareunia
4. Pressure, protrusions
5. Fatigue
6. Low backache
7. Symptoms may be worse after prolonged standing or deep penile penetration during intercourse.
C. Symptoms associated with cystocele
1. Incontinence or stress incontinence (dribbling with coughing or sneezing or any activity that increases intraabdominal pressure)
2. Urinary retention
3. Bladder infections (cystitis)
D. Symptoms associated with rectocele
1. Constipation
2. Hemorrhoids
3. Sense of pressure or need to defecate

Analysis (Nursing Diagnoses)

A. *Chronic pain* related to …
B. *Deficient knowledge* related to …
C. *Disturbed body image* related to …
D. *Alteration in bowel elimination* related to…
E. *Alteration in urine elimination* related to…

Nursing Plans and Interventions for Hysterectomy

A. Provide preoperative and postoperative care
B. Administer enema and douche as prescribed preoperatively.
C. Note amount and character of vaginal discharge. Postoperatively, there should be less than one saturated pad in 4 hours.
D. Avoid rectal thermometers or tubes, especially when A&P repair has been performed.
E. Check extremities for warmth and tenderness as indicators of thrombophlebitis.
F. Pain management postoperatively
1. Assess character of pain, and determine appropriate analgesic.
2. Administer analgesics as needed, and determine effectiveness.
G. Encourage ambulation as soon as possible.
H. Monitor urinary output (Foley catheter is usually inserted in surgery).
I. After catheter removal, assess voiding patterns; catheterize every 6 to 8 hours PRN.
J. Observe incision for bleeding.
K. Note abdominal distention; it may be a sign of gas (flatus) or internal bleeding.
L. Gradually increase diet from liquids to general.
M. Provide stool softeners before first bowel movement and thereafter as needed.
N. Instructions to client regarding follow-up care:
1. Limit tampon use.
2. Avoid douching.
3. Refrain from intercourse until approved by physician (usually 3 to 6 weeks).
4. Avoid heavy lifting (6 to 8 lb) or heavy housework for 4 to 6 weeks postoperatively.
O. Maintain adequate fluid intake (3 L/day).
P. Notify physician of complications:
1. Elevated temperature above 101° F (38.3° C)
2. Redness, pain, or swelling of suture line
3. Foul-smelling vaginal drainage
Q. Encourage verbalization of feelings.

Cancer of the Cervix

Description: Of cancers occurring in the cervix, 95% are squamous cell in origin. Some cervical cancers are directly linked to the human papillomavirus (HPV). Young women between the ages of 9 and 30 years of age are encouraged to be immunized with an intramuscular (IM) injection of quadrivalent HPV (types 6, 11, 16, 18) recombinant vaccine (Gardasil). All women should be tested for HPV, and women over 21 years of age and those who have engaged in sexual intercourse for at least 3 years should continue to have yearly Papanicolaou (Pap) tests.

A. Cancer of the cervix is easily detected early by the Pap test.
B. The precursor to cancer of the cervix is dysplasia.
C. Cancer of the cervix is subdivided into three stages.
1. Early dysplasia can be treated in a variety of ways, including:
    a. Cryosurgery
    b. LEEP (loop electrocautery excision procedure)
    c. Laser
    d. Conization
    e. Hysterectomy

HESI Hint • Laser therapy or cryosurgery is used to treat cervical cancer when the lesion is small and localized. Invasive cancer is treated with radiation, conization, hysterectomy, or pelvic exenteration (a drastic surgical procedure where the uterus, ovaries, fallopian tubes, vagina, rectum, and bladder are removed in an attempt to stop metastasis). Chemotherapy is not useful for this type of cancer.

   2. Early carcinoma can be treated by:
      a. Hysterectomy
      b. Intracavity radiation
   3. Late carcinoma (the tumor size and stage of invasion of surrounding tissues are greater) can be treated by:
      a. External beam radiation along with hysterectomy
      b. Antineoplastic chemotherapy; this is of limited use for cancers arising from squamous cells.
      c. Pelvic exenteration

HESI Hint • American College of Obstetricians and Gynecologists (ACOG) 2016[12] recommendations: Pap smears. In women aged 30–65 years, annual cervical cancer screening should not be performed. (Level A evidence) Patients should be counseled that annual well-woman visits are recommended even if cervical cancer screening is not performed at each visit. Every three years is the recommended time frame for Pap smears. Women ages 30 to 65 years should have a Pap smear with an HPV test every 5 years. Women over 65 do not need a Pap smear. Pap smears should not be performed for any woman under age 21 regardless of onset of sexual activity.

Care of the Client with Radiation Implants

A. Radiation implants are used to treat disease by delivering high-dose radiation seeds directly to the affected tissue.
B. The nurse must take certain precautions for protection of self as well as the client and visitors.
C. Follow specific guidelines provided by the agency. General care guidelines include:
   1. Remind the client that she is not radioactive; only the implants contain radioactivity.
   2. Remind the client that her isolation time is limited; isolation is not necessary indefinitely.
D. Assign client to a private room, and place a "Caution: Radioactive Material" sign on the door.
E. Do not permit pregnant caretakers or pregnant visitors into the room.
F. Keep a lead-lined container in the room for disposal of the implant should it become dislodged.
G. Client should remain in bed with as little movement as possible.
H. Be aware that all client secretions have the potential of being radioactive.
I. Wear latex gloves when handling potentially contaminated secretions.
J. Wear a dosimeter when providing care to clients with radiation implants.
   1. Badge is not to be worn outdoors.
   2. Badge is checked at regular intervals by health officials.
K. Provide nursing care in an efficient but caring manner.
   1. Plan care to limit overall time in the client's room. Time at the bedside is limited—each contact should last no more than 30 minutes. Staff is rotated to limit their exposure.
   2. Staff members should wear a dosimeter during every patient contact to monitor radiation exposure.
   3. When in the room, stand at the greatest possible distance away from the client to minimize exposure.
   4. Stop by frequently to check on the client from the door.
   5. Precautions for nurses' exposure include limit time, maintain distance, and wear protective shielding.
L. Keep all supplies and equipment the client might need within reach.

Ovarian Cancer

Description: Cancer of the ovaries can occur at all ages, including infancy and childhood. Early diagnosis is difficult because no useful screening test exists at present. Malignant germ cell tumors most common in women between 20 and 40 years of age and epithelial cancers occur most often in the perimenopausal age groups.

Nursing Assessment

A. It is asymptomatic in early stages.
B. Laparotomy is the primary tool for diagnosis and staging of the disease; ovarian cancer is surgically staged rather than clinically staged.
C. Advanced clinical manifestations include:
   1. Pelvic discomfort
   2. Low back pain and leg pain
   3. Weight change
   4. Abdominal pain
   5. Increased abdominal girth
   6. Nausea and vomiting
   7. Constipation
   8. Urinary frequency

Analysis (Nursing Diagnoses)

A. *Anticipatory grieving* related to …
B. *Chronic pain* related to …
C. *Readiness for enhanced self-care* (specify) related to …

Nursing Plans and Interventions

A. Provide the care required after any major abdominal surgery after laparotomy (see Nursing Plans and Interventions for Hysterectomy, p. 178).

B. Provide the care required for a client on chemotherapy (see Nursing Plans and Interventions for Immunosuppressed Clients, p. 174).

C. Teach client and family about disease and follow-up treatment.

D. Offer supportive care to client and family throughout diagnosis and treatment.

> **HESI Hint** • The major emphasis in nursing management of cancers of the reproductive tract is early detection.

Breast Cancer

Description: Cancer originating in the breast

A. Breast cancer is the leading cancer in women in the United States.

B. One in eight women will develop breast cancer in her lifetime.

C. Early detection is important to successful treatment.

D. Men can develop breast cancer. They account for less than 1% of reported cases.

E. Of all breast cancers, 90% to 95% are discovered through breast self-examination.

F. Risk factors include:
1. Positive family history
2. Menarche before 12 years of age and menopause after age 50
3. Nulliparous and those bearing first child after age 30
4. History of uterine cancer
5. Daily alcohol intake
6. Highest incidence: those age 40 to 49 and over 65

G. Breast cancer is generally adenocarcinoma, originating in epithelial cells, and it occurs in the ducts or lobes.

H. Tumors tend to be located in the upper outer quadrant of the breast and more often in the left breast than the right.

I. Early detection is important.
1. Every woman should perform a breast self-examination monthly, preferably as soon as menstrual bleeding ceases or if postmenopausal, the same date every month.

> **HESI Hint** • The importance of teaching female clients how to conduct a breast self-examination cannot be overemphasized. Early detection results in positive outcomes.

2. Mammography is very helpful in early detection of cancer of the breast.
   a. Baseline mammogram at approximately 35 to 40 years of age
   b. Mammogram every 1 to 2 years for women in their 40s
   c. Annual mammogram for women over 50 years of age

d. No use of lotions, talc powder, or deodorant under arms before procedure (may mimic calcium deposits on radiograph)

3. Physical examination by a professional skilled in examination of the breast should be done annually.

J. Tumors less than 4 cm are deemed curable.

K. Larger tumors require much more aggressive treatment (cure is difficult).

L. Definitive diagnosis of cancer of the breast is made by biopsy.

M. Common sites of metastasis (spread) are the axillary, supraclavicular, and mediastinal lymph nodes, followed by metastases to the lungs, liver, brain, and spine.

N. Bone metastasis is extremely painful.

O. Treatment is dependent on the stage of disease.
1. Mastectomy is commonly performed.
   a. Alternatives to mastectomy are lumpectomy/partial mastectomy.
   b. Axillary lymph node dissection often performed in conjunction with other surgery
2. Adjuvant treatment consists of radiation (either external beam or implants), antineoplastic chemotherapy, and hormonal therapy.
   a. Targeted therapy such as Estrogen inhibitors (tamoxifen) or trastuzumab.
   b. Aromatase inhibitors

> **HESI Hint** • The presence or absence of hormone receptors is paramount in selecting clients for adjuvant therapy.

Nursing Assessment

A. Hard lump (not freely movable and not painful)
B. Dimpling of skin
C. Retraction of nipple
D. Alterations in contour of breast
E. Change in skin color
F. Change in skin texture (peau d'orange)
G. Discharge from nipple
H. Pain and ulcerations (late signs)
I. Diagnostic tests include:
1. Mammogram
2. Biopsy and frozen section

Analysis (Nursing Diagnoses)

A. *Disturbed body image* related to …
B. *Anticipatory grieving* related to …
C. *Acute or chronic pain* related to …
D. *Readiness for enhanced self-care* (specify) related to …

Nursing Plans and Interventions

A. Assess lesion
1. Location
2. Size
3. Shape

4. Consistency
5. Fixation to surrounding tissues
6. Lymph node involvement

B. Preoperative
   1. Explore client's expectations of surgery and what the surgical site will look like postoperatively.
   2. Discuss skin graft if one is possible and cosmetic reconstruction that might be implemented with mastectomy or at a later time.

C. Postoperative
   1. Monitor bleeding; check under dressing, Hemovac, and under client's back (bleeding will run to back).
   2. Position arm on operative side on a pillow, slightly elevated.
   3. Avoid BP measurements, injections, and venipuncture in arm where surgery occurred.
   4. Instruct client to avoid injury such as burns or scrapes to affected arm.
   5. Encourage hand activity for the arm on the side where surgery occurred by squeezing a small rubber ball.
   6. Encourage client to perform activities that will use arm, like brushing hair.
   7. Teach postmastectomy exercises (wall climbing with affected arm and rope turning).

D. Encourage client to verbalize concerns.
   1. Cancer
   2. Death
   3. Loss of breast

E. Encourage client to discuss operation, diagnosis, feelings, concerns, and fears.

F. Be with client when she first looks at the operative site; offer emotional support.

G. Arrange for Reach to Recovery (American Cancer Society); physician prescription required.

H. Recognize the grief process.
   1. Allow client to cry, withdraw, etc.
   2. Help client to focus on the future while allowing discussions of loss.

I. If reconstruction was not discussed preoperatively, encourage client to discuss or explore these options postoperatively.

J. Discuss use of temporary and permanent prostheses.

Testicular Cancer

Description: Cancer of the testes is the leading cause of death from cancer in males 15 to 35 years of age. If untreated, death usually occurs within 2 to 3 years. If detected and treated early, there is a 90% to 100% chance of cure.

Nursing Assessment

A. Early signs are subtle and usually go unnoticed.
B. There is a feeling of heaviness or dragging sensation in lower abdomen and groin.

C. There is a lump or swelling (painless) on the testicle. Late signs include:
   1. Low back pain
   2. Weight loss
   3. Fatigue

Analysis (Nursing Diagnoses)

A. *Deficient knowledge* (specify) related to …
B. *Disturbed body image* related to …
C. *Anticipatory grieving* related to …

> **HESI Hint** • Men whose testes have not descended into the scrotum or whose testes descended after age 6 are at high risk for developing testicular cancer. The most common symptom is the appearance of a small, hard lump about the size of a pea on the front or side of the testicle. Testicular self-examination (TSE) should be done regularly at the same time every month by all males after age 14. It should be done after a shower by gently palpating the testes and cord to look for a small lump. Swelling may also be a sign of testicular cancer.

Nursing Plans and Interventions

A. Postoperative care after orchidectomy:
   1. Observe for hemorrhage.
   2. Active movement may be contraindicated.
B. Care for clients receiving radiation therapy.
C. Encourage genetic counseling (sperm banking is often recommended before surgery).
D. Counsel that sexual functioning is usually not affected because the remaining testis undergoes hyperplasia, producing sufficient testosterone to maintain sexual functioning. Although ejaculatory ability may be decreased, orgasm is still possible.

Cancer of the Prostate

Description: Prostate cancer rarely occurs before 40 years of age, but it is the second-leading cause of death from cancer in American men. High-risk groups include those with a history of multiple sexual partners, sexually transmitted diseases (STDs), certain viral infections, and family history.

Nursing Assessment

A. Asymptomatic if confined to gland
B. Symptoms of urinary obstruction
C. With metastasis: low back pain, fatigue, aching in legs, and hip pain
D. Elevated prostate-specific antigen (PSA)
   1. PSA test should be conducted before a digital rectal examination (DRE) so that manipulation of the prostate does not give a false-positive reading.
   2. Serial blood screening should be done to observe trends. A rise in PSA or consistently high PSA is more reliable than a single assay.

3. PSA levels can rise with inflammation, benign hypertrophy, or irritation, as well as in response to cancer.
E. Elevated prostatic acid phosphatase (PAP)
F. DRE revealing palpable nodule
G. Transrectal ultrasound (TRUS) visualizing nonpalpable tumors
H. Definitive diagnosis by biopsy

Analysis (Nursing Diagnoses)

A. *Deficient knowledge* (specify) related to …
B. *Altered body image* related to …
C. *Sexual dysfunction* related to…

Nursing Plans and Interventions

A. Teach the importance of early detection.
B. Suggest resources: local and national prostate cancer support groups; information is also available from the American Cancer Society (Man to Man program) and the Urology Care Foundation.
C. Prepare client for radiation therapy
1. External beam "teletherapy" radiation irradiates the prostate and pelvic region, and conformal techniques allow the delivery of a higher radiation dose without increasing the risk of complications by focusing the radiation and limiting the exposure of adjacent structures.
a. Explain how treatments help cancer.
(1) Need for repetitive treatments
(2) Attend all sessions for successful outcome.
b. Expected outcomes
c. Side effects
(1) Radiation-induced cystitis or proctitis
(2) Dysuria (discomfort with voiding): Subsides within 4 to 6 weeks; reduce intake of foods or beverages likely to irritate the bowel or bladder, including caffeine and heavily spiced or fatty foods.
(3) Daytime voiding frequency
(4) Increase in the number of times client awakens to void
(5) Suprapubic discomfort—may irritate the perineal skin; teach client to cleanse the perineal skin with a mild cleanser and lukewarm water, pay special attention to skin folds, and pat dry, wearing loose cotton clothing to help relieve skin irritation.
(6) Fatigue and loss of appetite: six small meals per day, foods that are high in protein and carbohydrates; a multivitamin should be taken daily throughout radiation therapy.
2. Proton beam radiotherapy combines conformal imaging and charged protons to target more specifically prostate cancer cells while limiting damage to the overlying skin or adjacent structures including the bladder and rectum (see External Beam Radiation).
3. Brachytherapy is the internal implantation of radioactive iodine-125 or palladium-103 seeds directly into the prostate, which emit highly localized radiation energy to kill localized cancer cells without excessive harm to nearby healthy cells.
a. Preparation includes bowel cleansing and administration of prophylactic antibiotics
b. A clear liquid diet 12 to 24 hours before the procedure
c. Rectal pressure or mild discomfort is felt when the ultrasound probe is placed, but pain is not associated with implantation of radioactive seeds.
d. A catheter is left in place that may be removed on the day of the procedure. Complete a voiding trial with removal of the catheter.
e. Seed implantation will cause inflammation of the prostate and may cause symptoms including daytime voiding frequency, an increase in nocturia, and difficulty initiating a urinary stream. These manifestations are typically transient and subside as prostatic inflammation diminishes.
f. Semen may have a brownish color over the first 1 to 2 months after implantation; intercourse should be avoided during this period and childbearing is contraindicated.
g. Monitor stool for passage of large volumes of bright red blood (rare), and advise client about how to manage radiation cystitis and proctitis.
h. Teach the client and partner the principles of radiation safety.
i. Avoid close contact with pregnant women and infants, refrain from having children (or adults) sit in their lap for a prolonged period during the first 2 months after therapy.
D. Provide preoperative bowel preparation to prevent fecal contamination of operative site.
1. Enemas and cathartics
2. Sulfasalazine (Azulfidine) or neomycin
3. Clear fluids only the day before surgery to prevent fecal contamination of operative site
E. Provide postoperative care.
1. Monitor for urine leaks, hemorrhage, and signs of infection.
2. Provide support dressing or supportive underwear to perineal incision.
3. Use donut cushion to relieve pressure on incision site while sitting.
4. Avoid rectal manipulation (rectal thermometers, rectal tubes, and hard suppositories).
5. Provide low-residue diet until wound healing is advanced.
6. Institute measures to prevent bowel action in the first postoperative week to prevent contamination of incision.

Sexually Transmitted Diseases (STDs)

Description: STDs are diseases that can be transmitted during intimate sexual contact.

A. STDs are the most prevalent communicable diseases in the United States.

B. Most cases of STDs occur in adolescents and young adults.

> **HESI Hint** • STDs in infants and children usually indicate sexual abuse and should be reported. The nurse is legally responsible to report suspected cases of child abuse.

Nursing Assessment

See Table 4-39.

Analysis (Nursing Diagnoses)

A. *Deficient knowledge* (specify) related to …

B. *Anxiety* related to …

C. *Anticipatory grieving* related to …

> **HESI Hint** • Chlamydia is the most commonly reported communicable disease in the United States.

Nursing Plans and Interventions

A. Use a nonjudgmental approach; be straightforward when taking history.

B. Reassure client that all information is strictly confidential. Obtain a complete sexual history, which should include:

1. The client's sexual orientation

TABLE 4-39 Sexually Transmitted Diseases and Treatment Options

STD	Symptoms	Treatment
Treponema pallidum, *Syphilis*		
Laboratory diagnosis: VDRL, FTA-ABS	**Primary (local):** up to 90 days postexposure • Chancre (red, painless lesions with indurated border) • Highly infectious **Secondary (systemic):** 6 weeks to 6 months postexposure • Influenza-type symptoms • Generalized rash that affects palms of hands and soles of feet • Lesions contagious **Tertiary:** 10-30 years postexposure • Cardiac and neurologic destruction	• Penicillin G IM (usually 2.4 million units) • If penicillin-allergic (adults), alternatives: tetracycline, or doxycycline, or ceftriaxone
Neisseria gonorrheae, *Gonorrhea*		
Laboratory diagnosis: smears, cultures	• Females: majority are asymptomatic • Males: dysuria, yellowish-green urethral discharge, urinary frequency	• Ceftriaxone sodium plus doxycycline hyclate or azithromycin • Cefixime plus doxycycline or azithromycin
Chlamydia trachomatis, *Chlamydia*		
Laboratory diagnosis: tissue culture; chlamydiazyme; MicroTrak	• Females: many asymptomatic, but may exhibit dysuria, urgency, vaginal discharge, oral temp >38.3, uterine or adnexal tenderness • Males: leading cause of nongonococcal urethritis	• Doxycycline hyclate or azithromycin • Cefoxitin Gentamycin
Trichomonas vaginalis, *Trichomoniasis*		
Laboratory diagnosis: wet slide	• Females: green, yellow, or white frothy foul-smelling vaginal discharge with itching • Males: asymptomatic	• Metronidazole (Flagyl) (male partners to be treated to prevent reinfection)
Candida albicans, *Candidiasis*		
Laboratory diagnosis: viral culture	• Females: odorless, white or yellow, cheesy discharge with itching • Males: asymptomatic	• Miconazole nitrate (Monistat) • Clotrimazole (Gyne-Lotrimin) • Nystatin (Mycostatin) • Fluconazole (Diflucan) PO single dose

Continued

TABLE 4-39 Sexually Transmitted Diseases and Treatment Options—cont'd

STD	Symptoms	Treatment
Herpes Simplex Virus 2, Herpes		

	• Vesicles in clusters that rupture and leave painful erosions that cause painful urination
	• Characterized by remissions and exacerbations
	• May be contagious even when asymptomatic
		• Acyclovir (Zovirax) partially controls symptoms
		• Famciclovir
		• Valacyclovir
		• Palliative care
		  • Viscous lidocaine topically to ease pain
		  • Keep lesions clean and dry

Human Papillomavirus (HPV)		
	• Multiple strains (>70), some of which are implicated in cervical cancer • Alarming rate increase in adolescent population • Lesions may be small, wartlike or clustered. • May be flat or raised	• Routine vaccination is recommended for select populations before onset of sexual activity. • Applied medications such as podophyllum resin (contraindicated in pregnancy) • Trichloroacetic acid (TCA) • Laser • Cryotherapy (freezing)
Human Immunodeficiency Virus (HIV), AIDS		
	(See Advanced Clinical Concepts)	

FTA-ABS, Fluorescent treponemal antibody absorption; *VDRL,* Venereal Disease Research Laboratory.

2. Sexual practices
  a. Penile-vaginal
  b. Penile-anal
  c. Penile-oral
  d. Oral-vaginal
  e. Anal-oral
3. Type of protection (barrier) used
4. Contraceptive practices
5. Previous history of STDs
C. Develop teaching plan and include:
  1. Signs and symptoms of STDs
  2. Mode of transmission of STDs
  3. Reminder that sexual contact should be avoided with anyone while infected
  4. Assess literacy level of client and if appropriate provide written instructions about treatment; request a return verbalization of these instructions to ensure the client has heard the instructions and understands them.
D. Encourage client to provide information regarding all sexual contacts.
E. Report incidents of STDs to appropriate health agencies and departments.
F. Instruct women of childbearing age about risks to a newborn:
  1. Gonorrheal conjunctivitis
  2. Neonatal herpes
  3. Congenital syphilis
  4. Oral candidiasis

HESI Hint • Pelvic inflammatory disease (PID) involves one or more of the pelvic structures. The infection can cause adhesions and eventually result in sterility. Manage the pain associated with PID with analgesics. Bed rest in a semi-Fowler position may increase comfort and promote drainage. Antibiotic treatment is necessary to reduce inflammation and pain and should be effective for N. Gonorrhea and C. trachomatis.

G. Teach safer sex.
  1. Reduce the number of sexual contacts.
  2. Avoid sex with those who have multiple partners.
  3. Examine genital area, and avoid sexual contact if anything abnormal is present.
  4. Wash hands and genital area before and after sexual contact.
  5. Use a latex condom as a barrier.
  6. Use water-based lubricants rather than oil-based lubricants.
  7. Use a vaginal spermicidal gel.
  8. Avoid douching before and after sexual contact; douching increases risk for infections because the body's normal defenses are reduced or destroyed.
  9. Seek attention from health care provider immediately if symptoms occur.

HESI Hint • A client comes into the clinic with a chancre on his penis. What is the usual treatment? IM dose of penicillin (such as benzathine penicillin G, 2.4 million units). Obtain a sexual history, including the names of his sex partners, so that they can receive treatment.

Review of Reproductive System

1. What are the indications for a hysterectomy in a client who has fibromas?
2. List the symptoms and conditions associated with a cystocele.
3. What are the most important nursing interventions for the postoperative client who has had a hysterectomy with an A&P repair?
4. Describe the priority nursing care for a client who has had radiation implants.
5. What screening tool is used to detect cervical cancer? What are the American Cancer Society's recommendations for the Pap smear screening for females under age 21?
6. Cite two nursing diagnoses for a client undergoing a hysterectomy for cervical cancer.
7. What are the three most important tools for early detection of breast cancer? How often should these tools be used?
8. Describe three nursing interventions to help decrease edema postmastectomy.
9. Name three priorities to include in a discharge plan for a client who has had a mastectomy.
10. What is the most common cause of nongonococcal urethritis?
11. What is the causative organism of syphilis?
12. Malodorous, frothy, greenish-yellow vaginal discharge is characteristic of which STD?
13. Which STD is characterized by remissions and exacerbations in both males and females?
14. Outline a teaching plan for a client with an STD.

Answers to Review

1. Severe menorrhagia leading to anemia, severe dysmenorrhea requiring narcotic analgesics, severe uterine enlargement causing pressure on other organs, severe low back and pelvic pain
2. Symptoms include incontinence or stress incontinence, urinary retention, and recurrent bladder infections. Conditions associated with cystocele include multiparity, trauma in childbirth, and aging.
3. Avoid taking rectal temperatures and rectal manipulation; manage pain; and encourage early ambulation.
4. Do not permit pregnant visitors or pregnant caretakers in room. Discourage visits by small children. Confine client to room. Nurse must wear radiation badge. Nurse limits time in room. Keep supplies and equipment within client's reach.
5. Females under the age of 21 should not have Pap smear screenings.
6. Altered body image related to uterine removal; pain related to postoperative incision
7. Breast self-examination monthly; mammogram baseline at age 35, followed by examinations every 1 to 2 years in 40s and every year after age 50; physical examination by a professional skilled in examination of the breast
8. Position arm on operative side on pillow. Avoid BP measurements, injections, and venipunctures in operative arm. Encourage hand activity and use.
9. Arrange for Reach to Recovery visit. Discuss the grief process with the client. Have physician discuss with client the reconstruction options.
10. Chlamydia trachomatis
11. Treponema pallidum (spirochete bacteria)
12. Trichomonas vaginalis
13. Herpes simplex type II
14. Signs and symptoms of STD; mode of transmission; avoiding sex while infected; providing concise written instructions regarding treatment, and requesting a return verbalization to ensure that the client understands; teaching safer sex practices

Burns

Description: Tissue injury or necrosis caused by transfer of energy from a heat source to the body
A. Categories
   1. Thermal
   2. Radiation
   3. Electrical
   4. Chemical
B. Tissue destruction results from
   1. Coagulation
   2. Protein denaturation
   3. Ionization of cellular contents
C. Critical systems affected include
   1. Respiratory
   2. Integumentary
   3. Cardiovascular
   4. Renal
   5. GI
   6. Neurologic
D. Severity is determined by burn depth (Fig. 4-10).
   1. First degree
      a. Superficial partial-thickness (e.g., sunburn)
      b. Injury to the epidermis

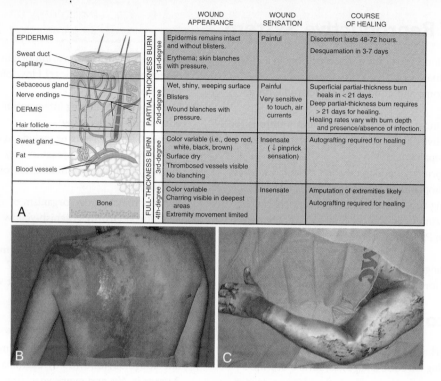

		WOUND APPEARANCE	WOUND SENSATION	COURSE OF HEALING
PARTIAL-THICKNESS BURN	1st-degree	Epidermis remains intact and without blisters. Erythema; skin blanches with pressure.	Painful	Discomfort lasts 48-72 hours. Desquamation in 3-7 days
	2nd-degree	Wet, shiny, weeping surface Blisters Wound blanches with pressure.	Painful Very sensitive to touch, air currents	Superficial partial-thickness burn heals in < 21 days. Deep partial-thickness burn requires > 21 days for healing. Healing rates vary with burn depth and presence/absence of infection.
FULL-THICKNESS BURN	3rd-degree	Color variable (i.e., deep red, white, black, brown) Surface dry Thrombosed vessels visible No blanching	Insensate (↓ pinprick sensation)	Autografting required for healing
	4th-degree	Color variable Charring visible in deepest areas Extremity movement limited	Insensate	Amputation of extremities likely Autografting required for healing

EPIDERMIS
Sweat duct
Capillary
Sebaceous gland
Nerve endings
DERMIS
Hair follicle
Sweat gland
Fat
Blood vessels
Bone

FIGURE 4-10 A, The tissues involved in burns of various depths. B, Partial-thickness burn injury. C, Full-thickness burn injury. (From Black JM, Hawks JH: *Medical-surgical nursing: clinical management for positive outcomes,* ed 8, St. Louis, 2009, Saunders.)

c. Leaves skin pink or red, but no blisters
d. Dry
e. Painful (relieved by cooling)
f. Slight edema
g. No scarring, and skin grafts are not required

2. Second degree
   a. Deep partial-thickness destruction of epidermis and upper layers of dermis
   b. Injury to deeper portions of the dermis
   c. Painful (sensitive to touch and cold air)
   d. Appears red or white, weeps fluid, blisters present
   e. Hair follicles intact (i.e., hair does not pull out easily)
   f. Very edematous
   g. Blanching followed by capillary refill
   h. Heals without surgical intervention, usually does not scar

3. Third degree
   a. Full-thickness and deep full-thickness; involves total destruction of dermis and epidermis
   b. Skin cannot regenerate
   c. Requires skin grafting
   d. Underlying tissue (fat, fascia, tendon, bone) may be involved
   e. Wound appears dry and leathery as eschar develops
   f. Painless

E. Severity is determined by extent of surface area burned.
   1. Rule of nines: head and neck 9%, upper extremities 9% each, lower extremities 18% each, front trunk

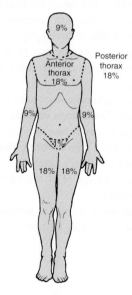

FIGURE 4-11 The rule of nines for estimating burn percentage. (From Black JM, Hawks JH: *Medical-surgical nursing: clinical management for positive outcomes,* ed 8, St. Louis, 2009, Saunders.)

18%, back trunk 18%, perineal area 1% for adults (Fig. 4-11)

   2. Lund and Browder method: Estimates the percentage of the body surface area burned; percentages are assigned to specific body parts based on the client's age; critical body areas are face, hands, feet, and perineum (Table 4-40).

TABLE 4-40 Lund and Browder Chart

Area	1 Year	1-4 Years	5-9 Years	10-14 Years	15 Years	Adult
Head	19	17	13	11	9	7
Neck	2	2	2	2	2	2
Anterior trunk	13	13	13	13	13	13
Posterior trunk	13	13	13	13	13	13
Right buttock	2½	2½	2½	2½	2½	2½
Left buttock	2½	2½	2½	2½	2½	2½
Genitalia	1	1	1	1	1	1
Right upper arm	4	4	4	4	4	4
Left upper arm	4	4	4	4	4	4
Right lower arm	3	3	3	3	3	3
Left lower arm	3	3	3	3	3	3
Right hand	2½	2½	2½	2½	2½	2½
Left hand	2½	2½	2½	2½	2½	2½
Right thigh	5½	6½	8	8½	9	9½
Left thigh	5½	6½	8	8½	9	9½
Right leg	5	5	5½	6	6½	7
Left leg	5	5	5½	6	6½	7
Right foot	½	3½	3½	3½	3½	3½
Left foot	3½	3½	3½	3½	3½	3½

F. Three stages of burn care
  1. Stage I: Resuscitative/emergent phase
     a. Begins at the time of injury and concludes with the restoration of capillary permeability, which typically reverses 48 to 72 hours after the injury.
     b. Is characterized by fluid shift from intravascular to interstitial and shock; focus of care is to preserve vital organ functioning.
     c. Expect to administer large volumes of fluid in this phase based on the client's weight and extent of injury.
     d. Fluid replacement formulas are calculated from the time of injury and not from the time of arrival at the hospital.
  2. Stage II: Acute phase
     a. Occurs from beginning of diuresis (48 to 72 hours after injury) to near completion of wound closure.
     b. Is characterized by fluid shift from interstitial to intravascular.
     c. Focus is on infection control, wound care and closure, pain management, nutritional support, and physical therapy.
  3. Stage III: Rehabilitation phase
     a. Occurs from major wound closure to return to optimal level of physical and psychosocial adjustment (approximately 5 years)
     b. Is characterized by grafting and rehabilitation specific to the client's needs

Nursing Assessment
A. Absence of bowel sounds indicating paralytic ileus
B. Radically decreased urinary output in the first 72 hours after injury, with increased specific gravity
C. Radically increased urinary output (diuresis) 72 hours to 2 weeks after initial injury
D. Signs of inadequate hydration
  1. Restlessness
  2. Disorientation
  3. Decreased urinary volume and urinary sodium and increased urine specific gravity
E. Signs of inhalation burn
  1. Red or burned face
  2. Singed facial and nasal hairs
  3. Circumoral burns
  4. Conjunctivitis
  5. Sooty nasal mucus or bloody sputum

6. Hoarseness
7. Asymmetry of chest movements with respirations and use of accessory muscles indicative of hypoxia
8. Rales, wheezing, and rhonchi denoting smoke inhalation
9. Impaired speech and drooling indicating laryngeal edema

F. Description of physiologic responses to burns (Fig. 4-12)
G. Preexisting conditions or illnesses that may influence recovery

---

HESI Hint • ABCs of Assessment
- Airway
- Breathing
- Circulation

Analysis (Nursing Diagnoses)

A. *Ineffective airway clearance* related to …
B. *Impaired gas exchange* related to …
C. *Decreased cardiac output* related to …
D. *Deficient fluid volume* related to …
E. *Ineffective tissue perfusion* (specify) related to …
F. *Impaired skin integrity* related to …
G. *Acute pain* related to …
H. *Disturbed body image* related to …
I. *Imbalanced nutrition: less than body requirements* related to …
J. *Risk for infection* related to …
K. *Impaired physical mobility* related to …

Nursing Plans and Interventions

A. Emergent phase: Efforts are directed toward stabilization with ongoing assessment.
   1. Assist with admission care.
      a. Extinguish source of burn (burning may continue with clothing attached to skin).
         (1) Thermal: Remove clothing, cool burns by immersion in tepid water, apply dry sterile dressings.
         (2) Chemical: Flush with water or normal saline.
         (3) Electrical: Separate client from electrical source.
      b. Provide an open airway; intubation may be necessary if laryngeal edema is a risk.
      c. Determine baseline data: vital signs, blood gases, weight.
      d. Determine depth and extent of burn.

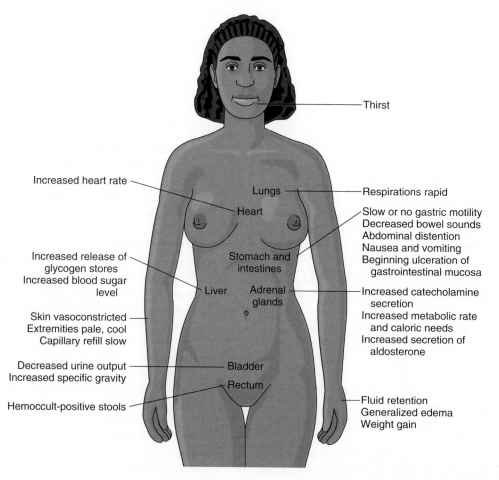

FIGURE 4-12 The physiologic actions of the sympathetic nervous system's compensatory responses to burn injury (early phase). (From Ignatavicius DD, Workman ML: *Medical-surgical nursing: patient-centered collaborative care,* ed 7, St. Louis, 2013, Saunders.)

e. Administer tetanus toxoid.

f. Initiate fluid and electrolyte therapy: Ringer's lactate solution with electrolytes and colloids adjusted according to laboratory results and fluid resuscitation formula used.

> **HESI Hint** • Massive volumes of IV fluids are given. It is not uncommon to give over 1000 mL/hr during various phases of burn care. Hemodynamic monitoring must be closely observed to be sure the client is supported with fluids but is not overloaded.

g. Insert NG tube to prevent vomiting, abdominal distention, and gastric aspiration.

h. Administer IV pain medication as prescribed.

2. Monitor hydration status.

a. Record urinary output hourly (30 to 100 mL/hr is normal range).

b. Maintain IV fluids titrated to keep urine output at 30 to 100 mL/hr.

c. Accurately record I&O.

d. Weigh daily.

e. Observe for signs of inadequate hydration:
(1) Restlessness
(2) Disorientation
(3) Hypothermia
(4) Decreased urine output

3. Monitor respiratory functioning.

a. Provide care for the intubated client.

b. Suction endotracheal or nasotracheal tube, when needed.

c. Monitor ABGs.

d. Observe for cyanosis, disorientation.

e. Administer O_2.

f. Encourage use of incentive spirometer, coughing, and deep breathing.

g. Elevate the head of the bed to 30 degrees or more for burns of the face and head.

4. Provide wound care.

a. Use strict aseptic technique.

> **HESI Hint** • Infection is a life-threatening risk for those with burns.

b. Perform débridement and dressing changes according to client's condition.

c. Change dressings in minimum time (very painful); premedicate client; maintain sterile technique.

d. Maintain room temperature above 90° F, humidified and free of drafts.

e. Monitor body temperature frequently; have hyperthermia blankets available.

5. Assess for paralytic ileus.

a. Absence of bowel sounds

b. Nausea and vomiting

c. Abdominal distention

6. Assist with management of pain.

a. Administer analgesics intravenously.

b. Teach distraction and relaxation techniques.

c. Teach use of guided imagery.

7. Assess for circulatory compromise in burns that constrict body parts. Prepare client for escharotomy.

8. Provide proper nutrition.

a. Maintain NPO status until bowel sounds are heard, and then advance to clear liquids as prescribed.

b. Provide a diet high in protein, carbohydrates, fats, and vitamins.

c. Monitor caloric intake.

B. Acute phase: Characterized by fluid shift from interstitial to intravascular (diuresis begins); occurs from 72 hours to 2 weeks after initial injury to near completion of wound closure.

1. Provide infection control, including the following:

a. Maintain protective isolation of entire burn unit.

b. Cover hair at all times.

c. Wear masks during dressing changes.

d. Use sterile technique for hydrotherapy, dressing change, and débridement.

e. Administer IV antibiotics if indicated.

f. Be sure any live plants and flowers are removed from room; they are prohibited.

2. Splint and position client to prevent contractures. Avoid use of pillows in cases of neck burns.

3. Perform ROM exercises; they are painful.

a. Administer pain medication immediately before performing ROM exercises.

b. Perform active ROM exercises for 3 to 5 minutes frequently during day.

c. Mobilize as soon as possible using splints designed for the client.

d. Encourage active ROM exercises when up and about.

4. Provide fluid therapy; may use colloids to keep fluid in vascular space.

a. Monitor serum chemistries at all times.

b. Keep an IV site available; a saline lock or peripherally inserted central catheter (PICC) for long-term use is helpful.

c. Maintain strict I&O.

d. Encourage oral intake of fluids.

5. Provide adequate nutrition.

a. Provide high-calorie (up to 5000 calories/day), high-protein, high-carbohydrate diet.

b. Give nutritional supplements via NG tube or enteral tube feeding at night if caloric intake is inadequate.

c. Keep accurate calorie counts.

d. Administer all medications with either milk or juice.

e. May require total parenteral nutrition (TPN)

f. Weigh daily.

> **HESI Hint** • Dressing changes are very painful! Medicate client before procedure!

6. Provide burn and wound care.
   a. Clean wound per agency routine (daily or up to three times a day) in hydrotherapy or shower.
   b. Apply silver sulfadiazine (Silvadene) or mafenide acetate (Sulfamylon), silver impregnated dressings like Acticoat can be left in place for 3 to 14 days or other antimicrobial agents to burn area as prescribed (Table 4-41).
   c. Cover with dressing (closed method) or leave open (open method), according to agency policy or physician's prescription.
   d. Prepare client for grafting when eschar has been removed.

e. Prepare client for autografts (use of client's own skin for grafting).

f. Use heat lamp to donor site after graft to allow the area to reepithelialize.

> **HESI Hint** • Preexisting conditions that might influence burn recovery are age, chronic illness (diabetes, cardiac problems, etc.), physical disabilities, disease, medications used routinely, and drug or alcohol abuse.

C. Rehabilitation phase: Characterized by the absence of infection risk
   1. Ongoing discharge planning occurs.
   2. Client may return home when the danger of infection has been eliminated.
   3. High-protein fluids with vitamin supplements are recommended.
   4. Pressure dressings such as Jobst garments may be worn continuously to prevent hypertrophic scarring and contractures.

TABLE 4-41 Topical Antimicrobial Agents

Drugs	Indications	Adverse Reactions	Nursing Implications
• Mafenide acetate	• Treatment of burns • Usually used with open method of wound care	• Painful • Causes mild acidosis	• Administer pain medication *before* dressing change. • Penetrates wound rapidly
• Silver sulfadiazine	• Treatment of burns • Usually used with open method of wound care • Used to avoid acid–base complications • Keeps eschar soft, making débridement easier	• Penetrates wound slowly	• Administer pain medication *before* dressing change.

Review of Burns

1. List four categories of burns.
2. Burn depth is a measure of severity. Describe the characteristics of superficial partial-thickness, deep partial-thickness, and full-thickness burns.
3. Describe fluid management in the emergent phase, acute phase, and rehabilitation phase of the burned client.
4. Describe pain management of the burned client.
5. Outline admission care of the burned client.
6. Nutritional status is a major concern when caring for a burned client. List three specific dietary interventions used with burned clients.
7. Describe the method of extinguishing each of the following burns: thermal, chemical, and electrical.
8. List four signs of an inhalation burn.
9. Why is the burned client allowed no "free" water?
10. Describe an autograft.

Answers to Review

1. Thermal, radiation, chemical, electrical
2. Superficial partial-thickness, first degree: pink to red skin (e.g., sunburn), slight edema, and pain relieved by cooling; deep partial-thickness, second degree: destruction of epidermis and upper layers of dermis; white or red, very edematous, sensitive to touch and cold air, hair does not pull out easily
3. Full-thickness, third degree: total destruction of dermis and epidermis; reddened areas do not blanch with pressure; not painful; inelastic; waxy white skin to brown, leathery eschar
4. Stage I (emergent phase): Replacement of fluids is titrated to urine output.

5. Stage II (acute phase): Patent infusion site is maintained in case supplemental IV fluids are needed; saline lock is helpful; colloids may be used.

6. Stage III (rehabilitation phase): No extra fluids are needed, but high-protein drinks are recommended.

7. Administer pain medication, especially before dressing wound. Teach distraction and relaxation techniques. Teach use of guided imagery.

8. Provide a patent airway because intubation may be necessary. Determine baseline data. Initiate fluid and electrolyte therapy. Administer pain medication. Determine depth and extent of burn. Administer tetanus toxoid. Insert NG tube.

9. High-calorie, high-protein, high-carbohydrate diet; medications with juice or milk; no "free" water; tube feeding at night. Maintain accurate, daily calorie counts. Weigh client daily.

10. Thermal: Remove clothing, immerse in tepid water. Chemical: Flush with water or saline. Electrical: Separate client from electrical source.

11. Singed nasal hairs, circumoral burns; sooty or bloody sputum, hoarseness, and pulmonary signs, including asymmetry of respirations, rales, or wheezing

12. Water may interfere with electrolyte balance. Client needs to ingest food products with highest biologic value.

13. Use of client's own skin for grafting.

References

1. World Health Organization, as adopted by the International Health conference NY 19-22 June 1946, signed on 22 July 1946 by the representatives of 61 states (official records of the EHO, no 2p100) and entered into force on 7 April 1948. The definition has not been amended since 1948.

2. Pulchaski CM. In Riley JB, *Communication in Nursing*, ed 7, St. Louis, 2013, Mosby.

3. Riley JB: *Communication in Nursing*, ed 7, St. Louis, 2013, Mosby.

4. Complementary and Alternative Medicine in the United States. 2005. http://www.nationalacademies.org/hmd/Reports/Complementary-and Alternative. Institute of Medicine.

5. Reid, R. (2014). Premenstrual syndrome. Accessed on 28 April 2016 at www.endotext.org.

6. Bartlett (1999). In Buckle J: *Clinical Aromatherapy: Essential Oils in Practice (revised)*, ed 2, St. Louis, 2003, Elsevier.

7. Bartlett (1999). In Buckle J: *Clinical Aromatherapy: Essential Oils in Practice (revised)*, ed 2, St. Louis, 2003, Elsevier.

8. Arnold E, Boggs K: *Interpersonal Relationships: Professional Communication Skills for Nurses*, ed 7, St. Louis, 2016, Saunders.

9. Varcarolis EM: *Essentials of Psychiatric Mental Health Nursing (revised)*, ed 2, St. Louis, 2013, Saunders. Revised reprint.

10. Centers for Disease Control.

11. Centers for Disease Control.

12. ACOG Practice Guideline for Pap Smear Screening (January 2016).

Growth and Development

Description: Growth and development follow an orderly yet individual pattern. Nurses should assess growth and the emergence of developmental skills in all pediatric clients. Knowledge of psychosocial, cognitive, and moral developmental abilities allows a nurse to adapt teaching to the level of the child. Knowledge of appropriate toys and interests of children at different ages enables the nurse to use play to facilitate the child's development and minimize problems caused by the hospitalization and illness.

Infant (Birth to 1 Year)

A. Developmental milestones (Fig. 5-1)
   1. Birth weight doubles by 6 months, triples by 12 months
   2. Birth length increases by 50% at 12 months
   3. Explores environment by motor and oral means
B. Nursing implications
   1. During hospitalization, the infant's emerging skills may disappear.
   2. If the parents are not able to be with the infant, the baby may be inconsolable due to separation anxiety (usually beginning around 6 months to 30 months).
   3. The nurse should plan to have the parents be part of the infant's care and should encourage them to do so.
   4. Respect the infant's schedule at home by implementing usual routine when possible.
   5. Preparation and teaching should be directed to the family. However, the nurse should always speak to the infant and console the infant, especially while performing painful or stressful procedures.
   6. Toys for hospitalized infants include mobiles, rattles, squeaking toys, picture books, balls, colored blocks, and activity boxes.

Toddler (1 to 3 Years)

A. Developmental milestones
   1. Birth weight quadruples by 30 months
   2. Achieves 50% of adult height by 2 years
   3. Growth velocity slows
B. Nursing implications
   1. Give simple, brief explanations immediately before procedures, keeping in mind that a 1-year-old does not benefit from the same explanation as that given to a 3-year-old.
   2. During hospitalization, enforced separation from parents is the greatest threat to the toddler's

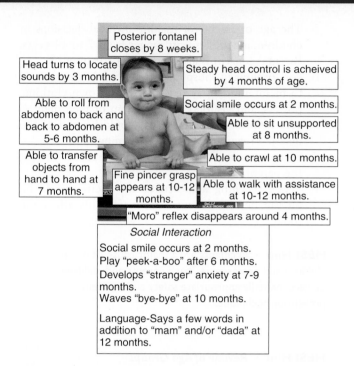

Posterior fontanel closes by 8 weeks.

Head turns to locate sounds by 3 months.

Steady head control is acheived by 4 months of age.

Able to roll from abdomen to back and back to abdomen at 5-6 months.

Social smile occurs at 2 months.

Able to sit unsupported at 8 months.

Able to transfer objects from hand to hand at 7 months.

Fine pincer grasp appears at 10-12 months.

Able to crawl at 10 months.

Able to walk with assistance at 10-12 months.

"Moro" reflex disappears around 4 months.

Social Interaction

Social smile occurs at 2 months.
Play "peek-a-boo" after 6 months.
Develops "stranger" anxiety at 7-9 months.
Waves "bye-bye" at 10 months.

Language-Says a few words in addition to "mam" and/or "dada" at 12 months.

FIGURE 5-1 Infant milestones (Modified from Hockenberry M, Wilson D. *Wong's nursing care of infants and children*, ed 9. St. Louis, Elsevier/Mosby, 2011. Multimedia Enhanced Version.)

psychological and emotional integrity.

3. Security objects or favorite toys from home should be provided for a toddler.
4. Teach parents to explain their plans to the child (e.g., "I will be back after your nap").
5. Respect the child's routine and implement when possible.
6. Expect regression (e.g., bedwetting).
7. Toys for the hospitalized toddler include board and mallet, push-pull toys, toy telephones, stuffed animals, and storybooks with pictures, depending on the reason for hospitalization. Toddlers benefit from being taken to the hospital playroom when able because mobility is very important to their development.
8. Toddlers are learning to name body parts and are concerned about their bodies.
9. Very basic explanations should be given to toddlers about procedures.
10. Autonomy should be supported by providing guided choices when appropriate.

Preschool Child (3 to 6 Years)

A. Developmental milestones
1. Each year, a child gains about 5 pounds and grows 2½ to 3 inches.
2. A child stands erect with more slender posture.
3. A child learns to run, jump, skip, and hop.
4. Handedness is established.
5. A 3 year old can ride a tricycle.

6. A child uses scissors at 4 years.
7. A child ties shoelaces at 5 years.
8. A child learns colors and shapes.
9. Visual acuity approaches 22/20.
10. A child learns sexual identity (curiosity and masturbation are common).
11. Imaginary playmates and fears are common.
12. Aggressiveness at 4 years is replaced by more independence at 5 years.

B. Nursing implications
1. Nursing care for hospitalized preschoolers should emphasize understanding of the child's egocentricity. Explain that he or she did not cause the illness and that painful procedures are not a punishment for misdeeds.
2. The child's questions should be answered at the child's level. Use simple words that will be understood by the child.
3. Therapeutic play or medical play that allows the child to act out his or her experiences is helpful.
4. Fear of mutilation by procedures is common. A Band-Aid may be quite helpful in restoring body integrity.
5. Toys and play for the hospitalized preschooler include coloring books, puzzles, cutting and pasting, dolls, building blocks, clay, and toys that allow the preschooler to work out hospitalization experiences, depending on the reason for hospitalization.
6. The preschooler needs preparation for procedures. He or she should understand what is and what is not going to be "fixed." Simple explanations and basic pictures are helpful. Let the child handle equipment or models of the equipment.

HESI Hint • Use facts and principles related to growth and development in planning teaching interventions. For example: What task could a 5-year-old child with diabetes expect to accomplish by himself or herself? One correct answer would be to let the child choose the injection sites. This is possible for a preschooler to do and gives the child some sense of control

HESI Hint • Knowledge of normal growth and developmental milestones are important in the delivery of care of an infant. If there appears to be a discrepancy in the infant's development, this will warrant the health care professionals to further investigate the possible cause of the delay.

School-Age Child (6 to 12 Years)

A. Developmental milestones
B. Nursing implications
1. The hospitalized school-age child may need more support from parents than the child wishes to admit.

2. Maintaining contact with peers and school activities is important during hospitalization.
3. Explanation of all procedures is important. They can learn from verbal explanations, pictures, and books and by handling equipment.
4. Privacy and modesty are important and should be respected during hospitalization (e.g., close curtains during procedures, allow privacy during baths).
5. Participation in care and planning with staff fosters a sense of involvement and accomplishment.
6. Toys for the school-age child include board games, card games, and hobbies, such as stamp collecting, puzzles, and video games.

> **HESI Hint** • School-age children are in Erikson's stage of industry, meaning they like to do and accomplish things. Peers are also becoming important for children of this age.

> **HESI Hint** • Tanner Stages of Pubertal Development
> **Girls:** Breast changes, rapid increase in height and weight, growth of pubic hair, appearance of axillary hair, menstruation, abrupt deceleration of linear growth.
> **Boys:** Enlargement of testicles; growth of pubic hair, axillary hair, facial hair, and body hair; rapid increase in height; changes in larynx and voice; nocturnal emissions; abrupt deceleration of linear growth.

Adolescent (12 to 19 Years)

A. Developmental milestones
   1. Girls' growth spurts during adolescence begin earlier than boys' (may begin as early as 9½ years for girls).
   2. Boys catch up at around 14 and continue to grow.
   3. Girls finish growth at around 15, boys at around 17.
   4. Secondary sex characteristics develop.
   5. Adultlike thinking begins around 15. They can problem-solve and use abstract thinking.
   6. Family conflicts develop.
B. Erikson's theory: Developing a sense of identity (identity versus role confusion)
C. Nursing implications
   1. Hospitalization of adolescents disrupts school and peer activities; they need to maintain contact with both.
   2. They should share a room with other adolescents.
   3. Illnesses, treatments, and procedures that alter the adolescent's body image can be viewed by the adolescent as devastating.
   4. Teaching about procedures should include time without the parents being present. It is important to direct questions to the adolescent when the parents are present.

5. The age of assent for making medical decisions in children and adolescents ranges from 7 to 14 years. Parental consent is also needed for treatment.
6. For prolonged hospitalizations, adolescents need to maintain identity (e.g., have their own clothing, posters, and visitors). A teen room or teen night is very helpful. The adolescent should be part of the decision regarding a parent's rooming-in.
7. Some assessment questions should be asked without the parents' presence.
8. When teaching adolescents, the focus should be on the here and now—"How will this affect me today?"

> **HESI Hint** • Accidents are a major cause of death in children and adolescents. Teach parents and children developmentally appropriate safety and accident-prevention techniques.

> **HESI Hint** • *Review of Age Groups*
> Frequently tested content areas on the NCLEX-RN® examination:
> - When does birth length double? Answer: by 4 years.
> - When does the child sit unsupported? Answer: 8 months.
> - When does a child achieve 50% of adult height? Answer: 2 years.
> - When does a child throw a ball overhand? Answer: 18 months.
> - When does a child speak two- to three-word sentences? Answer: 2 years.
> - When does a child use scissors? Answer: 4 years.
> - When does a child tie his or her shoes? Answer: 5 years.
> - Be aware that a girl's growth spurt during adolescence begins earlier than a boy's (as early as 10 years of age).
> - Temper tantrums are common in the toddler (i.e., they are considered normal or average behavior).
> - Be aware that adolescence is a time when the child forms his or her identity and that rebellion against family values is common for this age group.

> **HESI Hint** • Age groups' concepts of bodily injury:
> - Infants: After 6 months, their cognitive development allows them to remember pain.
> - Toddlers: They fear intrusive procedures.
> - Preschoolers: They fear body mutilation.
> - School-age children: They fear loss of control of their bodies.
> - Adolescents: Their major concern is change in body image.

Pain Assessment and Management in the Pediatric Client

Description: Historically, pain in the pediatric population has been unrecognized or undertreated. Research has shown that children, including neonates and infants, experience pain. Untreated pain may lead to complications, such as delayed recovery, alterations in sleep patterns, and alterations in nutrition.

The pediatric client's signs and symptoms of pain manifest in different ways. The infant and/or toddler who is unable to verbalize the experience of pain may display pain through actions and mannerisms.

Different tools have been developed to help health care providers recognize and identify if the infant/toddler is experiencing pain. See the following charts that are normally used in the health care setting.

Pain assessment is often referred to as the *fifth vital sign*.

Nursing Assessment

A. Verbal report by the child. Children as young as 3 years of age are able to report the location and degree of pain they are experiencing.
B. Observe for nonverbal signs of pain, such as grimacing, irritability, restlessness, and difficulty in sleeping or feeding.
C. Include the child's parents in the assessment.
D. Observe for physiologic responses to pain, such as increased heart rate, increased respiratory rate, diaphoresis, and decreased oxygen levels.
E. Physiologic responses to pain are most often seen in response to acute pain rather than in response to chronic pain.

0	1 or 2	2 or 4	3 or 6	4 or 8	5 or 10
No hurt	Hurts little bit	Hurts little more	Hurts even more	Hurts whole lot	Hurts worst

FIGURE 5-2 Wong-Baker FACES Pain Rating Scale (From Wong-Baker FACES Foundation [2016]. Wong-Baker FACES® Pain Rating Scale. Retrieved June 3, 2016 with permission from http://www.WongBakerFACES.org.)

Analysis (Nursing Diagnoses)

A. *Acute pain* related to …
B. *Anxiety* related to …
C. *Disturbed sleep pattern* related to …
D. *Ineffective infant feeding pattern* related to …

Nursing Plans and Interventions

A. A pain rating scale appropriate for the child's age and developmental level should be used.
   1. CRIES can be used with infants 32 to 60 weeks of gestational age.
   2. Pain Rating Scale (PRS) can be used with all children of any age.
      a. FACES Pain Rating Scale and the Poker Chip Scale can be used by children of preschool age and older (Fig. 5-2).
      b. Numeric Pain Scale can be used by children 9 years of age and older.
      c. The Oucher Pain Scale is a scale used for children 3 to 12 years of age with culturally specific photographs showing different levels of pain and discomfort.
      d. The FLACC pain assessment tool can be used by the nonverbal child. The nurse evaluates the child's **F**acial expression, **L**eg movement, **A**ctivity, **C**ry, and **C**onsolability.
   3. Documentation of a child's self-report of pain is essential to effectively treat the child's pain.
B. Nonpharmacologic interventions
   1. Should be used according to the child's age and developmental level.
   2. Infants may respond best to pacifiers, holding, and rocking.
   3. Toddlers and preschoolers may respond best to distraction. Distraction may be provided through books, music, television, and bubble blowing.
   4. School-aged children and adolescents may use guided imagery.
   5. Other interventions may include massage, application of heat or cold, and deep-breathing exercises.

C. Pharmacologic interventions
   1. Before administering a pain medication to a pediatric client, verify that the prescribed dose is safe for the child on the basis of the child's weight (mg/kg).
   2. Monitor the child's vital signs after administration of opioid medications.
   3. Children as young as 5 years of age may be taught to use a patient-controlled analgesia (PCA) pump.
   4. Children may deny pain if they fear receiving an intramuscular (IM) injection.

> **HESI Hint** • Child Health Promotion
> Description: Immunization of children against communicable diseases is one of the greatest accomplishments of modern medicine. Childhood mortality and morbidity rates have greatly decreased. Protection against disease should begin in infancy according to the recommendations of the American Academy of Pediatrics and the U.S. Public Health Service (Table 5-1). Recommendations can be found at http://www.cdc.gov/vaccines/schedules/hcp/child-adolescent.html

Communicable Diseases of Childhood

The nursing care of children with communicable diseases is virtually the same for all, regardless of the particular disease.
A. Rubeola (measles)
   1. A highly contagious viral disease that can lead to neurologic problems or death
   2. Transmitted by direct contact with droplets from infected persons
   3. Contagious mainly during the prodromal period, which is characterized by fever and upper respiratory symptoms
   4. Classic symptoms include the following:
      a. Photophobia
      b. Koplik spots on the buccal mucosa
      c. Confluent rash that begins on the face and spreads downward
B. Paramyxovirus (mumps)
   1. Incubation: 14 to 21 days
   2. Symptoms: Fever, headache, malaise, parotid gland swelling and tenderness; manifestations include submaxillary and sublingual infection, orchitis, and meningoencephalitis
   3. Transmitted by direct contact or droplet spread
   4. Analgesics used for pain and antiseptics for fever
   5. Bed rest maintained until swelling subsides
C. Rubella (German measles)
   1. Common viral disease that has teratogenic effects on fetus during the first trimester of pregnancy
   2. Transmitted by droplet and direct contact with infected person
   3. Discrete red maculopapular rash that starts on face and rapidly spreads to entire body
   4. Rash disappears within 3 days

D. Pertussis (whooping cough)
   1. Acute infectious respiratory disease usually occurring in infancy
   2. Caused by a gram-negative bacillus
   3. Begins with upper respiratory symptoms
   4. Paroxysmal stage characterized by prolonged coughing and crowing or whooping upon inspiration; lasts from 4 to 6 weeks
   5. Transmitted by direct contact, droplet spread, or freshly contaminated objects
   6. The vaccine for pertussis is recommended for all people.
   7. CDC recommends infants and children to receive doses at 2, 4, 6, and 15 to 18 months and another between 4 and 6 years of age.
E. Varicella (chickenpox)
   1. Viral disease characterized by skin lesions
   2. Lesions that begin on the trunk and spread to the face and proximal extremities
   3. Progresses through macular, papular, vesicular, and pustular stages
   4. Transmitted by direct contact, droplet spread, or freshly contaminated objects
   5. Communicable prodromal period to the time all lesions have crusted
   6. CDC recommends two doses of varicella vaccine for everyone
   7. Children should receive their first dose between 12 and 15 months of age and their second dose at 4 to 6 years of age

Nursing Care for Children with Communicable Diseases

A. Isolate child during period of communicability.
B. Treat fever with *nonaspirin* product.
C. Report occurrence to the health department.
D. Prevent child from scratching skin (e.g., cut nails, apply mittens, and provide soothing baths).
E. Administer diphenhydramine HCl (Benadryl) as prescribed for itching.
F. *Wash hands* after caring for child and handling secretions or child's articles.
G. Administer vaccinations using the recommended CDC schedule.

> **HESI Hint** • Children with German measles pose a serious threat to their unborn siblings. The nurse should counsel all expectant mothers, especially those with young children, to be aware of the serious consequences of exposure to German measles during pregnancy.

> **HESI Hint** • Common childhood problems are encountered by nurses caring for children in the community or hospital settings. The child's age directly influences the severity and management of these problems.

TABLE 5-1 **Vaccines**

Type of Vaccine	Description
MMR Vaccine	
• Measles, mumps, rubella (MMR) • Offers protection against these three diseases	• It is generally administered at 12–15 mo of age and repeated at 4–6 yr or by 11–12 yr. • In times of measles epidemics, it is possible to give measles protection at 6 mo and repeat the MMR at 15 mo. • Measles vaccine is contraindicated for persons with history of anaphylactic reaction to neomycin or eggs, those with known altered immunodeficiency, and pregnant women. It may be given to those with human immunodeficiency virus (HIV) and to breastfeeding women. • Administer subcutaneously at separate sites. • Child may have a light, transient rash 2 wk after administration of vaccine.

HESI Hint • Pertinent history should be obtained before administering certain immunizations because reactions to previous immunizations or current health conditions may contraindicate current immunizations:
• DTaP: History of reactions, seizures, neurologic symptoms after previous vaccine, or systematic allergic reactions
• MMR: History of anaphylactic reaction to eggs or neomycin

Type of Vaccine	Description
DTaP Vaccine	

• Diphtheria, pertussis, tetanus
• Offers protection against these diseases
	• Beginning at age 2 mo, administer three doses at 2-mo intervals.
	• Booster doses given at 15–18 mo and at 4–6 yr.
	• Administer IM (separate site from other vaccine).
	• Not given to children past the seventh birthday; they receive Td, which contains full-strength protection against tetanus and lesser-strength diphtheria protection.
	• When pertussis vaccine is contraindicated, give DT, full-strength diphtheria, and tetanus without pertussis vaccine, until seventh birthday.
	• Contraindications to pertussis vaccine include:
	  • Encephalopathy within 7 days of previous dose of DTaP
	  • History of seizures
	  • Neurologic symptoms after receiving the vaccine
	  • Systemic allergic reactions to the vaccine
	• Parents should be instructed to begin acetaminophen (Tylenol) administration after the immunization (normal dosage is 10–15 mg/kg).
	• Instruct parents to report immediately any side effects of the immunization to the primary caregiver.

Polio Vaccine	
• Inactive polio vaccine (IPV)	• Recommended for all persons under 18 yr • Administer at 2 mo of age and again at 4 mo of age. Boosters are given at 6–18 mo and at 4–6 yr. • Administer IPV subcutaneously or IM at separate site. • IPV is contraindicated for those with history of anaphylactic reaction to neomycin or streptomycin. • May give with all other vaccines

Continued

TABLE 5-1 Vaccines—cont'd

Type of Vaccine	Description
Hib (Haemophilus influenzae type B) Vaccine	
• Offers protection against bacteria that cause serious illness (epiglottitis, bacterial meningitis, septic arthritis) in small children and those with chronic illnesses such as sickle cell disease	• Three conjugate vaccines have been recommended for administration to infants: PRP-OPMs can be given beginning as early as 2 mo of age. DTaP/Hib combinations should not be used as primary immunizations at ages 2, 4, or 6 mo. • Vaccines have different series administration schedules; the schedules cover children through 5 yr of age. • Children at high risk who were not immunized previously should be immunized after the age of 5. • Administer intramuscularly. • There are no contraindications.
Hepatitis B	
• Offers protection against hepatitis B • May be given to newborns before hospital discharge • All children up to 18 yr of age should be vaccinated.	• Is contraindicated for persons with anaphylactic reaction to common baker's yeast
Varicella	
• Offers protection against chickenpox • Is a school entry requirement in almost all states • Is safe for children with asymptomatic HIV infection	• Administer at 12–18 mo of age (must be at least 12 mo). • Give MMR and varicella on same day or >30 days apart (separate site).
Tuberculosis (TB) Skin Testing	

• Offers screening for exposure to TB	• Screening is usually done using one of the following:
	  • Mantoux test with PPD (tuberculin purified protein derivative) injected intradermally on the forearm; standard method for identifying infection with *Mycobacterium tuberculosis*
	  • Tine test (OT, old tuberculin), which consists of four prongs pressed into the forearm. These multiple puncture tests are unreliable and should not be used to determine the presence of a TB infection.
	• A positive reaction represents exposure to *M. tuberculosis*.
	• Screening can be initiated at 12 mo.

HESI Hint • Subcutaneous injection, rather than intradermal injection, invalidates the Mantoux test.

HESI Hint • The common cold is not a contraindication for immunization.

HESI Hint • After immunization, what teaching should the nurse provide to the parents?
• Irritability, fever 102° F (38.8° C), redness, and soreness at injection site for 2 to 3 days are normal side effects of DTaP and IPV administration.
• Call health care provider if seizures, high fever, or high-pitched crying occurs.
• A warm washcloth on the thigh injection site and "bicycling" the legs with each diaper change decreases soreness.
• Acetaminophen (Tylenol) is administered orally every 4 to 6 hours (10–15 mg/kg).

HESI Hint • Pertussis fatalities continue to occur in nonimmunized infants in the United States.

Pediatric Nutritional Assessment

Description: Profile of the child's and family's eating habits

A. Iron deficiency occurs most commonly in children 12 to 36 months old, in adolescent females, and in females during their childbearing years.
   1. Recommended amount of vitamin D is 400 IU/day.
   2. If a mother is not taking enough vitamin D, it is recommended that the infant receive an oral dose of 400 IU/daily.
B. The vitamins most often consumed in less-than-appropriate amounts by preschool and school-age children are:
   1. Vitamin A
   2. Vitamin C
   3. Vitamin B_6
   4. Vitamin B_{12}

Nursing Plans and Interventions

A. Determine dietary history.
   1. The 24-hour recall: Ask the family to recall all food and liquid intake during the past 24 hours.
   2. Food diary: Ask the family to keep a 3-day record (2 weekdays and 1 weekend day) of all food and liquid intake and the amount of each.
   3. Food frequency record: Provide a questionnaire and ask family to record information regarding the number of times per day, week, or month a child consumes items from the four food groups.
B. Perform a clinical examination.
   1. Assess skin, hair, teeth, lips, tongue and eyes
   2. Use anthropometry: measurement of height, weight, body mass index (BMI), head circumference in young children, proportion, skinfold thickness, and arm circumference.
      a. Height and head circumference reflect past nutrition.
      b. Weight, skinfold thickness, and arm circumference reflect present nutritional status (especially protein and fat reserves).
      c. Skinfold thickness provides a measurement of the body's fat content (half of the body's total fat stores are directly beneath the skin).
   3. Obtain biochemical analysis.
      a. Plasma, blood cells, urine, or tissues from liver, bone, hair, or fingernails can be used to determine nutritional status.
      b. Laboratory testing of Hgb, Hct, albumin, creatinine, and nitrogen is commonly used to determine nutritional status.
C. Implement appropriate nursing interventions, including client and family teaching, to correct identified nutritional deficits (Table 5-2).

Diarrhea

Description: Increased number or decreased consistency of stools

A. Diarrhea can be a serious or fatal symptom, especially in infancy.
B. Causes include but are not limited to:
   1. Infections: bacterial, viral, parasitic
   2. Malabsorption problems
   3. Inflammatory diseases
   4. Dietary factors
C. Conditions associated with diarrhea are:
   1. Dehydration
   2. Metabolic acidosis
   3. Shock

Nursing Assessment

A. Usually occurs in infants
B. History of exposure to pathogens, contaminated food, dietary changes
C. Signs of dehydration
   1. Poor skin turgor/tenting of skin
   2. Absence of tears
   3. Dry and sticky mucous membranes
   4. Weight loss (5%–15%)
   5. Depressed fontanel
   6. Decreased urinary output, increased specific gravity
   7. Acidotic state
D. Laboratory signs of acidosis:
   1. Loss of bicarbonate (serum pH <7.35)
   2. Loss of sodium and potassium through stools
   3. Elevated hematocrit (Hct)
   4. Elevated blood urea nitrogen (BUN)
E. Signs of shock
   1. Decreased blood pressure
   2. Rapid, weak pulse
   3. Skin: mottled to gray color; cool and clammy to touch
   4. Delayed capillary refill greater than (+) 4 seconds
   5. Changes in mental status

HESI Hint • Because the infant's hands may be acrocyanotic, it is best to check capillary refill on the infant's sternum.

Analysis (Nursing Diagnoses)

A. *Diarrhea* related to …
B. *Risk for deficient fluid volume* related to …

Nursing Plans and Interventions

A. Assess hydration status and vital signs frequently.
B. Monitor intake and output.
C. Do *not* take temperature rectally.
D. Rehydrate as prescribed with fluids and electrolytes.
E. Calculate intravenous (IV) hydration to include maintenance and replacement fluids.
F. Collect specimens to aid in diagnosis of cause.
G. Check stools for pH, glucose, and blood.
H. Administer antibiotics as prescribed.

TABLE 5-2 Nutritional Assessment

Nutrient	Signs of Deficiency	Food Sources
• Iron	• Anemia • Pale conjunctiva • Pale skin color • Atrophy of papillae on tongue • Brittle, ridged, spoon-shaped nails • Thyroid edema	• Iron-fortified formula • Infant high-protein cereal • Infant rice cereal • Liver • Beef • Pork • Eggs
• Vitamin B₂ (riboflavin)	• Redness and fissuring of eyelid corners; burning, itching, tearing eyes; photophobia • Magenta-colored tongue, glossitis • Seborrheic dermatitis, delayed wound healing	• Prepared infant formula • Liver • Cow's milk • Cheddar cheese • Some green leafy vegetables (broccoli, green beans, spinach) • Enriched cereals
• Vitamin A (retinol)	• Dry, rough skin • Dull cornea; soft cornea; Bitot spots • Night blindness • Defective tooth enamel • Retarded growth; impaired bone formation • Decreased thyroxine formation	• Liver • Sweet potatoes • Carrots • Spinach • Peaches • Apricots
• Vitamin C (ascorbic acid)	• Scurvy • Receding gums that are spongy and prone to bleeding • Dry, rough skin; petechiae • Decreased wound healing • Increased susceptibility to infection • Irritability, anorexia, apprehension	• Strawberries • Oranges and orange juice • Tomatoes • Broccoli • Cabbage • Cauliflower • Spinach
• Vitamin B₆ (pyridoxine)	• Scaly dermatitis • Weight loss • Anemia • Irritability • Convulsions • Peripheral neuritis	• Meats, especially liver • Cereals (wheat and corn) • Yeast • Soybeans • Peanuts • Tuna • Chicken • Bananas

HESI Hint • Teach proper cooking and storage methods to preserve potency (e.g., cook vegetables in small amounts of liquid).
• Store milk in opaque container.

I. Check urine for specific gravity.
J. Institute careful isolation precautions; *wash hands.*
K. Teach home care of child with diarrhea:
   1. Provide child with oral rehydration solution such as Pedialyte or Lytren.
   2. Child may temporarily need lactose-free diet.
   3. Children should not receive antidiarrheals (e.g., Imodium A-D).
   4. Do not give child grape juice, orange juice, apple juice, cola, or ginger ale. These solutions have high osmolality.

HESI Hint • It is important to document the method used for taking the temperature (e.g., axillary, tympanic, etc.).
   Also when obtaining the temperature, ensure the tympanic probe fits properly in the ear canal; also ensure the client does not have otitis media.

HESI Hint • Antibiotics are not recommended for diarrhea. They are only prescribed if the child has diarrhea caused by a bacterial, fungal, or parasitic infection.

HESI Hint • Add potassium to IV fluids *only* when the client has an adequate urine output.

Standard intravenous fluids used to treat pediatric dehydration are isotonic (e.g., Ringer's lactate [LR]) or normal saline (NS). The amount is a fluid bolus of 20 mL/kg.

Burns

Description: Tissue injuries caused by heat, electricity, chemicals, or radiation

A. Burns are a major cause of accidental death in children younger than 15 (after automobile accidents).

B. It is estimated that 75% of burns are preventable.

C. Scald burns:

1. Children younger than 5 are one of the two highest risk groups.

2. Ranked top cause of burns (accidentally or purposeful) to children younger than 4 years old.

3. Hot water heater temperature greater than 140 degrees can cause a third-degree burn on a child in 15 seconds and is responsible for 17% of childhood admissions for scald burns.

D. Children younger than age 2 have a higher mortality rate due to:

1. Greater central body surface area. In a child younger than 2, a greater part of the body surface area is concentrated in the head and trunk compared with an older child or an adult; therefore the younger child is more likely to have serious effects from burns to the trunk and head (see Fig. 5-3).

2. Greater fluid volume (proportionate to body size)

3. Less effective cardiovascular responses to fluid volume shifts

E. In childhood, a partial-thickness burn is considered a major burn if it involves more than 25% of body surface.

F. A full-thickness burn is considered major if it involves more than 10% of body surface.

G. Because of the changing proportions of the child, especially the infant, the rule of nines cannot be used to assess the percentage of burn (Fig. 5-3).

H. An assessment tool such as the Lund-Browder chart, which takes into account the changing proportions of the child, should be used.

I. Fluid needs should be calculated from the time of the burn.

J. The Parkland formula is a commonly used guideline for calculating fluid replacement and maintenance. It is based on child's body surface area and should include volume for burn losses and maintenance.

K. Adequacy of fluid replacement is determined by evaluating urinary output.

HESI Hint • Urinary output for infants and children should be 1 to 2 mL/kg/hr.

L. Specific gravity should be less than 1.025.

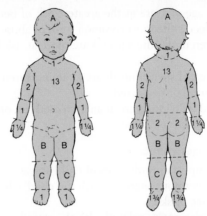

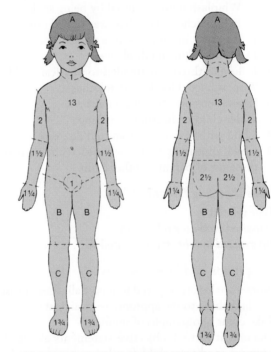

RELATIVE PERCENTAGES OF AREAS AFFECTED BY GROWTH

A

AREA	BIRTH	AGE 1 YR	AGE 5 YR
A = ½ of head	9½	8½	6½
B = ½ of one thigh	2¾	3¼	4
C = ½ of one leg	2½	2½	2¾

RELATIVE PERCENTAGES OF AREAS AFFECTED BY GROWTH

B

AREA	AGE 10 YR	AGE 15 YR	ADULT
A = ½ of head	5½	4½	3½
B = ½ of one thigh	4½	4½	4¾
C = ½ of one leg	3	3¼	3½

FIGURE 5-3 Estimated distribution of burns in children. **(A)** Children from birth to age 5 years. **(B)** Older children. (From Hockenberry M: *Wong's nursing care of infants and children*, ed 8, St. Louis, 2007, Mosby. In Betz C, Sowden L. *Mosby's pediatric nursing reference*, ed 6. Mosby.)

Child Abuse

Description: Intentional or nonintentional physical and mental injury, sexual abuse, and emotional and physical neglect of a child under the age of 18 years old who is under the care of an adult. It is believed that 25% of children will experience some form of abuse in their lifetime. Children under the age of 1 are at the greatest risk of being abused. Child neglect is the most common form of abuse (80%).

A. Children under the age of 4 are more at risk for being a victim.
B. Children of special needs are at an increased risk of being abused or neglected.
C. Abused individuals are at an increased risk of becoming a perpetrator of abuse.

Nursing Assessment

A. Most important indicators of child abuse:
 1. Injuries not congruent with the child's developmental age or skills
 2. Injuries not correlated with the stated cause
   a. Bruises in unusual places and in various stages of healing
   b. Bruises, welts caused by belts, cords, etc.
   c. Burns (cigarette, iron); immersion burns (symmetrical in shape)
   d. Whiplash injuries caused by being shaken
   e. Bald patches where hair was pulled out
   f. Fractures in various stages of healing
 3. Delay in seeking medical care
 4. Failure to thrive, unattended-to physical problems
 5. Torn, stained, bloody underclothes
 6. Lacerations of external genitalia
 7. Older child bedwetting or soiling
 8. Child with sexually transmitted diseases
 9. Child appearing frightened and withdrawn in the presence of parent or other adult

Analysis (Nursing Diagnoses)

A. *Fear* related to . . .
B. *Impaired parenting* related to . . .
C. *Interrupted family process* related to . . .

Nursing Plans and Interventions

A. Nurses are legally required to report all cases of suspected child abuse to the appropriate local or state agency.
B. Take color photographs of injuries.
C. Document factual, objective statements about child's physical condition, child–family interactions, and interviews with family.
D. Establish trust, and care for the child's physical problems; these are the primary and immediate needs of these children.
E. Recognize own feelings of anger toward the parents.
F. Utilize principles of crisis intervention.
G. Assist child and family to develop self-esteem.
H. Teach basic child development and parenting skills to family.
I. Support the need for family therapy.

> **HESI Hint** • Abused children have difficulty establishing trust. Select only one nurse to care for an abused child because the child will be less anxious with a consistent caregiver.

Poisonings

Description: Ingesting, inhaling, or absorbing a toxic substance
A. Poisoning, particularly by ingestion, is a common cause of childhood injury and illness.
B. Most poisonings occur in children younger than 6 years, with a peak at age 2 years.
C. The exploratory behavior, curiosity, and oral motor activity of early childhood place the child at risk for poisonings.
D. About 90% of poisonings occur in the home.

Nursing Assessment

A. Child found near source of poison
B. Gastrointestinal (GI) disturbance: nausea, abdominal pain, diarrhea, vomiting
C. Burns of mouth, pharynx
D. Respiratory distress
E. Seizures, changes in level of consciousness
F. Cyanosis
G. Shock

Analysis (Nursing Diagnoses)

A. *Risk for poisoning* related to …
B. *Deficient knowledge* (*home safety*) related to …

Nursing Plans and Interventions

A. Identify the poisonous agent quickly!
B. Assess the child's respiratory, cardiac, and neurologic status.
C. Instruct parent to bring any emesis, stool, etc., to the emergency department.
D. Determine the child's age and weight.

> **HESI Hint** • Use of syrup of ipecac is no longer recommended by the American Academy of Pediatrics. Teach parents that it is *not* recommended to induce vomiting in any way because it may cause more damage.

E. Poison removal and care may require gastric lavage, activated charcoal, N-acetylcysteine, or naloxone HCl.
F. Teach home safety.
 1. Poison-proof and child-proof the home
   a. Identify location of poisons: under the sink (cleaning supplies, drain cleaners, bug poisons); medicine cabinets; storage rooms (paints, varnishes); garages (antifreeze, gasoline); poisonous plants (philodendron, dieffenbachia).
   b. Put locks on cabinets.
   c. Use safety containers: do *not* place poisonous materials in other nonsafe containers.
   d. Discard unused medications.
 2. Make sure child is always under adult supervision.
 3. Post telephone number for local poison control center next to telephone.
 4. Examine the environment from the child's viewpoint (the height to which a 2- to 5-year-old can reach).
 5. Be aware of changes in the child's environment because of house guests or visiting a relative or friends.

G. Contact community health nurse or child welfare agency if necessary.

> **HESI Hint** • Common household products that are poisonous to children if ingested: perfume and aftershave, sunburn relief products, alcohol, cigarettes or any type of tobacco products, and mouthwash.

Lead Poisoning

Description: It is estimated that ½ million children between 1 and 5 years of age living in the United States have blood levels of lead greater than 5 mcg/dL (level CDC uses to encourage public health action). There is no established "safe" level of lead for children. Every system in the human body can be affected by lead exposure. Lead exposure and elevated levels have been linked to decreased IQs.

A. Children 6 years of age and younger are most vulnerable to the effects of lead because children tend to put things in their mouths.
B. Although numerous sources of lead can result in exposure in young children, the major cause of lead poisoning is deteriorating lead-based paint.
C. Lead enters the body through ingestion, inhalation, or, in the case of an unborn child, placental transfer when the mother is exposed. The most common route is ingestion either from hand-to-mouth behavior via contaminated hands, fingers, toys, or pacifiers or, less often, from eating sweet-tasting loose paint chips found in a home built before the 1950s or in a play area.
D. The renal, neurologic, and hematologic systems are the most seriously affected by lead.
E. The blood lead level (BLL) test is currently used for screening and diagnosis.
F. Erythrocyte protoporphyrin (EP) test (a good indicator of early toxic effects of lead) remains useful as a clinical tool, along with the BLL test, to help estimate the potential body burden of lead in a child.

Nursing Assessment

A. Screen for lead poisoning using CDC guidelines of blood lead surveillance and other risk factor data collected over time to establish the status and risk of children throughout the state.
B. In areas without available data, universal screening is recommended.
   1. All children should have a BLL test at the ages of 1 and 2 years.
      a. Collect blood in a capillary tube and send to the laboratory.
      b. During collection, avoid contamination of blood specimen and lead on the skin.
   2. Any child between 3 and 6 years of age who has not been screened should also be tested.
C. Obtain a history of possible sources of lead in the child's environment.

D. Physical assessment
   1. General signs
      a. Anemia
      b. Acute cramping; abdominal pain
      c. Vomiting
      d. Constipation
      e. Anorexia
      f. Headache
      g. Lethargy
      h. Impaired growth
   2. Central nervous system (CNS) signs (early)
      a. Hyperactivity
      b. Aggression
      c. Impulsiveness
      d. Decreased interest in play
      e. Irritability
      f. Short attention span
   3. CNS signs (late)
      a. Mental retardation
      b. Paralysis
      c. Blindness
      d. Convulsions
      e. Coma
      f. Death

Analysis (Nursing Diagnoses)

A. *Risk for poisoning* related to …
B. *Interrupted family processes* related to …
C. *Risk for injury* related to …
D. *Risk for decreased cognitive ability* related to …

Nursing Plans and Interventions

A. Identify sources of lead in the environment to prevent further exposure.
B. Administer prescribed chelating agents to reduce high BLL levels.
   1. It is important to ask if the child is allergic to peanuts. Children who have peanut allergies should not be given chelating agents such as dimercaprol (also called *BAL* [British anti-Lewisite]), *D-penicillamine*, or *calcium disodium EDTA.*
D. IM and IV administration
   1. Calcium disodium EDTA is generally administered IM.
   2. Dimercaprol (also called *BAL*) is given in conjunction with calcium disodium EDTA (may contain peanut oil) to help in efficacy of treatment.
   3. Considerations for administration.
      a. Rotate injection sites if chelating agent is given intramuscularly.
      b. Reassure child that injections are a treatment, not a punishment.
      c. Administer the local anesthetic procaine with IM injection of calcium disodium EDTA to reduce discomfort.
      d. Apply EMLA cream over puncture site 2½ hours before the injection to reduce discomfort.

HESI Hint • Monitor client's renal functioning and complete blood count (CBC) while client is receiving chelating agents.

E. Avoid giving iron during chelation because of possible interactive effects.
F. If home oral chelation therapy is used, teach family proper administration of medication.
G. Administer prescribed cleansing enemas or cathartic for acute lead ingestion.
H. Assist family to obtain sources of help for removing lead from the environment.

1. Do not vacuum hard-surfaced floors or windowsills or window wells in homes built before 1960 because this spreads dust.
2. Wash and dry child's hands and face frequently, especially before the child eats.
3. Wash toys and pacifiers frequently.
4. Make sure that home exposure is not occurring from parental occupations or hobbies.

HESI Hint • More lead is absorbed on an empty stomach. Hot water can contain higher levels of lead because it dissolves lead more quickly than cold water, so use only cold water for consumption (drinking, cooking, and especially for making infant formula).

Review of Child Health Promotion

1. List two contraindications to live virus immunization.
2. List three classic signs and symptoms of measles.
3. List the signs and symptoms of iron deficiency.
4. Identify food sources of vitamin A.
5. What disease occurs with vitamin C deficiency?
6. What measurements reflect present nutritional status?
7. List the signs and symptoms of dehydration in an infant.
8. List the laboratory findings that can be expected in a dehydrated child.
9. How should burns in children be assessed?
10. How can the nurse best evaluate the adequacy of fluid replacement in children?
11. How should a parent be instructed to childproof a house?
12. What interventions should the nurse perform first in caring for a child who has ingested a poison?
13. What early signs should the nurse assess for if lead poisoning is suspected?

Answers to Review

1. Immunocompromised child or a child in a household with an immunocompromised individual
2. Photophobia, confluent rash that begins on the face and spreads downward, and Koplik spots on the buccal mucosa
3. Anemia; pale conjunctiva; pale skin color; atrophy of papillae on tongue; brittle, ridged, or spoon-shaped nails; and thyroid edema
4. Liver, sweet potatoes, carrots, spinach, peaches, and apricots
5. Scurvy
6. Weight, skinfold thickness, and arm circumference
7. Poor skin turgor, absence of tears, dry mucous membranes, weight loss, depressed fontanel, and decreased urinary output
8. Loss of bicarbonate/decreased serum pH, loss of sodium (hyponatremia), loss of potassium (hypokalemia), elevated Hct, and elevated BUN
9. By using the Lund-Browder chart, which takes into account the changing proportions of the child's body
10. By monitoring urine output
11. By being taught to lock all cabinets, to safely store all toxic household items in locked cabinets, and to examine the house from the child's point of view
12. Assessment of the child's respiratory, cardiac, and neurologic status
13. Anemia, acute cramping, abdominal pain, vomiting, constipation, anorexia, headache, lethargy, hyperactivity, aggression, impulsiveness, decreased interest in play, irritability, short attention span

Respiratory Disorders

Important Signs in Children

A. Normal pulse and respiratory rates (Table 5-3)
B. Signs of respiratory distress in children
 1. Cardinal signs of respiratory distress
  a. Restlessness
  b. Increased respiratory rate
  c. Increased pulse rate
  d. Diaphoresis
 2. Other signs of respiratory distress
  a. Flaring nostrils
  b. Retractions
  c. Grunting
  d. Adventitious breath sounds (or absent breath sounds)
  e. Use of accessory muscles, head bobbing

TABLE 5-3 Normal Pulse and Respiratory Rates for Children

Age	Pulse	Respirations	Nursing Implications
Newborn	100–160	30–60	These ranges are averages only and vary with the sex, age, and condition of child. Always note whether the child is crying, febrile, or in some distress.
1–11 mo	100–150	25–35	
1–3 yr (toddler)	80–130	20–30	
3–5 yr (preschooler)	80–120	20–25	
6–10 yr (school age)	70–110	18–22	
10–16 yr (adolescent)	60–90	16–20	

f. Alterations in blood gases: decreased P_{O_2}, elevated P_{CO_2}
g. Cyanosis and pallor
h. Alterations in mental status

HESI Hint • Symptoms of hypoxia
Early: Restlessness, anxiety, tachycardia/tachypnea
Late: Bradycardia, extreme restlessness, severe dyspnea
Pediatrics: Difficulty feeding, inspiratory stridor, nares flaring, grunting with expirations, sternal retractions

---

C. Nursing implications
  1. A pediatric client often goes into respiratory failure before cardiac failure.
  2. The nurse should know the signs of respiratory distress.

Asthma

Description: Inflammatory reactive airway disease that is commonly chronic
A. The airways become edematous.
B. The airways become congested with mucus.
C. The smooth muscles of the bronchi and bronchioles constrict.
D. Air trapping occurs in the alveoli.

Nursing Assessment

A. History of asthma in the family
B. History of allergies and/or eczema
C. Home environment containing pets or other allergens
D. Tight cough (nonproductive cough) usually occurs and/or worsens at nighttime
E. Breath sounds: coarse expiratory wheezing, rales, crackles
F. Chest diameter enlarges (late sign and symptom)
G. Increased number of school days missed during past 6 months
H. Signs of respiratory distress

Analysis (Nursing Diagnoses)

A. *Impaired gas exchange* related to ...
B. *Ineffective breathing pattern* related to ...

Nursing Plans and Interventions

A. Monitor carefully for increasing respiratory distress.

B. Administer rapid-acting bronchodilators and steroids for acute attacks.
C. Maintain hydration (oral fluids or IV).
D. Monitor blood gas values for signs of respiratory acidosis (see Advanced Clinical Concepts, Fluid, and Electrolyte Balance).
E. Administer oxygen or nebulizer therapy as prescribed.
F. Monitor pulse oximetry as prescribed (usually >95% is normal).
G. Monitor beta-adrenergic agonists, as well as antiinflammatory corticosteroids, which are commonly used medications (Table 5-4); and see Table 4-4).
H. Teach home care program, including:
  1. Identifying precipitating factors
  2. Eliminating triggers
  3. Reducing allergens in the home
  4. Using metered-dose inhaler/nebulizer
  5. Monitoring peak expiratory flow rate at home
  6. Doing breathing exercises
  7. Monitoring drug actions, dosages, and side effects
  8. Managing acute episode and when to seek emergency care
I. Refer child and family for emotional and psychological counseling.

Cystic Fibrosis

A. Description: An autosomal-recessive disease that causes dysfunction of the exocrine glands.
  1. Lung insufficiency (most critical problem)
  2. Pancreatic insufficiency
  3. Increased loss of sodium and chloride in sweat

Nursing Assessment

A. Most often found in a white infant or child
B. Meconium ileus at birth (10%–20% of cases)
C. Recurrent respiratory infection
D. Pulmonary congestion
E. Steatorrhea (excessive fat, greasy stools)
F. Foul-smelling bulky stools
G. Delayed growth and poor weight gain
H. Skin that tastes salty when kissed (caused by excessive secretions from sweat glands)
I. End stages: cyanosis, nail-bed clubbing, congestive heart failure (CHF)

TABLE 5-4 Adrenergics

Drugs/Route	Indications	Adverse Reactions	Nursing Implications
• Epinephrine HCl INH, subcutaneous, IM, IV	• Rapid-acting bronchodilator • Drug of choice for acute asthma attack	• Tachycardia • Hypertension • Tremors • Nausea	• Give subcutaneously, intravenously, via nebulizer • May be repeated in 20 min

HESI Hint • When calculating a pediatric dosage, the nurse must often change the child's weight from pounds to kilograms. 2.2 lb = 1 kg (divide pounds by 2.2).
a. If the child's weight is in pounds, convert the pounds directly to kilograms.
b. If the child's weight is in pounds and ounces, convert the ounces to the nearest tenth of a pound and add this to the total pounds. Then convert the total pounds to kilograms to the nearest tenth.

HESI Hint • Weight expressed in kilograms should always be a smaller number than the weight expressed in pounds.

Analysis (Nursing Diagnoses)

A. *Ineffective airway clearance* related to …
B. *Imbalanced nutrition: less than body requirements* related to …

Nursing Plans and Interventions

A. Monitor respiratory status.
B. Assess for signs of respiratory infection.
C. Administer IV antibiotics as prescribed; manage vascular access.
D. Administer pancreatic enzymes (Cotazym-S, Pancrease: for infants, with applesauce, rice, or cereal; for an older child, with food).
E. Administer fat-soluble vitamins (A, D, E, K) in water-soluble form.
F. Administer oxygen (Box 5-1) and nebulizer treatments (recombinant human deoxyribonuclease or dornase alfa as prescribed).
G. Evaluate effectiveness of respiratory treatments.
H. Teach family percussion and postural-drainage techniques.
I. Teach dietary recommendations: high in calories, high in protein, moderate to high in fat (more calories per volume), and moderate to low in carbohydrates (to avoid an increase in CO_2 drive).

HESI Hint • A child needs 150% of the usual calorie intake for normal growth and development.

J. Provide age-appropriate activities.
K. Refer family for genetic counseling.

HESI Hint • Cystic fibrosis is now screened with tests performed after birth. The diagnosis is made in the child's first month of life before signs and symptoms occur.

Epiglottitis

Description: Severe life-threatening infection of the epiglottis is a medical emergency

---

BOX 5-1 Respiratory Client

Administration of Oxygen
• Oxygen hood: Used for infants.
• Nasal prongs: Provide low to moderate concentrations of oxygen (up to 4–6 L).
• Tents: Provide mist and oxygen. Monitor child's temperature. Keep edges tucked in. Keep child dry.

Measurement of Oxygenation
• Pulse oximetry measures oxygen saturation (SaO_2) of arterial hemoglobin noninvasively via a sensor that is usually attached to the finger or toe or, in an infant, to sole of foot.
• Nurse should be aware of the alarm parameters signaling decreased SaO_2 (usually <95%).
• Blood gas evaluation is usually monitored in respiratory clients through arterial sampling.
• Norms: PO_2: 80 to 100 mm Hg; PcO_2: 35 to 45 mm Hg for children (not infants and newborns)

A. Epiglottitis progresses rapidly, causing acute airway obstruction.
B. The organism usually responsible for epiglottitis is *Haemophilus influenzae* (primarily type B).

Nursing Assessment

A. Sudden onset
B. Restlessness
C. High fever
D. Sore throat, dysphagia
E. Drooling
F. Muffled voice
G. Child assuming upright sitting position with chin out and tongue protruding ("tripod position")

Analysis (Nursing Diagnoses)

A. *Ineffective breathing pattern* related to …
B. *Anxiety* related to …

Nursing Plans and Interventions

A. Encourage prevention with Hib vaccine B. Maintain child in upright sitting position.
C. Prepare for intubation or tracheostomy.
D. Administer IV antibiotics as prescribed.
E. Prepare for hospitalization in intensive care unit (ICU).
F. Restrain as needed to prevent extubation.
G. Employ measures to decrease agitation and crying.

Bronchiolitis

Description: Viral infection of the bronchioles that is characterized by thick secretions

A. Bronchiolitis is usually caused by respiratory syncytial virus (RSV) and is found to be readily transmitted by close contact with hospital personnel, families, and other children.
B. Bronchiolitis occurs primarily in young infants.

Nursing Assessment

A. History of upper respiratory symptoms
B. Irritable, distressed infant
C. Paroxysmal coughing
D. Poor eating
E. Nasal congestion
F. Nasal flaring
G. Prolonged expiratory phase of respiration
H. Wheezing, rales can be auscultated
 I. Deteriorating condition that is often indicated by shallow, rapid respirations

Analysis (Nursing Diagnoses)

A. *Impaired gas exchange* related to …
B. *Ineffective airway clearance* related to …

Nursing Plans and Interventions

A. Isolate child (isolation of choice for RSV is contact isolation).
B. Assign nurses to clients with RSV who have no responsibility for any other children to prevent transmission of the virus.
C. Monitor respiratory status; observe for hypoxia.
D. Clear airway of secretions using a bulb syringe for suctioning.
E. Provide care in mist tent; administer oxygen as prescribed.
F. Maintain hydration (oral and IV fluids).
G. Evaluate response to respiratory therapy treatments.
H. Administer palivizumab to provide passive immunity against RSV in high-risk children (younger than 2 years of age with a history of prematurity, lung disease, or congenital heart disease).

> **HESI Hint** • In planning and providing nursing care, a patent airway is always the priority, regardless of age!

Otitis Media

Description: Inflammatory disorder of the middle ear

A. Otitis media may be suppurative or serous.
B. Anatomic structure of the ear predisposes young child to ear infections.
C. There is a risk for conductive hearing loss if untreated or incompletely treated.

Nursing Assessment

A. Fever, pain; infant may pull at ear
B. Enlarged lymph nodes
C. Discharge from ear (if drum is ruptured)
D. Upper respiratory symptoms
E. Vomiting, diarrhea

Analysis (Nursing Diagnoses)

A. *Risk for infection* related to …
B. *Acute pain* related to …

Nursing Plans and Interventions

A. Administer antibiotics if prescribed.
B. Reduce body temperature (can be very high, with risk for seizures).
　　1. Tepid baths
　　2. Acetaminophen (Tylenol) if prescribed
C. Position child on affected side.
D. Provide comfort measure: warm compress on affected ear.
E. Teach home care.
　　1. Teach to finish all prescribed antibiotics.
　　2. Encourage follow-up visit.
　　3. Monitor for hearing loss.
　　4. Teach preventive care: avoid exposure to secondhand smoke and discourage bottle feeding when the child is in supine position.
F. Tympanostomy tubes placement:

> **HESI Hint** • Respiratory disorders are the primary reason most children and their families seek medical care. Therefore these disorders are frequently tested on the NCLEX-RN. Knowing the normal parameters of respiratory rates and the key signs of respiratory distress in children is essential!

Tonsillitis

Description: Inflammation of the tonsils

A. Tonsillitis may be viral or bacterial.
B. Tonsillitis may be related to infection by a *Streptococcus* species.
C. If related to strep, treatment is *very important* because of the risk for developing acute glomerulonephritis or rheumatic heart disease.

Nursing Assessment

A. Sore throat and may have difficulty swallowing that lasts longer than 48 hours
B. Fever

C. Enlarged tonsils (may have purulent discharge on tonsils)
D. Breathing may be obstructed (tonsils touching, called *kissing tonsils*)
E. Throat culture to determine viral or bacterial cause

Analysis (Nursing Diagnoses)

A. *Impaired swallowing* related to …
B. *Risk for injury* related to …

Nursing Plans and Interventions

A. Collect throat culture if prescribed.
B. Instruct parents in home care.
1. Encourage warm saline gargles.
2. Provide ice chips.
3. Administer antibiotics if prescribed.
4. Manage fever with acetaminophen.
C. If a tonsillectomy is indicated:
1. Provide preoperative teaching and assessment.
2. Monitor for signs of postoperative bleeding.
a. Frequent swallowing
b. Vomiting fresh blood
c. Clearing throat
3. Encourage soft foods and oral fluids (avoid red fluids, which mimic signs of bleeding); do not use straws.
4. Provide comfort measures: ice collar helps with pain and with vasoconstriction.
5. Teach that the highest risk for hemorrhage is during the first 24 hours and 5 to 10 days *after* surgery.

HESI Hint • Teach parents why it is important to administer pain medication as prescribed. (Pain medication for this procedure generally has a cough suppressant property to suppress coughing. Coughing may loosen sutures, if used, or clots, at the surgical site causing active bleeding.)

HESI Hint • Removal of ingested sharp objects is a medical emergency.

Review of Respiratory Disorders

1. Describe the purpose of bronchodilators.
2. What are the physical assessment findings for a child with asthma?
3. What nutritional support should be provided for a child with cystic fibrosis?
4. Why is genetic counseling important for the family of a child with cystic fibrosis?
5. List seven signs of respiratory distress in a pediatric client.
6. Describe the care of a child in a mist tent.
7. What position does a child with epiglottitis assume?
8. Why are IV fluids important for a child with an increased respiratory rate?
9. Children with chronic otitis media are at risk for developing what problem?
10. What is the most common postoperative complication after a tonsillectomy? Describe the signs and symptoms of this complication.

Answers to Review

1. To help open the airways by relaxing the bronchial muscles
2. Expiratory wheezing, rales, tight cough, and signs of altered blood gases
3. Pancreatic enzyme replacement; fat-soluble vitamins; and a moderate- to low-carbohydrate, high-protein, moderate- to high-fat diet
4. Because the disease is autosomal recessive in its genetic pattern
5. Restlessness, tachycardia, tachypnea, diaphoresis, flaring nostrils, retractions, and grunting
6. Monitor child's temperature, keep tent edges tucked in, keep clothing dry, assess respiratory status, look at child inside tent
7. Upright sitting, with chin out and tongue protruding ("tripod position")
8. The child is at risk for dehydration and acid-base imbalance.
9. Hearing loss
10. Hemorrhage; frequent swallowing, vomiting fresh blood, and clearing throat

Cardiovascular Disorders

Congenital Heart Disorders

Description: Heart anomalies that develop in utero and manifest at birth or shortly thereafter (Table 5-5)
A. Congenital heart disorders occur in 4 to 10 children per 1000 live births.
B. They may be categorized as:
1. Acyanotic
a. Left-to-right shunts or increased pulmonary blood flow
b. Obstructive defects
2. Cyanotic
a. Right-to-left shunts or decreased blood flow
b. Mixed blood flow

TABLE 5-5 **Congenital Heart Disorders**

Congenital Heart Defects	Conditions	Hemodynamics	Classical Symptoms
ACYANOTIC L → R shunt	ASD VSD PDA	Increased pulmonary blood flow	Increase fatigue Murmur Increase risk endocarditis CHF Growth retardation
	Coarctation/stenosis of aorta	Obstructive pulmonary blood flow	
CYANOTIC R → L shunt	Tetralogy of Fallot	Decreased pulmonary blood flow	Squatting Cyanosis Clubbing Syncope
	TGV TA	Mixed pulmonary blood flow	

C. Hemodynamic classification may used.
1. Increased pulmonary blood flow defects (ASD, VSD, PDA)
2. Obstructive defects (coarctation of aorta, AS)
3. Decreased pulmonary blood flow defects (tetralogy of Fallot)
4. Mixed defects (TGA, TA)

Acyanotic Heart Defects

Ventricular Septal Defect (VSD; Increased Pulmonary Blood Flow)

A. There is a hole between the ventricles.
B. Oxygenated blood from left ventricle is shunted to right ventricle and recirculated to the lungs.
C. Small defects may close spontaneously.
D. Large defects cause Eisenmenger syndrome or CHF and require surgical closures (Fig. 5-4).

Atrial Septal Defect (ASD; Increased Pulmonary Blood Flow)

A. There is a hole between the atria.
B. Oxygenated blood from the left atrium is shunted to the right atrium and lungs.
C. Most defects do not compromise children seriously.
D. Surgical closure is recommended before school age. It can lead to significant problems, such as CHF or atrial dysrhythmias later in life if not corrected (Fig. 5-5).

Patent Ductus Arteriosus (PDA; Increased Pulmonary Blood Flow)

A. There is an abnormal opening between the aorta and the pulmonary artery.
B. It usually closes within 72 hours after birth.
C. If it remains patent, oxygenated blood from the aorta returns to the pulmonary artery.
D. Increased blood flow to the lungs causes pulmonary hypertension.
E. It may require medical intervention with indomethacin (Indocin) administration or surgical closure (Fig. 5-6).
F. Characteristic machinelike murmur

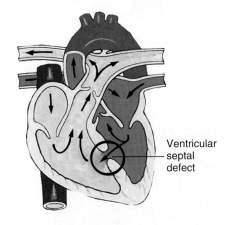

FIGURE 5-4 Ventricular septal defect. (From Hockenberry MJ, Wilson D. *Wong's nursing care of infants and children,* ed 9, St. Louis, 2011, Mosby.)

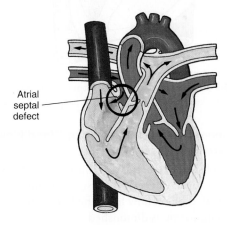

FIGURE 5-5 Atrial septal defect. (From Hockenberry MJ, Wilson D. *Wong's nursing care of infants and children,* ed 9, St. Louis, 2011, Mosby.)

Coarctation of the Aorta (Obstruction of Blood Flow from Ventricles)

A. There is an obstructive narrowing of the aorta.
B. The most common sites are the aortic valve and the aorta near the ductus arteriosus.
C. A common finding is hypertension in the upper extremities and decreased or absent pulses in the lower extremities.
D. It may require surgical correction (Fig. 5-7).

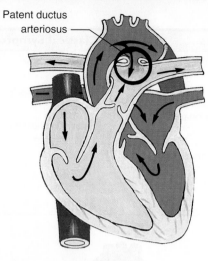

FIGURE 5-6 Patent ductus arteriosus. (From Hockenberry MJ, Wilson D. *Wong's nursing care of infants and children,* ed 9, St. Louis, 2011, Mosby.)

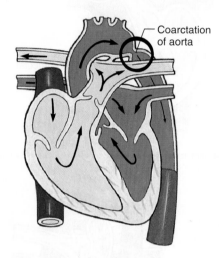

FIGURE 5-7 Coarctation of the aorta. (From Hockenberry MJ, Wilson D. *Wong's nursing care of infants and children,* ed 9, St. Louis, 2011, Mosby.)

Aortic Stenosis (AS; Obstruction of Blood Flow from Ventricles)

A. It is an obstructive narrowing immediately before, at, or after the aortic valve. (It is most commonly valvular.)
B. Oxygenated blood flow from the left ventricle into systemic circulation is diminished.
C. Symptoms are caused by low cardiac output.
D. It may require surgical correction (Fig. 5-8).

The Traditional Three Ts of Cyanotic Heart Disease

Tetralogy of Fallot (Decreased Pulmonary Blood Flow)

A. Combination of four defects:
1. VSD
2. Aorta placed over and above the VSD (overriding aorta)

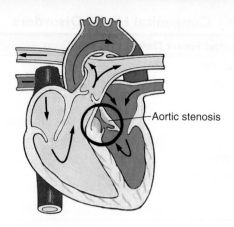

FIGURE 5-8 Aortic stenosis. (From Hockenberry MJ, Wilson D. *Wong's nursing care of infants and children,* ed 9, St. Louis, 2011, Mosby.)

3. Pulmonary stenosis (PS) obstructs right ventricular outflow
4. Right ventricular hypertrophy (the severity of the pulmonary stenosis is related to the degree of right ventricular hypertrophy and the extent of shunting)

The child experiences "tet" spells, or hypoxic episodes; they are relieved by the child's squatting or being placed in the knee-chest position.

Tetralogy of Fallot requires staged surgery for correction (Fig. 5-9).

> **HESI Hint** • Polycythemia is common in children with cyanotic defects.

Truncus Arteriosus (Mixed Blood Flow)

A. Pulmonary artery and aorta do not separate; one artery (truncus), rather than two arteries (aorta and pulmonary artery), arises from both ventricles.
B. One main vessel receives blood from the left and right ventricles together.
C. Blood mixes in right and left ventricles through a large VSD, resulting in cyanosis.
D. Increased pulmonary resistance results in increased cyanosis.
E. This congenital defect requires surgical correction; only the presence of the large VSD allows for survival at birth (Fig. 5-10).

Transposition of the Great Vessels (Mixed Blood Flow)

A. The great vessels are reversed; the pulmonary artery leaves the left ventricle, and the aorta exits from the right ventricle.
B. The pulmonary circulation arises from the left ventricle, and the systemic circulation arises from the right ventricle.
C. This is incompatible with life unless coexisting VSD, ASD, and/or PDA is present.
D. The diagnosis is a *medical emergency.* The child is given prostaglandin E (PGE) to keep the ductus open (Fig. 5-11).

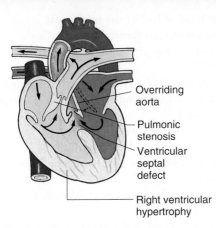

FIGURE 5-9 Tetralogy of Fallot. (From Hockenberry MJ, Wilson D. *Wong's nursing care of infants and children,* ed 9, St. Louis, 2011, Mosby.)

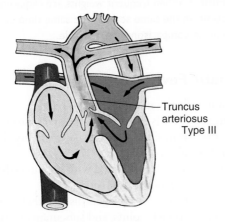

FIGURE 5-10 Truncus arteriosus. (From Hockenberry MJ, Wilson D. *Wong's nursing care of infants and children,* ed 9, St. Louis, 2011, Mosby.)

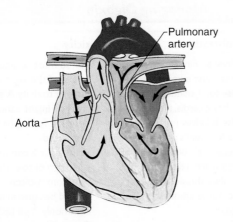

FIGURE 5-11 Transposition of the great vessels. (From Hockenberry MJ, Wilson D. *Wong's nursing care of infants and children,* ed 9, St. Louis, 2011, Mosby.)

Care of Children with Congenital Heart Disease (CHD)

Nursing Assessment

A. Manifestations of CHD
  1. Murmur (present or absent; thrill or rub)
  2. Cyanosis, clubbing of digits (usually after age 2)
  3. Poor feeding, poor weight gain, failure to thrive (FTT)
  4. Frequent regurgitation
  5. Frequent respiratory infections
  6. Activity intolerance, fatigue
B. The following are assessed:
  1. Heart rate and rhythm and heart sounds
  2. Respiratory status/difficulty
  3. Pulses (quality and symmetry)
  4. Blood pressure (upper and lower)
  5. Feeding difficulties; tires easily

> **HESI Hint** • For normal cardiac rates in children, see "Respiratory Disorders" and Table 5-7 in this chapter. The heart rate of a child increases with crying or fever.

Analysis (Nursing Diagnoses)

A. *Decreased cardiac output* related to …
B. *Activity intolerance* related to …
C. *Delayed growth and development* related to …

Nursing Plans and Interventions

A. Provide care for the child with cardiovascular dysfunction.

> **HESI Hint** • Infants may require tube feeding to conserve energy. Infants being tube-fed need to continue to satisfy sucking needs.

  1. Maintain hydration (polycythemia increases risk for thrombus formation).
  2. Maintain neutral thermal environment.
  3. Monitor frequently for fever.
  4. Plan frequent rest periods.
  5. Organize activities so as to disturb child only as indicated.
  6. Administer digoxin and diuretics as prescribed.
  7. Monitor for signs of deteriorating condition or CHF.
  8. Teach family the need for prophylactic antibiotics before any dental or invasive procedures due to risk for endocarditis.
B. Assist with diagnostic tests, and support family during diagnosis.
  1. Electrocardiogram (ECG)
  2. Echocardiography
C. Prepare family and child for cardiac catheterization (conducted when surgery is probable or as an intervention for certain procedures).
  1. Risks of catheterization are similar to those for a child undergoing cardiac surgery:
    a. Arrhythmias
    b. Bleeding
    c. Perforation
    d. Phlebitis
    e. Arterial obstruction at the entry site

2. Child requires reassurance and close monitoring after catheterization:
   a. Vital signs
   b. Pulses
   c. Incision site
   d. Cardiac rhythm
3. Prepare family and child (as able) for surgical intervention if necessary.
D. Prepare child as appropriate for age
   1. Show to ICU.
   2. Explain chest tubes, IV lines, monitors, dressings, and ventilator.
   3. Show family and child waiting area for families.
   4. Use a doll or a drawing for explanations.
   5. Provide emotional support.
   6. Include and incorporate family as much as possible in client teachings.

> **HESI Hint** • Basic differences between cyanotic and acyanotic defects:
> - Acyanotic: Has abnormal circulation; however, all blood entering the systemic circulation is oxygenated.
> - Cyanotic: Has abnormal circulation with unoxygenated blood entering the systemic circulation.

Congestive Heart Failure

Congestive Heart Failure (CHF) is more often associated with acyanotic defects.
Description: Condition in which the heart is unable to pump effectively the volume of blood that is presented to it.

> **HESI Hint** • CHF is a common complication of CHD. It reflects the increased workload of the heart caused by shunts or obstructions. The two objectives in treating CHF are to reduce the workload of the heart and increase cardiac output.

Nursing Assessment

A. Tachypnea, shortness of breath
B. Tachycardia
C. Difficulty feeding
D. Cyanosis
E. Grunting, wheezing, pulmonary congestion
F. Edema (face, eyes of infants), weight gain
G. Diaphoresis (especially head)
H. Hepatomegaly

Analysis (Nursing Diagnoses)

A. *Decreased cardiac output* related to …
B. *Impaired gas exchange* related to …

Nursing Plans and Interventions

A. Monitor vital signs frequently, and report signs of increasing distress.
B. Assess respiratory functioning frequently.

C. Elevate head of bed or use infant seat.
D. Administer oxygen therapy as prescribed.
E. Administer digoxin and diuretics as prescribed (Box 5-2).
F. Weigh frequently (may be every shift for infants).
G. Maintain strict input and output (I&O); weigh diapers (1 g = 1 mL).
H. Report any unusual weight gains.
I. Provide low-sodium diet or formula.
J. Gavage-feed infants if unable to get adequate nutrition by mouth.
K. Continue care for infant or child with a congenital defect as indicated.
L. See Nursing Plans and Interventions, Cyanotic Heart Defects.

> **HESI Hint** • When frequent weights are required, weigh client on the same scale at the same time of day so that accurate comparisons can be made.

Rheumatic Fever

Description: Inflammatory disease
A. Rheumatic fever is the most common cause of *acquired* heart disease in children. It usually affects the aortic and mitral valves of the heart.
B. Rheumatic fever is associated with an antecedent beta-hemolytic streptococcal infection.
C. Rheumatic fever is a collagen disease that injures the heart, blood vessels, joints, and subcutaneous tissue.

BOX 5-2 *Managing Digoxin*	
Administration	**Toxicity**

• Before administering digoxin, nurse must take child's apical pulse for 1 minute to assess for bradycardia. Hold dose if pulse is below normal heart rate for child's age.
• Therapeutic blood levels of digoxin are 0.8 to 2.0 ng/mL.
• Families should be taught safe home administration of digoxin:
  • Administer on a regular basis; do not skip or make up for missed doses.
  • Give 1 hour before or 2 hours after meals. Do not mix with formula or food.
• Take child's pulse before administration, and know when to call the caregiver.
• Keep in safe place (e.g., a locked cabinet).
	• Nurse must be acutely aware of the signs of digoxin toxicity. A small child or infant cannot describe feeling bad or nauseated.
	• Vomiting is a common early sign of toxicity. This symptom is often overlooked because infants commonly "spit up."
	• Other GI symptoms include anorexia, diarrhea, and abdominal pain.
	• Neurologic signs include fatigue, muscle weakness, and drowsiness.
	• Hypokalemia can increase digoxin toxicity.

Nursing Assessment

A. Chest pain, shortness of breath (carditis)
B. Tachycardia, even during sleep
C. Migratory large-joint pain
D. Chorea (irregular involuntary movements)
E. Rash (erythema marginatum)
F. Subcutaneous nodules over bony prominences
G. Fever
H. Laboratory findings:
    1. Elevated erythrocyte sedimentation rate (ESR)
    2. Elevated ASO (antistreptolysin O) titer

Analysis (Nursing Diagnoses)

A. *Decreased cardiac output* related to …
B. *Risk for injury* related to …

Nursing Plans and Interventions

A. Monitor vital signs.
B. Assess for increasing signs of cardiac distress.
C. Encourage bed rest (as needed during febrile illness).
D. Assist with ambulation.
E. Reassure child and family that chorea is temporary.
F. Administer prescribed medications.
    1. Penicillin or erythromycin
    2. Aspirin for antiinflammatory and anticoagulant actions
G. Teach home care program.
    1. Explain the necessity for prophylactics.
       a. Antibiotics taken either orally or IM
       b. IM penicillin G each month (Table 5-6)
    2. Inform dentist and other health care providers of diagnosis so they can evaluate the necessity for prophylactic antibiotics.

Kawasaki Disease (Mucocutaneous Lymph Node Syndrome)

Description: Kawasaki disease is an acute systemic vasculitis that can cause damage to vessels, including the coronary arteries that supply blood flow to the heart. This disease also affects the mucous membrane lining of the mouth, nose, and throat, as well as the lymph nodes and skin. The disease causes permanent damage to the main arteries to the heart, resulting in the formation of an aneurysm of the coronary artery.
A. Cause of disease is unknown
B. Usually seen in children younger than 5 years of age
C. Has three phases: acute, subacute, and convalescent
D. Leading cause of acquired heart disease in children
E. Early treatment is essential to decrease chances of permanent heart damage

Assessment (Data Collection)

A. Acute phase
    1. High fever 39° C (102.2° F or higher) for more than 5 days
    2. Conjunctival redness without discharge, cracked and dried lips, and strawberry tongue
    3. Swollen lymph nodes of the neck
    4. Rash present on trunk and genital area
    5. Red, swollen hands and feet
B. Subacute phase
    1. Peeling of hands and feet
    2. Cardiovascular manifestations may be seen
    3. GI manifestations: abdominal pain, vomiting, and diarrhea
    4. Skeletal joint pain.
C. Convalescent (last) phase starts when all signs are gone and ends when laboratory values have returned to normal.
D. Extreme irritability is seen in the child during the disease process.

Analysis (Nursing Diagnoses)

A. *Impaired skin integrity* related to…
B. *Decreased cardiac output* related to…

Nursing Plan and Interventions

A. Administer intravenous immunoglobulin (IVIG) and aspirin (salicylate therapy) as prescribed to treat the disease process, not to treat the fever.
B. Treat high fevers with acetaminophen as prescribed.
C. Monitor cardiac status by documenting the child's:
    1. Intake and output
    2. Daily weights
D. Minimize skin discomfort with lotions and cool compresses.
E. Initiate meticulous mouth care.
F. Monitor intake of clear liquids and soft foods.
G. Support family as they comfort child during periods of irritability.
H. Provide discharge teaching and home referral.

TABLE 5-6 Antiinfective

Drug/Route	Indications	Adverse Reactions	Nursing Implications
• Penicillin G IM	• Prophylaxis for recurrence of rheumatic fever	• Allergic reactions ranging from rashes to anaphylactic shock and death	• Penicillin G is released very slowly over several weeks, giving sustained levels of concentration. • Have emergency equipment available wherever medication is administered. • *Always* determine existence of allergies to penicillin and cephalosporins; check chart and record and inquire of client and family.

Review of Cardiovascular Disorders

1. Differentiate between a right-to-left and a left-to-right shunt in cardiac disease.
2. List the four defects associated with tetralogy of Fallot.
3. List the common signs of cardiac problems in an infant.
4. What are the two objectives in treating CHF?
5. Describe nursing interventions to reduce the workload of the heart.
6. What position would best relieve the child experiencing a tet spell?
7. What are the common signs of digoxin toxicity?
8. List five risks in cardiac catheterization.
9. What cardiac complications are associated with rheumatic fever?
10. What medications are used to treat rheumatic fever?

Answers to Review

1. A right-to-left shunt bypasses the lungs and delivers unoxygenated blood to the systemic circulation, causing cyanosis. A left-to-right shunt moves oxygenated blood back through the pulmonary circulation.
2. VSD, overriding aorta, pulmonary stenosis, and right ventricular hypertrophy
3. Poor feeding, poor weight gain, respiratory distress and infections, edema, and cyanosis
4. Reduce the workload of the heart and increase cardiac output.
5. Give small, frequent feedings or gavage feedings. Plan frequent rest periods. Maintain a neutral thermal environment. Organize activities to disturb child only as indicated.
6. Knee-chest position or squatting
7. Diarrhea, fatigue, weakness, nausea, and vomiting; the nurse should check for bradycardia before administration
8. Arrhythmia, bleeding, perforation, phlebitis, and obstruction of the arterial entry site
9. Aortic valve stenosis and mitral valve stenosis
10. Penicillin, erythromycin, and aspirin

Neuromuscular Disorders

Down Syndrome

Description: Most common chromosomal abnormality in children
A. Down syndrome is evidenced by various physical characteristics and by cognitive impairment (Fig. 5-12).
B. Down syndrome occurs when cell division is abnormal; as a result there is extra genetic material from chromosome 21 and, in less than 5% of cases, a translocation of chromosome 21.
D. Common associated problems
   1. Cardiac defects
   2. Respiratory infections
   3. Feeding difficulties
   4. Delayed developmental skills
   5. Mental retardation (low IQ range of 20–70)
   6. Skeletal defects
   7. Altered immune function
   8. Endocrine dysfunctions; hypothyroidism; diabetic muscular infarction (DMI)

Analysis (Nursing Diagnoses)

A. *Delayed growth and development* related to …
B. *Risk for impaired parenting* related to …

Nursing Plans and Interventions

A. Assist and support parents during the diagnostic process and management of child's associated problems.

A. Common physical characteristics

HEAD to TOE	
1.	Small head
2.	Flat, wide nasal bridge
3.	Inner epicanthal eye fold
4.	Upward, outward slant of eyes
5.	Brushfield spots on the iris (white spots)
6.	Small, irregularly shaped ears; low-set
7.	Small mouth and protruding tongue
8.	Short neck.
9.	Short, stubby hands with a single crease in palm (Simian crease)
10.	Short arms and legs in comparison to their body
11.	Short in stature
12.	Hypotonic flexibility
13.	Atlantoaxial instability
14.	Short, stubby toes with an enlarged space between the big toe and other toes.
15.	Hyperextensible and lax joint (hypotonia)

FIGURE 5-12 Head-to-toe common characteristics of Down syndrome (Adapted by Katherine T. Ralph MSN, RN, Elsevier/HESI.)

B. Assess and monitor growth and development.
C. Teach use of bulb syringe for suctioning nares.
D. Teach signs of respiratory infection.
E. Assist family with feeding problems.
F. Feed to back and side of mouth.
G. Monitor for signs of cardiac difficulty or respiratory infection.

H. Refer family to early intervention program.
I. Refer to other specialists as indicated: nutritionist, speech therapist, physical therapist, and occupational therapist.

> **HESI Hint** • The nursing goal in caring for a child with Down syndrome is to help the child reach his or her optimal level of functioning.

Cerebral Palsy (CP)

Description: Nonprogressive injury to the motor centers of the brain causing neuromuscular problems of spasticity or dyskinesia (involuntary movements). This injury can occur to a healthy infant during uterine development, the birthing process, or exposure to an infection such as meningitis during the early years of development; it is irreversible. The extent of the damage is dependent on the location of trauma to the brain; the symptoms either worsen or improve over time.
A. Associated problems may include cognitive impairment and seizures.
B. Causes include:
   1. Anoxic injury before, during, or after birth
   2. Maternal infections
   3. Kernicterus
   4. Low birth weight (major risk factor)

Nursing Assessment

A. Persistent neonatal reflexes (Moro, tonic neck) after 6 months
B. Delayed developmental milestones
C. Apparent early preference for one hand
D. Poor suck, tongue thrust
E. Spasticity (may be described as "difficulty with diapering" by mother or caregiver)
F. Scissoring of legs (legs are extended and crossed over each other, feet are plantar flexed; a common characteristic of spastic CP)
G. Involuntary movements
H. Seizures

Analysis (Nursing Diagnoses)

A. *Delayed growth and development* related to …
B. *Risk for imbalanced nutrition: less than body requirements* related to …

Nursing Plans and Interventions

A. Identify CP through follow-up of high-risk infants such as premature infants, breech births, cardiac and/or respiratory distress during birth, low Apgar scores, a product of multiple pregnancies, and/or severe jaundiced.
B. Refer to community-based agencies.
C. Coordinate with physical therapist, occupational therapist, speech therapist, nutritionist, orthopedic surgeon, and neurologist

> **HESI Hint** • Feed infant or child with CP using nursing interventions aimed at preventing aspiration. Position child upright, and support the lower jaw.

D. Support family through grief process at diagnosis and throughout the child's life. Caring for severely affected children is very challenging.
E. Administer anticonvulsant medications such as phenytoin (Dilantin) if prescribed (Table 5-7).
F. Administer diazepam (Valium) for muscle spasms if prescribed (see Table 7-4).

Attention-Deficit Disorder, Attention-Deficit/Hyperactivity Disorder

Description: Attention-Deficit Disorder, Attention Deficit/Hyperactivity Disorder (ADD/ADHD) are classified in the DSM5 as neurodevelopmental disorders (see Chapter 7 Psychiatric Nursing). However, recent studies indicate that these disorders may be linked to genetics. Children up to 16 years old are identified as having attention-deficit disorder if they exhibit a minimum of six of the inattention symptoms.

Spina Bifida

Description: Malformation of the vertebrae and spinal cord resulting in varying degrees of disability and deformity depending on the location of the malformation (Fig. 5-13). It is often referred to as a *neural tube defect*.
A. Types of spina bifida
   1. Spina bifida occulta is a defect of vertebrae only. No sac is present, and it is usually a benign condition, although bowel and bladder problems may occur.
   2. With meningocele and myelomeningocele, a sac is present at some point along the spine.
   3. Meningocele contains only meninges and spinal fluid and has less neurologic involvement than a myelomeningocele.
   4. Myelomeningocele is more severe than meningocele because the sac contains spinal fluid, meninges, and nerves.
B. Prevention
   1. Women in childbearing years before and during pregnancy should consume a minimum 400 mcg of folic acid daily, whether from a supplement or folic-enriched foods such as egg yolks, dark green vegetables, citrus fruits, juices, or beans.
D. Every child with a history of spina bifida should be screened for latex allergies.

Nursing Assessment

A. Spina bifida occulta: dimple with or without hair tuft at base of spine
B. Presence of sac in myelomeningocele is usually lumbar or lumbosacral

TABLE 5-7 Anticonvulsants

Drugs/Routes	Indications	Adverse Reactions	Nursing Implications
• Phenobarbital PO, IM, IV	• Tonic-clonic and partial seizures • Is the longest acting of common barbiturates • Usually combined with other drugs	• Drowsiness • Nystagmus • Ataxia • Paradoxic excitement	• Therapeutic levels: 15-40 mcg/mL • Avoid rapid IV infusion. • Monitor blood pressure during IV infusion.
• Phenytoin PO, IV	• Tonic-clonic and partial seizures	• Gingival hyperplasia • Dermatitis • Ataxia • Nausea, anorexia • Bone marrow depression • Nystagmus	• Therapeutic levels: 10–20 mcg/mL • Monitor any drug interactions. • Do not administer with milk. • Ensure meticulous oral hygiene. • Monitor CBC. • Report to physician if any rash develops. • For IV administration, flush IV line before and after with normal saline *only*.
• Fosphenytoin sodium IM, IV	• Generalized convulsive status epilepticus • Prevention and treatment of seizures during neurosurgery • Short-term parenteral replacement for phenytoin oral (Dilantin)	• Rapid IV infusion can cause hypotension. • Severe: ataxia, CNS toxicity, confusion, gingival hyperplasia, irritability, lupus erythematosus, nervousness, nystagmus, paradoxic excitement, Stevens-Johnson syndrome, toxic epidural necrosis	• Use for short-term parenteral use (IV infusion or IM injection) only. • Should always be prescribed and dispensed in phenytoin sodium equivalents (PEs) • Before IV infusion, dilute in D_5W or NS to administer. • Infuse at IV rate of no more than 150 mg PE/min.
• Valproic acid PO	• Absence seizures • Myoclonic seizures	• Hepatotoxicity, especially in children less than 2 yr • Prolonged bleeding times • GI disturbances	• Monitor liver function. • Potentiates phenobarbital and Dilantin, altering blood levels • Therapeutic levels: 50–100 mEq/mL
• Carbamazepine PO	• Tonic-clonic, mixed seizures • Drowsiness • Ataxia	• Hepatitis • Agranulocytosis	• Monitor liver function while on therapy. • Therapeutic levels: 6–12 mcg/mL
• Lamotrigine PO	• Partial seizures • Tonic-clonic seizures • Absence seizures	• Dizziness • Headache • Nausea • Rash	• Withhold drug if rash develops. • Do not discontinue abruptly.
• Clonazepam PO	• Absence seizures • Myoclonic seizures	• Drowsiness • Hyperactivity • Agitation • Increased salivation	• Therapeutic levels: 20–80 mcg/mL • Do not abruptly discontinue drug. • Monitor liver function, CBC, and renal function periodically.

C. Flaccid paralysis and limited or no feeling below the defect

D. Head circumference at variance with norms on growth grids

E. Associated problems:
1. Hydrocephalus (90% with myelomeningocele)
2. Neurogenic bladder, poor anal sphincter tone
3. Congenital dislocated hips
4. Club feet

5. Skin problems associated with anesthesia below the defect

6. Scoliosis

Analysis (Nursing Diagnoses)

A. *Risk for infection* related to …

B. *Impaired urinary elimination patterns* related to …

C. *Impaired physical mobility* related to …

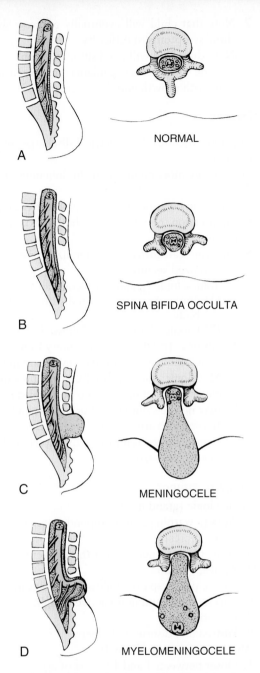

FIGURE 5-13 Midline defects of osseous spine with varying degrees of neural herniations. **(A)** Normal. **(B)** Spina bifida occulta. **(C)** Meningocele. **(D)** Myelomeningocele. (From Hockenberry MJ, Wilson D. *Wong's essentials of pediatric nursing,* ed 9, St. Louis, 2013, Mosby.)

Nursing Plans and Interventions

A. Preoperative: Place infant in prone position.
  1. Keep sac free of stool and urine.
  2. Cover sac with moist sterile dressing.
  3. Elevate foot of bed, and position child on his or her abdomen, with legs abducted.
  4. Measure head circumference at least every 8 hours or every shift; check fontanel.
  5. Assess neurologic function.
  6. Monitor for signs of infection.
  7. Empty bladder using Credé method, or catheterize if needed.
  8. Promote parent–infant bonding.
B. Postoperative: Place infant in prone position.
  1. Make same assessments as preoperatively.
  2. Assess incision for drainage and infection.
  3. Assess neurologic function.
C. Long-term care.
  1. Teach family catheterization program when child is young.
  2. Help older children to learn self-catheterization.
  3. Administer propantheline (Pro-Banthine) or bethanechol (Urecholine) as prescribed to improve continence.
  4. Develop bowel program.
    a. High-fiber diet
    b. Increased fluids
    c. Regular fluids
    d. Suppositories as needed
  5. Assess skin condition frequently.
  6. Assist with range-of-motion (ROM) exercises, ambulation, and bracing, if client is able.
  7. Coordinate with team members: neurologist, orthopedist, urologist, physical therapist, and nutritionist.
D. Support independent functioning of child.
E. Assist family to make realistic developmental expectations of child.

Hydrocephalus

Description: Condition characterized by an abnormal accumulation of cerebrospinal fluid (CSF) within the ventricles of the brain that does not drain properly from the cranium
A. It is usually caused by an obstruction in the flow of CSF between the ventricles.
B. Results in enlargement of the ventricles, which causes pressure on the brain tissue.
C. Hydrocephalus is most often associated with spina bifida; it can be a complication of meningitis.

> **HESI Hint** • Infants with hydrocephalus have enlarged head circumference as a result of widening fontanels that compensate for accumulating cerebral spinal fluid and that help relieve pressure of the developing brain.

> **HESI Hint** • The signs of increased intracranial pressure (ICP) are the opposite of those of shock:
> • Shock: increased pulse, decreased blood pressure
> • Increased ICP: decreased pulse, increased blood pressure

Nursing Assessment

A. Toddlers and older children show classic signs of ICP
  1. Change in level of consciousness (LOC)
  2. Irritability

3. Vomiting
4. Headache on awakening
5. Motor dysfunction
6. Unequal pupil response
7. Seizures
8. Decline in academics
9. Change in personality

B. Signs of increased ICP in infants
1. Irritability, lethargy
2. Increasing head circumference
3. Bulging fontanels
4. Widening suture lines
5. "Sunset" eyes
6. High-pitched cry
7. Feeding difficulties
8. Decreased muscle tone and strength.

> **HESI Hint** • Baseline data on the child's usual behavior and level of development are essential so changes associated with increased ICP can be detected early.

Analysis (Nursing Diagnoses)

A. *Delayed growth and development* related to …
B. *Risk for injury* related to …

Nursing Plans and Interventions

A. Prepare infant and family for diagnostic procedures.
B. Monitor for signs of increased ICP.
C. Maintain seizure precautions.
D. Elevate head of bed.
E. Prepare parents for surgical procedure (e.g., ventricular shunt placement)
F. Purpose of the shunt is to drain the excess fluid off the brain.
G. Postoperative care
1. Assess for signs of shunt malfunction.
   a. Infant
      (1) Change in size, signs of bulging, tenseness in fontanels, and separation of suture lines
      (2) Irritability, lethargy, or seizure activity
      (3) Altered vital signs and feeding behavior
   b. Older child: Increase in ICP
      (1) Change in LOC
      (2) Complaint of headache
      (3) Changes in customary behavior (sleep patterns, developmental capabilities)
2. Assess for signs of infection (meningitis).
   a. Increase fever greater than 38.6° C (100.5° F).
   b. Shunt tract appears reddened, tender, and swollen; drainage may be present.
   c. Decrease feeding/increase vomiting.
   d. Stiff neck and headache.
3. Monitor I&O closely.
4. Assess surgical sites (head and abdomen)
H. Teach home care program.
1. Teach to watch for signs of increased ICP or infection.

2. Note that child will eventually outgrow shunt and show symptoms of difficulty.
3. Note that child will need shunt revision.
4. Provide anticipatory guidance for potential problems with growth and development.

Seizures

Description: Uncontrolled electrical discharges of neurons in the brain

A. Seizures are more common in children under the age of 2 years.
B. Seizures can be associated with immaturity of the CNS, fever, infection, neoplasms, cerebral anoxia, and metabolic disorders.
C. Seizures are categorized as generalized or partial.
1. Generalized seizures are:
   a. Tonic-clonic (grand mal): consciousness is lost
      (1) Tonic phase: generalized stiffness of entire body
      (2) Clonic phase: spasm followed by relaxation
   b. Absence (petit mal): momentary LOC, posture is maintained; has minor face, eye, hand movements
   c. Myoclonic: sudden, brief contractures of a muscle or group of muscles, no postictal state, may or may not be symmetrical or include LOC
2. Partial seizures arise from a specific area in the brain and cause limited symptoms. Examples are focal and psychomotor seizures.

Nursing Assessment

A. Tonic-clonic (grand mal)
1. Aura (a warning sign of impending seizure)
2. LOC
3. Tonic phase: generalized stiffness of entire body
4. Apnea, cyanosis
5. Clonic phase: spasms followed by relaxation
6. Pupils dilated and nonreactive to light
7. Incontinence
8. Postseizure: disoriented, sleepy
B. Absence seizures (petit mal)
1. Onset between 4 and 12 years of age
2. Last 5 to 10 seconds
3. Child appears to be inattentive, daydreaming
4. Poor performance in school

> **HESI Hint** • Medication noncompliance is the most common cause of increased seizure activity.

Analysis (Nursing Diagnoses)

A. *Risk for injury: trauma* related to …
B. Redirection for enhanced self health …

Nursing Plans and Interventions

A. Maintain airway during seizure: Turn client on side to aid ventilation.

B. Do not restrain client.
C. Protect client from injury during seizure, and support head (avoid neck flexion).
D. Document seizure, noting all data in assessment.
E. Maintain seizure precautions.
   1. Reduce environmental stimuli as much as possible.
   2. Pad side rails or crib rails.
   3. Have suction equipment and oxygen quickly accessible; set up at the bedside/crib side. Tape oral airway to the head of the bed.

> **HESI Hint** • Do *not* use tongue blade, padded or not, during a seizure. It can cause traumatic damage to the oral cavity.

F. Support during diagnostic tests: electroencephalogram (EEG), computed tomography (CT) scan
G. Support during workup for infections such as meningitis
H. Administer anticonvulsant medications as prescribed (see Table 5-7).
   1. For tonic-clonic seizures: phenytoin, carbamazepine, phenobarbital, and fosphenytoin
   2. For absence seizures: ethosuximide, valproic acid
I. Monitor therapeutic drug levels.
J. Teach family about drug administration: dosage, action, and side effects.

Bacterial Meningitis

Description: Bacterial inflammatory disorder of the meninges that cover the brain and spinal cord
A. Meningitis is usually caused by Haemophilus influenzae type B (less prevalent), Streptococcus pneumoniae, or Neisseria meningitidis.
B. The usual source of bacterial invasion is the middle ear or the nasopharynx.
C. Other sources of bacteria from wounds include fractures of the skull, lumbar punctures, and shunts.
D. Exudate covers brain, and cerebral edema occurs.
E. Lumbar puncture shows
   1. Increased white blood cells (WBCs)
   2. Decreased glucose
   3. Elevated protein
   4. Increased ICP
   5. Positive culture for meningitis

> **HESI Hint** • Decreased glucose and elevated protein occur because bacteria present in the CSF consume the glucose and then defecate the protein.

Nursing Assessment

A. Older children
   1. Classic signs of increased ICP (see Hydrocephalus)
   2. Fever, chills
   3. Neck stiffness, opisthotonos
   4. Photophobia
   5. Positive Kernig sign (inability to extend leg when thigh is flexed anteriorly at hip)
   6. Positive Brudzinski sign (neck flexion causing adduction and flexion movements of lower extremities)
B. Infants and young children (3 months to 2 years old)
   1. Absence of classic signs
   2. Ill, with generalized symptoms
   3. Poor feeding
   4. Vomiting, irritability
   5. Bulging fontanel (an important sign)
   6. Seizures
C. Neonates (birth to 2 months)
   1. Very difficult to diagnose.
   2. Temperature nonspecific: may be normal, hypothermia or hyperthermia.
   3. Symptoms can appear a few days after birth.
   4. Infant has difficulty eating and refuses to eat when prompted.
   5. Weak cry.
   6. Vomiting and diarrhea may be present.
   7. Movement decreases, along with tone.
   8. Restless, sleep pattern changes.
   9. Late sign: bulging and tense fontanel.

Analysis (Nursing Diagnoses)

A. *Nausea* (specify) related to …
B. *Risk for trauma* related to …

Nursing Plans and Interventions

A. Administer antibiotics (usually ampicillin, ceftriaxone, or chloramphenicol) and antipyretics as prescribed.
B. Isolate for at least 24 hours.
C. Monitor vital signs and neurologic signs.
D. Keep environment quiet and darkened to prevent overstimulation.
E. Implement seizure precautions.
F. Position for comfort: head of the bed slightly elevated, with client on side if prescribed.
G. Measure head circumference daily in infants.
H. Monitor I&O closely.
I. Administer Hib vaccine to protect against *H. influenzae* infection (see Table 5-1).

> **HESI Hint** • Monitor hydration status and IV therapy carefully. With meningitis, there may be inappropriate antidiuretic hormone (ADH) secretions causing fluid retention (cerebral edema) and dilutional hyponatremia.

Reye Syndrome

Description: Acute, rapidly progressing encephalopathy and hepatic dysfunction
A. Causes include antecedent viral infections, such as influenza or chickenpox.
B. Occurrence is often associated with aspirin use.

C. Disease is staged according to the clinical manifestations to reflect the severity of the condition.

Nursing Assessment

A. Usually occurs in school-age children
B. Lethargy, rapidly progressing to deep coma (marked cerebral edema)
C. Vomiting
D. Elevated aspartate aminotransferase (AST), alanine aminotransferase (ALT), lactate dehydrogenase, serum ammonia, decreased PT
E. Hypoglycemia

Analysis (Nursing Diagnoses)

A. *Excess fluid volume* related to …
B. *Ineffective breathing pattern* related to …

Nursing Plans and Interventions

A. Provide critical care early in syndrome.
B. Monitor neurologic status: frequent noninvasive assessments and invasive ICP monitoring.
C. Maintain ventilation.
D. Monitor cardiac parameters (i.e., invasive cardiac monitoring system).
E. Administer mannitol, if prescribed, to increase blood osmolality (Table 5-8).
F. Monitor I&O accurately.
G. Care for Foley catheter.
H. Provide family with emotional support.

Brain Tumors

Description: Third most common cancer in children after leukemia and lymphomas
A. Most pediatric brain tumors are infratentorial, making them difficult to excise surgically.
B. Tumors usually occur close to vital structures.
C. Medulloblastomas are the most common childhood brain tumors.

Nursing Assessment

A. Headache

> **HESI Hint** • Headache upon awakening is a common presenting symptom of brain tumor in children.

B. Vomiting (usually in the morning), often without nausea
C. Loss of concentration

D. Change in behavior or personality
E. Vision problems, tilting of head
F. In infants: widening sutures, increasing frontal occipital circumference, tense fontanel

Analysis (Nursing Diagnoses)

A. *Ineffective tissue perfusion* (cerebral) related to …
B. *Risk for trauma* related to …
C. *Risk for infection* (postoperative) related to …

Nursing Plans and Interventions

A. Identify baseline neurologic functioning.
B. Support child and family during diagnostic workup and treatment.
C. If surgery is treatment of choice, provide preoperative teaching:
   1. Explain that head will be shaved.
   2. Describe ICU, dressings, IV lines, etc.
   3. Identify child's developmental level, and plan teaching accordingly.
D. Assess family's response to the diagnosis, and treat family appropriately.
E. After surgery, position client as prescribed by the health care provider.

> **HESI Hint** • Most postoperative clients with infratentorial tumors are prescribed to lie flat or turn to either side. A large tumor may require that the child *not* be turned to the operative side.

F. Monitor IV fluids and output carefully. Overhydration can cause cerebral edema and increased ICP.
G. Administer steroids and osmotic diuretics as prescribed (see Table 5-12).
H. Support child and family to promote optimum functioning postoperatively.

> **HESI Hint** • Suctioning, coughing, straining, and turning cause increased ICP.

Muscular Dystrophy

Description: Inherited disease of the muscles, causing muscle atrophy and weakness
A. The most serious and most common of the dystrophies is Duchenne muscular dystrophy, an X-linked recessive disease affecting primarily males.

TABLE 5-8 Diuretic

Drug/Route	Indications	Adverse Reactions	Nursing Implications

• Mannitol IV	• Osmotic diuretic used to reduce:
	  • Cerebral edema
	  • Postoperative swelling or trauma
		• Circulatory overload
		• Confusion
		• Hypokalemia
		• Hyponatremia
			• Use in-line filter for IV administration, and avoid extravasation.
			• Monitor I&O.
			• Furosemide (Lasix) may also be prescribed.

B. Duchenne muscular dystrophy appears in early childhood (ages 3 to 5 years) (children appear normal at birth until signs and symptoms of the disease manifest).

C. By the age of 9 to 11 years old, the child loses the ability to walk independently.

Nursing Assessment

A. Waddling gait, lordosis
B. Increasing clumsiness, muscle weakness
C. Gowers sign: difficulty rising to standing position; has to "walk" up legs, using hands
D. Pseudohypertrophy of muscles (especially noted in calves) due to fat deposits
E. Muscle degeneration, especially the thighs, and fatty infiltrates (detected by muscle biopsy); cardiac muscle also involved
F. Delayed cognitive development
G. Later in disease: scoliosis, respiratory difficulty, and cardiac difficulties
H. Eventual wheelchair dependency, confinement to bed

Analysis (Nursing Diagnoses)

A. *Impaired physical mobility* related to …
B. *Chronic low self-esteem* related to …

Nursing Plans and Interventions

A. Provide supportive care.
B. Provide exercises (active and passive).
C. Prevent exposure to respiratory infection.
D. Encourage a balanced diet to avoid obesity.
E. Support family's grieving process.
F. Support participation in the Muscular Dystrophy Association.
G. Coordinate with health care team: physical therapist, occupational therapist, nutritionist, neurologist, orthopedist, and geneticist.

> **HESI Hint** • Encourage the parents of children who are diagnosed with any type of neuromuscular disease to allow the child to do as much as possible as he or she can for himself or herself to try to maintain muscle function and independence.

Review of Neuromuscular Disorders

1. What are the physical features of a child with Down syndrome?
2. Describe scissoring.
3. What are two nursing priorities for a newborn with myelomeningocele?
4. List the signs and symptoms of increased ICP in older children.
5. What teaching should parents of a newly shunted child receive?
6. State the three main goals in providing nursing care for a child experiencing a seizure.
7. What are the side effects of Dilantin?
8. Describe the signs and symptoms of a child with meningitis.
9. What antibiotics are usually prescribed for bacterial meningitis?
10. How is a child usually positioned after brain tumor surgery?
11. Describe the function of an osmotic diuretic.
12. What nursing interventions increase intracranial pressure?
13. Describe the mechanism of inheritance of Duchenne muscular dystrophy.
14. What is the Gowers sign?

Answers to Review

1. Simian creases in palms, hypotonia, protruding tongue, and upward-outward slant of eyes
2. A common characteristic of spastic CP in infants; legs are extended and crossed over each other; feet are plantar flexed
3. Prevention of infection of the sac and monitoring for hydrocephalus (measure head circumference, check fontanel, assess neurologic functioning)
4. Irritability, change in LOC, motor dysfunction, headache, vomiting, unequal pupil response, and seizures
5. Information about signs of infection and increased ICP; understanding that shunt should not be pumped and that child will need revisions with growth; guidance concerning growth and development
6. Maintain patent airway, protect from injury, and observe carefully.
7. Gingival hyperplasia, dermatitis, ataxia, GI distress
8. Fever, irritability, vomiting, neck stiffness, opisthotonos, positive Kernig sign, positive Brudzinski sign; infant may not show all classic signs even though very ill
9. Ampicillin, ceftriaxone, or chloramphenicol
10. Flat or on either side
11. Osmotic diuretics remove water from the CNS to reduce cerebral edema
12. Suctioning and positioning, turning
13. Duchenne muscular dystrophy is inherited as an X-linked recessive trait.
14. Gowers sign is an indicator of muscular dystrophy; to stand, the child has to "walk" hands up legs.

Renal Disorders

Acute Glomerulonephritis (AGN)

Description: Immune complex response to an antecedent beta-hemolytic streptococcal infection of skin or pharynx; antigen–antibody complexes become trapped in the membrane of the glomeruli, causing inflammation and decreased glomerular filtration.

Nursing Assessment

A. Recent streptococcal infection (e.g., strep throat)
B. Mild to moderate edema (often confined to face)
C. Irritability, lethargy
D. Hypertension
E. Dark-colored urine (hematuria)
F. Slight to moderate proteinuria
G. Elevated antistreptolysin (ASO) titer, elevated BUN and creatinine
H. Oliguria
I. Edematous face, especially around the eyes, abdomen, hands, and feet

Analysis (Nursing Diagnoses)

A. *Excess fluid volume* related to …
B. *Risk for trauma* related to …

Nursing Plans and Interventions

A. Provide supportive care.
B. Monitor vital signs (especially blood pressure) frequently.
C. Monitor I&O closely.
D. Weigh daily.
E. Provide low-sodium diet with no added salt; low potassium, if oliguric.
F. Encourage bed rest during acute phase (usually 4 to 10 days).
G. Administer antihypertensives if prescribed.
H. Monitor for seizures (hypertensive encephalopathy).
I. Monitor for signs of CHF.
J. Monitor for signs of renal failure (uncommon).

> **HESI Hint** • Decreased urinary output is the first sign of renal failure.

Nephrotic Syndrome

Description: A disorder in which the basement membrane of the glomeruli becomes permeable to plasma proteins; most often idiopathic in nature
A. It usually occurs between the ages of 2 and 3 years.
B. Its course may involve exacerbations and remissions over several years.
C. Refer to Table 5-9

TABLE 5-9 Comparison of Acute Glomerulonephritis and Nephrotic Syndrome

Variable	Acute Glomerulonephritis	Nephrotic Syndrome
Causes	Follows streptococcal infection	Usually idiopathic
Edema	Mild, usually around eyes	Severe, generalized
Blood pressure	Elevated	Normal
Urine	Dark, tea-colored (hematuria) Slight or moderate proteinuria	Dark, frothy yellow Massive proteinuria
Blood	Normal serum protein Positive ASO titer	Decreased serum protein Negative ASO titer

Nursing Assessment

A. Edema that begins insidiously becomes severe and generalized
B. Lethargy
C. Anorexia
D. Pallor
E. Frothy-appearing urine
F. Massive proteinuria
G. Decreased serum protein (hypoproteinemia)
H. Elevated serum lipids

Analysis (Nursing Diagnoses)

A. *Excess fluid volume* related to …
B. *Imbalanced nutrition: less than body requirements* related to …

Nursing Plans and Interventions

A. Provide supportive care.
B. Monitor temperature; assess for signs of infection.
C. Protect from persons with infections.
D. Provide skin care (edematous areas are vulnerable).
E. Maintain bed rest during edematous phase.
F. Administer steroids such as prednisone and cholinergics such as bethanechol (Urecholine) as prescribed (Table 5-10).
G. Monitor I&O.
H. Measure abdominal girth daily.
I. Administer cyclophosphamide (Cytoxan) if prescribed (used if nonresponsive to prednisone).
J. Provide small, frequent feedings of a normal-protein, low-salt diet. Client is commonly prescribed IV albumin followed by diuretic.
K. Teach home care:
  1. Instruct to weigh child daily.
  2. Describe medication side effects.

TABLE 5-10 Medications Used in Renal Disorders

Drugs/Route	Indications	Adverse Reactions	Nursing Implications

• Bethanechol chloride PO, IM, IV	• Cholinergic used to treat:
	  • Urinary retention
	  • Neurogenic bladder
	  • Gastric reflux
		• Orthostatic hypotension
		• Flushing
		• Asthmatic reaction
		• GI distress
			• *Do not give IV or IM (may cause circulatory collapse).*
			• Monitor vital signs.
			• Preferably give on empty stomach.

• Prednisone PO	• Adrenocorticosteroid used to treat:
	  • Immunosuppression (acts as an antiinflammatory)
	  • Edema (promotes diuresis in nephritic syndrome)
		• Mood changes
		• Increased susceptibility to infection
		• Cushingoid appearance (moon face and buffalo hump)
		• Acne
		• GI distress
		• Thrombocytopenia
		• Edema
		• Potassium loss
		• *Growth failure in children*
			• In children, every other day administration is best to avoid growth failure when drug is taken long term.
			• Discontinuing this drug requires tapering dose.
			• Avoid live virus vaccines in children receiving prednisone.

• Oxybutynin PO, transdermal
• Tolterodine PO
	• Genitourinary smooth-muscle relaxants (antispasmodics) used to treat:
	  • Uninhibited neurogenic bladder
	  • Reflex urogenic bladder
	• Both are characterized by voiding symptoms of urgency, frequency, nocturia, and incontinence.
		• Increased susceptibility to UTI
		• GI distress
		• Dry eyes
		• Dry mouth
		• Vision changes
		• Dizziness
		• Chest pain
		• Drowsiness
			• Administered orally; available in extended-release forms.
			• Do not administer with other medications that have anticholinergic effects.
			• May exacerbate reflux esophagitis.
			• Contraindicated in clients with untreated glaucoma or any GI narrowing (GI obstruction may occur).
			• Safety for use with children has not been established.

3. Describe signs of relapse (see "Nursing Assessment" earlier).
4. Train to prevent infection.

Urinary Tract Infection (UTI)

Description: Bacterial infection anywhere along the urinary tract (most ascend).

Nursing Assessment

A. In infants
   1. Vague symptoms
   2. Fever
   3. Irritability
   4. Poor food intake
   5. Diarrhea, vomiting, jaundice
   6. Strong-smelling urine
B. In older children
   1. Urinary frequency
   2. Hematuria
   3. Enuresis
   4. Dysuria
   5. Fever

Analysis (Nursing Diagnoses)

A. *Impaired urinary elimination patterns* related to …
B. *Deficient knowledge* (medications) related to …

Nursing Plans and Interventions

A. Suspect and assess for UTI in infants who are ill.
B. Assess for recurrent UTI. In infants and young boys, UTI may indicate structural abnormalities of the urinary system.
C. Collect clean voided or catheterized specimen, as prescribed (Table 5-11).
D. Administer antibiotics as prescribed.
E. Teach home program:
   1. Instruct to finish all prescribed medication.
   2. Note that follow-up specimens are needed.
   3. Teach to avoid bubble baths.
   4. Teach to increase acidic oral fluids (e.g., apple juice, cranberry juice).
   5. Instruct to void frequently.

TABLE 5-11 Collection of Urine Specimens

Method	Description for Children and Infants
Clean catch	• Best obtained by using a urine bag to catch the specimen. • Apply from side to side or back to front. Diaper should be applied over the bag. • Check child frequently to note urination.
Catheterization	• Sterile feeding tube is often used to catheterize small children and infants.
Sterile specimen	• In small infants it is best collected by the physician performing a bladder tap. Urine is aspirated through a needle inserted directly into the bladder. The nurse is responsible for making sure infant is appropriately hydrated and restrained during the procedure.

6. Teach to clean genital area from front to back.
7. Note symptoms of recurrence.

Vesicoureteral Reflex

Description: Result of valvular malfunction and backflow of urine into the ureters (and higher) from the bladder (severe cases are associated with hydronephrosis)

Nursing Assessment

A. Recurrent UTI
B. Reflux (common with neurogenic bladder)
C. Reflux noted on voiding cystourethrogram (VCUG)

Analysis (Nursing Diagnoses)

A. *Risk for infection* related to …
B. *Risk for trauma* related to …

Nursing Plans and Interventions

A. Teach home program for prevention of UTI.
B. Teach family the importance of medication compliance, which usually leads to resolution of mild cases.
C. Provide support for children and families requiring surgery.
D. Explain the goal of ureteral reimplantation: to stop reflux and prevent kidney damage.
E. Monitor postoperative urinary drainage (may be suprapubic or urethral).
   1. Measure output from both catheters.
   2. Assess dressing and incision for drainage.
   3. Restrain child's hands as necessary.
F. Maintain hydration with IV or oral fluids.
G. Manage pain relief postoperatively.
   1. Surgical pain
   2. Bladder spasms

Wilms Tumor (Nephroblastoma)

Description: Malignant renal tumor
A. A Wilms tumor is embryonic in origin.
B. This tumor is encapsulated.
C. It occurs in preschool children.
D. Usually one kidney is affected.
E. The prognosis is good with early detection, surgery, and adjuvant chemotherapy, as well as postoperative radiation therapy.

Nursing Assessment

A. Fever
B. Pallor, lethargy
C. Elevated blood pressure (excess renin secretion)
D. Hematuria (rare)

Analysis (Nursing Diagnoses)

A. *Risk for injury: trauma* related to …
B. *Fear* related to …

Nursing Plans and Interventions

A. Support family during diagnostic period.
B. Protect child from injury; place a sign on bed stating "no abdominal palpation" (to prevent accidental fragmentation and dislodging into the abdominal cavity).
C. Prepare family and child for imminent nephrectomy.
D. Provide postoperative care.
   1. Monitor for increased blood pressure.
   2. Monitor kidney function: I&O, urine specific gravity.
   3. Provide care for abdominal surgery client.
      a. Maintain nasogastric tube.
      b. Check for bowel sounds.
   4. Support child and family during chemotherapy or radiation therapy.

Hypospadias

Description: Congenital defect of urethral meatus in males; urethra opens on ventral side of penis behind the glans.

Nursing Assessment

A. Abnormal placement of meatus
B. Altered voiding stream
C. Presence of chordee
D. Undescended testes and inguinal hernia (may occur concurrently)

Analysis (Nursing Diagnoses)

A. *Impaired urinary elimination* related to …
B. *Disturbed body image* related to …

Nursing Plans and Interventions

A. Prepare child and family for surgery (no circumcision before surgery).
B. Assess circulation to tip of penis postoperatively.

C. Monitor urinary drainage after urethroplasty:
  1. Foley catheter
  2. Suprapubic tube
  3. Urethral stent
D. Restrain child's arms and legs as necessary.
E. Maintain hydration (IV and oral fluids).

F. Teach home care.
  1. Teach care of catheters.
  2. Teach how to empty drainage bag.
  3. Teach prevention of catheter displacement or blockage.
  4. Instruct to increase oral fluids.
  5. Describe signs of infection.

Review of Renal Disorders

1. Compare the signs and symptoms of AGN with those of nephrosis.
2. What antecedent event occurs with AGN?
3. Compare the dietary interventions for AGN and nephrosis.
4. What is the physiologic reason for the laboratory finding of hypoproteinemia in nephrosis?

5. Describe safe monitoring of prednisone administration and withdrawal.
6. What interventions can be taught to prevent urinary tract infections in children?
7. Describe the pathophysiology of vesicoureteral reflux.
8. What are the priorities for a client with a Wilms tumor?
9. Explain why hypospadias correction is performed before the child reaches preschool age.

Answers to Review

1. AGN: gross hematuria, recent strep infection, hypertension, and mild edema; nephrosis: severe edema, massive proteinuria, frothy-appearing urine, anorexia
2. Beta-hemolytic streptococcal infection
3. AGN: low-sodium diet with no added salt; nephrosis: high-protein, low-salt diet
4. Hypoproteinemia occurs because the glomeruli are permeable to serum proteins.
5. Long-term prednisone should be given every other day. Signs of edema, mood changes, and GI distress should be noted and reported. The drug should be tapered, not discontinued suddenly.

6. Avoid bubble baths; void frequently; drink adequate fluids, especially acidic fluids such as apple or cranberry juice; and clean genital area from front to back.
7. A malfunction of the valves at the end of the ureters, allowing urine to reflux out of the bladder into the ureters and possibly into the kidneys
8. Protect the child from injury to the encapsulated tumor. Prepare the family and child for surgery.
9. Preschoolers fear castration, achieving sexual identity, and acquiring independent toileting skills.

Gastrointestinal Disorders

Cleft Lip or Palate

Description: Malformations of the face and oral cavity that seem to be multifactorial in hereditary origin (Fig. 5-14)
A. Cleft lip is readily apparent.
B. Cleft palate may not be identified until the infant has difficulty with feeding.
C. Initial closure of cleft lip is performed when infant weighs approximately 10 pounds (4.54 kg) and has an Hgb of 10 g/dL.
D. Closure of palate defect is usually performed at 1 year of age to minimize speech impairment.

Nursing Assessment

A. Failure of fusion of the lip, palate, or both
B. Difficulty sucking and swallowing
C. Parent reaction to facial defect

Analysis (Nursing Diagnoses)

A. *Imbalanced nutrition: less than body requirements* related to …
B. *Risk for impaired attachment* related to …

Nursing Plans and Interventions

A. Promote family bonding and grieving during newborn period.
B. Inform family that successful corrective surgery is available.
C. In newborn period, assist with feeding.
  1. Feed in upright position.
  2. Feed slowly, with frequent burping.
  3. Use soft, large nipples; lamb's nipple; prosthetic palate; or rubber-tipped Asepto syringe.
  4. Support mother's breastfeeding if possible.
  5. Consider the ESSR method for feeding: Enlarge nipple opening; stimulate the child to Suck, Swallow normally, and Rest. *Use caution to prevent the infant from aspirating.*

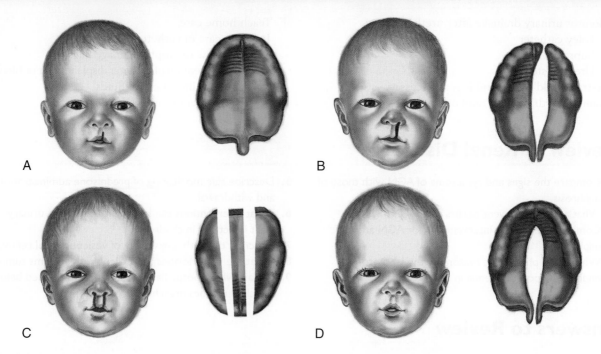

FIGURE 5-14 Variations in clefts of lip and palate at birth. **(A)** Notch in vermilion border. **(B)** Unilateral cleft lip and cleft palate. **(C)** Bilateral cleft lip and cleft palate. **(D)** Cleft palate. (From Hockenberry MJ, Wilson D. *Wong's nursing care of infants and children*, ed 9, St. Louis, 2011, Mosby.)

D. Provide postoperative care:
1. Maintain patent airway and proper positioning.
   a. Cleft lip: Place client on side or upright in infant seat (not prone).
   b. Cleft palate: Place client on side or abdomen.
   c. Remove oral secretions carefully with bulb syringe or Yankauer suction set.
2. Protect surgical site.
   a. Minimize crying to prevent strain on lip suture line.
   b. Maintain Logan bow to lip if applied.
3. Provide care for restrained child.
   a. Provide age-appropriate stimulation.
4. Resume feeding as prescribed. Cleanse suture site with sterile water after feeding; formula remaining on suture line may impede healing and lead to infection.
5. Encourage family participation in care and feeding.
   a. Fluids are taken by a cup or an Asepto syringe with a rubber tip (gravity feeder).
   b. The diet progresses from a clear to a full liquid diet.
   c. The child may go home on a soft diet (nothing harder than mashed potatoes).
E. Usually for cleft palate: Coordinate long-term care with other team members: plastic surgeon, ear/nose/throat (ENT) specialist, nutritionist, speech therapist, orthodontist, pediatrician, nurse.

HESI Hint • Typical parent and family reactions to a child with an obvious malformation such as cleft lip or palate are guilt, disappointment, grief, sense of loss, and anger.

It is helpful to families to provide pictures before and after surgical repair of children with cleft lip or cleft palate.

Esophageal Atresia with Tracheoesophageal Fistula (TEF)

Description: Congenital anomaly in which the esophagus does not fully develop (Fig. 5-15)
A. Most common: upper esophagus ends in a blind pouch, and the lower part of the esophagus is connected to the trachea.
B. This condition is a clinical and surgical *emergency.*

Nursing Assessment

A. Three Cs of TEF in the newborn:
   1. Choking
   2. Coughing
   3. Cyanosis
B. Excess salivation
C. Respiratory distress
D. Aspiration pneumonia

Analysis (Nursing Diagnoses)

A. *Risk for aspiration* related to …
B. *Imbalanced nutrition: less than body requirements* related to …

Nursing Plans and Interventions

A. Provide preoperative care.
   1. Monitor respiratory status.
   2. Remove excess secretions (suction is usually continuous to blind pouch).
   3. Elevate infant into antireflux position of 30 degrees.
   4. Provide oxygen as prescribed.
   5. Maintain NPO.
   6. Administer IV fluids as prescribed.

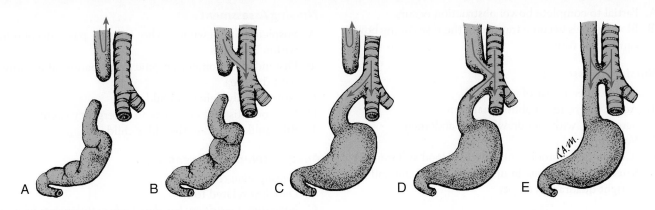

FIGURE 5-15 Five most common types of esophageal atresia and tracheoesophageal fistula. (From Hockenberry MJ, Wilson D. *Wong's essentials of pediatric nursing*, ed 9, St. Louis, 2013, Mosby.)

B. Provide postoperative care.
   1. Maintain NPO.
   2. Administer IV fluids.
   3. Monitor I&O.
   4. Provide gastrostomy tube care and feedings as prescribed.
   5. Provide pacifier to meet developmental needs.
   6. Monitor child for postoperative stricture of the esophagus.
      a. Poor feeding
      b. Dysphagia
      c. Drooling
      d. Regurgitating undigested food
C. Promote parent–infant bonding for high-risk infant.

Pyloric Stenosis

Description: A thickening of the pylorus that results in stricture at the gastric outlet. It occurs as a result of hypertrophied or spastic muscle fibers surrounding the opening failing to relax sufficiently to allow food to pass easily from the stomach to the duodenum.[1,2]

Nursing Assessment

A. Usually occurs in first-born males
B. Vomiting (free of bile) usually begins around the third to sixth week of life (rarely seen in children over 3 years old). Projectile vomiting occurs within minutes after eating.
C. Hungry, fretful infant
D. Weight loss, failure to gain weight
E. Dehydration with decreased sodium and potassium
F. Metabolic alkalosis (decreased serum chloride, increased pH and bicarbonate or CO_2 content)
G. Palpable olive-shaped mass in upper-right quadrant of the abdomen
H. Visible peristaltic waves

Analysis (Nursing Diagnoses)

A. *Imbalanced nutrition: less than body requirements* related to …
B. *Deficient fluid volume* related to …

> **HESI Hint** • Children with cleft lip or palate and those with pyloric stenosis both have a nursing diagnosis of "Alteration in nutrition; less than body requirements."
> • Cleft lip or palate is related to decreased ability to suck.
> • Pyloric stenosis is related to frequent vomiting.

Nursing Plans and Interventions

A. Preoperative care
   1. Assess for dehydration.
   2. Administer IV fluids and electrolytes as prescribed.
   3. Weigh daily; monitor I&O.
   4. Provide small, frequent feedings if prescribed.
B. Prepare family for surgery by teaching that:
   1. The hypertrophied wall is surgically corrected to allow proper drainage from the stomach into the small intestines.
   2. Prognosis is excellent.
C. Postoperative care
   1. Continue IV fluids as prescribed.
   2. Provide small oral feedings with electrolyte solutions or glucose (usually 4 to 6 hours postoperative).
   3. Position on *right* side in semi-Fowler position after feeding.
   4. Burp frequently to avoid stomach becoming distended and putting pressure on surgical site.
   5. Weigh daily; monitor I&O.

Intussusception

Description: Telescoping of one part of the intestine into another part of the intestine, usually the ileum into the colon (called *ileocolic*)

A. Partial to complete bowel obstruction occurs.
B. Blood vessels become trapped in the telescoping bowel, causing necrosis.

Nursing Assessment

A. Child under 1 year of age
B. Acute, intermittent abdominal pain
C. Screaming, with legs drawn up to abdomen
D. Vomiting
E. "Currant jelly" stools (mixed with blood and mucus)
F. Sausage-shaped mass in upper right quadrant and lower-right quadrant is empty

Analysis (Nursing Diagnoses)

A. *Ineffective tissue perfusion* (bowel) related to …
B. *Risk for deficient fluid volume* related to …

Nursing Plans and Interventions

A. Monitor carefully for shock and bowel perforation.
B. Administer IV fluids as prescribed.
C. Monitor I&O.
D. Prepare family for emergency intervention.
E. Prepare child for barium enema (which provides hydrostatic reduction). Two of three cases respond to this treatment; if not, surgery is necessary.
F. Provide postoperative care for infants who require abdominal surgery.

HESI Hint • Nutritional needs and fluid and electrolyte balance are key problems for children with GI disorders. The younger the child, the more vulnerable he or she is to fluid and electrolyte imbalances and the greater the need for the caloric intake required for growth.

Congenital Aganglionic Megacolon (Hirschsprung Disease)

Description: Congenital absence of autonomic parasympathetic ganglion cells in a distal portion of the colon and rectum

A. There is a lack of peristalsis in the area of the colon where the ganglion cells are absent.
B. Fecal contents accumulate above the aganglionic area of the bowel.
C. Correction usually involves a series of surgical procedures:
1. A temporary colostomy until 12 months of age.
2. Later, a reanastomosis and closure of the colostomy

Nursing Assessment

A. Suspicion in newborn who fails to pass meconium within 24 hours
B. Distended abdomen, chronic constipation alternating with diarrhea
C. Nutritionally deficient child
D. Enterocolitis that occurs as an emergency event
E. Ribbonlike stools in the older child

Analysis (Nursing Diagnoses)

A. *Constipation* related to …
B. *Diarrhea* related to …
C. *Imbalanced nutrition: less than body requirements* related to …

Nursing Plans and Interventions

A. Provide preoperative care.
1. Begin preparation for abdominal surgery.
2. Provide bowel-cleansing program as prescribed.
3. Insert rectal tube if prescribed.
4. Observe for symptoms of bowel perforation.
a. Abdominal distention (measure abdominal girth)
b. Vomiting
c. Increased abdominal tenderness
d. Irritability
e. Dyspnea and cyanosis
5. Initiate preoperative teaching regarding colostomy.
B. Provide postoperative care.
1. Check vital signs, axillary temperature.

HESI Hint • Take axillary temperature in children with congenital megacolon.

---

2. Administer IV fluids as prescribed.
3. Monitor I&O.
4. Care for nasogastric tube with connection to intermittent suction.
5. Check abdominal and perineal dressings.
6. Assess bowel sounds and bowel function.
C. Prepare family for home care.
1. Teach care of temporary colostomy.
2. Teach skin care.
3. Refer family to enterostomal therapist and social services.
D. Prepare child and family for closure of temporary colostomy.
E. After closure, encourage family to be patient with child when toileting.
F. Teach family to begin toilet training after age 2.

Review of Gastrointestinal Disorders

1. Describe feeding techniques for a child with cleft lip or palate.
2. List the signs and symptoms of esophageal atresia with TEF.
3. What nursing actions are initiated for the newborn with suspected esophageal atresia with TEF?
4. Describe the postoperative nursing care for an infant with pyloric stenosis.
5. Describe why a barium enema is used to treat intussusception.
6. Describe the preoperative nursing care for a child with Hirschsprung disease.
7. What care is needed for a child with a temporary colostomy?
8. What are the signs of anorectal malformation?
9. What are the priorities for a child undergoing abdominal surgery?

Answers to Review

1. Use lamb's nipple or prosthesis. Feed child upright, with frequent bubbling.
2. Choking, coughing, cyanosis, and excess salivation
3. Maintain NPO immediately, and suction secretions.
4. Maintain IV hydration, and provide small, frequent oral feedings of glucose or electrolyte solutions or both within 4 to 6 hours. Gradually increase to full-strength formula. Position infant on right side in semi-Fowler position after feeding.
5. A barium enema reduces the telescoping of the intestine through hydrostatic pressure without surgical intervention.
6. Check vital signs and take axillary temperatures. Provide bowel cleansing program, and teach about colostomy. Observe for bowel perforation; measure abdominal girth.
7. Family needs education about skin care and appliances. Referral to an enterostomal therapist is appropriate.
8. A newborn who does not pass meconium within 24 hours; meconium appearing through a fistula or in the urine; an unusual-appearing anal dimple
9. Maintain fluid balance (I&O, nasogastric suction, monitor electrolytes); monitor vital signs; care for drains, if present; assess bowel function; prevent infection of incisional area and other postoperative complications; and support child and family with appropriate teaching.

Hematologic Disorders

Iron Deficiency Anemia

Description: Hemoglobin levels below normal range because of the body's inadequate supply, intake, or absorption of iron
A. Iron deficiency anemia is the leading hematologic disorder in children.
B. The need for iron is greater in children than in adults because of accelerated growth.
C. Anemia may be caused by the following:
   1. Inadequate stores during fetal development
   2. Deficient dietary intake
   3. Chronic blood loss
   4. Poor utilization of iron by the body

Nursing Assessment

A. Pallor, paleness of mucous membranes
B. Tiredness, fatigue
C. Usually seen in infants 6 to 24 months old (times of growth spurt); toddlers and female adolescents most affected
D. Overweight "milk baby"
E. Dietary intake low in iron
F. Milk intake greater than 32 oz/day
G. Pica habit (eating nonfood substances)
H. Laboratory values:
   1. Decreased Hgb
   2. Low serum iron level
   3. Elevated total iron binding capacity (TIBC)

> **HESI Hint** • Remember the Hgb norms:
> • Newborn: 14 to 24 g/dL
> • Infant: 10 to 17 g/dL
> • Child: 9.5 to 15.5 g/dL

Analysis (Nursing Diagnoses)

A. *Ineffective tissue perfusion* (specify) related to …
B. *Activity intolerance* related to …

Nursing Plans and Interventions

A. Support child's need to limit activities.
B. Provide rest periods.
C. Administer oral iron (ferrous sulfate) as prescribed.

HESI Hint • Teach family about administration of oral iron:
- Give on empty stomach (as tolerated, for better absorption).
- Give with citrus juices (vitamin C) for increased absorption.
- Use dropper or straw to avoid discoloring teeth.
- Teach that stools will become tarry.
- Teach that iron can be fatal in severe overdose; keep away from other children.
- Do not give with any dairy products.

D. Teach family nutritional facts concerning iron deficiency.
1. Limit milk intake to less than 32 oz/day.
2. Teach about dietary sources of iron:
   a. Meat
   b. Green, leafy vegetables
   c. Fish
   d. Liver
   e. Whole grains
   f. Legumes
   g. For infants: iron-fortified cereals and formula
3. Teach about appropriate nutrition for child's age.
E. Be aware of family's income and cultural food preferences.
F. Refer family to nutritionist.
G. Refer to Women, Infants, and Children's (WIC) nutrition program, if available to family.

Hemophilia

Description: Inherited bleeding disorder
A. Most bleeding disorders are transmitted by an X-linked recessive chromosome (mother is the carrier; her sons may express the disease). A normal individual has between 50% and 200% factor activity in blood; the hemophiliac has from 0% to 25% activity.
B. The affected individual usually is missing either factor VIII (classic, 75% of cases) or factor IX.

Nursing Assessment

A. Male child: First red flag may be prolonged bleeding at the umbilical cord or injection site (vitamin K), or after circumcision.
B. Prolonged bleeding with minor trauma
C. Hemarthrosis (most frequent site of bleeding)
D. Spontaneous bleeding into muscles and tissues (less severe cases have fewer bleeds)
E. Loss of motion in joints
F. Pain
G. Laboratory values:
1. PTT is prolonged.
2. Factor assays less than 25%

Analysis (Nursing Diagnoses)

A. *Risk for trauma* related to …
B. *Deficient knowledge (home care)* related to …

Nursing Plans and Interventions

A. Administer fresh-frozen plasma, cryoprecipitate of fresh plasma, or lyophilized (freeze-dried) concentrate as prescribed.
B. Administer pain medication as prescribed (analgesics containing *no* aspirin).
C. Follow blood precautions: risk for hepatitis.
D. Teach child and family home care.
1. Teach to recognize early signs of bleeding into joints.
2. Teach local treatment for minor bleeds (pressure, splinting, ice).
3. Teach administration of factor replacement (clients receiving routine treatments of the clotting factors usually have a Port-a-cath).
4. Discuss dental hygiene: Use soft toothbrushes.
5. Provide protective care: Give child soft toys; use padded bed rails.
6. Have child wear MedicAlert identification.
E. Refer family for genetic counseling.
F. Support child and family during periods of growth and development when increased risk for bleeding occurs (e.g., learning to walk, tooth loss).

HESI Hint • Inherited bleeding disorders (hemophilia and sickle cell disease) are often used to test knowledge of genetic transmission patterns. Remember:
- Autosomal recessive: Both parents must be heterozygous, or carriers of the recessive trait, for the disease to be expressed in their offspring. With each pregnancy, there is a one in four chance that the infant will have the disease. However, all children of such parents can get the disease—not just 25% of them. This is the transmission pattern of sickle cell disease, cystic fibrosis, and phenylketonuria (PKU).
- X-linked recessive trait: The trait is carried on the X chromosome; therefore it usually affects male offspring, as in hemophilia. With each pregnancy of a woman who is a carrier, there is a 25% chance of having a child with hemophilia. If the child is male, he has a 50% chance of having hemophilia. If the child is female, she has a 50% chance of being a carrier.

Sickle Cell Disease (SCD)

Description: A genetic disorder that results in the formation of abnormal Hgb chains.
A. It occurs in less than 1% of African American newborns; approximately 8% of African Americans carry the gene. SCD also affects certain people whose ancestors are from India, the Mediterranean region, and the Middle East.[3,4]
B. It usually appears after 6 months of age.
C. Hemoglobin S (HgbS) replaces all or part of the normal Hgb, which causes the red blood cells to sickle when oxygen is released into the tissues.

A Normal red blood cells

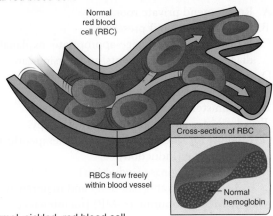

B Abnormal, sickled, red blood cell
(sickle cells)

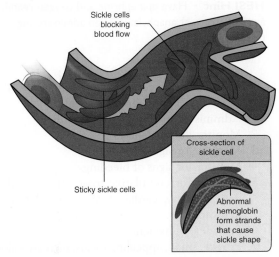

FIGURE 5-16 Normal red cells and sickle red cells. **(A)** Normal red blood cells flowing freely in a blood vessel. The inset image shows a cross-section of a normal red blood cell with normal hemoglobin. **(B)** Abnormal, sickled red blood cells blocking blood flow in a blood vessel. The inset image shows a cross-section of a sickle cell with abnormal (sickle) hemoglobin forming abnormal stiff rods. (From NIH: National Heart, Lung, and Blood Institute assessed at **http://www.nhlbi.nih.gov/health/health-topics/topics/sca**.)

1. Sickled cells cannot flow through capillary beds (Fig. 5-16).
2. Dehydration promotes sickling.
3. Increased sickling episodes occur with cold because cold causes constriction of the vessels.

> **HESI Hint** • Hydration is very important in the treatment of sickle cell disease because it promotes hemodilution and circulation of red cells through the blood vessels.

D. HgbS has a less-than-normal life span (fewer than 40 days), which leads to chronic anemia.
E. Tissue ischemia causes widespread pathologic changes in spleen, liver, kidney, bones, and CNS.

> **HESI Hint** • Important terms
> - Heterozygous gene (*HgbAS*)—sickle cell trait
> - Homozygous gene (*HbSS*)—sickle cell disease
> - Abnormal hemoglobin (*HgbS*)—disease and trait

Nursing Assessment
A. Children of African descent, usually over 6 months of age
B. Parents with sickle cell trait or sickle cell disease
C. Laboratory diagnosis: Hgb electrophoresis (differentiates trait from disease)
D. Frequent infections (nonfunctional spleen)
E. Tiredness
F. Chronic hemolytic anemia
G. Delayed physical growth
H. Vasoocclusive crisis; the classic signs:
   1. Fever
   2. Severe abdominal pain
   3. Hand–foot syndrome (infants); painful edematous hands and feet
   4. Arthralgia
I. Leg ulcers (adolescents)
J. Cerebrovascular accidents (increased risk with dehydration)

Analysis (Nursing Diagnoses)
A. *Acute pain* related to …
B. *Risk for infection* related to …
C. *Deficient knowledge (crisis prevention)* related to …

Nursing Plans and Interventions
A. Teach family that to prevent crisis (hypoxia), they should:
   1. Keep child from exercising strenuously.
   2. Keep child away from high altitudes.
   3. Avoid letting child become infected, and seek care at first sign of infection.
   4. Use prophylactic penicillin if prescribed.
   5. Keep child well hydrated.
   6. Not withhold fluids at night because enuresis is a complication of both the disease and the treatment.
B. For a child hospitalized with a vasoocclusive crisis:
   1. Administer IV fluids (one to two times maintenance levels) and electrolytes, as prescribed, to increase hydration and treat acidosis.
   2. Monitor I&O.
   3. Administer blood products as prescribed.
   4. Administer analgesics, including parenteral morphine for severe pain, as prescribed.
   5. Use warm compresses (not ice).
   6. Administer prescribed antibiotics to treat infection.
C. Administer pneumococcal vaccine, meningococcal vaccine, and Hib vaccine as prescribed.
D. Administer hepatitis B vaccine as prescribed (for child at risk because of transfusions).

E. Refer family for genetic counseling.

F. Support child and family experiencing chronic disease.

> **HESI Hint** • Supplemental iron is not given to clients with sickle cell disease. The anemia is not caused by iron deficiency. Folic acid is given orally to stimulate red blood cell (RBC) synthesis.

Acute Lymphocytic Leukemia

Description: Cancer of the blood-forming organs

A. Acute lymphocytic leukemia accounts for about 80% of childhood leukemia.

B. It is noted for the presence of lymphoblasts (immature lymphocytes), which replace normal cells in the bone marrow.

C. Blast cells are also seen in the peripheral blood.

D. Acute lymphocytic leukemia is classified according to whether it involves:

1. T lymphocytes
2. B lymphocytes
3. Null cells (neither T cells nor B cells)

E. More than 75% of children with acute lymphocytic leukemia have the null cell type, which has the best prognosis.

F. The signs and symptoms of leukemia result from the replacement of normal cells by leukemic cells in the bone marrow and extramedullary sites.

G. Treatment has four phases:

1. Induction
2. Sanctuary
3. Consolidation
4. Maintenance

Nursing Assessment

A. Pallor, tiredness, weakness, lethargy due to anemia

B. Petechia, bleeding, bruising due to thrombocytopenia

C. Infection, fever due to neutropenia

D. Bone joint pain due to leukemic infiltration of bone marrow

E. Enlarged lymph nodes; hepatosplenomegaly

F. Headache and vomiting (signs of CNS involvement)

G. Anorexia, weight loss

H. Laboratory data: bone marrow aspiration that reveals 80% to 90% immature blast cells

Analysis (Nursing Diagnoses)

A. *Risk for infection* related to …

B. *Fear* related to …

C. *Deficient knowledge (disease process and chemotherapy)* related to …

Nursing Plans and Interventions

A. Recommend private room.

B. Reverse isolation if prescribed.

C. Provide child with age-appropriate explanations for diagnostic tests, treatments, and nursing care.

D. Examine child for infection of skin, needle-stick sites, dental problems.

E. Administer blood products as prescribed.

F. Administer antineoplastic chemotherapy.

G. Monitor for side effects of chemotherapeutic agents.

1. Vincristine (induction)
2. L-Asparaginase (induction)
3. Methotrexate (sanctuary and maintenance)
4. Mercaptopurine (6-MP) (maintenance)

> **HESI Hint** • Have epinephrine and oxygen readily available to treat anaphylaxis when administering L-asparaginase.

H. Provide care directed toward managing side effects and toxic effects of antineoplastic agents.

1. Administer antiemetics as prescribed.
2. Monitor fluid balance.
3. Monitor for signs of infection.
4. Monitor for signs of bleeding.
5. Monitor for cumulative toxic effects of drugs: hepatic toxicity, cardiac toxicity, renal toxicity, and neurotoxicity.
6. Provide oral hygiene.
7. Provide small, appealing meals; increase calories and protein; refer to nutritionist.
8. Promote self-esteem and positive body image if child has alopecia, severe weight loss, or other disturbance in body image.
9. Provide care to prevent infection.

I. Provide emotional support for family in crisis.

J. Encourage family's and child's input and control in determining plans and treatment.

> **HESI Hint** • Prednisone is frequently used in combination with antineoplastic drugs to reduce the mitosis of lymphocytes. Allopurinol, a xanthine oxidase inhibitor, is also administered to prevent renal damage caused by uric acid buildup and cellular lysis.

Review of Hematologic Disorders

1. Describe the information families should be given when a child is receiving oral iron preparations.
2. List dietary sources of iron.
3. What is the genetic transmission pattern of hemophilia?
4. Describe the sequence of events in a vasoocclusive crisis in sickle cell disease.
5. Explain why hydration is a priority in treating sickle cell disease.
6. What should families and clients do to avoid triggering sickling episodes?
7. Nursing interventions and medical treatments for a child with leukemia are based on what three physiologic problems?
8. Nursing interventions and medical treatments for a child with retinoblastoma are based on what type of treatment and if inherited?

Answers to Review

1. Give oral iron on an empty stomach and with vitamin C. Use straws to avoid discoloring teeth. Tarry stools are normal. Increase dietary sources of iron.
2. Meat, green leafy vegetables, fish, liver, whole grains, legumes
3. It is an X-linked recessive chromosomal disorder transmitted by the mother and expressed in male children.
4. A vasoocclusive crisis is caused by the clumping of RBCs, which blocks small blood vessels; therefore the cells cannot get through the capillaries, causing pain and tissue and organ ischemia. Lowered oxygen tension affects HgbS, which causes sickling of the cells.
5. Hydration promotes hemodilution and circulation of the RBCs through the blood vessels.
6. Keep child well hydrated. Avoid known sources of infections. Avoid high altitudes. Avoid strenuous exercise.
7. Anemia (decreased erythrocytes); infection (neutropenia); bleeding thrombocytopenia (decreased platelets)
8. The nursing interventions and medical treatment are dependent on the type of treatment. Children with inherited blastoma need to be screened throughout their lives for development of other forms of cancer.

Metabolic and Endocrine Disorders

Congenital Hypothyroidism

Description: Congenital condition resulting from inadequate thyroid tissue development in utero. Cognitive impairment and growth failure occur if it is not detected and treated in early infancy.

Nursing Assessment

A. Newborn screening reveals low T_4 (thyroxine) and high thyroid-stimulating hormone (TSH).
B. Symptoms in the newborn:
   1. Long gestation (>42 weeks)
   2. Large hypoactive infant
   3. Delayed meconium passage
   4. Feeding problems (poor suck)
   5. Prolonged physiologic jaundice
   6. Hypothermia
C. Symptoms in early infancy if untreated with thyroxine:
   1. Large, protruding tongue
   2. Coarse hair/hairline will appear low
   3. Lethargy, sleepiness
   4. Flat expression
   5. Constipation
   6. Hypotonia
   7. Delay of serum phenylalanine testing will lead to CNS damage, including mental retardation.

D. Prognosis is good if the condition is recognized and treated. The infant's intelligence is usually not affected if treatment is initiated within the first month of life.

> **HESI Hint** • An infant with hypothyroidism is often described as a good, quiet baby by the parents.

Analysis (Nursing Diagnoses)

A. *Delayed growth and development* related to …
B. *Deficient knowledge (medication program)* related to …

Nursing Plans and Interventions

A. Perform newborn screening programs before discharge.
B. Assess newborn for signs of congenital hypothyroidism.
C. Once identified, teach family about replacement therapy with thyroid hormone:
   1. Explain that child will have a lifelong need for the therapy.
   2. Tell parents to give child a single dose in the morning.
   3. Teach family to check child's pulse daily before giving thyroid medication.
   4. Signs of overdose include rapid pulse, irritability, fever, weight loss, and diarrhea.
   5. Signs of underdose include lethargy, fatigue, constipation, and poor feeding.
   6. Periodic thyroid testing is necessary.

Phenylketonuria (PKU)

Description: Rare autosomal-recessive disorder in which the body cannot metabolize the essential amino acid phenylalanine, which accumulates in the blood after the infant begins consuming breast milk or formula. PKU is usually detected early through newborn screenings 24 hours after the infant's first ingested meal and subsequent tests 2 to 3 weeks after birth. Individuals diagnosed with PKU must limit their intake of phenylalanine-containing foods throughout their lives.

Nursing Assessment (if Undetected and/or Untreated)

A. Newborn screening using the Guthrie test; positive result; serum phenylalanine level of 4 mg/dL
B. Frequent vomiting, failure to gain weight
C. Irritability
D. Musty odor of urine
 3. Delayed growth and development
 4. Signs of failure to thrive
 5. Unpleasant peculiar body odor and urine
 6. Often fair-skinned blonde and blue-eyed children; however, other racial and ethnic groups are also susceptible
 7. May have microcephaly
B. Mothers diagnosed with PKU disease who do not maintain a low-phenylalanine diet during pregnancy can cause problems for their children who do inherit PKU. Those infants are at risk for:
 1. Cognitive impairment
 2. Microcephaly
 3. Birth weight below 2500 grams
 4. Disrupted growth and development
 5. Congenital heart anomalies

> **HESI Hint** • Early detection of hypothyroidism and PKU is essential for preventing cognitive impairment in infants. Knowledge of normal growth and developmental patterns is important because a lack of attainment can be used to detect the presence of a disease and to evaluate the treatment's effects.

Analysis (Nursing Diagnoses)

A. *Delayed growth and development* related to …
B. *Deficient knowledge (disease process and diet)* related to …

Nursing Plans and Interventions

A. Perform newborn screening as close to discharge as possible and no later than seven days after birth. Obtain a subsequent sample by 2 weeks of age if the initial specimen is collected before the newborn is 24 hours old.
 1. Screen infants born at home who have no hospital contact, as well as infants adopted internationally.

B. Once identified, teach family dietary management.
 1. Stress the importance of strict adherence to prescribed low-phenylalanine diet.
 2. Instruct family to provide special formulas for infant: Lofenalac, Phenex-1.
 3. Instruct family to provide phenyl-free milk substitute after the age of 2 years.
 4. Teach family to avoid foods high in phenylalanine, that is, high-protein foods, such as meat, milk, dairy products, and eggs.
 5. Teach family to offer foods low in phenylalanine, that is, vegetables, fruits, juices, cereals, breads, and starches.
 6. Encourage family to work with nutritionist.
 7. Teach that diet must be maintained at least until brain growth is complete (ages 6 to 8 years) to limit cognitive deficits.
C. Refer for genetic counseling.

> **HESI Hint** • NutraSweet (aspartame) contains phenylalanine and therefore should not be given to a child with PKU.

Insulin-Dependent Diabetes Mellitus (IDDM), or Type 1 Diabetes

Description: Metabolic disorder in which the insulin-producing cells of the pancreas are nonfunctioning as a result of some insult (see Medical-Surgical Nursing: Diabetes Mellitus).

A. Heredity, viral infections, and autoimmune processes are implicated in diabetes mellitus (DM).
B. Diabetes causes altered metabolism of carbohydrates, proteins, and fats.
C. Insulin replacement, dietary management, and exercise are the recommended treatments.

Nursing Assessment

A. Classic three Ps:
 1. Polydipsia
 2. Polyphagia
 3. Polyuria, enuresis (bedwetting) in previously continent child
B. Irritability, fatigue
C. Weight loss
D. Abdominal complaints, nausea, and vomiting
E. Usually occurs in school-age children but can occur even in infancy
F. See Table 4-27.

Analysis (Nursing Diagnoses)

A. *Imbalanced nutrition: less than body requirements* related to …
B. *Deficient knowledge (home program for diabetes)* related to …

HESI Hint • DM in children was typically diagnosed as insulin-dependent diabetes (type 1) until recently. Adolescence frequently causes difficulty in management because growth is rapid, and the need to be like peers makes compliance difficult. Remember to consider the child's age, cognitive level of development, and psychosocial development when answering NCLEX-RN questions.

Nursing Plans and Interventions

A. Assist with diagnosis (fasting blood sugar >120 mg/dL glucose).
B. If child is in ketoacidosis, provide care for seriously ill child (may be unconscious).
  1. Monitor vital signs and neurologic status.
  2. Monitor blood glucose, pH, serum electrolytes.

HESI Hint • When a child is in ketoacidosis, administer regular insulin IV in normal saline as prescribed.

  3. Administer IV fluids, insulin, and electrolytes as prescribed.
  4. Assess hydration status.
  5. Maintain strict I&O.
C. Initiate home teaching program as soon as possible; involve child and family.
  1. Teach insulin administration.
    a. Child usually receives multiple doses daily.
    b. May be administered subcutaneously or via insulin pump.
  2. Teach dietary management (carbohydrate counting preferred).
    a. Meals and snacks
    b. Growth and exercise needs
    c. Four basic food groups, no concentrated sweets
    d. Advice from nutritionist
  3. Teach about exercise.
    a. Regular, planned activities
    b. Diet modification; snacks before or during exercise
  4. Teach about home glucose monitoring and urine testing.
  5. Teach the signs and symptoms of hyperglycemia and hypoglycemia.
  6. Teach sick-day management
  7. Ensure that the parents involve the school nurse and/or daycare in daily management.
D. Initiate program for school-age child, as appropriate.
  1. Identify issues specific to school.
    a. Physical education class and exercise
    b. Scheduled times for meals and snacks
    c. Cooperation with teachers and school nurse
    d. Need to be like peers
  2. Teach that a school-age child should be responsible for most management.
  3. Instruct the child to wear a MedicAlert ID bracelet.

HESI Hint • There has been an increase in the number of children diagnosed with type 2 diabetes. The increasing rate of obesity in children is thought to be a contributing factor. Other contributing factors include lack of physical activity and a family history of type 2 diabetes.

Review of Metabolic and Endocrine Disorders

1. How is congenital hypothyroidism diagnosed?
2. What are the symptoms of congenital hypothyroidism in early infancy?
3. What are the outcomes of untreated congenital hypothyroidism?
4. What are the metabolic effects of PKU?
5. What two formulas are prescribed for infants with PKU?
6. List foods high in phenylalanine.
7. What are the three classic signs of diabetes?
8. Differentiate the signs of hypoglycemia and hyperglycemia.
9. Describe the nursing care of a child with ketoacidosis.
10. Describe developmental factors that would affect the school-age child with diabetes.
11. What is the relationship between hypoglycemia and exercise?

Answers to Review

1. Newborn screening revealing a low T_4 and a high TSH
2. Large, protruding tongue; coarse hair; lethargy; sleepiness; and constipation
3. Mental retardation and growth failure
4. CNS damage, mental retardation, and decreased melanin
5. Lofenalac and Phenex-1
6. Meat, milk, dairy products, and eggs
7. Polydipsia, polyphagia, and polyuria

Answers to Review—cont'd

8. Hypoglycemia: tremors, sweating, headache, hunger, nausea, lethargy, confusion, slurred speech, anxiety, tingling around mouth, nightmares. Hyperglycemia: polydipsia, polyuria, polyphagia, blurred vision, weakness, weight loss, and syncope

9. Provide care for an unconscious child, administer regular insulin IV in normal saline, monitor blood gas values, and maintain strict I&O.

10. Need to be like peers; assuming responsibility for own care; modification of diet; snacks and exercise in school

11. During exercise, insulin uptake is increased and the risk for hypoglycemia occurs.

Skeletal Disorders

Fractures

Description: Traumatic injury to bone. Younger children diagnosed with fractures may be at risk for child abuse (85% under the age of 3 and 69% under the age of 1). It is important that the story of the incident matches the injury and sounds plausible.

A. Fractures can be classified according to type (see Table 4-29).
   1. Complete fractures: Bone fragments are completely separate.
   2. Incomplete fractures: Bone fragments remain attached (e.g., greenstick, bends, buckles).
   3. Comminuted fractures: Bone fragments from the fractured shaft break free and lie in the surrounding tissue. This type of fracture is rare in children.
   4. Spiral fractures: Fracture line results from twisting force; forms a spiral encircling the bone.
B. Fractures that occur in the epiphyseal plate (growth plate) may affect growth of the limb.

> **HESI Hint** • Fractures in older children are common because they fall during play and are involved in motor vehicle accidents.
> • Spiral fractures (caused by twisting) and fractures in infants may be related to child abuse.
> • Fractures involving the epiphyseal plate (growth plate) can have serious consequences in terms of the growth of the affected limb.

Nursing Assessment

A. General condition
   1. Visible bone fragments
   2. Misalignment of the limb
   3. Pain
   4. Swelling
   5. Contusions
   6. Child guarding or protecting the extremity
   7. Limited range of motion

B. Possibility of being able to use fractured extremity due to intact periosteum
C. The five Ps (may indicate the presence of ischemia):
   1. Pain
   2. Pallor
   3. Pulselessness
   4. Paresthesia
   5. Paralysis

Analysis (Nursing Diagnoses)

A. *Ineffective tissue perfusion (peripheral)* related to …
B. *Acute pain* related to …

Nursing Plans and Interventions

A. Obtain baseline data, and frequently perform neurovascular assessments.
   1. Pulses: Check pulses distal to the injury to assess circulation.
   2. Color: Check injured extremity for pink, brisk, capillary refill.
   3. Movement and sensation: Check injured extremity for nerve impairment; compare for symmetry with uninjured extremity (child may guard injury).
   4. Temperature: Check extremity for warmth.
   5. Swelling: Check for an increase in swelling. Elevate extremity to prevent swelling.
   6. Pain: Monitor for severe pain that is not relieved by analgesics (Table 5-12).
   7. Newly fractured sites are generally splinted and braced until swelling goes down. Once the swelling has subsided, a cast is applied to the affected extremity.
B. Report abnormal assessment promptly! Compartment syndrome may occur; it results in permanent damage to the nerves and vasculature of the injured extremity due to compression.
C. Compromised circulation with abnormal neurovascular checks are the result of compartment syndrome. Compartment syndrome is progressive decrease of tissue perfusion occurring as a result of increased pressure from edema or swelling that presses on the tissues and vessels.

TABLE 5-12 Medications Used in Skeletal Disorders

Drugs/Route	Indications	Adverse Reactions	Nursing Implications
• Infliximab IV • Methocarbamol PO, IM, IV • Cyclobenzaprine PO	• Nonnarcotics to treat pain, stiffness, and discomfort	• Nausea • Vomiting • Fever • Chills • Dizziness • Drowsiness • Chest pain • Allergic response: rash, difficulty breathing, etc.	• Review history: heart disease (all); thyroid disorders, and use of MAOIs • Remicade use can worsen TB.

D. Maintain traction if prescribed. Note bed position, type of traction, weights, pulleys, pins, pin sites, adhesive strips, Ace wraps, splints, and casts.
   1. Skin traction: Force is applied to skin.

> **HESI Hint** • Skin traction for fracture reduction should *not* be removed unless health care provider prescribes its removal.

    a. Buck extension traction: lower extremity, legs extended, no hip flexion
    b. Dunlop traction: two lines of pull on the arm
    c. Russell traction: two lines of pull on the lower extremity, one perpendicular, one longitudinal
    d. Bryant traction: both lower extremities flexed 90 degrees at hips (rarely used because extreme elevation of lower extremities causes decreased peripheral circulation)
   2. Skeletal traction: Pin or wire applies pull directly to the distal bone fragment.
    a. Ninety-degree traction: 90-degree flexion of hip and knee; lower extremity is in a boot cast; can also be used on upper extremities.
    b. Dunlop traction: may be used as skeletal traction

> **HESI Hint** • Pin sites can be a source of infection. Monitor for signs of infection. Cleanse and dress pin sites as prescribed.

> **HESI Hint** • When moving the client in bed, with either skin or skeletal traction, it is necessary for someone to hold and move the weights of the traction as the client changes position to avoid additional tension on the traction and fracture sites.

E. Maintain child in proper body alignment; restrain if necessary.
F. Monitor for problems of immobility.
G. Provide age-appropriate play and toys.
H. Prepare child for cast application; use age-appropriate terms when explaining procedures.
I. Provide routine cast care after application; petal cast edges.
J. Teach home cast care to family, including:
   1. Neurovascular assessment of casted extremity.
   2. Not to get cast wet.
   3. Teach that in the presence of a hip spica, family may use a Bradford frame under a small child to help with toileting; they must *not* use abduction bar to turn child.
   4. Teach to seek follow-up care with health care provider.

> **HESI Hint** • Skeletal disorders affect the infant's or child's physical mobility, and typical NCLEX-RN questions focus on appropriate toys and activities for the child who is confined to bed rest and who is immobilized.

Developmental Dysplasia of Hip (DDH)

Description: Abnormal development of the femoral head in the acetabulum, usually diagnosed at birth.
A. Contributing factors:
   1. Breech position in utero
   2. Familial history of DDH
   3. Oligohydraminos
B. Treatment

Nursing Assessment

A. Infant
   1. Positive Ortolani sign ("clicking" with abduction; is the sound heard when the health care provider maneuvers the femoral head and it slips back into the acetabulum)
   2. Positive Barlow maneuver ("feel" the dislocation as the femur leaves the acetabulum when the health care provider adducts and extends the hips while stabilizing the pelvis; Fig. 5-17).
B. Older child
   1. Limp on affected side
   2. Trendelenburg sign

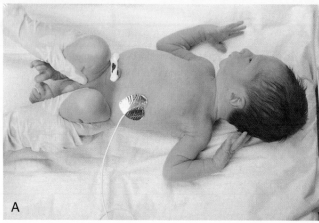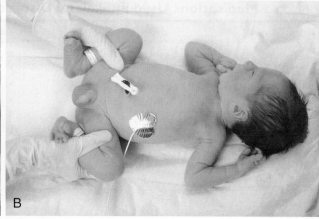

FIGURE 5-17 Assessment of the hips. A, Barlow test: adduct the hips and apply gentle pressure down and back with the thumbs. In hip dysplasia, the examiner can feel the femoral head move out of the acetabulum. B, Ortolani test: abduct the thighs and apply gentle pressure forward over the greater trochanter. A "clunking" sensation indicates a dislocated femoral head moving into the acetabulum. A hip click is normal from ligament movement. (From McKinney ES, James SR, Murray SS, Nelson KA, Ashwill JW. *Maternal-child nursing*, ed 4, St. Louis, 2013, Saunders.)

Analysis (Nursing Diagnoses)

A. *Impaired physical mobility* related to …
B. *Deficient knowledge (home care)* related to …

Nursing Plans and Interventions

A. Perform newborn assessment at birth.
B. Apply abduction device or splint (Pavlik harness; Frejka or von Rosen splint) as prescribed. Therapy involves positioning legs in flexed abducted position.
C. Teach parents home care.
 1. Teach application and removal of device (worn 24 hours a day).
 2. Teach skin care and bathing (physician may allow parents to remove device for bathing).
 3. Teach diapering.
 4. Teach that follow-up care involves frequent adjustments because of growth.
D. Teach how to provide care for an infant in Bryant traction (used if splinting is ineffective).
 1. Instruct to maintain hips in 90-degree flexion.
 2. Instruct to elevate buttocks off bed.
 3. Instruct to monitor circulation to feet.
 4. Instruct to meet developmental needs of an immobilized infant.
 5. Incorporate family in care.
 6. Prepare family for spica cast application.
E. Provide nursing care for a child requiring surgical correction.
 1. Perform preoperative teaching of child and family, including cast application.
 2. Perform postoperative care.
 a. Assess vital signs.
 b. Check cast for drainage and bleeding.
 c. Perform neurovascular assessment of extremities.
 d. Promote respiratory hygiene.

 e. Administer narcotic analgesics or morphine either IV (preferred) or IM.
 f. Teach family cast care when child gets home, including checking the cast for "hot spots" (possibly indicative of infection)

> **HESI Hint** • Children do not like injections and will deny pain to avoid "shots."

Scoliosis

Description: Lateral curvature of the spine that generally occurs during rapid growth spurts in adolescents. Hereditary conditions, neuromuscular diseases, congenital spinal defects, and trauma or infections to the spine may factor in the development of scoliosis. Treatment depends on the curvature of the spine:

Nursing Assessment

A. Occurs most commonly in adolescent females (10 to 15 years old)
 1. Elevated shoulder or hip
 2. Head and hips not aligned
 3. While child is bending forward, a rib hump is apparent. (Ask child to bend forward from the hips with arms hanging free, and examine child for a curve of the spine, rib hump, and hip asymmetry.)

Analysis (Nursing Diagnoses)

A. *Impaired physical mobility* related to …
B. *Disturbed body image* related to …

Nursing Plans and Interventions

A. Screen all adolescent children, especially females, during growth spurt.

BOX 5-3 *Log Rolling*

- Usually requires two or more persons, depending on the size of the client.
- Client is carefully moved on a draw sheet to the side of the bed away from which he or she is to be turned (moved to the left if he or she is to face to the right).
- Client is then turned in a simultaneous motion (log-rolled), maintaining the spine in a straight position.
- Pillows are arranged for support and comfort, and they assist the client to maintain alignment.
- Sitting upright should begin with log rolling and then moving the entire torso to an upright position in one movement from a side-lying log roll position.

B. Prepare child and family for conservative treatment, such as the use of a brace.
 1. Teach application of brace (Boston, Wilmington, and Milwaukee are the most common braces used) to include:
  a. Wearing 23 hours a day.
  b. Wearing a T-shirt under brace to decrease skin irritation.
  c. Checking skin for areas of irritation or breakdown.
 2. Suggest clothing modifications to camouflage brace.
 3. Reinforce prescribed exercise regimen for back and abdominal muscles.
 4. Plan ways of improving self-concept with the adolescent.
 5. Teach family that severe, untreated scoliosis can cause respiratory difficulty.

HESI Hint • A brace does not correct the spine's curve in a child with scoliosis; it only stops or slows the progression.

C. Prepare child and family for surgical correction if required.
 1. Teach child and family log-rolling technique.
 2. Teach how to practice respiratory hygiene.
 3. Orient child to ICU.
 4. Discuss postoperative tubes: Foley, nasogastric tube, and chest tube (if anterior fusion is performed).
 5. Describe postoperative pain management; PCA may be used.
 6. Obtain a baseline neurologic assessment.
D. Provide postoperative care.
 1. Perform frequent neurologic assessments.
 2. Log-roll for 5 days (Box 5-3).
 3. Administer IV fluids and analgesics as prescribed.
 4. Perform oral hygiene (client NPO).
 5. Monitor nasogastric tube and bowel sounds.
 6. Assist with ambulation, provide body jacket, progressively ambulate.

7. Teach child and family that body jacket will be worn for several months until the bone fusion is stable.
8. Determine the need for a teacher in the home.
9. Encourage child's participation in care to promote self-esteem.

Juvenile Arthritis (JA) or Juvenile Idiopathic Arthritis (JIA)

Description: Chronic inflammatory disorder of the joint synovium is considered one of the most common rheumatoid conditions occurring in children under the age of 17. JIA is diagnosed when the client presents with the following symptoms for a minimum of 6 weeks:
A. Continuous arthritic pain in single or multiple joints.
B. Repetitive fevers up to 39.44° C (103° F)
C. Systematic indications appearing as pinkish/reddish rash on the legs, arms, and trunk.
D. The exact cause is unknown; the child's immune system attacks the synovial lining of the joints

Nursing Assessment

A. Joint swelling and stiffness (usually large joints)
B. Painful joints
C. Generalized symptoms: fever, malaise, and rash
D. Periods of exacerbations and remissions
E. Varying severity: mild and self-limited or severe and disabling
F. Laboratory data: latex fixation test (usually negative) and elevated ESR
G. Poorest prognosis:
 1. Positive rheumatoid factor
 2. Polyarticular systemic onset

Analysis (Nursing Diagnoses)

A. *Impaired physical mobility* related to …
B. *Chronic pain* related to …

Nursing Plans and Interventions

A. Plan home program of prescribed exercise, splinting, and activity.
B. Assist in identifying adaptations in routine (e.g., Velcro fasteners, frequent rest periods).
C. Support the maintaining of school schedule and activities appropriate for age.
D. Teach about medication regimen; combination drugs are used (see Medical-Surgical Nursing).
 1. Nonsteroidal antiinflammatory drugs
  a. Aspirin
  b. Tolmetin sodium
  c. Ibuprofen
  d. Naproxen
 2. Antirheumatic drugs
 3. Corticosteroids (prednisone)
 4. Cytotoxic drugs (cyclophosphamide, methotrexate)

E. Teach child and family about side effects and toxic effects of prescribed drugs.
F. Inform child and family that the optimum antiinflammatory effects of drugs may take a month to achieve.
G. Encourage periodic eye examinations for early detection of iridocyclitis so as to prevent vision loss.
H. Encourage family to allow child's independence.

> **HESI Hint** • Corticosteroids are used in the short term in low doses during exacerbations. Long-term use is avoided because of side effects and their adverse effects on growth.

Review of Skeletal Disorders

1. List normal findings in a neurovascular assessment.
2. What is compartment syndrome?
3. What are the signs and symptoms of compartment syndrome?
4. Why are fractures of the epiphyseal plate a special concern?
5. How is skeletal traction applied?
6. What discharge instructions should be included concerning a child with a spica cast?
7. What are the signs and symptoms of congenital dislocated hip in infants?
8. How would the nurse conduct a scoliosis screening?
9. What instructions should a child with scoliosis receive about a skeletal brace?
10. What care is indicated for a child with juvenile rheumatoid arthritis?

Answers to Review

1. Warm extremity, brisk capillary refill, free movement, normal sensation of the affected extremity, and equal pulses
2. Damage to nerves and vasculature of an extremity due to compression
3. Abnormal neurovascular assessment: cold extremity, severe pain, inability to move the extremity, and poor capillary refill
4. Fractures of the epiphyseal plate (growth plate) may affect the growth of the limb.
5. Skeletal traction is maintained by pins or wires applied to the distal fragment of the fracture.
6. Check child's circulation. Keep cast dry. Do not place anything under cast. Prevent cast soilage during toileting or diapering. Do not turn child using an abductor bar.
7. Unequal skin folds of the buttocks, Ortolani sign, limited abduction of the affected hip, and unequal leg lengths
8. Ask the child to bend forward from the hips, with arms hanging free. Examine the child for a curve in the spine, a rib hump, and hip asymmetry.
9. The child should be instructed to wear the brace 23 hours per day; wear a T-shirt under brace; check skin for irritation; perform back and abdominal exercises; and modify clothing. The child should be encouraged to maintain normal activities as able.
10. Prescribed exercise to maintain mobility; splinting of affected joints; and teaching about medication management and side effects of drugs.

For more review, go to http://evolve.elsevier.com/HESI/RN for HESI's online study examinations.

References

1. Fuller J. *Surgical technology: principles and practice*, ed 6. Saunders; 2013.
2. Price SA. *Pathophysiology: clinical concepts of disease processes*, ed 6. Mosby; 2003.
3. deWit S, Kumagai C. *Medical-surgical nursing: concepts & practice*, ed 2. Saunders, 2013.
4. Ignatavicius D, Workman M. *Medical-surgical nursing: patient-centered collaborative care*, ed 7. Saunders, 2013.

MATERNITY NURSING

Anatomy and Physiology of Reproduction

The Menstrual Cycle

Description: Most women have ovulatory cycles within 24 months after menarche (first menstruation) (Fig. 6-1). Pregnancy can occur after the very first menstrual cycle; a sexually active girl may conceive before her first menstrual cycle. The mean age for menarche in the United States is 12.87 years, or 1 to 3 years after breast budding. The menstrual cycle is composed of four phases.

Phases of the Menstrual Cycle

A. Menstrual phase: Days 1 to 5 of cycle
   1. Shedding of the endometrium occurs in the form of uterine bleeding.
B. Proliferation (follicular) phase: Day 5 to ovulation
   1. Begins the first day of menstruation and ends 14 days later in a 28-day cycle
   2. In this preovulatory phase, follicle-stimulating hormone (FSH) is secreted by the anterior pituitary.
   3. Preovulatory surge of luteinizing hormone (LH) converts the follicle to a corpus luteum, which produces progesterone.
C. Ovulatory phase
   1. About 2 days prior to ovulation there is a marked rise in LH and FSH, slight decrease in production of follicular estrogen, and a rise in progesterone secretion.
   2. Final maturation of a single follicle and release of its mature ovum occurs.
   3. Ovulation marks the beginning of the luteal phase (occurs about 14 days into the menstrual cycle).
   4. A mature follicle ruptures and the ovum is released from the ovary.
   5. The ovum is picked up by the fimbriated end of the fallopian tube and transported to the uterus.
D. Luteal phase: Begins immediately after ovulation and ends with menstruation.
   1. Postovulatory phase requires 13-15 days.
   2. Corpus luteum reaches its peal of functional activity 8 days after ovulation, secreting estrogen and progesterone.

3. The fertilized ovum is implanted in the endometrium.
   4. In the absence of implantation the corpus luteum regresses, estrogen and progesterone levels decrease, and the endometrium is shed via menstruation.
E. Endometrial Cycle
   1. Menstrual phase: periodic vasoconstriction in upper layers of endometrium initiates shedding of functional 2/3 of the endometrium
   2. Proliferative phase: depends on estrogen
   3. Secretory phase: includes the day of ovulation to 3 days prior to next menstrual period.
   4. Ischemic phase:
      a. blood supply to the functional endometrium is blocked and necrosis occurs.
      b. functional layer separates from basal layer and menstruation begins (day 1 of the next cycle).

HESI Hint • The menstrual phase varies in length in most women.

HESI Hint • Ovulation occurs approximately 14 days before the next menstrual cycle.

HESI Hint • To avoid pregnancy a woman should abstain from unprotected sexual intercourse during her fertile days. The most fertile days for pregnancy are the day before ovulation and the day of ovulation. The fertile period begins 4-5 days prior to ovulation and ends 24-48 hours after ovulation. A couple must avoid unprotected intercourse for several days before an anticipated ovulation and for 3 days after ovulation to prevent pregnancy because sperm can live in a woman's body approximately 4 to 5 days and eggs live approximately 24-48 hours after being released.

Fertilization

A. Indications of ovulation
   1. A slight drop in temperature occurs 1 day before ovulation (basal body temperature may be less than 37°; a rise of 0.5 degree to 1 degree in temperature occurs at ovulation). Temperature remains elevated for approximately 10 to 12 days.

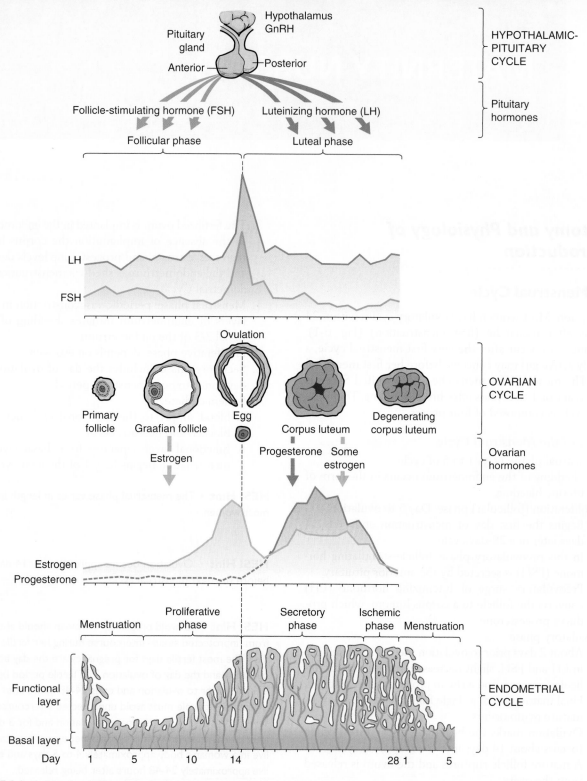

FIGURE 6-1 Menstrual cycle: hypothalamic-pituitary, ovarian, and endometrial. (From Lowdermilk DL, Perry SE: *Maternity and women's health care*, ed 10, St. Louis, 2012, Mosby.)

2. Preovulatory and postovulatory mucus is thick (viscous) to discourage sperm penetration.
3. At ovulation cervical mucus is abundant, watery, thin, clear (it looks, feels, and stretches like egg white, called spinnbarkeit)

4. Cervical os dilates slightly, softens, and rises in the vagina.
5. Some women have localized abdominal pain called mittelschmerz that coincides with ovulation.
6. Ferning is seen under microscope.

B. Conditions for fertilization
   1. Postcoital test demonstrates live, motile, normal sperm present in cervical mucus.
   2. Fallopian tubes are patent.
   3. Endometrial biopsy indicates adequate progesterone and secretory endometrium.
   4. Semen is supportive to pregnancy: 2 mL semen; at least 20 million sperm per mL; >60% are normal; and >50% are motile (moving forward).
C. Implantation
   1. Fertilization takes place in ampulla (outer third) section of the fallopian tube.
   2. The zygote (fertilized ovum) takes 3 to 4 days to enter the uterus.
   3. It takes 7 to 10 days to complete the process of nidation (implantation).
D. Fetal development
   1. Zygote
      a. 12 to 14 days after fertilization
      b. From the time the ovum is fertilized until it is implanted in the uterus
   2. Embryo
      a. 3 to 8 weeks after fertilization
      b. Embryo most vulnerable to teratogens (viruses, drugs, radiation, or infections), which can cause major congenital anomalies
   3. Fetus
      a. 9 weeks after fertilization to term (38 + weeks)
      b. Fewer major anomalies (Fig. 6-2) caused by teratogens

Maternal Physiologic Changes during Pregnancy

A. Pregnancy length: counted from the first day of last menstrual period (LMP)
   1. 280 days (approximately)
   2. 40 weeks
   3. 10 lunar months (perfect 28-day months)
   4. 9 calendar months
B. Pregnancy divided into three 13-week trimesters:
   1. First trimester: from the first day of LMP through 13 weeks
   2. Second trimester: 14 weeks through 26 weeks
   3. Third trimester: 27 weeks to 40 weeks

HESI Hint • Some women do not realize they are pregnant because they experience implantation bleeding or spotting.

Fetal and Maternal Changes

8 Weeks
A. Fetal development
   1. Rapid development
   2. Major divisions of brain are discernible

3. Heart begins to pump blood.
   4. Facial features are discernible.
   5. Limb buds are well developed.
   6. Ears develop from skin folds.
   7. Tiny muscles form beneath the skin embryo.
   8. Weight is 2 g.
B. Maternal changes
   1. Nausea persists up to 12 weeks.
   2. Uterus changes from pear to globular shape.
   3. Hegar sign occurs (softening of the isthmus of cervix).
   4. Goodell sign occurs (softening of cervix).
   5. Cervix flexes.
   6. Leukorrhea increases.
   7. Ambivalence about pregnancy may occur.
   8. There is no noticeable weight gain.
   9. Chadwick sign (bluing of vagina) is a presumptive sign appearing as early as 4 weeks.
C. Nursing interventions
   1. Teach prevention of nausea.
      a. Suggest eating dry crackers before getting out of bed in the morning.
      b. Suggest eating small, frequent meals; avoiding fatty foods; and avoiding skipping meals.
   2. Teach safety.
      a. Avoid hot tubs, saunas, and steam rooms throughout pregnancy (increases risk for neural tube defects in first trimester; hypotension may cause fainting).
   3. Prepare client for pregnancy.
      a. Discuss attitudes toward pregnancy.
      b. Discuss value of early pregnancy classes that focus on what to expect during pregnancy.
      c. Provide information about childbirth preparation classes.
      d. Include partner and family in preparation for childbirth (expectant partners experience many of the same feelings and conflicts experienced by the expectant mother).
      e. A doula is a trained labor support person employed by the mother to provide emotional and physical labor support.

12 Weeks
A. Fetal development
   1. Embryo becomes a fetus.
   2. Heart is discernible by ultrasound.
   3. Lower body develops.
   4. Sex is determinable.
   5. Kidneys produce urine.
   6. Fetus weighs 907.18 to 1814.4 g (2 to 4 lb)
B. Maternal changes
   1. Uterus rises above pelvic brim.
   2. Braxton Hicks contractions are possible (continue throughout pregnancy).
   3. Potential for urinary tract infection (UTI) increases (exists throughout pregnancy).

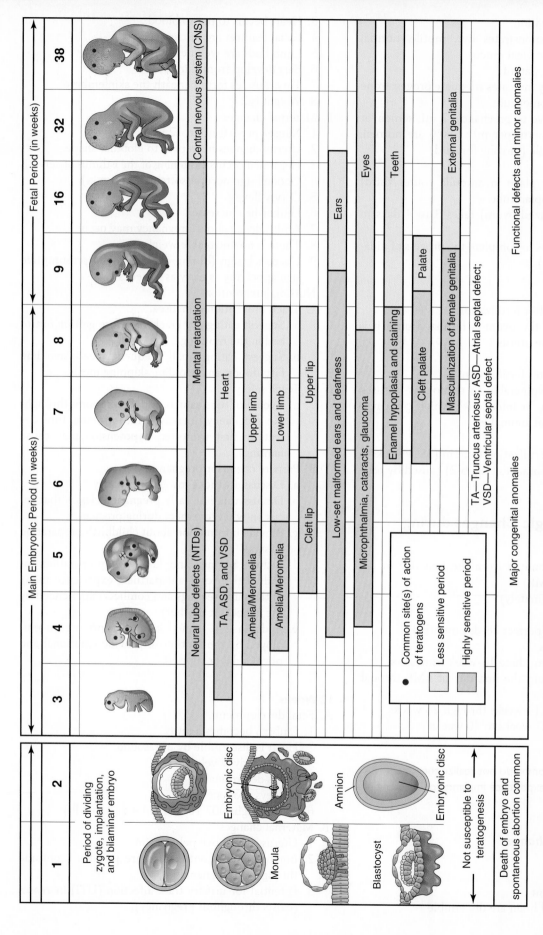

FIGURE 6-2 Sensitive or critical periods in human development. Purple denotes highly sensitive periods; green indicates stages that are less sensitive to teratogens. (Moore KL: *Before we are born: essentials of embryology and birth defects*, ed 8. Philadelphia, 2013, W. B. Saunders Company.)

4. Weight gain is 2 to 4 lb during the first trimester.
5. Placenta is fully functioning and producing hormones.

C. Nursing interventions
   1. Teach prevention of urinary tract infections.
      a. Encourage adequate fluid intake (3 L/day).
      b. Instruct to void frequently (every 2 hours while awake).
      c. Encourage to void before and after intercourse.
      d. Teach to wipe from front to back.
   2. Discuss nutrition and exercise.
      a. Increase caloric intake by 300 calories per day.
      b. Stress the value of regular exercise.
   3. Discuss possible effects of pregnancy on sexual relationship. Recognize father's role as he labors to incorporate the parental role into his self-identity.

16 Weeks

A. Fetal development
   1. Head still dominant, but face looks human and arm/leg ratio is proportionate
   2. Scalp hair appears
   3. Meconium in bowel, and anus open
   4. Most bones and joint cavities seen on ultrasound, and muscular movements detected
   5. Heart muscle well developed, and blood formation active in spleen
   6. Elastic fibers appear in lungs and terminal; respiratory bronchioles appear
   7. Kidneys in position
   8. Cerebral lobes delineated, and cerebellum assumes some prominence
   9. General sense organs differentiated
   10. Testes in position for descent into scrotum or vagina open

B. Maternal changes
   1. Quickening, the mother's first perception of fetal movement, may be noted between weeks 16 and 20.
   2. Colostrum, the creamy white to yellowish premilk, may be expressed from the nipples as early as 16 weeks of gestation.
   3. Serum cholesterol increases from 16 to 32 weeks of pregnancy and remains at this level until after birth.
   4. By 14 to 16 weeks, the placenta is clearly defined.
   5. Insulin resistance begins as early as 14 to 16 weeks of gestation and continues to rise until it stabilizes during the last few weeks of pregnancy.
   6. Approximate weight gain of 1 lb per week beginning in the second trimester and continuing until delivery.

C. Nursing interventions
   1. Explain the screening test, and obtain blood sample for maternal serum alpha-fetoprotein (MSAFP) between 15 and 22 weeks of gestation, ideally between 16 and 18 weeks of gestation.
      a. Elevated levels are associated with open neural tube defects and multiple gestations.
      b. Low levels are associated with Down syndrome. Abnormal levels are followed by second-trimester ultrasonography for more in-depth investigation.
   2. Explain the multiple-marker, or triple-screen, blood test, and obtain a specimen for screening between 16 and 18 weeks of gestation to measure the MSAFP, human chorionic gonadotropin (hCG), and unconjugated estriol, the levels of which are combined to yield one value.
      a. Low levels may be associated with Down syndrome and other chromosomal abnormalities.

20 Weeks

A. Fetal development
   1. Vernix protects the body.
   2. Lanugo (fine hair) covers the body and protects the body.
   3. Eyebrows, eyelashes, and head hair develop.
   4. Fetus sleeps, sucks, and kicks.
   5. Fetus weighs 200 to 400 g (11 to 14 oz).

B. Maternal changes
   1. Fundus reaches level of umbilicus.
   2. Breasts begin secreting colostrum; areolae darken.
   3. Amniotic sac holds approximately 400 mL of fluid.
   4. Postural hypotension may occur.
   5. Fetal movement felt (quickening); pregnancy becomes "real."
   6. Nasal stuffiness may begin.
   7. Leg cramps may begin.
   8. Varicose veins may develop.
   9. Constipation may develop.

C. Nursing interventions
   1. Teach comfort measures.
      a. Encourage to remain active.
      b. Encourage to sit with feet elevated when possible.
      c. Teach to avoid pressure on lower thighs.
      d. Teach that use of support stockings may be helpful.
      e. Teach to dorsiflex foot to relieve leg cramps.
      f. Suggest applying heat to muscles affected by cramps.
      g. Suggest that cool-air vaporizer or saline nasal spray may help with nasal stuffiness.
   2. Teach measures to avoid constipation.
      a. Encourage to eat raw fruits, vegetables, cereals with bran.
      b. Encourage to drink 3 L of fluid per day.
      c. Encourage to exercise frequently.

24 Weeks

A. Fetal development
   1. Body fairly well proportioned; skin red and wrinkled; sweat glands forming
   2. Blood formation increases in bone marrow and decreases in liver.
   3. Alveolar ducts and sacs present, and lecithin begins to appear in amniotic fluid (weeks 26 to 27).

4. Neuronal proliferation in cerebral cortex ends.
5. Can hear
6. Testes at inguinal ring in descent to scrotum
B. Maternal changes
   1. Uterus rises to the level of the umbilicus.
   2. Diastolic blood pressure (BP) gradually increases at 24 to 32 weeks, after having decreased in the first trimester, and returns to prepregnancy levels by term. Systolic BP usually remains the same as the prepregnancy level.
C. Nursing interventions
   1. Explain and obtain a blood sample for a glucose challenge that is usually done between 24 and 28 weeks' gestation.
   2. At between 24 and 32 weeks' gestation, two or three ultrasound measurements may be taken 2 weeks apart to compare against standard fetal growth curves.

28 Weeks

A. Fetal development
   1. Fetus can breathe, swallow, and regulate temperature.
   2. Surfactant forms in lungs.
   3. Fetus can hear.
   4. Fetus's eyelids open.
   5. Period of greatest fetal weight gain begins.
   6. Fetus weighs 1100 g (2½ lb).
B. Maternal changes
   1. Fundus is halfway between umbilicus and xiphoid process.
   2. Thoracic breathing replaces abdominal breathing.
   3. Fetal outline is palpable.
   4. Woman becomes more introspective and concentrates interest on the unborn child.
   5. Heartburn may begin.
   6. Hemorrhoids may develop.
C. Nursing interventions
   1. Teach treatment of hemorrhoids.
      a. Suggest sitz baths.
      b. Suggest topical anesthetic agents.
      c. Suggest taking stool softeners as prescribed.
   2. Teach comfort measures.
      a. Encourage woman to elevate legs when sitting.
      b. Suggest that woman assume side-lying position when resting.
   3. Teach measures to avoid heartburn.
      a. Teach woman to eat small, frequent meals.
      b. Teach avoidance of fatty foods.
      c. Encourage woman to avoid lying down after meals.
      d. Teach that antacids may be prescribed.
      e. Teach woman to avoid sodium bicarbonate.
   4. Prepare woman for delivery and parenthood.
      a. Discuss mother's, father's, and family's expectations of labor and delivery.
      b. Discuss mother's, father's, and family's expectations about caring for infant.
      c. Encourage woman to start childbirth-preparation classes.

32 Weeks

A. Fetal development
   1. Brown fat deposits develop beneath skin to insulate baby after birth.
   2. Fetus is 15 to 17 inches in length.
   3. Fetus begins storing iron, calcium, and phosphorus.
   4. Fetus weighs 1800 to 2200 g (4 to 5 lb).
B. Maternal changes
   1. Fundus reaches xiphoid process.
   2. Breasts are full and tender.
   3. Urinary frequency returns.
   4. Swollen ankles may occur.
   5. Sleeping problems may develop.
   6. Dyspnea may develop.
C. Nursing interventions
   1. Teach measures to decrease edema.
      a. Encourage woman to elevate legs one or two times per day for approximately 1 hour.
   2. Teach comfort measures.
      a. Encourage woman to wear well-fitting supportive bra.
      b. Encourage woman to maintain proper posture.
      c. Teach woman to use semi-Fowler position at night for dyspnea.
   3. Prepare woman for childbirth.
      a. Review signs of labor.
      b. Discuss plans for other children (if any).
      c. Discuss plans for transportation to agency.
      d. Assess father's (family member's) role during childbirth.

36 to 40 Weeks

A. Fetal development
   1. Fetus occupies entire uterus; activity is restricted.
   2. Maternal antibodies are transferred to fetus (provide immunity for approximately 6 months, until infant's own immune system can take over).
   3. L/S (lecithin/sphingomyelin) ratio is 2:1 and phosphatidylglycerol (PG) is present.
   4. Fetus weighs 3200+ g
B. Maternal changes
   1. Lightening occurs.
   2. Placenta weighs approximately 519-567 g
   3. Mother is eager for birth, may have burst of energy.
   4. Backaches increase.
   5. Urinary frequency increases.
   6. Braxton Hicks contractions intensify (cervix and lower uterine segment prepare for labor).
C. Nursing interventions
   1. Teach safety measures.
      a. Teach to wear low-heeled shoes or flats.
      b. Instruct to avoid heavy lifting.
      c. Encourage sleeping on side to relieve bladder pressure and urinating frequently.
   2. Encourage preparation for delivery.
      a. Teach woman to do pelvic tilt exercises.
      b. Encourage packing a suitcase.

c. Encourage couple to tour labor and delivery area.

d. Discuss postpartum circumstances: circumcision, rooming-in, possibility of postpartum blues, birth control, need for adequate rest, father's role.

Antepartum Nursing Care

Psychosocial Responses to Pregnancy

Maternal Responses

A. First trimester
  1. Ambivalence: Whether pregnancy is planned or unplanned, ambivalence is normal.
  2. Financial worries about increased responsibility are normal.
  3. Career concerns may arise.
B. Second trimester
  1. Quickening occurs and pregnancy becomes real.
  2. Pregnant woman accepts pregnancy.
  3. Ambivalence wanes.
C. Third trimester
  1. Pregnant woman becomes introverted and self-absorbed.
  2. Pregnant woman begins to ignore partner (may strain the relationship).
D. Throughout pregnancy
  1. Wide mood swings (joy, anticipation, fear) occur.
  2. Pregnant woman is ultrasensitive.
  3. Strained relationship with partner may occur.

> **HESI Hint** • Signs of healthy psychosocial maternal-fetal bonding include massaging the abdomen, nicknaming the fetus, and talking to the fetus in utero.

Paternal Responses

A. Announcement phase, acceptance of the biologic fact of pregnancy
  1. At the confirmation of pregnancy, men may react with joy or dismay, depending on whether the pregnancy is desired or unplanned or unwanted.
  2. Ambivalence in the early stages of pregnancy is common.
  3. Some men experience pregnancylike symptoms, such as nausea, weight gain, and other physical symptoms; this is known as *couvade syndrome.*
  4. May last from a few hours to a few weeks
B. Moratorium phase: the period of adjustment to the reality of pregnancy
  1. Accepts the pregnancy
  2. May put conscious thought of the pregnancy aside for a time and become more introspective by engaging in many discussions about his philosophy of life, religion, childbearing, and childrearing practices and relationships with family members, particularly with his father

  3. This phase may be relatively short or persist until the last trimester, depending on the father's readiness for the pregnancy.
C. Focusing phase, active involvement in both the pregnancy and his relationship with his child
  1. Negotiates with the mother the role he is to play in labor and to prepare for parenthood
  2. Concentrates on his experience of the pregnancy and begins to think of himself as a father
  3. Begins in the last trimester

Activities during First Prenatal Visit

A. Obtain history.
  1. Medical history
  2. Obstetrical history can be determined by two common methods:
    a. Two digits: G/P only records the gravida and para of a client.
      (1) *Gravida* refers any pregnancy; as well as to the number of times a woman has been pregnant (regardless of the duration or outcome) including the pregnancy in progress.
      (2) *Para* refers to the number of pregnancies that have reached 20 weeks or greater gestation. When calculating parity, multiple births count only as (1) after pregnancy has reached 20 weeks and before birth. Any pregnancy loss occurring before 20 weeks is counted as an abortion (whether spontaneous or elective termination) and adds only to a client's gravidity, not parity.
      (3) Age of viability occurs by 20 weeks' gestation when the function of the lungs has matured enough for the fetus to survive outside the uterus.
    b. Five digits: GTPAL (Gravidity, Term Births, Preterm Births, Abortions and Miscarriages, Living Children) provides information of the client's obstetrical history.
      (1) **G**ravidity – number of pregnancies
      (2) **T**erm – term births or pregnancies delivered (full term is a fetus at 38-40 weeks' gestation).
      (3) **P**reterm – pregnancy that has reached 20 weeks of gestation but ends before completion of 37 weeks of gestation
      (4) **A**bortions and Miscarriages – pregnancy that does not reach 20 weeks of gestation.
      (5) **L**iving children – infants that have survived birth
  3. History and status of current pregnancy

> **HESI Hint** • For many women, battering (emotional or physical abuse) begins during pregnancy. Women should be assessed for abuse in private, away from the partner, by a nurse who is familiar with local resources and knows how to determine the safety of the client.

HESI Hint • Practice determining gravidity and parity. A woman who is 6 weeks pregnant has the following maternal history:

- She has healthy 2-year-old male fraternal twins
- She had a miscarriage at 22 weeks
- She had an elective abortion at 6 weeks, 5 years earlier.
- With this pregnancy she is gravida 4 para 2, only 2 deliveries after 20 weeks' gestation, and twins are two living
- GTPAL is 4 1-1-1-21 (G-4 pregnancies (twins, miscarriage, electrive abortion, current pregnancy; T-1 (twins count as one birth); P-1 (22 week miscarriage); A-1 (elective abortion at 6 weeks); L-2 (twins).

B. Assist with physical examination.
C. Calculate gestational age: estimated date of birth (EDB) using the Nägele rule:
1. Count back 3 months from the first day of the last normal menstrual period, and add 7 days.
2. For example: If the LMP was March 23, the EDB would be December 30.

HESI Hint • Practice calculating EDB. If the first day of a woman's last normal menstrual period was December 9, what is her EDB, using the Nägele rule? Answer: September 16. Count back 3 months and add 7 days (always give February 28 days).

D. Vital signs
1. BP should rise no more than 30 points systolic and 15 points diastolic from previous baseline normal. Average BP is 90 to 140 mm Hg systolic and 60 to 90 mm Hg diastolic.
2. Average pulse is 60 to 90 beats per minute (bpm).
3. Average respiration is 16 to 24 breaths per minute (breaths/min).
4. 36.1° to 37.7° C
E. Future office visits
1. Low-risk client's schedule is:
   a. Every 4 weeks until 28 weeks
   b. Every 2 weeks from 28 weeks until 36 weeks
   c. Every week from 36 weeks until delivery
2. High-risk client's schedule is determined by client's needs; visits are scheduled as necessary.
F. Obtain laboratory data (see Appendix C).
1. Hgb: values during pregnancy >1 at least 11 g/dL first trimester and 10.5 g/dL 2nd trimester
2. Hct: values during pregnancy >33% 1st and 3rd trimesters and at least 32% in 2nd trimester

HESI Hint • At approximately 28 to 32 weeks' gestation, a plasma volume increase of 25% to 40% occurs, resulting in normal hemodilution of pregnancy and Hct values.

above 38% or hemoglobin levels above 13g/dL are associated with gestational hypertension. High Hct values may look good, but in reality they represent a gestational hypertension disorder and a depleted vascular space.

3. White blood cell (WBC) and differential
4. Hgb electrophoresis (sickle cell)
5. Pap smear and cytology (gonorrhea and chlamydia)
6. Antibody screens
   a. Human immunodeficiency virus (HIV)
   b. Hepatitis B
   c. Toxoplasmosis
   d. Rubella (>1:10 = immunity)
   e. Syphilis (rapid plasma regain [RPR], Venereal Disease Research Laboratory [VDRL])
   f. Cytomegalovirus
7. Tuberculin skin testing (purified protein derivative [PPD])
8. Rh and blood type
9. Urinalysis

HESI Hint • Hgb and Hct data can be used to evaluate nutritional status. Example: A 22-year-old primigravida at 12 weeks' gestation has an Hgb of 9.6 g/dL and an Hct of 31%. She has gained 3 pounds during the first trimester. A weight gain of 907.18 to 1814.4 g. (2 to 4 lb) during the first trimester is recommended. Since this client is anemic supplemental iron and a diet higher in iron are needed.
   Foods high in iron:
- Fish and red meats
- Cereals and yellow vegetables
- Green leafy vegetables and citrus fruits
- Egg yolks and dried fruits

Activities during Subsequent Visits

A. Check urine.
1. Albumin: no more than a trace in a normal finding (related to preeclampsia)
2. Glucose: no more than 1+ in a normal finding (related to gestational diabetes)
3. Protein: A trace amount of protein may be present in the urine; a higher presence may indicate contamination by vaginal secretions, kidney disease, or preeclampsia. ≥30 mg/dL (≥1 +) on dipstick (mild preeclampsia); 2+ to 3+ protein on dipstick (severe preeclampsia).
B. Graph weight gain.
1. 907.18 to 1814.4 g (2 to 4 lb) weight gain in the first trimester is recommended.
2. 1 lb per week weight gain thereafter is recommended (>2 lb/week related to preeclampsia-edema).
3. Total weight gain during the pregnancy should be between 11340 and 15876 g (25 to 35 lb)

C. Check fundal height (Fig. 6-3).
   1. 12 to 13 weeks: Fundus rises above symphysis.
   2. From gestational weeks 18 to 32, the height of the fundus, measured in centimeters and with an empty bladder, is approximately the same as the number of weeks of gestation. Example: 24 weeks' gestation should be 24 cm when measured from the symphysis pubis to the top of the fundus.

> **HESI Hint** • As pregnancy advances, the uterus presses on abdominal vessels (vena cava and aorta). Teach the woman that a left side-lying position relieves supine hypotension and increases perfusion to uterus, placenta, and fetus.

D. Check fetal heart rate (FHR).
   1. 10 to 12 weeks: detectable by using Doppler
   2. 15 to 20 weeks: detectable by using fetoscope
   3. 110 to 160 bpm: normal range

> **HESI Hint** • The normal FHR is 110 to 160 bpm. Changes in FHR are the first and most important indicators of compromised blood flow to the fetus; these changes require action! Fetal well-being is determined by assessing fundal height, fetal heart tones and rate, fetal movement, and uterine activity (contractions).

E. Teach the importance of continuing prenatal care.
F. Provide anticipatory guidance: first trimester
   1. Discomforts such as nausea, fatigue, and urinary frequency subside after 13 weeks.
   2. Sleep needs increase to 8 hr/day.
   3. Rest periods should be planned.
   4. Exercise is fine as long as woman is able to converse easily while exercising. If not, she should slow down.

   5. Work is acceptable if there is no exposure to hazardous chemicals or toxins.
   6. Bathing is acceptable until membranes rupture (usually within hours of delivery).
   7. Travel by car is acceptable, but woman will need frequent breaks and must wear seat belt.
   8. Air travel is acceptable, but policies vary with airline. Advise woman to remain well hydrated and to move about frequently to minimize the risk for thrombophlebitis
   9. It is best to ingest no medications and no alcohol and to stop smoking.
G. Provide anticipatory guidance: second trimester
   1. Sexual needs and desires may change for better or for worse. Encourage communication with partner regarding adjustments.
   2. Encourage woman to have regular dental check-ups, to maintain dental hygiene (gum hypertrophy is common), and to delay radiographs and major dental work if possible.
H. Provide anticipatory guidance: third trimester
   1. Encourage woman to schedule childbirth classes.
   2. Note that urinary frequency and dyspnea return.
   3. Review interventions for leg cramps (dorsiflex foot), nasal stuffiness, varicose veins, and constipation.
   4. Teach safety related to balance.
   5. Teach about positioning with pillows for comfort.
   6. Note that round-ligament pain will occur.
   7. Instruct client to come to hospital when contractions are occurring regularly 5 minutes apart.
   8. Provide information on feeding methods.
   9. Encourage choosing a pediatrician and clinic.
   10. Reinforce nutritional needs because third trimester is a period of rapid fetal growth.
   11. Teach the risks and symptoms of preterm labor.

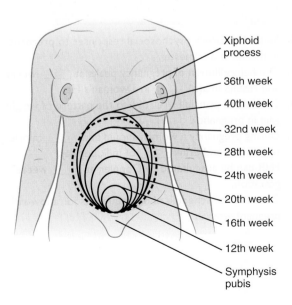

FIGURE 6-3 Fundal height assessment.

Labels (top to bottom): Xiphoid process, 36th week, 40th week, 32nd week, 28th week, 24th week, 20th week, 16th week, 12th week, Symphysis pubis

> **HESI Hint** • Early intervention can optimize maternal and fetal outcome. Teach clients to report immediately any of the following danger signs. Possible indications of preeclampsia and eclampsia are:
> - Visual disturbances
> - Swelling of face, fingers, or sacrum
> - Severe, continuous headache
> - Persistent vomiting
> - Epigastric pain
> - Infection:
>   - Chills
>   - Temperature over 38° C
>   - Dysuria
>   - Pain in abdomen
> - Fluid discharge or bleeding from vagina (anything other than normal leukorrhea)
> - Change in fetal movement or increased FHR

Nutrition

Nursing Assessment

A. Diet
   1. Ask client to recall diet for past 24 hours.
   2. Use a questionnaire to determine individual deficiencies.
   3. Determine body mass index (BMI).
   4. Note symptoms of malnutrition:
      a. Glossitis
      b. Cracked lips
      c. Dry, brittle hair
B. Dental caries, periodontitis
C. Weight (those who weigh [44 kg or 88 kg] <100 lb or >200 lb are at risk)

Analysis (Nursing Diagnoses)

A. *Imbalanced nutrition: less than/more than body requirements* related to …
B. *Deficient knowledge* (specify) related to …

Nursing Plans and Interventions

A. Teach about minimum nutritional increases. Teach that client should:
   1. Increase intake by 300 calories above basal and activity needs.
   2. Increase protein by 30 g/day.
   3. Increase intake of iron and folic acid through diet and supplements as directed by health care provider.
   4. Increase intake of vitamin A, vitamin C, and calcium through diet.
   5. Drink a total of 8 to 10 glasses of fluid per day; 4 to 6 glasses should be water.

> **HESI Hint** • Most providers prescribe prenatal vitamins to ensure that the client receives an adequate intake of vitamins. However, only the health care provider can prescribe prenatal vitamins. It is the nurse's responsibility to teach about proper diet and about taking prescribed vitamins as they have been prescribed by the health care provider.

B. Relate recommended weight gain by trimester to fetal growth and fetal health.
   1. Record weight at each visit, using graph.
   2. Advise client to maintain steady weight gain of 1 lb/week in second and third trimesters.
C. Provide a copy of daily food guide to post on refrigerator (consider cultural food patterns in choices given). Include the following:
   1. Three servings from dairy group (milk, cheese)
   2. Five servings of protein (meats, eggs, legumes)
   3. Five servings of vegetables (green and deep yellow vegetables are good sources of vitamin C)
   4. Six servings of breads or cereals
   5. Four servings of fruit
D. Advise regarding vitamin and iron supplementation.
E. Explain that poor nutrition can lead to anemia, preterm labor, obesity, and intrauterine growth restriction (IUGR).

> **HESI Hint** • It is recommended that pregnant women consume the equivalent of 3 cups of milk or yogurt per day. This will ensure that the daily calcium needs are met and help alleviate the occurrence of leg cramps.

Review of Anatomy and Physiology of Reproduction and Antepartum Nursing Care

1. State the objective signs that signify ovulation.
2. Ovulation occurs how many days before the next menstrual period?
3. State three ways to identify the chronological age of a pregnancy (gestation).
4. What maternal position provides optimum fetal and placental perfusion during pregnancy?
5. Name the major discomforts of the first trimester and one suggestion for amelioration of each.
6. If the first day of a woman's last normal menstrual period was February 3, what is the EDB using the Nägele rule?
7. At 20 weeks' gestation, the fundal height would be _____; the fetus would weigh approximately _____ and would look like _____.
8. State the normal psychosocial responses to pregnancy in the second trimester.
9. The hemodilution of pregnancy peaks at _____ weeks and results in a(n) _____ in a woman's Hct.
10. State three principles relative to the pattern of weight gain in pregnancy.
11. During pregnancy a woman should add _____ calories to her diet and drink _____ of milk per day.
12. FHR can be auscultated by Doppler at _____ weeks' gestation.
13. Describe the schedule of prenatal visits for a low-risk pregnant woman.

Answers to Review

1. Abundant, thin, clear cervical mucus; Spinnbarkeit (egg-white stretchiness) of cervical mucus; open cervical os; slight drop in basal body temperature and then 0.5 degree to 1 degree F rise; ferning under the microscope
2. 14 days
3. 10 lunar months; 9 calendar months consisting of three trimesters of 3 months each; 40 weeks; 280 days
4. The knee-chest position, but the ideal position of comfort for the mother, which supports fetal, maternal, and placental perfusion, is the side-lying position (removes pressure from the abdominal vessels [vena cava, aorta]).
5. Nausea and vomiting: crackers before rising; fatigue: rest periods and naps and 7 to 8 hours of sleep at night
6. Count back 3 months and add 7 days: November 10 (always give February 28 days).
7. At the umbilicus; 300 to 400 g; a baby—with hair, lanugo, and vernix, but without any subcutaneous fat
8. Ambivalence wanes and acceptance of pregnancy occurs; pregnancy becomes "real"; signs of maternal-fetal bonding occur.
9. 28 to 32 weeks; decrease
10. Total gain should average 11340 and 15876 g (25 to 35 lb). Gain should be consistent throughout pregnancy. An average of 1 lb/week should be gained in the second and third trimesters.
11. 300; 236.5 ml (8 ounce) glasses per day
12. 10 to 12
13. Once every 4 weeks until 28 weeks; every 2 weeks from 28 to 36 weeks; then once a week until delivery

Fetal and Maternal Assessment Techniques

Description: Techniques used to obtain data regarding fetal and maternal physiologic status
A. Maternal risk factors include but are not limited to:
   1. Age under 17 or over 34
   2. High parity (>5)
   3. Pregnancy (3 months since last delivery)
   4. Hypertension, preeclampsia in current pregnancy
   5. Anemia, history of hemorrhage, or current hemorrhage
   6. Multiple gestations
   7. Rh incompatibility
   8. History of dystocia or previous operative delivery
   9. A height of 60 inches (5 feet) or less
   10. Malnutrition (15% under ideal weight) or extreme obesity (20% over ideal weight)
   11. Medical disease during pregnancy (diabetes, hyperthyroidism, hyperemesis, clotting disorders such as thrombocytopenia)
   12. Infection in pregnancy: toxoplasmosis, other agents, rubella, cytomegalovirus, herpes simplex (TORCH diseases); influenza; HIV; *Chlamydia;* human papillomavirus (HPV)
   13. History of family violence, lack of social support
B. Various techniques are used to determine fetal and maternal well-being.

HESI Hint • In some states, screening for neural tube defects by testing either maternal serum alpha-fetoprotein (AFP) levels or amniotic fluid AFP levels is mandated by state law. This screening test is highly associated with both false positives and false negatives.

Ultrasonography

Description: High-frequency sound waves are beamed onto the abdomen; echoes are returned to a machine that records the fetus's location and size.
A. Used in the first trimester to determine:
   1. Number of fetuses
   2. Presence of fetal cardiac movement and rhythm
   3. Uterine abnormalities
   4. Gestational age
B. Used in the second and third trimesters to determine:
   1. Fetal viability and gestational age
   2. Size-date discrepancies
   3. Amniotic fluid volume
   4. Placental location and maturity
   5. Uterine anomalies and abnormalities
   6. Results of amniocentesis
C. Findings
   1. Fetal heart activity is apparent as early as 6 to 7 weeks' gestation.
   2. Serial evaluation of biparietal diameter and limb length can differentiate between wrong dates and true IUGR.
   3. A biophysical profile (BPP) is made to ascertain fetal well-being.
      a. Five variables are assessed: fetal breathing movements, gross body movements, fetal tone, reactivity of FHR, and amniotic fluid volume.
      b. A score of 2 or 0 can be obtained for each variable. An overall score of 10 designates that the fetus is well on the day of the examination.
D. Nursing care
   1. Instruct the woman to drink 3 to 4 glasses of water before coming for examination and not to urinate. When the fetus is very small (in the first and second trimesters), the client's bladder must be full during the examination in order for the uterus to be supported for imaging. (A full bladder is not needed if ultrasound is done transvaginally instead of abdominally.)

2. Position the woman with pillows under neck and knees to keep pressure off bladder; late in the third trimester, place wedge under right hip to displace uterus to the left.
3. Position display so woman can watch if she wishes.
4. Have bedpan or bathroom immediately available.

E. Complications
1. There are no known complications.
2. There is controversy regarding routine use of ultrasound in pregnancy.

> **HESI Hint** • Gestational age is best determined by an early sonogram rather than a later one.

Chorionic Villi Sampling (CVS)

Description: Removal of a small piece of villi during the period between 8 and 12 weeks' gestation under ultrasound guidance (cannot replace amniocentesis completely because no sample of amniotic fluid can be obtained for AFP or Rh disease testing)

A. Findings
1. The test determines genetic diagnosis early in the first trimester.
2. The results are obtained in 1 week.

B. Nursing care
1. Have informed consent signed before any procedure.
2. Place woman in lithotomy position using stirrups.
3. Warn of slight sharp pain upon catheter insertion.
4. Results should not be given over the phone.

C. Complications
1. Spontaneous abortion (5%)
2. Controversy regarding fetal anomalies (limb)

Amniocentesis

Description: Removal of amniotic fluid sample from the uterus

A. Is used to determine:
1. Fetal genetic diagnosis (usually in the first trimester)
2. Fetal lung maturity (last trimester)
3. Fetal well-being

B. Performed only when uterus rises above the symphysis (between 12 and 13 weeks) and amniotic fluid has formed (see Fig. 6-3).

C. Usually takes 10 days to 2 weeks to develop cultured cell karyotype. Therefore woman could be well into second trimester before diagnosis is made, making choice for abortion more dangerous.

D. Findings
1. Genetic disorders
   a. Karyotype: determines Down syndrome (trisomy 21), other trisomies, and sex chromatin (sex-linked disorders)
   b. Biochemical analysis: determines more than 60 types of metabolic disorders (Tay-Sachs)
   c. AFP: Elevations may be associated with neutral tube defects; low levels may indicate trisomy 21.

2. Fetal lung maturity
   a. L/S ratio: 2:1 ratio indicates fetal lung maturity unless mother is diabetic or has Rh disease or fetus is septic.
   b. L/S ratio and presence of PG: most accurate determination of fetal maturity. PG is present after 35 weeks' gestation.
   c. Lung maturity is the best predictor of extrauterine survival.
   d. Creatinine: renal maturity indicator >1.8
   e. Orange-staining cells: Lipid-containing exfoliating sebaceous gland maturity; >20% stained orange means 35 weeks or more.

3. Fetal well-being
   a. Bilirubin delta optical density (OD) assessment should be performed in mother previously sensitized to the fetal Rh+ red blood cells (RBCs) and having antibodies to the Rh+ circulating cells. The delta OD test measures the change in OD of the amniotic fluid caused by staining with bilirubin. Performed at 24 weeks' gestation.
   b. Meconium in amniotic fluid may indicate fetal distress.

E. Nursing care
1. Obtain baseline vital signs and FHR.
2. Place client in supine position with hands across chest.
3. If prescribed, shave area and scrub with povidone-iodine (Betadine).
4. Draw maternal blood sample for comparison with postprocedure blood sample to determine maternal bleeding.
5. Provide emotional support, explain procedure, stay with the client (do not leave her alone).
6. Label samples; if bilirubin test is prescribed, darken room and immediately cover the tubes with aluminum foil or use opaque tubes.
7. After specimen is drawn, wash abdomen; assist woman to empty bladder. A full bladder can irritate the uterus and cause contractions.
8. Monitor FHR for 1 hour after procedure, and assess for uterine contractions and irritability.
9. Instruct woman to report any contractions, change in fetal movement, or fluid leaking from vagina.

F. Complications
1. Spontaneous abortion (1%)
2. Fetal injury
3. Infection

> **HESI Hint** • When an amniocentesis is done in early pregnancy, the bladder must be full to help support the uterus and to help push the uterus up in the abdomen for easy access. When an amniocentesis is performed in late pregnancy, the bladder must be empty so it will not be punctured.

Electronic Fetal Monitoring

Variables Measured by Fetal Monitoring

A. Contractions
1. Beginning, peak (acme), and end of each contraction
2. Duration: length of each contraction from beginning to end
3. Frequency: beginning of one contraction to beginning of the next (three to five contractions must be measured)
4. Intensity: measured not by external monitoring but in mm Hg by internal (intrauterine) monitoring after amniotic membranes have ruptured; ranges from 30 mm Hg (mild) to 70 mm Hg (strong) at peak

B. Baseline FHR
1. The range of FHR (average 110 to 160 bpm) between contractions, monitored over a 10-minute period
2. The balance between parasympathetic and sympathetic impulses usually produces no observable changes in the FHR during uterine contractions (with a healthy fetus, a healthy placenta, and good uteroplacental perfusion; Fig. 6-4).

Nursing Actions Based on Fetal Heart Rate

A. Baseline FHR
1. Normal rhythmicity
2. Average FHR 110 to 160 bpm
3. Description
   a. The FHR results from the balance between the parasympathetic and the sympathetic branches of the autonomic nervous system.
   b. It is the most important indicator of the health of the fetal central nervous system (CNS).

B. Variability
1. A characteristic of the baseline FHR and described as normal irregularity of the cardiac rhythm.
2. There are four categories of variability:
   a. Absent: amplitude range undetectable
   b. Minimal: amplitude range detectable up to and including 5 beats/min
   c. Moderate: amplitude range of 6 to 25 beats/min
   d. Marked: amplitude range >25 beats/min

C. Nursing actions
1. Assess contractions using monitor strip.
2. Assess FHR for normal baseline range and variability.

D. Periodic changes
1. FHR changes in relation to uterine contractions (Fig. 6-5).
2. Description:
   a. Accelerations
      (1) Caused by sympathetic fetal response
      (2) Occur in response to fetal movement
      (3) Indicative of a reactive, healthy fetus
   b. Early decelerations (Fig. 6-6)
      (1) Benign pattern caused by parasympathetic response (head compression)
      (2) Heart rate slowly and smoothly decelerates at beginning of contraction and returns to baseline at end of contraction

E. Nursing actions for early decelerations
1. No nursing interventions are required except to monitor the progress of labor.
2. Document the processes of labor.

Nonreassuring Warning Signs

A. Variability (Fig. 6-7)
1. FHR is absent or minimal.

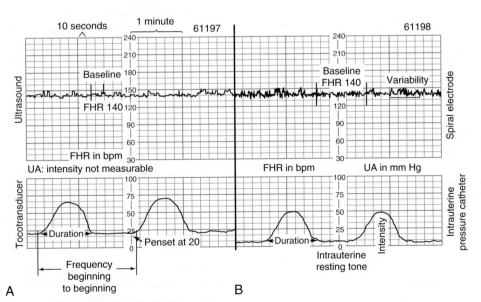

FIGURE 6-4 Display of fetal heart rate and uterine activity on chart paper. **A,** External mode with ultrasound and tocotransducer as signal course. **B,** Internal mode with spiral electrode and intrauterine catheter as signal source. Frequency of contractions is measured from the beginning of one contraction to the beginning of the next. Peak-to-peak measurement is sometimes used when electronic uterine activity monitoring is done. (From Miller L, Tucker SM: *Pocket guide to fetal monitoring and assessment,* ed 7, St. Louis, 2013, Mosby.)

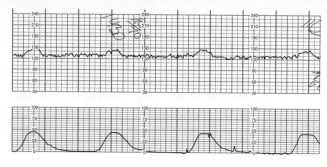

FIGURE 6-5 Periodic accelerations with uterine contractions. (From Miller L, Tucker SM: *Pocket guide to fetal monitoring and assessment*, ed 7, St. Louis, 2013, Mosby.)

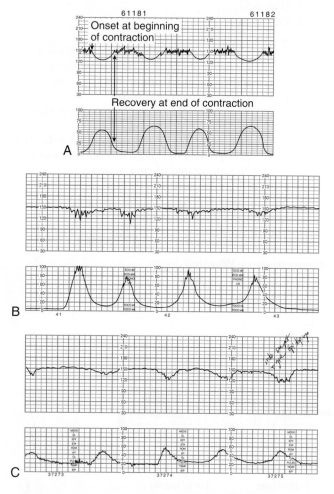

FIGURE 6-6 A, Early deceleration (illustration, with key points identified). **B** and **C,** Early decelerations (actual tracings). (From Miller L, Tucker SM: *Pocket guide to fetal monitoring and assessment*, ed 7, St. Louis, 2013, Mosby.)

2. Causes:
   a. Hypoxia (asphyxia)
   b. Acidosis
   c. Maternal drug ingestion (narcotics, CNS depressants such as magnesium sulfate)
   d. Fetal sleep

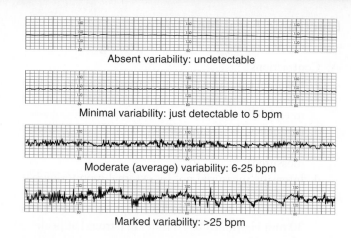

FIGURE 6-7 Classification of variability. (From Miller L, Tucker SM: *Pocket guide to fetal monitoring and assessment*, ed 7, St. Louis, 2013, Mosby.)

B. Bradycardia
   1. Baseline FHR is below 110 bpm (assessed between contractions) for 10 minutes (as differentiated from a periodic change).
   2. Causes:
      a. Late manifestation of fetal hypoxia
      b. Medication-induced (narcotics, $MgSO_4$)
      c. Maternal hypotension
      d. Fetal heart block
      e. Prolonged umbilical cord compression
C. Tachycardia
   1. Baseline FHR is above 160 bpm (assessed between contractions) for 10 minutes
   2. Causes:
      a. Early sign of fetal hypoxia
      b. Fetal anemia
      c. Dehydration
      d. Maternal infection, maternal fever
      e. Maternal hyperthyroid disease
      f. Medication-induced (atropine, terbutaline, hydroxyzine)
D. Nursing actions for decreased variability, bradycardia, and tachycardia:
   1. Treatment is based on cause.
E. Variable deceleration pattern (Fig. 6-8)
   1. It is the most common periodic pattern.
   2. It occurs in 40% of all labors and is caused mainly by cord compression, but can also indicate rapid fetal descent. It is characterized by an abrupt transitory decrease in the FHR that is variable in duration, depth of fall, and timing relative to the contraction cycle.
   3. An occasional variable is usually benign.
F. Nursing actions for variable decelerations:
   1. Change maternal position.
   2. Stimulate fetus if indicated.
   3. Discontinue oxytocin (Pitocin) if infusing.
   4. Administer oxygen at 10 L by tight facemask.

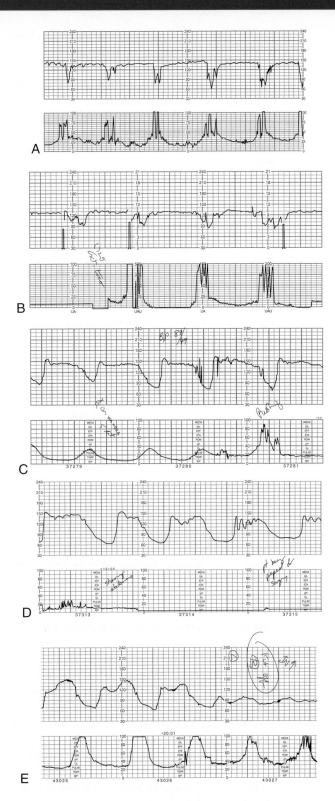

FIGURE 6-8 Variable decelerations. Note the progression in severity from panel **A** to panel **E**, with overshoots and decreasing variability and eventually a prolonged and smooth deceleration (actual tracings). (From Miller L, Tucker SM: *Pocket guide to fetal monitoring and assessment*, ed 7, St. Louis, 2013, Mosby.)

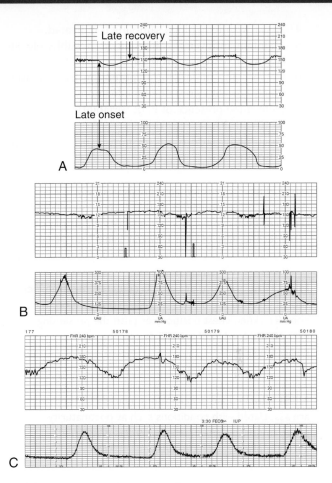

FIGURE 6-9 A, Late decelerations (illustration, with key points identified). **B** and **C,** Late decelerations (actual tracings). (From Miller L, Tucker SM: *Pocket guide to fetal monitoring and assessment*, ed 7, St. Louis, 2013, Mosby.)

    5. Perform a vaginal examination to check for cord prolapse.
    6. Report findings to physician and document.

Nonreassuring (Ominous) Signs

A. Severe variable decelerations
    1. FHR below 70 bpm lasting longer than 30 to 60 seconds
    2. Slow return to baseline
    3. Decreasing or absent variability
B. Late decelerations (Fig. 6-9)
    1. An ominous and potentially disastrous nonreassuring sign
    2. Indicative of uteroplacental insufficiency (UPI)
    3. The shape of the deceleration is uniform, and the FHR returns to baseline after the contraction is over.
    4. The depth of the deceleration does not indicate severity; rarely falls below 100 bpm.
C. Nursing actions
    1. Immediately turn client onto left side.
    2. Discontinue oxytocin (Pitocin) if infusing.
    3. Administer oxygen at 10 L by tight facemask.

4. Assist with fetal blood sampling if indicated.
5. Maintain intravenous line, and if possible, elevate legs to increase venous return.
6. Correct any underlying hypotension by increasing IV rate or with prescribed medications.
7. Determine presence of FHR variability.
8. Notify health care provider.
9. Document pattern and response to each nursing action.

HESI Hint • Check for labor progress if early decelerations are noted (Fig. 6-10A). Early decelerations caused by head compression and fetal descent usually occur in the second stage of labor between 4 and 7 cm dilation.

HESI Hint • If cord prolapse is detected, the examiner should position the mother to relieve pressure on the cord (i.e., knee-chest position) or push the presenting part off the cord until immediate cesarean delivery can be accomplished.

HESI Hint • Late decelerations indicate UPI and are associated with conditions such as postmaturity, preeclampsia, diabetes mellitus, cardiac disease, and abruptio placentae (Fig. 6-10B).

HESI Hint • The situation is ominous (potentially dangerous) and requires immediate intervention and fetal assessment when deceleration patterns (late or variable) are associated with decreased or absent variability and tachycardia.

HESI Hint • A decrease in uteroplacental perfusion results in late decelerations; cord compression results in a pattern of variable decelerations (Fig. 6-10C). Nursing interventions should include changing maternal position, discontinuing oxytocin (Pitocin) infusion, administering oxygen, and notifying the health care provider.

Additional Antepartum Tests

A. Nonstress test
   1. Description
      a. It is used to determine fetal well-being in high-risk pregnancy and is especially useful in postmaturity (notes response of the fetus to its own movements).
      b. A healthy fetus will usually respond to its own movement by means of an FHR acceleration of 15 beats, lasting for at least 15 seconds after the movement, twice in a 20-minute period.

c. The fetus that responds with the 15/15 acceleration is considered "reactive" and healthy.
   2. Nursing care
      a. Apply fetal monitor, ultrasound, and tocodynamometer to maternal abdomen.
      b. Give mother handheld event marker, and instruct her to push the button whenever fetal movement is felt or recorded as fetal movement on the FHR strip.
      c. Monitor client for 20 to 30 minutes, observing for reactivity.
      d. Suspect fetus is sleeping if there is no fetal movement. Stimulate fetus acoustically or physically or have mother move fetus around and begin test again.
B. Contraction stress test (CST) or oxytocin challenge test (OCT)
   1. Description
      a. The fetus is challenged with the stress of labor by the induction of uterine contractions, and the fetal response to physiologically decreased oxygen supply during uterine contractions is noted.
      b. An unhealthy fetus will develop nonreassuring FHR patterns in response to uterine contractions; late decelerations are indicative of UPI.
      c. Contractions can be induced by nipple stimulation or by infusing a dilute solution of oxytocin.
   2. Nursing care
      a. Assess for contraindications: prematurity, placenta previa, hydramnios, multiple gestation, previous uterine classical scar, rupture of membranes (ROM).
      b. Place external monitors on abdomen (FHR ultrasound monitor and tocodynamometer).
      c. Record a 20-minute baseline strip to determine fetal well-being (reactivity) and presence or absence of contractions.
      d. To assess for fetal well-being, a recording of at least three contractions in 10 minutes must be obtained.
      e. If nipple stimulation is attempted, have woman apply warm, wet washcloths to nipples and roll the nipple of one breast for 10 minutes. Begin rolling both nipples if contractions do not begin in 10 minutes. Proceed with oxytocin infusion if unsuccessful with nipple stimulation.
      f. Exogenous oxytocin can be used to stimulate uterine contractions.
      g. A negative test suggests fetal well-being (i.e., no occurrence of late decelerations).

HESI Hint • With nipple stimulation there is no control of the "dose" of oxytocin delivered by the posterior pituitary. The chance of hyperstimulation or tetany (contractions lasting over 90 seconds or contractions with less than 30 seconds in between) is increased.

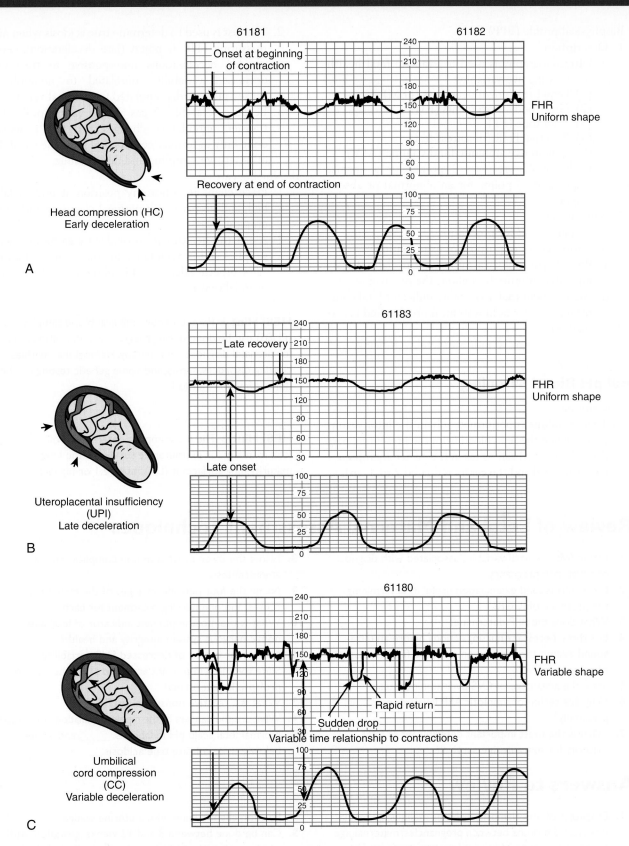

FIGURE 6-10 Review of fetal variability. **A,** Early decelerations caused by head compression. **B,** Late decelerations caused by uteroplacental insufficiency. **C,** Variable decelerations caused by cord compression. (From Miller L, Tucker SM: *Pocket guide to fetal monitoring and assessment,* ed 7, St. Louis, 2013, Mosby.)

C. Biophysical profile (BPP)
1. Description
   a. Ultrasonography is used to evaluate fetal health by assessing five variables:
      (1) Fetal breathing movements (FBM)
      (2) Gross body movements (FM)
      (3) Fetal tone (FT)
      (4) Reactive FHR (nonstress test)
      (5) Qualitative amniotic fluid volume (AFV)
   b. Each variable receives 2 points for a normal response or 0 points for an abnormal or absent response.
2. Nursing care
   a. Prepare client for procedure.
   b. Inform client of purpose of examination.
   c. Provide psychological support, especially if testing will continue throughout the pregnancy.
   d. Advise client that a low score indicates fetal compromise that would warrant more detailed investigation.
   e. A score of 8 to 10 indicates fetal well-being.

Fetal pH Blood Sampling

A. Description
1. This technique is performed only in the intrapartum period when the fetal blood from the presenting part (breech or scalp) can be taken (i.e., when membranes have ruptured and the cervix is dilated 2 to 3 cm).

2. The test is used to determine true acidosis when non-reassuring FHR is noted (late decelerations, severe variable decelerations unresponsive to treatment, decreased variability unrelated to nonasphyxial causes, tachycardia unrelated to maternal variables).
3. Because fetal blood gas values vary rapidly with transient circulatory changes, this test is usually done only in tertiary centers that have the capability of repetitive sampling and rapid results.

B. Nursing care
1. Place client in lithotomy position at end of labor bed, and prepare with perineal cleansing and sterile draping.
2. Assist the health care provider by gathering sterile supplies and providing ice in cup or emesis basin to carry pipette filled with blood to unit's pH machine or to laboratory.

> **HESI Hint** • Percutaneous umbilical blood sampling (PUBS) can be done during pregnancy under ultrasound for prenatal diagnosis and therapy. Hemoglobinopathies, clotting disorders, sepsis, and some genetic testing can be done using this method.

> **HESI Hint** • The most import determinant of fetal maturity for extrauterine survival is the lung maturity:lung surfactant (L/S) ratio (2:1 or higher).

Review of Fetal and Maternal Assessment Techniques

1. Name five maternal variables associated with diagnosis of a high-risk pregnancy.
2. Is one ultrasound examination useful in determining the presence of IUGR?
3. What does the BPP determine?
4. List three necessary nursing actions before an ultrasound examination for a woman in the first trimester of pregnancy.
5. State the advantage of CVS over amniocentesis.
6. Why are serum or amniotic AFP levels done prenatally?
7. What is the most important determinant of fetal maturity for extrauterine survival?
8. Name the three most common complications of amniocentesis.
9. Name the four periodic changes of the FHR, their causes, and one nursing treatment for each.
10. What is the most important indicator of fetal autonomic nervous system integrity and health?
11. Name four causes of decreased FHR variability.
12. State the most important action to take when a cord prolapse is determined.
13. What is a reactive nonstress test?
14. What are the dangers of the nipple-stimulation stress test?
15. Normal fetal scalp pH in labor is _____, and values below _____ indicate true acidosis.

Answers to Review

1. Diagnosis of preeclampsia, diabetes mellitus, or cardiac disease; <3 months between pregnancies; maternal age (under 17 or over 34 years of age); parity (over 5)
2. No. Serial measurements are needed to determine IUGR.
3. Fetal well-being
4. Have client fill bladder. Do not allow client to void.

Position client supine with a uterine wedge.
5. Can be done between 8 and 12 weeks' gestation, with results returned within 1 week, which allows for decision about termination while still in first trimester.
6. To determine AFP levels: elevated AFP may indicate the presence of neural tube defects; or low AFP levels may indicate trisomy 21.

7. L/S ratio (lung maturity, lung surfactant development)

8. Spontaneous abortion, fetal injury, infection

9. Accelerations are reassuring and require no treatment because they are caused by a burst of sympathetic activity. Early decelerations are caused by head compression; they are benign and alert the nurse to monitor for labor progress and fetal descent. Variable decelerations are caused by cord compression; change of position should be tried first. Late decelerations are caused by UPI and should be treated by placing client on her side and administering oxygen.

10. FHR variability

11. Hypoxia, acidosis, drugs, fetal sleep

12. Examiner should position mother to relieve pressure on the cord or push the presenting part off the cord with fingers until emergency delivery is accomplished.

13. FHR acceleration of 15 bpm for 15 seconds in response to fetal movement

14. The inability to control oxytocin "dosage" and the chance of tetany/hyperstimulation

15. 7.25 to 7.35; 7.2

Intrapartum Nursing Care

Description: Begins with true labor and consists of four stages

A. First stage of labor: From the beginning of regular contractions or ROM to 10 cm of dilatation and 100% effacement (Table 6-1)

B. Second stage of labor: 10 cm to delivery of the fetus

C. Third stage of labor: Delivery of the fetus to delivery of the placenta

D. Fourth stage of labor: Arbitrarily lasts about 2 hours after delivery of the placenta (recovery)

Initial Examination

> **HESI Hint** • Be able to differentiate true labor from false labor.
>
> ***True Labor***
> - Pain in lower back that radiates to abdomen
> - Pain accompanied by regular rhythmic contractions
> - Contractions that intensify with ambulation
> - Progressive cervical dilatation and effacement
>
> ***False Labor***
> - Discomfort localized in abdomen
> - No lower back pain
> - Contractions decrease in intensity or frequency with ambulation

Nursing Assessment

A. Prodromal labor signs include the following:
   1. Lightening (fetus drops into true pelvis)
   2. Braxton Hicks contractions (practice contractions)
   3. Cervical softening and slight effacement
   4. Bloody show or expulsion of mucous plug
   5. Burst of energy, "nesting instinct"

B. Determine the following:
   1. Gravidity and parity >5 (grand multiparity)
   2. Gestational age 38 to 40 weeks (term gestation)
   3. FHR best heard over fetal back (Fig. 6-11 and Box 6-1)
   4. Maternal vital signs
   5. Contraction frequency, intensity, and duration

C. Perform vaginal examination to determine:
   1. Fetal presentation and position
   2. Cervical dilatation, effacement, position, and consistency
   3. Fetal station

D. Assess the client for:
   1. Status of membranes (ruptured or intact)
   2. Urine glucose and albumin data
   3. Comfort level
   4. Labor and delivery preparation
   5. Presence of support person
   6. Presence of true or false labor

Vaginal Examination

A. It is preceded by antiseptic cleansing with client in modified lithotomy position.
   1. Sterile gloves are worn.
   2. Examinations are not done routinely. They are sharply curtailed after membranes rupture so as to prevent infection.
   3. Examinations are performed:
      a. Before analgesia and anesthesia
      b. To determine the progress of labor
      c. To determine whether second-stage pushing can begin

B. The purpose of a vaginal examination is to determine:
   1. Cervical dilation: Cervix opens from 0 to 10 cm.
   2. Cervical effacement: Cervix is taken up into the upper uterine segment; expressed in percentages from 0% to 100%. Cervix is "shortened" from 3 cm to <0.5 cm in length; often called *thinning of the cervix,* which is a misnomer.
   3. Cervical position: Cervix can be directly anterior and palpated easily or posterior and difficult to palpate.
   4. Cervical consistency: It is firm to soft.

C. Fetal station: Location of presenting part in relation to midpelvis or ischial spines; expressed as cm above or below the spines (Fig. 6-12).
   1. Station 0 is engaged.
   2. Station −2 is 2 cm above the ischial spines.

TABLE 6-1 First Stage of Labor

Phase	Description	Psychological and Physical Responses
Latent	From beginning of true labor until 3-4 cm cervical dilatation	• Mildly anxious, conversant • Able to continue usual activities • Contractions mild, initially 10-20 min apart, 15-20 sec duration; later 5-7 min apart, 30-40 sec duration
Active	From 4-7 cm cervical dilatation	• Increased anxiety • Increased discomfort • Unwillingness to be left alone • Contractions moderate to severe, 2-3 min apart, 30-60 sec duration

Transition	From 8-10 cm cervical dilatation	• Changed behavior:
		  • Sudden nausea, hiccups
		  • Extreme irritability and unwillingness to be touched, although desirous of companionship
		  • Contractions severe, 1½ min apart, 60-90 sec duration

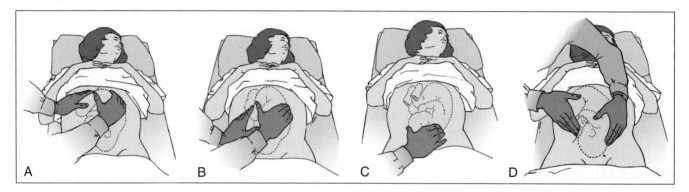

FIGURE 6-11 Leopold maneuvers. (From Lowdermilk DL, Perry SE: *Maternity nursing,* ed 9, St. Louis, 2010, Mosby.)

BOX 6-1 *Leopold Maneuvers*

Description: Abdominal palpations used to determine fetal presentation, lie, position, and engagement

A. With client in supine position, place both cupped hands over fundus and palpate to determine whether breech (soft, immovable, large) or vertex (hard, movable, small).

B. Place one hand firmly on side and palpate with other hand to determine presence of small parts or fetal back. (FHR is heard best through fetal back.)

C. Facing client, grasp the area over the symphysis with the thumb and fingers and press to determine the degree of descent of the presenting part. (A ballotable or floating head can be rocked back and forth between the thumb and fingers.)

D. Facing the client's feet, outline the fetal presenting part with the palmar surface of both hands to determine the degree of descent and attitude of the fetus. (If cephalic prominence is located on the same side as small parts, assume the head is flexed.)

D. Fetal presentation: The part of the fetus that presents to the inlet (Fig. 6-13):
　1. Vertex (head, cephalic)
　2. Shoulder (acromion)
　3. Breech (buttocks)
　4. Other variations include brow (sinciput) and chin (mentum)

E. Fetal position: The relationship of the point of reference (occiput, sacrum, acromion) on the fetal presenting part (vertex, breech, shoulder) to the mother's pelvis. Most common is LOA (left occiput anterior). The point of reference on the vertex (oc-

ciput) is pointed up toward the symphysis and directed toward the left side of the maternal pelvis (Fig. 6-14).

F. Fetal lie: The relationship of the long axis (spine) of the fetus to the long axis (spine) of the mother. It can be longitudinal (up and down), transverse (perpendicular), or oblique (slanted; see Fig. 6-13).

G. Fetal attitude
　1. Relationship of the fetal parts to one another
　2. Flexion or extension
　3. Flexion is desirable so that the smallest diameters of the presenting part move through the pelvis.

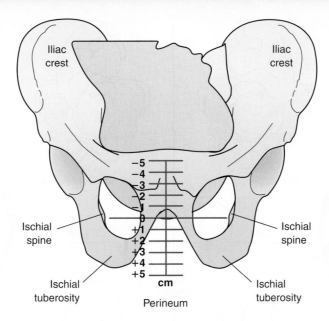

FIGURE 6-12 Fetal stations. Stations of presenting part, or degree of descent. The lowermost portion of the presenting part is at the level of the ischial spines, station 0. (From Lowdermilk DL, Perry SE: *Maternity nursing,* ed 9, St. Louis, 2010, Mosby.)

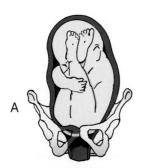

Frank breech

Lie: Longitudinal or vertical
Presentation: Breech (incomplete)
Presenting part: Sacrum
Attitude: Flexion, except for legs at knees

A

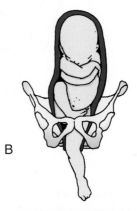

Single footling breech

Lie: Longitudinal or vertical
Presentation: Breech (incomplete)
Presenting part: Sacrum
Attitude: Flexion, except for one leg extended at hip and knee

B

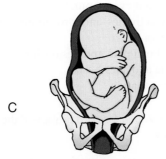

Complete breech

Lie: Longitudinal or vertical
Presentation: Breech (sacrum and feet presenting)
Presenting part: Sacrum (with feet)
Attitude: General flexion

C

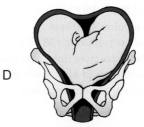

Shoulder presentation

Lie: Transverse or horizontal
Presentation: Shoulder
Presenting part: Scapula
Attitude: Flexion

D

FIGURE 6-13 Fetal presentations. **A, B, C,** Breech (sacral) presentation. **D,** Shoulder presentation. (From Lowdermilk DL, Perry SE: *Maternity nursing,* ed 9, St. Louis, 2010, Mosby.)

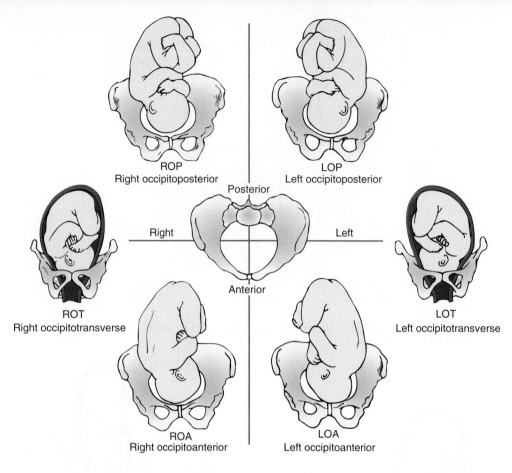

Lie: Longitudinal or vertical
Presentation: Vertex
Reference point: Occiput
Attitude: General flexion

FIGURE 6-14 Fetal positions. Examples of fetal vertex (occiput) presentations in relation to front, back, or side of maternal pelvis. (From Lowdermilk DL, Perry SE: *Maternity nursing,* ed 9, St. Louis, 2010, Mosby.)

Analysis (Nursing Diagnoses)

A. *Deficient knowledge (labor/delivery)* related to …
B. *Acute pain* related to …
C. *Anxiety* related to …

> **HESI Hint** • It is important to know the normal findings for a client in labor:
> - Normal FHR in labor: 110 to 160 bpm
> - Normal maternal BP: <140/90
> - Normal maternal pulse: <100 bpm
> - Normal maternal temperature: <38.0° C
> - Slight elevation in temperature may occur because of dehydration and the work of labor. Anything higher indicates infection and must be reported immediately.

Nursing Plans and Interventions

A. Determine FHR (auscultation schedule).
  1. FHR every 30 minutes in early latent stage
  2. FHR every 15 to 30 minutes in midactive stage
  3. FHR every 15 minutes in transition stage
B. Assess maternal vital signs.
  1. Take BP *between* contractions, in side-lying position, at least every hour unless abnormal (BP increases during contractions).
  2. Take temperature every 4 hours until membranes rupture, then every hour.
C. Explain all activities and procedures to mother and support person.
D. Determine birth plan and desires for:
  1. Analgesia and anesthesia
  2. Delivery situation

> **HESI Hint** • Watch for cord prolapse if the infant's head is floating.

E. Assess urine every 8 hours unless abnormal. Normal findings:
  1. Protein (< trace)
  2. Glucose (1+ or less)

F. Assess contractions when assessing FHR.
 1. *Frequency.* Time contractions from beginning of one contraction to the beginning of the next (measured in minutes apart).
 2. *Duration.* Time the length of the entire contraction (from beginning to end).
 3. *Strength.* Assess the intensity of strongest part (peak) of contraction. It is measured by clinical estimation of the indentability of the fundus (use gentle pressure of fingertips to determine it):
  a. Very indentable (mild)
  b. Moderately indentable (moderate)
  c. Unindentable (firm)
 4. *Norms.* Contraction frequency, duration, and intensity vary with the stage of labor.
G. If membranes or bag of waters (BOW) has ruptured:
 1. Nitrazine paper turns black or dark blue.
 2. Vaginal fluid ferns under microscope.
 3. Color and amount of amniotic fluid should be noted.
 4. Woman should be allowed to ambulate during labor only if the FHR is within a normal range and if the fetus is engaged (zero station). If the fetus is not engaged, there is an increased risk that a prolapsed cord will occur.
H. Begin graph of labor progress (Friedman graph; Fig. 6-15).
 1. Prolonged latent phase lasts >20 hours in primigravida, >14 hours in multipara.
 2. A primigravida dilates an average of 1.2 cm/hr in the midactive phase; a multipara, 1.5 cm/hr.

HESI Hint • Meconium-stained fluid is yellow-green or gold-yellow and may indicate fetal stress.

I. Take client to bathroom or offer bedpan at least every 2 hours during labor (a full bladder can impede labor progress).
J. Assist woman with use of psychoprophylactic coping techniques, such as breathing exercises and effleurage (abdominal massage).

HESI Hint • Breathing techniques, such as deep chest, accelerated, and cued, are not prescribed by the stage and phase of labor but by the discomfort level of the laboring woman. If coping is decreasing, switch to a new technique.

K. Provide mouth care, ice chips, and hard candy as needed for dry mouth.

HESI Hint • Hyperventilation results in respiratory alkalosis that is caused by blowing off too much CO_2.
 Symptoms include:
 • Dizziness
 • Tingling of fingers
 • Stiff mouth
 Have woman breathe into her cupped hands or a paper bag in order to rebreathe CO_2.

L. Maintain asepsis in labor by means of frequent perineal care and by changing linen and underpads.
M. Allow sips of clear fluid if no general anesthesia is anticipated.
N. Offer anesthesia or analgesia in midactive phase of labor.
 1. If given too early, they may retard the progress of labor.
 2. If given too late, narcotics increase the risk of neonatal respiratory depression.
O. Monitor fetus continuously if any high-risk situation occurs.
P. Notify health care provider if any of the following occurs:
 1. Labor progress is retarded.
 2. Maternal vital signs are abnormal.
 3. Fetal distress noted.

Second Stage of Labor

Description: Heralded by the involuntary need to push, 10 centimeters of cervical dilatation, rapid fetal descent, and birth
A. The second stage of labor averages 1 hour for a primigravida, 15 minutes for a multipara.
B. The addition of abdominal force to the uterine contraction force enhances the cardinal movements of the fetus: engagement, descent, flexion, internal rotation, extension, restitution, and external rotation (Fig. 6-16).

Nursing Assessment

A. Assess BP and pulse every 5 to 15 minutes.
B. Determine FHR with every contraction.
C. Observe perineal area for the following:
 1. Increase in bloody show
 2. Bulging perineum and anus
 3. Visibility of the presenting part
D. Palpate bladder for distention.
E. Assess amniotic fluid for color and consistency.

Analysis (Nursing Diagnoses)

A. *Acute pain* related to …
B. *Risk for injury* related to …
C. *Deficient knowledge* (specify) related to …

Nursing Plans and Interventions

A. Document maternal BP and pulse every 15 minutes between contractions.
B. Check FHR with each contraction or by continuous fetal monitoring.
C. Continue comfort measures: mouth care, linen change, positioning.
D. Decrease outside distractions.
E. Teach mother positions such as squatting, side-lying, or high-Fowler/lithotomy for pushing.

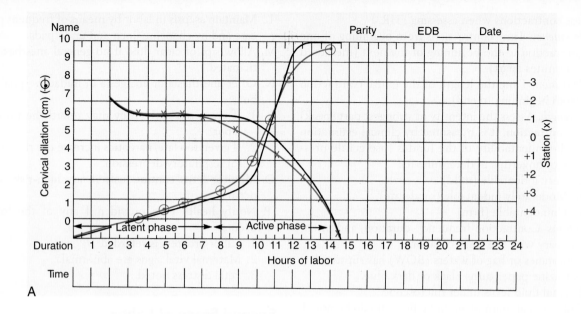

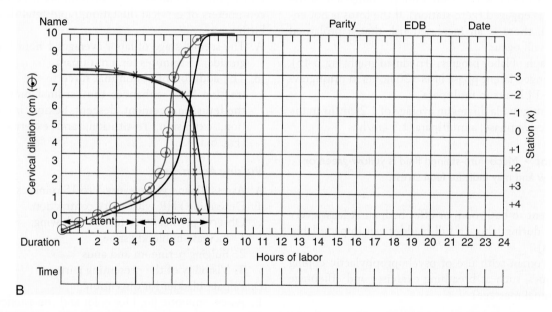

FIGURE 6-15 Labor graph. Partogram for assessment of patterns of cervical dilatation and descent. Individual woman's labor patterns *(colored)* are superimposed on labor graph *(black)* for comparison. **A,** Nulliparous labor. **B,** Multiparous labor. The rate of cervical dilatation is indicated by the symbol O. A line drawn through the symbols depicts the slope of the curve. Station is indicated by an X. A line drawn through the Xs reveals the pattern of descent. (From Lowdermilk DL, Perry SE: *Maternity nursing,* ed 9, St. Louis, 2010, Mosby.)

F. Teach mother to exhale when pushing or use "gentle" pushing technique (pushing down on vagina while constantly exhaling through open mouth, followed by deep breath).

> **HESI Hint** • Determine cervical dilatation before allowing client to push. Cervix should be completely dilated (10 cm) before the client begins pushing. If pushing starts too early, the cervix can become edematous and never fully dilate.

G. If delivering in another room or setting:
1. Transfer multipara at 8 to 9 cm, +2 station.
2. Transfer primigravida at 10 cm, with presenting part visible between contractions *and* during contractions.
H. Set up delivery table, including bulb syringe, cord clamp, and sterile supplies.
I. Perform perineal cleansing.
J. At crowning, put gentle counterpressure against the perineum. Do not allow rapid delivery over woman's perineum.
K. Make sure client and support person can visualize delivery if they so desire. If siblings are present, make sure

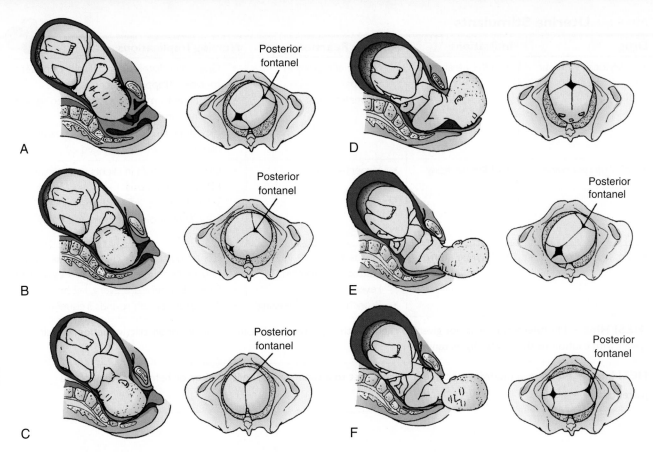

FIGURE 6-16 Cardinal movements of the mechanism of labor. Left occipitoanterior (LOA) position. Pelvic figures show the position of the fetal head as seen by the birth attendant. **A,** Engagement and descent. **B,** Flexion. **C,** Internal rotation to occipitoanterior position (OA). **D,** Extension. **E,** External rotation beginning (restitution). **F,** External rotation. (From Lowdermilk D, Perry S, Cashion M, Alden K: *Maternity and women's health care,* ed 10. St. Louis, 2012, Mosby.)

they are closely attended to by support person explaining that their mom is all right.

L. Record *exact* delivery time (complete delivery of baby).

Third Stage of Labor

Description: From complete expulsion of the baby to complete expulsion of the placenta

A. Average length of third stage of labor is 5 to 15 minutes.

B. The longer the third stage of labor, the greater the chance for uterine atony or hemorrhage to occur.

Nursing Assessment

A. Signs of placental separation:
   1. Lengthening of umbilical cord outside vagina
   2. Gush of blood
   3. Uterus changes from oval (discoid) to globular.

B. Mother describes a "full" feeling in vagina.

C. Firm uterine contractions continue.

Analysis (Nursing Diagnoses)

A. *Risk for deficient fluid volume* related to …

B. *Anxiety* related to …

Nursing Plans and Interventions

> **HESI Hint •** Give the oxytocin (Pitocin) after the placenta is delivered because the drug will cause the uterus to contract. If the oxytocic drug is administered before the placenta is delivered, it may result in a retained placenta, which predisposes the client to hemorrhage and infection.

A. Place hand under drape and palpate fundus of uterus for firmness and placement at or below the umbilicus. At signs of placental separation, instruct mother to push gently.

B. Take maternal BP before and after placental separation.

C. Check patency and site integrity of infusing IV.

D. Administer oxytocic medication immediately after delivery of the placenta (Table 6-2).

E. Observe for blood loss and ask physician for estimate of blood loss (EBL).

F. Dry and suction infant, perform Apgar assessment, place blanket on mother's abdomen or allow skin-to-skin contact with mother after delivery.

G. Place stockinette cap on newborn's head or cover head to prevent heat loss.

TABLE 6-2 Uterine Stimulants

Drug	Indications	Adverse Reactions	Nursing Implications
• Oxytocin, synthetic	• Uterine atony	• Severe afterpains in multipara • Hypertension	• Give immediately after delivery of placenta to avoid "trapped" placenta. • Continue to monitor vaginal bleeding and uterine tone. • May stimulate let-down milk reflex and flow of milk when engorged
• Methylergonovine maleate	• Uterine atony	• Hypertension	• Use with caution in clients with elevated BP or preeclampsia. • Take BP before administration and if 140/90 or above, withhold and notify physician.
• Prostaglandin F_2	• Uterine atony	• Headache • Nausea and vomiting • Fever • Bronchospasm, wheezing	• Contraindicated for clients with asthma. • May be given intramyometrially by provider. • Check temperature every 1-2 hr. • Auscultate breath sounds frequently.

HESI Hint • Methylergonovine is not given to clients with hypertension because of its vasoconstrictive action. Pitocin is given with caution to those with hypertension.

HESI Hint • Never give methylergonovine or carboprost to a client while she is in labor or before delivery of the placenta.

H. Allow father or other support person to hold infant during repair of episiotomy.
I. Allow any siblings present to hold new family member.
J. Gently cleanse vulva and apply sterile perineal pad.

HESI Hint • *Application of Perineal Pads after Delivery*
• Place two on perineum.
• Do not touch inside of pad.
• Do apply from front to back, being careful not to drag pad across the anus.

K. Remove both legs simultaneously if legs are in stirrups.
L. Provide clean gown and warm blanket.
M. Lock bed before moving mother, and raise side rails during transfer.

Fourth Stage of Labor

Description: The fourth stage of labor is the first 1 to 4 hours after delivery of placenta.

Nursing Assessment

A. Review antepartum and labor and delivery records for possible complications.
   1. Postpartum hemorrhage
   2. Uterine hyperstimulation
   3. Uterine overdistention
   4. Dystocia
   5. Antepartum hemorrhage
   6. Magnesium sulfate therapy
   7. Bladder distention
B. Routine postpartum physical assessment
C. Mother–infant bonding

Analysis (Nursing Diagnoses)

A. *Risk for deficient fluid volume* related to …
B. *Risk for injury* related to …
C. *Risk for impaired parenting* related to …

Nursing Plans and Interventions

A. Maintain bed rest for at least 2 hours to prevent orthostatic hypotension.
B. Assess BP, pulse, and respirations every 15 minutes for 1 hour, then every 30 minutes until stable (BP <140/90, pulse <100, and respiration <24).
C. Assess temperature at beginning of fourth stage and before discharge to postpartum room. If >38° C, report it to physician and monitor hourly.
D. Assess fundal firmness and height, bladder, lochia, and perineum every 15 minutes for 1 hour, then every 30 minutes for 2 hours.
   1. Fundus: firm, midline, at or below the umbilicus. Massage if soft or boggy. Suspect full bladder if above umbilicus and to the right side of abdomen.

HESI Hint • Full bladder is one of the most common reasons for uterine atony or hemorrhage in the first 24 hours after delivery. If the nurse finds the fundus soft, boggy, and displaced above and to the right of the umbilicus, what action should be taken first? First, perform fundal massage; then have the client empty her bladder. Recheck fundus every 15 minutes for 1 hour, then every 30 minutes for 2 hours.

2. Lochia: rubra (red), moderate, and clots <2 cm to 3 cm. Suspect undetected laceration if fundus is firm and bright-red blood continues to trickle. Always check perineal pad *and* under buttocks.
3. Perineum: intact, clean, and slightly edematous. Suspect hematomas if very tender or discolored or if pain is disproportionate to vaginal delivery.

E. Report to health care provider:
1. Abnormal vital signs
2. Uterus not becoming firm with massage
3. Second perineal pad soaked in 15 minutes
4. Signs of hypovolemic shock: pale, clammy, tachycardic, lightheaded, hypotensive

F. Monitor infusion of intravenous oxytocin (Pitocin). (Check health care provider's prescription and hospital policy.)

G. Change perineal pads and cleanse vulva and perineum with each change.

H. Prevent the discomfort of afterpains.
1. Keep bladder empty. Catheterize only if absolutely necessary.
2. Place warm blanket on abdomen.
3. Administer analgesics as prescribed (usually codeine, acetaminophen, or ibuprofen).

HESI Hint • If narcotic analgesics are given, raise side rails and place call light within reach. Instruct client not to get out of bed or ambulate without assistance. Caution client about drowsiness as a side effect.

I. Offer oral fluids when the woman is alert and able to swallow.
J. Apply ice pack to perineum to minimize edema, especially if a third- or fourth-degree episiotomy has been performed or if lacerations are present.
K. Apply witch hazel compresses to perineum for comfort.

HESI Hint • A first-degree tear involves only the epidermis. A second-degree tear involves dermis, muscle, and fascia. A third-degree tear extends into the anal sphincter. A fourth-degree tear extends up the rectal mucosa. Tears cause pain and swelling. Avoid rectal manipulations.

L. Support parental emotional needs and promote bonding.
1. Allow extended time with newborn.
2. Openly share in the joy and excitement of childbirth; also grieve with parents experiencing loss.
3. Encourage initiation of breastfeeding.
4. Provide a warm, darkened environment so newborn will open eyes.
5. Withhold eye prophylaxis for up to 1 hour.
6. Perform newborn admission and routine procedures in room with parents.

Newborn Care (Delivery Room)

Description: Care provided to newborn, usually performed by the nurse

Nursing Assessment

A. Maternal history and labor data indicating potential problems with newborn
B. Apgar scores
C. Findings of brief physical examination performed in delivery room

Analysis (Nursing Diagnoses)

A. *Risk for ineffective airway clearance* related to …
B. *Risk for injury* related to …

Nursing Plans and Interventions

A. Immediately dry infant under warmer or skin to skin with mother; suction mouth and nose with bulb syringe; keep head slightly lower than body; and assess airway status.
1. Assess for five symptoms of respiratory distress.
   a. Retractions
   b. Tachypnea (rate >60)
   c. Dusky color, circumoral cyanosis
   d. Expiratory grunt
   e. Flaring nares
2. Do not hyperextend the newborn neck at any time (may close glottis). Place infant in "sniff" position (neck slightly extended as if sniffing the air) to open airway.

B. Obtain Apgar score at 1 and 5 minutes (Table 6-3).
C. Continue to allow maternal/parent contact if newborn is stable.
D. Keep neonate's head covered.
E. Do quick gestational age assessment (Table 6-4).
1. Sole creases
2. Breast tissue bud
3. Skin, vessels, and peeling
4. Genitalia
5. Resting posture

F. Examine cord for presence of three vessels (two arteries, one vein), and document.
G. Make sure cord blood is collected for analysis and sent to laboratory.
1. Rh
2. Blood type
3. Hct
4. Possible cord blood gases

TABLE 6-3 Apgar Assessment

Performed at exactly 1 and 5 minutes after birth.
Cannot just eyeball; must have hands-on examination. Score:
- → 7-10: Good
- → 4-6: Needs moderate resuscitative efforts
- → 0-3: Severe need for resuscitation

HESI Hint • Do not wait until a 1-minute Apgar is assigned to begin resuscitation of the compromised neonate.

Heart rate	Absent = 0; <100 = 1; ≥100 = 2
Respiratory effort	No cry = 0; weak cry = 1; vigorous cry = 2
Muscle tone	Flaccid = 0; some flexion = 1; total flexion = 2
Reflex irritability	No response to foot tap = 0; slight response to foot tap (grimace) = 1; quick foot removal = 2
Color	Dusky, cyanotic = 0; acrocyanotic = 1; totally pink = 2

HESI Hint • Apgar scores of 6 or lower at 5 minutes require an additional Apgar assessment at 10 minutes.

TABLE 6-4 Gestational Age Assessment

28 Weeks	• No nipple bud • Testes in the inguinal canal or labia majora widely separated, with labia minora prominent, open, and equal in size • Vernix (cheesy coating) over the entire body • Lanugo (fine, downy hair) over the entire body • Full extension of extremities in resting posture
40 Weeks	• Raised nipple with a tissue bud underneath • Descended testes with large rugae (folds) on the scrotum • Labia majora large and covering the minora • Vernix only in the creases • Lanugo perhaps only over the shoulders • Hypertonic flexion of extremities in resting posture

H. Document passage of meconium or urine after delivery.
I. Place two identity bands on neonate and one on mother.
J. Obtain newborn footprints and maternal thumb and fingerprint. Follow institutional policy regarding identification procedures.
K. Perform brief physical examination of newborn.
   1. Check for gross anomalies: spina bifida, hydrocephaly, and cleft lip or palate.
   2. Elicit reflexes: Moro (startle) and rooting (suck).
   3. Examine cord clamp for closure, absence of blood oozing from cord; again check for presence of three vessels.
L. May instill eye prophylaxis in delivery room (Table 6-5).
M. If parents desire an open-eye bonding period, may delay eye prophylaxis for up to 1 hour. The Centers for Disease Control and Prevention (CDC) states that a delay of up to 1 hour is safe.

Labor with Analgesia or Anesthesia

A. Analgesia and anesthesia are usually withheld until the midactive phase of labor.
   1. If given in the early latent phase of the first stage of labor, it may retard the progress of labor.
   2. If given late in transition or in the second stage, it may depress the newborn (some narcotic analgesics).
B. Most drugs used for systematic pain relief and relaxation cause CNS depression, which can slow labor and harm fetus.
C. Regional blocks (epidural, caudal, and subarachnoid) cause a temporary interruption of nerve impulses (especially pain) but also cause vasodilation in area below block, causing pooling of blood and hypotension.

Nursing Assessment

A. Acute pain is experienced during active labor.
B. Birth plan includes use of analgesic and anesthetic agents.
C. Decreased coping and increased anxiety are observed.
D. Assess the client and obtain the following data:
   1. Vital signs and FHR
   2. Labor progress (e.g., cervical dilatation and effacement, fetal position and lie)
   3. Last time and amount of food or fluids ingested
   4. Laboratory values (Hgb, Hct, clotting time)
   5. Hydration status
   6. Signs and symptoms of infection

Analysis (Nursing Diagnoses)

A. *Acute pain* related to …
B. *Ineffective coping* related to …
C. *Risk for injury (mother or fetus)* related to …

Nursing Plans and Interventions

A. Administration of analgesic drugs in labor
   1. Document baseline maternal vital signs and FHR before administration of narcotics or sedatives (Table 6-6).

TABLE 6-5 **Newborn Prophylactic Eye Care**

Drugs	Indications	Adverse Reactions	Nursing Implications
Ointments			
Erythromycin	Prevention of ophthalmia neonatorum and *Chlamydia trachomatis* conjunctivitis	• Most commonly used agents • None known, except puffy eyes resulting from manipulation	• Place a thin line of ointment along the entire lower lid in conjunctival sac. • Use only one tube per baby and *discard*. • Manipulate upper lids to ensure complete eye coverage. • After 1 min, may wipe excess from around eyes.

TABLE 6-6 **Analgesics**

Drugs	Indications	Adverse Reactions	Nursing Implications
• Fentanyl • Morphine sulfate • Hydromorphone	• Narcotic used to produce analgesia, euphoria, and sedation in labor • Analgesia during labor	• Fetal narcosis, distress • Hypotension • Itching • Urinary retention • Respiratory depression	• Record use accurately. • *Do not* administer if respirations <12/min. • Have narcotic antagonist available (Narcan). • Monitor respirations, pulse, BP closely.
• Butorphanol tartrate • Nalbuphine	• Opioid agonist/antagonist • Provision of analgesia in labor • Narcotic analgesic	• Woman with preexisting narcotic dependency will experience withdrawal symptoms immediately (abstinence syndrome).	• Give IV or IM. • Obtain drug history before administration. • Monitor respirations, pulse.
• Naloxone HCl	• Narcotic antagonist used to counteract narcotic effects on mother/fetus	• Decreased respirations rarely occur	• Monitor respirations closely because drug action is shorter than the narcotic (may need to readminister). • Pain returns after administration to mother. • Can be administered to newborn after delivery to counteract narcotic depression

2. Assess phase and stage of labor.
3. Obtain physician's order for medication.
4. Determine client's and family's desires regarding analgesics, and verbally praise informed choice.
5. Do *not* give PO medications. Labor retards gastrointestinal activity and absorption.
6. Administer medications IV when possible, IM if necessary.

HESI Hint • IV administration of analgesics is preferred to IM administration for a client in labor because the onset and peak occur more quickly and the duration of the drug is shorter. It is important to know the following:

IV Administration
- Onset: 5 minutes
- Peak: 30 minutes
- Duration: 1 hour

IM Administration
- Onset: within 30 minutes
- Peak: 1 to 3 hours after injection
- Duration: 4 to 6 hours

---

7. Push IV bolus into line *slowly*, at the beginning of a contraction (i.e., give medication during contraction, when uterine blood vessels are constricted, so less analgesic reaches the fetus).
8. Explain the purpose of the drug to the laboring woman, but do not promise results.

B. After drug administration:
1. Record the woman's response and level of pain relief.
2. Monitor maternal vital signs, FHR, and characteristics of uterine contractions every 15 minutes for 1 hour after administration.
3. Monitor bladder for distention and retention (medication can decrease perception of bladder filling).
4. Decrease environmental stimuli: Darken room, reduce number of visitors, turn off TV.
5. Note on delivery record the time between drug administration and birth of baby.
6. If baby delivers during peak drug absorption time, notify pediatrician or neonatologist for delivery room assistance and possible use of naloxone (Narcan) for neonate (see Table 6-6).

C. General anesthesia is rarely used in today's obstetric units. It might be used in emergency deliveries or when regional block anesthesia is contraindicated or refused.
1. Administer drugs to reduce gastric secretions (e.g., famotidine [Pepcid] or clear [nonparticulate]) antacids to neutralize gastric acid. (The most common cause of maternal death is aspiration of gastric contents into the lung.)

> **HESI Hint** • Tranquilizers (ataractics and phenothiazines), such as promethazine and hydroxyzine, are used in labor as analgesic-potentiating drugs to decrease the amount of narcotic needed and to decrease maternal anxiety.

> **HESI Hint** • Agonist narcotic drugs (morphine) produce narcosis and have a higher risk for causing maternal and fetal respiratory depression. Antagonist drugs (butorphanol, nalbuphine) have less respiratory depression but must be used with caution in a mother with preexisting narcotic dependency because withdrawal symptoms occur immediately.

2. Assist with speedy delivery. (General anesthesia may depress fetus if delivery is not accomplished quickly.)
3. Assess closely for uterine atony; check fundal firmness and uterine contraction. (General anesthesia is associated with postpartum uterine atony.)

Regional Block Anesthesia

A. Local anesthesia:
1. Is used for pain relief during episiotomy and perineal repair
2. Is safe for mother and infant
B. Regional blocks:
1. Used for relief of perineal and uterine pain
2. Usually safe for mother and infant unless severe hypotension occurs
3. Types of regional blocks
   a. Pudendal block: given in second stage to deaden pudendal nerve plexus, thus deadening pain in the perineum and vagina
      (1) Has no effect on pain of uterine contractions
      (2) Is safe for mother and infant
   b. Peridural (epidural, caudal) block: given in first or second stage of labor to block nerve impulses from T10 to S5, thereby deadening pain of contractions
      (1) Used in conjunction with local or pudendal block for delivery; or given to deaden perineum for delivery
      (2) May be given in single dose or continuously through catheter threaded into epidural space
      (3) Is moderately associated with hypotension, which can cause maternal and fetal distress

(4) Epidural block associated with prolonged second stage due to decreased effectiveness of pushing
   c. Intradural (subarachnoid, spinal) block: given in second stage of labor to deaden uterine and perineal pain
      (1) Rapid onset, but highly associated with maternal hypotension, which can cause maternal and fetal distress
      (2) Client must remain flat for 6 to 8 hours after delivery.
C. Contraindications to subarachnoid and peridural blocks:
1. Client's refusal or fear
2. Anticoagulant therapy or presence of bleeding disorder
3. Presence of antepartum hemorrhage causing acute hypovolemia
4. Infection or tumor at injection site
5. Allergy to -caine drugs
6. CNS disorders, previous back surgery, or spinal anatomic abnormality

> **HESI Hint** • Pudendal block and subarachnoid (saddle) block are used only in the second stage of labor. Peridural and epidural blocks may be used during all stages of labor.

Nursing Assessment

A. No contraindications to regional block anesthesia
B. Experiencing severe pain
C. Possible need for cesarean delivery
D. BP before block >100/70 mm Hg
E. Status of maternal-fetal unit

Analysis (Nursing Diagnoses)

A. *Risk for injury (fetus/client)* related to …
B. *Urinary retention* related to …

Nursing Plans and Interventions

A. Ensure that the health care provider has explained the procedures, the risks, the benefits, and the alternatives.
B. Prehydrate client to counteract possible hypotension: 500 to 1000 mL IV fluid (isotonic) are infused over 20 to 30 minutes before initiation of regional block.
C. Place client in a modified Sims position or sitting on side of bed with head flexed.
D. Ask client to describe symptoms after test dose of medication is given.
1. Metallic taste in mouth and ringing in ears denote possible injection of medication into bloodstream.
2. Nausea and vomiting are among the first signs of hypotension.

> **HESI Hint** • The first sign of a block's effectiveness is usually warmth and tingling in the ball of the foot or the big toe.

E. Determine BP every 1 to 2 minutes for 15 minutes after injection of anesthetic drug, and initiate continuous fetal monitoring.

F. Determine BP every 15 minutes during continuous regional block infusion.

G. Assist client to keep bladder empty.

H. Assess level of pain relief using the sharp-dull technique, and record return of pain sensation.

I. Report return of pain sensation, incomplete anesthesia, or uneven anesthesia to anesthesiologist.

J. If hypotension occurs, do the following:
1. Immediately turn client onto left side.
2. Increase IV infusion.
3. Begin O_2 at 10 L/min by facemask.
4. Notify health care provider stat and have ephedrine available at bedside.
5. Assess FHR.

K. Assist client in the pushing technique once complete dilatation has been achieved.

> **HESI Hint** • Stop continuous infusion at end of stage I or during transition to increase effectiveness of pushing.

> **HESI Hint** • *Regional Block Anesthesia and Fetal Presentation*
> - Internal rotation is harder to achieve when the pelvic floor is relaxed by anesthesia; this results in a persistent occiput-posterior position of fetus.
> - Monitor fetal position. Remember, the mother cannot tell you she has back pain, which is the cardinal sign of persistent posterior fetal position.
> - Regional blocks, especially epidural and caudal blocks, commonly result in assisted (forceps or vacuum) delivery because of the inability to push effectively during the second stage.

Review of Intrapartum Nursing Care

1. List five prodromal signs of labor the nurse might teach the client.
2. How is true labor discriminated from false labor?
3. State two ways to determine whether the membranes have truly ruptured.
4. Are psychoprophylactic breathing techniques prescribed for use according to the stage and phase of labor?
5. Identify two reasons to withhold anesthesia and analgesia until the midactive phase of stage I labor.
6. Hyperventilation often occurs in the laboring client. What results from hyperventilation, and what actions should the nurse take to relieve the condition?
7. Describe the maternal changes that characterize the transition phase of labor.
8. When should a laboring client be examined vaginally?
9. Define cervical effacement.
10. Where is the FHR best heard?
11. Normal FHR during labor is _____.
12. Normal maternal BP during labor is _____.
13. Normal maternal pulse during labor is _____.
14. Normal maternal temperature during labor is _____.
15. List four nursing actions for the second stage of labor.
16. List three signs of placental separation.
17. When should the postpartum dosage of oxytocin be administered? Why is it administered?
18. State one contraindication to the use of ergot drugs (methylergonovine).
19. State five symptoms of respiratory distress in the newborn.
20. If meconium was passed in utero, what action must the nurse take in the delivery room?
21. What is considered a good Apgar score?
22. What is the purpose of eye prophylaxis in the newborn?
23. What is the danger associated with regional blocks?
24. What is the major cause of maternal death when general anesthesia is administered?
25. Why are PO medications avoided in labor?
26. State the best way to administer IV drugs during labor.
27. When is it dangerous to administer butorphanol, an agonist/antagonist narcotic?
28. Hypotension commonly occurs after the laboring client receives a regional block. What is one of the first signs the nurse might observe?
29. State three actions the nurse should take when hypotension occurs in a laboring client.
30. How is the fourth stage of labor defined?
31. What actions can the nurse take to assist in preventing postpartum hemorrhage?
32. To promote comfort, what nursing interventions are used for a third-degree episiotomy that extends into the anal sphincter?
33. What nursing interventions are used to enhance maternal-infant bonding during the fourth stage of labor?
34. List three nursing interventions to ease the discomfort of afterpains.
35. List the symptoms of a full bladder that might occur in the fourth stage of labor.
36. What action should the nurse take first when a soft, boggy uterus is palpated?
37. What are the symptoms of hypovolemic shock?
38. How often should the nurse check the fundus during the fourth stage of labor?

Answers to Review

1. Lightening, Braxton Hicks contractions, increased bloody show, loss of mucous plug, burst of energy, and nesting behaviors.
2. True labor: regular, rhythmic contractions that intensify with ambulation, pain in the abdomen sweeping around from the back, and cervical changes. False labor: irregular rhythm, abdominal pain (not in back) that decreases with ambulation
3. Nitrazine testing: Paper turns dark blue or black. Demonstration of fluid ferning under microscope
4. No. Clients should use these techniques according to their discomfort level and should change techniques when one is no longer working for relaxation.
5. If analgesia and anesthesia are given too early, they can retard labor; if given too late, they can cause fetal distress.
6. Respiratory alkalosis occurs; it is caused by blowing off CO_2 and is relieved by breathing into a paper bag or cupped hands.
7. Irritability and unwillingness to be touched, but does not want to be left alone; nausea, vomiting, and hiccupping
8. Vaginal examinations should be done before analgesia and anesthesia to rule out cord prolapse, to determine labor progress if it is questioned, and to determine when pushing can begin.
9. The taking up of the lower cervical segment into the upper segment; the shortening of the cervix expressed in percentages from 0% to 100%, or complete effacement.
10. Through the fetal back in vertex, OA positions
11. 110 to 160 bpm
12. <140/90
13. <100 bpm
14. 38° C
15. Make sure cervix is completely dilated before pushing is allowed. Assess FHR with each contraction. Teach woman to hold breath for no longer than 10 seconds. Teach pushing technique.
16. Gush of blood, lengthening of cord, and globular shape of uterus
17. Give immediately after placenta is delivered to prevent postpartum hemorrhage and atony.
18. Hypertension
19. Tachypnea, dusky color, flaring nares, retractions, and grunting
20. Arrange for immediate endotracheal tube observation to determine the presence of meconium below the vocal cords (prevents pneumonitis and meconium aspiration syndrome).
21. 7 to 10
22. To prevent ophthalmia neonatorum, which results from exposure to gonorrhea in the vagina
23. Hypotension resulting from vasodilatation below the block, which pools blood in the periphery, reducing venous return
24. Aspiration of gastric contents
25. Gastric activity slows or stops in labor, decreasing absorption from PO route; it may cause vomiting.
26. At beginning of contraction, push a little medication in while uterine blood vessels are constricted, thereby reducing dose to fetus.
27. When the client is an undiagnosed drug abuser of narcotics, it can cause immediate withdrawal symptoms.
28. Nausea
29. Turn client to left side. Administer O_2 by mask at 10 L/min. Increase speed of intravenous infusion (if it does not contain medication).
30. The first 1 to 4 hours after delivery of placenta
31. Massage the fundus (gently) and keep the bladder emptied.
32. Ice pack, witch hazel compresses, and no rectal manipulation
33. Withhold eye prophylaxis for up to 1 hour. Perform newborn admission and routine procedures in room with parents. Encourage early initiation of breastfeeding. Darken room to encourage newborn to open eyes.
34. Keep bladder empty. Provide a warm blanket for abdomen. Administer analgesics prescribed by health care provider.
35. Fundus above umbilicus, dextroverted (to the right side of abdomen), increased bleeding (uterine atony)
36. Perform fundal massage.
37. Pallor, clammy skin, tachycardia, lightheadedness, and hypotension
38. Every 15 minutes for 1 hour; every 30 minutes for 2 hours if normal

Normal Puerperium (Postpartum)

Description: Period after pregnancy and delivery (usually 6 weeks) when the body returns to the nonpregnant state
A. Care during this period is focused on wellness and family integrity.
B. Teaching must be initiated early to cover the physical self-care needs and the emotional needs of the mother, infant, and family.

Normal Puerperium Changes

A. Reproductive system
   1. Uterus
      a. Myometrial contractions occur for 12 to 24 hours postdelivery due to high oxytocin levels (prominent in multiparas, breastfeeding women, and women who have experienced overdistention of the uterus).

b. Involution occurs (1 to 2 cm/day).
  (1) First day: at or 1 to 2 cm above umbilicus
  (2) 7 to 10 days: decreases to 12-week size, slides back under symphysis pubis
c. Placenta site contracts and heals without scarring.

2. Cervix
  a. Becomes parous, with a transverse slit
  b. Heals within 6 weeks

3. Vagina
  a. Rugae (folds) reappear within 3 weeks.
  b. Walls are thin and dry.

4. Breasts
  a. Nonlactating
    (1) Nodules are palpable.
    (2) Engorgement may occur 2 to 3 days postpartum.
  b. Lactating
    (1) Milk sinuses (lumps) are palpable.
    (2) Colostrum (yellowish fluid) is expressed first, then milk (bluish-white).
    (3) Breasts may feel warm, firm, tender for 48 hours.

B. Cardiovascular system
  1. At delivery
    a. Maternal vascular bed is reduced by 15%.
    b. Pulse may decrease to 50 (normal puerperal bradycardia).
    c. These changes are hypothesized to result in client's "shivering."
    d. BP and pulse should quickly return to prepregnant levels.
  2. First 72 hours
    a. 24 to 48 hours postpartum, cardiac output remains elevated (returns to nonpregnant levels in 2 to 3 weeks).
    b. Plasma loss > RBC loss; reverses hemodilution of pregnancy (Hct rises)
    c. Diaphoresis (especially at night) helps restore normal plasma volume.

C. Hematologic system
  1. Hct rises.
  2. WBC count is elevated (12,000 to 25,000).
  3. It is difficult to use WBC for determination of infection.
  4. Blood-clotting factors are elevated; increases risk for thromboembolism.

D. Urinary system
  1. Diuresis occurs; woman excretes up to 3000 mL/day of urine.
  2. Bladder distention and incomplete emptying are common.
  3. Persistent dilation of ureter and renal pelvis increase risk for UTI.
  4. Urine glucose, creatinine, and blood urea nitrogen (BUN) levels are normal after 7 days.

E. Gastrointestinal system
  1. Excess analgesia and anesthesia may decrease peristalsis.
  2. No bowel movements are expected for 2 to 3 days.

F. Integumentary system
  1. Chloasma and hyperpigmentation areas (linea nigra, areolae) regress; some areas may remain permanently darker.
  2. Palmar erythema declines quickly.
  3. Spider nevi fade; some in legs may remain.

G. Musculoskeletal system
  1. Pelvic muscles regain tone in 3 to 6 weeks.
  2. Abdominal muscles regain tone in 6 weeks unless diastasis recti (separation of rectus abdominis muscles) occurs.

HESI Hint • Assessments should be made before notifying the health care provider about any abnormal finding. Assess fundal height and firmness; assess perineal integrity; check for signs and symptoms of thromboembolism; assess pulse, respirations and BP; assess client's subjective description of symptoms (e.g., burning on urination, pain in leg, excessive tenderness of uterus).

Normal leukocytosis of pregnancy averages 12,000 to 15,000 mm^3. During the first 10 to 12 days postbirth, values of 25,000 mm^3 are common. Elevated WBC and the normal elevated erythrocyte sedimentation rate (ESR) may confuse interpretation of acute postpartal infections. For example, if a client's temperature is 38.2° C on the second postpartum day, what assessment should be made?

HESI Hint • Client and family teaching is a common subject of NCLEX-RN® questions. Remember that when teaching the first step is to assess the clients' (parents') level of knowledge and to identify their readiness to learn. Client teaching regarding lochia changes, perineal care, breastfeeding, and sore nipples are subjects that are commonly tested.

Nursing Assessment

A. Review prenatal, antepartum, L&D (labor and delivery), and early postpartum records for status, laboratory data, and possible complications.
B. Review newborn's record for Apgar scores, sex, possible complications, and relevant psychosocial information (adoption, single parent, etc.)
C. Assess postpartum status (Table 6-7): vital signs, fundal height and firmness, lochia, urination, perineum, bowel sounds, presence of thrombophlebitis.
D. Assess maternal-infant bonding and identify teaching needs of mother and family.

Analysis (Nursing Diagnoses)

A. *Acute pain* related to …
B. *Risk for infection* related to …

TABLE 6-7 Normal Postpartal Vital Signs

Vital Sign	Description
Temperature	May rise to 100.4° F due to dehydrating effects of labor. Any higher elevation may be due to infection and must be reported.
Pulse	May decrease to 50 (normal puerperal bradycardia). Pulse >100 may indicate excessive blood loss or infection.
Blood pressure	Should be normal. Suspect hypovolemia if it decreases, preeclampsia if it increases.
Respirations	Rarely change. If respirations increase significantly, suspect pulmonary embolism, uterine atony, or hemorrhage.

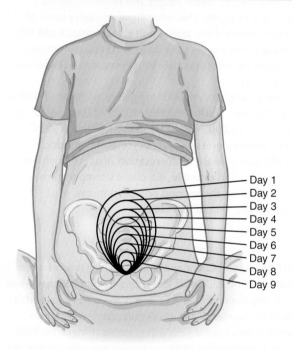

- Day 1
- Day 2
- Day 3
- Day 4
- Day 5
- Day 6
- Day 7
- Day 8
- Day 9

FIGURE 6-17 Involution of the uterus. Height of the uterine fundus decreases by approximately 1 cm per day. (From Murray SS, McKinney ES: *Foundations of maternal-newborn and women's health nursing*, ed 5, St. Louis, 2010, Saunders.)

C. *Urinary retention* related to …

D. *Deficient knowledge* (specify) related to …

E. *Risk for situational low self-esteem* related to …

Nursing Plans and Interventions

A. Monitor vital signs every 4 hours for 24 hours, then every 8 hours.

B. Check fundal height and firmness:
1. On the first postpartum day (first day after birth), the top of the fundus is located approximately 1 cm below the umbilicus (Fig. 6-17).
2. The fundus should be midline and firm immediately after delivery.
3. Massage the fundus if it is soft or boggy by stabilizing the bottom of the uterus before applying pres-

sure; teach mother the procedure but advise against overstimulation, which can lead to atony.
4. Teach about the normalcy of afterpains.

C. Assess and document lochia:
1. Lochia rubra: blood-tinged discharge, including shreds of tissue and decidua; lochia rubra lasts 2 to 3 days postpartum
2. Lochia serosa: pale pinkish to brownish discharge lasting 1 week postpartum
3. Lochia alba: thicker, whitish-yellowish discharge with leukocytes and degenerated cells; lochia alba lasts up to 4 weeks postpartum

> **HESI Hint** • After the first postpartum day, the most common cause of uterine atony is retained placental fragments. The nurse must check for the presence of fragments in lochial tissue.

4. Subinvolution: placental site does not heal; lochia persists, with brisk periods of lochia rubra; a dilation and curettage (D&C) may be necessary.
5. Document amount of lochia.
   a. Scant: <1-inch (2.54-cm) stain on pad
   b. Small: <4-inch (10.16-cm) stain on pad
   c. Moderate: <6-inch (15.24-cm) stain on pad
   d. Heavy: saturated pad within 1 hour
   e. Clots: <2 to 3 cm (1 to 2 inches)
   f. Odor: fleshy, not foul
6. Teach client about normal lochia changes.

> **HESI Hint** • Women can tolerate blood loss, even slightly excessive blood loss, in the postpartal period because of the 40% increase in plasma volume during pregnancy. In the postpartal period, a woman can void up to 3000 mL/day to reduce the volume increase that occurred during pregnancy.

D. Assess perineum and episiotomy site.
1. Place woman in lateral Sims position, don gloves, and use flashlight to increase accuracy of visualization.
2. Check for redness, edema, intactness, and presence of hematomas; teach self-inspection with mirror.
3. Teach hygiene and comfort and healing measures.
   a. Instruct to change pad as needed and with every voiding and defecation.
   b. Instruct to wipe perineum front to back.
   c. Instruct to use good handwashing technique.
   d. Teach about use of ice packs, sitz baths, using a squeeze bottle for perineal lavage, and topical application of anesthetic spray and pads (Box 6-2).

E. Examine breasts.
1. Assess nipples for cracks, fissures, redness, and tenderness.
2. For breastfeeding mothers (see Table 6-18):

a. Assess breasts for engorgement

b. Teach mothers how to prevent engorgement

3. Palpate breasts for lumps and nodules.
4. Determine woman's motivation to breastfeed or bottlefeed.
5. If not breastfeeding, teach woman nonpharmacologic measures of milk suppression: supportive bra or binder, ice packs, and avoiding breast stimulation.
6. Teach breast self-examination (see Box 6-2).

HESI Hint • Client should void within 4 hours of delivery. Monitor client closely for urine retention. Suspect retention if voiding is frequent and <100 mL per voiding.

HESI Hint • Women often have a syncopal (fainting) spell on the first ambulation after delivery (usually related to vasomotor changes, orthostatic hypotension). The astute nurse will check the client's Hgb and Hct for anemia and BP, sitting and lying down, to ascertain orthostatic hypotension.

F. Assist mother and infant with breastfeeding (Table 6-8).

G. Assess bladder and urine output.
1. Palpate for spongy, full feeling over symphysis.
2. Check urge to void when bladder is palpated.
3. Assist client to ambulate for first void (orthostatic hypotension may occur); measure if possible.

BOX 6-2 *Postpartum Teaching*

Breast Self-Examination
- Begin with inspection in a mirror. Place both hands at sides and observe; then look again with hands overhead and bending forward. Assess for:
  - Change in size and shape
  - Dimpling, puckering, scaling, redness, swelling of any part of breast
- Lie flat with right hand under head and pillow or towel under right shoulder.

- Use left hand to palpate using concentric circles around right breast, feeling for lumps, nodules, or thickening.
- Repeat with left breast.

Episiotomy Care
- Perineal care
- Fill a squeeze bottle with warm water and, if prescribed, an ounce of povidone-iodine solution.
- Lavage perineum with several squirts and blot dry instead of rubbing; avoid anal area.

TABLE 6-8 **Teaching Breastfeeding**

Topics to Include	Data Related to Topics
Advantages of breast-feeding	• Low cost • Distinct immunologic advantages for newborn
Milk production	• Stimulated by the decrease in postpartum estrogen production, which allows release of prolactin from the pituitary
Let-down reflex (milk ejection)	• Caused by action of oxytocin released from posterior pituitary, which stimulates myoepithelial cells around milk ducts and sinuses
Breast size	• Has no relationship to successful breastfeeding
Inverted and retracted nipples	• Women with inverted or retracted nipples can wear shields, which may help the infant latch on to the nipple.
Diet during breastfeeding and lactation	• Avoid dieting. • Add 500 calories to prepregnancy intake. • Drink 2 quarts (8 glasses) of noncaffeinated beverages daily.
Avoid	• Smoking and the intake of drugs, alcohol, and caffeine • Stress, which is the most common reason for decreased milk supply.
Encourage	• Rest
Care of breasts and nipples	• Newborn should remain on first breast 10 min, then switch to second breast and suckle until satisfied (it is no longer recommended to limit breastfeeding time to 2-3 min first day, 5 min second day, etc.). • Use warm water, not drying soap, on nipples. • Let nipples air-dry for 15 min two to three times daily. • Breast creams should not be routinely used; colostrum may be expressed and rubbed on nipples.

TABLE 6-8 **Teaching Breastfeeding—cont'd**

Topics to Include	Data Related to Topics
• Engorgement	• Nurse more frequently, and manually express milk to soften areola before feeding.
	• Wear supportive bra.
	• Take warm or hot showers (water over breasts promotes milk flow).
	• Watch for symptoms of mastitis (commonly occurs when breasts are not emptied).
	• Teach the mother to wash her breasts with water not soap, to allow nipples to air dry, wear breast-feeding pads, and to frequently change the breastfeeding position used to hold the infant.
	• To reduce possibility of breast engorgement the mother should start breastfeeding as soon as possible to after birth to allow the infant to learn breastfeeding prior to the breasts becoming full and firm.
	• To prevent engorgement the mother should use the breast pump or express milk by hand to remove milk remaining after the infant is satiated.
	• Assess breasts for engorgement.
	• Signs of engorgement are: swollen, firm, and painful breasts. If left untreated the affected breast becomes more swollen, hard, shiny, and slightly lumpy when palpated. The nipple may retract into the areola.
	• Mother may complain of fatigue, loss of appetite, weakness and chills.
	• Fever (39^0 or less) occurs in approximately 10% to 15% of mothers.
	• To alleviate the pain of engorgement the following interventions can be used: teach mother ways to alleviate discomfort by wearing a supportive bra, taking analgesics, or applying warm compresses or ice packs or washed cabbage leaves to the breasts (Fig. 6-18) to reduce the pain of engorgement
	• A complementary and alternative (CAM) intervention for engorgement is the application of washed green cabbage leaves (chilled or room temperature) to breasts between feedings for 20 minutes up to three times per day. Applications should cease as soon as engorgement begins to subside because the intervention can decrease breast milk supply.
• Incorrect positioning	• Incorrect positioning of baby on breast is most common reason for sore nipples.
	• Make sure baby has as much of areola as possible in mouth.
	• Break suction with insertion of little finger into the baby's mouth.

4. Run warm water over perineum or place spirit of peppermint in bedpan to relax urethra if necessary.
5. Catheterize only if necessary.
6. Teach symptoms of UTI: dysuria, frequency, and urgency.
7. Promote retoning of perineal muscles by Kegel exercises.

> **HESI Hint** • Kegel exercises increase the integrity of the introitus and improve urine retention. Teach client to alternate contraction and relaxation of the pubococcygeal muscles.

H. Assess bowel and anal area:
1. Inspect for hemorrhoids; describe size and number.
2. Administer antihemorrhoidal cream, ointment, or suppositories as prescribed.
3. Auscultate bowel sounds; check abdominal distention.
4. Document flatus and bowel movement.
5. Encourage early ambulation.
6. Encourage increased fluids and use of roughage and bulk in diet.
7. Administer stool softeners (docusate sodium, enemas, or suppositories) as prescribed (Table 6-9).

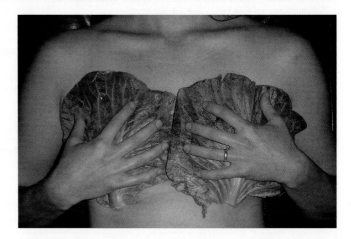

FIGURE 6-18 Cabbage leaves to treat breast engorgement. Engorgement can be painful to the mother and distention of the nipple and areola make it difficult for the infant to successfully latch for breastfeeding. (From Lowdermilk D, Perry S, Cashion M, Alden M: *Maternity and women's health care,* ed 10. St. Louis, 2012, Mosby.)

8. Avoid rectal manipulation if third- or fourth-degree episiotomy was performed.
I. Prevent thrombophlebitis.
1. Encourage early ambulation.
2. Encourage foot paddling and ankle rolling after general anesthesia.

TABLE 6-9 Postpartum Drugs

Drugs	Indications	Adverse Reactions	Nursing Implications
Bisacodyl	• Constipation	• Abdominal cramping	• Insert suppository into anus past internal rectal sphincter. • Because it is a contact laxative that stimulates rectal mucosa directly, there may be some burning. • Usually effective in 15 min-1 hr
Docusate sodium	• Constipation • Painful defecation due to fourth-degree tear	• Abdominal cramping	• Encourage increased fluid intake. • Results usually occur within 1-3 days of continual use.

Rho(D) immune globulin (RhoGAM)	• Prevention of Rh isoimmunization with next pregnancy	• None known	• Given to Rh-negative women after miscarriage, abortion, or any procedure or complication that increases the risk for maternal-fetal blood exchange (amniocentesis, PUBS, abdominal trauma)
			• Routinely given at 28 wk gestation to Rh-negative mothers with a negative antibody titer
			• Given postpartally to Rh-negative mother after delivery or abortion when fetus is Rh-positive
			• Never given to an infant or father
			• Must be given within 72 hr of delivery
			• Always given IM
			• Is a blood product:
			  • Must be checked by two nurses
			  • Syringe must be returned to laboratory with label
			  • Not given to a mother with positive indirect Coombs; she is already sensitized to fetal cells and has developed antibodies.

Rubella vaccine	• Rubella titer of ≤1:10 or enzyme immunoassay (EIA) of ≤0.10	• Transient benign arthralgia • Transient rash • Hypersensitivity if allergic to duck eggs • Slight elevation in temperature	• Given subcutaneously before hospital discharge to nonimmune women • Woman may breastfeed. • Do not give if woman or other family members are immunocompromised. • Requires informed consent • Teach about contraception; women should avoid pregnancy for 2-3 mo after immunization.

HESI Hint • Remember, RhoGAM is given to an Rh-negative mother who delivers an Rh-positive fetus and has a negative direct Coombs test. If the mother has a positive Coombs test, there is no need to give RhoGAM because the mother is already sensitized.

HESI Hint • Because Rh immune globulins suppress the immune system, the client who receives both RhoGAM and the rubella vaccine should be tested for rubella immunity at 3 months.

> **HESI Hint** • Assess for thromboembolism: Examine legs of postpartum client daily for pain, warmth, and tenderness or a swollen vein that is tender to the touch.

J. Determine the need for RhoGAM (see Table 6-9).
K. Determine the need for a rubella vaccine.
L. Assess maternal psychological adaptation. Reva Rubin identified three distinct emotional stages after delivery:
   1. Taking in: dependency behaviors for 24 to 48 hours; asking for help on the simplest of tasks
   2. Taking hold: less focus on physical discomforts, beginning confidence with infant caretaking. Not uncommon for mother to feel inadequate caring for infant; the astute nurse will not take over but will praise efforts of parents. At this time, new parents are usually most receptive to teaching about infant care.
   3. Letting go: total separation of newborn from self; confident in caretaking activities of self and newborn
M. Assess mother–infant bonding behaviors:
   1. Eye contact between mother and neonate
   2. Exploration of infant from head to toe
   3. Stroking, kissing, and fondling the neonate
   4. Smiling, talking, singing to the neonate
   5. Use of claiming expressions (e.g., "He's got my feet.")
   6. Absence of negative statements such as "She just doesn't like me."
   7. Naming the newborn quickly and calling the infant by name
N. Promote mother–infant bonding.
   1. Ensure mother is comfortable: Provide pain relief, hygiene, and adequate rest.
   2. If possible, have baby room-in; include family in teaching; praise and reinforce all positive parenting behaviors.
   3. Teach about neonatal behavioral traits.
   4. Assure normalcy of comparing idealized child to looks and sex of real child, but prevent long-term

disappointment by encouraging verbalization of those feelings now.
   5. Teach responses to cues from the baby.
      a. Pick baby up when he or she is crying (reciprocity).
      b. Soothe with calm, interactive responses until baby returns to quiet, active state (synchrony).
   6. Encourage verbalization of feelings; offer support in nonjudgmental manner.

> **HESI Hint** • "Postpartum blues" are usually normal, especially 5 to 7 days after delivery (unexplained tearfulness, feeling down, and having a decreased appetite). Encourage use of support persons to help with housework for first 2 postpartum weeks. Refer to community resources.

O. Instruct client to notify health care provider or clinic promptly of:
   1. Heavy vaginal bleeding with clots
   2. Temperature of (38° C) or higher lasting 24 hours or longer
   3. A red, warm lump in breast
   4. Pain on urination
   5. Tenderness in calf
P. Teach self-care for discharge.
   1. Instruct to continue perineal care and pad changes.
   2. Encourage balanced diet and fluid intake.
   3. Encourage client to rest or nap when newborn does.
   4. Teach to abstain from sexual intercourse until lochia has ceased.
   5. Inform that first sexual experience may not be pleasant because of vaginal dryness.
Q. Counsel about sibling rivalry, especially if there is a toddler (age 18 months to 3 years) at home.
   1. Alert parents that sibling may regress.
   2. Suggest taking a present to toddler from the newborn, and encourage mother to hug toddler.
   3. Encourage client to plan time alone with siblings.
R. Assist client with choice of contraceptive method. Teach use, risks, and technique before discharge (Table 6-10).

Review of Normal Puerperium (Postpartum)

1. A nurse discovers a postpartum client with a boggy uterus that is displaced above and to the right of the umbilicus. What nursing action is indicated?
2. Which women experience afterpains more than others?
3. Upon admission to the postpartum room, 3 hours after delivery, a client has a temperature of 37.5° C. What nursing actions are indicated?
4. A client feels faint on the way to the bathroom. What nursing assessments should be made?
5. What factor places the postpartum client at risk for thromboembolism?
6. A breastfeeding mother complains of very tender nipples. What nursing actions should be taken?
7. Three days postpartum, a lactating mother has full, warm, taut, tender breasts. What nursing actions should be taken?
8. What information should be given to a client regarding resumption of sexual intercourse after delivery?
9. A woman has decided to take birth control pills as her contraceptive method. What should she do if she misses taking the pill for 2 consecutive days?
10. A woman asks why she is urinating so much in the postpartum period. The nurse bases the response on what information?
11. A woman's white blood count is 17,000; she is afebrile and has no symptoms of infection. What nursing action is indicated?

12. What is the most common cause of uterine atony in the first 24 hours postpartum?

13. What is the purpose of giving docusate sodium to the postpartum client?

14. What should the fundal height be at 3 days postpartum for a woman who has had a vaginal delivery?

15. List three signs of positive bonding between parents and newborn.

Answers to Review

1. Perform immediate fundal massage. Ambulate to the bathroom or use bedpan to empty bladder because cardinal signs of bladder distention are present.

2. Breastfeeding women, multiparas, and women who experienced overdistention of the uterus

3. Temperature is probably elevated due to dehydration and work of labor; force fluids and retake temperature in an hour; notify physician if above 38° C.

4. Assess BP sitting and lying; assess Hgb and Hct for anemia.

5. Increased clotting factors

6. Have her demonstrate infant position on breast (incorrect positioning often causes tenderness). Leave bra open to air-dry nipples for 15 minutes three times daily. Express colostrum and rub on nipples.

7. She is engorged; have newborn suckle frequently; take measures to increase milk flow: warm water, breast massage, and supportive bra.

8. Avoid until postpartum examination. Use water-soluble jelly. Expect slight discomfort due to vaginal changes.

9. Take two pills for 2 days and use an alternative form of birth control.

10. Up to 3000 mL per day can be voided because of the reduction in the 40% plasma volume increase during pregnancy.

11. Continue routine assessments; normal leukocytosis occurs during postpartal period because of placental site healing.

12. A full bladder

13. To soften the stool in mothers with third- or fourth-degree episiotomies, hemorrhoids, or cesarean section delivery.

14. Three fingerbreadths/cm below the umbilicus.

15. Calling infant by name, exploring newborn head to toe, using en face position.

TABLE 6-10 Methods of Contraception

Method	Use, Risk, and Technique
Diaphragm	• Used with spermicide • Must be fitted by a nurse practitioner or doctor • Must be left in place for 6 hr after intercourse • Must be refitted if excessive weight gain or loss occurs • Must be checked for integrity • Can irritate urethra
Cervical cap	• Used with spermicide • Contraindicated if cervical anomalies exist • Associated with cervical changes • Pap smear recommended 3 mo after use
Condom (with spermicide)	• Used with spermicide to increase effectiveness • Recommended if any suspicion of STD • Penis must be withdrawn while erect or condom may fall off. • Petroleum jelly can deteriorate rubber; water-soluble jelly should be used.

Symptothermal, prothermal, or fertility awareness	• Signs of ovulation should be taught:
	  • Cervical mucus assessment
	  • Basal body temperature assessment
	  • Mittelschmerz (abdominal pain in the region of an ovary during ovulation)

IUD (intrauterine device)	• Contraindications: diabetes, anemia, abnormal Pap, history of pelvic infections • High association with dysmenorrhea and infection

TABLE 6-10 Methods of Contraception—cont'd

Method	Use, Risk, and Technique
*Oral contraceptives	• Estrogen in pills prevents pituitary secretion of FSH, preventing ovulation. • Woman still menstruates. • Lowest failure rate of methods • Contraindications: history of coagulation problems, thromboembolism, liver disease, reproductive cancer, coronary artery disease • Compliance is a problem because pill must be taken every day. • If one pill is missed, it should be taken as soon as remembered and the next one taken at the usual time. • If two pills are missed, two pills should be taken for 2 days and an alternative method of contraception should be used for next 7 days. • If more than two pills are missed in the third week, or three or more pills are missed at any time, pills for that cycle should not be taken; alternative method of contraception should be used. Pills should be resumed on fifth day of menstruation.
Ethinyl estradiol/norelgestromin (Ortho Evra) transdermal contraceptive patch	• Mechanism of action, efficacy, contraindications, and side effects are similar to those of oral contraceptives. • Delivers continuous levels of progesterone and estradiol • Can be applied to lower abdomen, upper outer arm, buttock, or upper torso (except the breasts) • To be applied on the same day once a week for 3 wk, followed by 1 wk without patch
Norplant (levonorgestrel implant)	• Sustained-release, subdermal, progestin-only contraceptive • Consists of six thin, flexible capsules made of soft Silastic tubing • Placed in a fanlike pattern just beneath the skin of the upper arm • Effective within 24 hr after insertion; effective for approximately 5 yr • Efficacy is not dependent on client compliance once inserted. • Reversible with return to previous level of fertility after removal • Side effects include menstrual pattern changes, headache, nervousness. • Works by suppression of ovulation, as well as by thickening of cervical mucus • Efficacy challenged; not available in United States; two-rod implant approved by Food and Drug Administration
Depo-Provera	• IM injection every 3 mo for contraception • Administered during the first 5 days of menstrual cycle • New mothers may be given the injection during the postpartum period, before discharge. • Efficacy of 99% • Protection from pregnancy is immediate after injection • Most women experience weight gain and irregular or unpredictable menstrual bleeding (after 1 yr use, many women stop having menstrual periods altogether). • Must monitor for signs and symptoms of thrombophlebitis • Contraindications: history of breast cancer, stroke, blood clots, liver disease • Side effects: nervousness, dizziness, GI disturbances, headaches, and fatigue; may also increase risk for osteoporosis
Ethinyl estradiol/etonogestrel (NuvaRing)	• A 2-in-diameter ring is an ethylene vinyl acetate complex impregnated with ethinyl estradiol and etonogestrel. • Continuous slow absorption of estrogen/progestin allows for lower estrogen dosing than with oral contraceptives. • The ring is placed deep into the vagina once every 3 wk and is removed on day 21, then, after a 7-day drug-free interval, a new ring is inserted for an additional 21 days. • Requires an additional form of contraception for the first 7 days of therapy. • The vaginal ring estrogen/progestin administration has the same risks, adverse effects, contraindications, precautions, and drug interactions as oral contraceptives.

The Normal Newborn

Description: During the immediate transitional period (first 6 to 8 hours of life) and the early newborn period (first few days of life), the nurse assesses, plans, and provides nursing interventions based on the outcomes of the individual newborn's examination.

Nursing Assessment

A. Review L&D report of neonatal history to determine risks during newborn transition caused by medical and obstetric complications.
   1. Cesarean delivery; missing of vaginal squeeze
   2. Prematurity or postmaturity
   3. Diabetic mother
   4. Prolonged ROM >24 hours: sepsis workup
   5. Rh+ isoimmunization (positive direct Coombs test)
   6. Traumatic (forceps or vacuum suction) delivery
B. Review L&D report of neonatal history to determine risks during newborn transition caused by drugs and anesthesia during labor and delivery.
   1. Magnesium sulfate during labor: Hypermagnesemia in neonate causes depressed respirations, hypocalcemia, and hypotonia.
   2. Narcosis (late administration of narcotic analgesics); causes decreased respirations and hypotonia.
C. Review L&D report of neonatal history to determine risks during newborn transition caused by degree of birth asphyxia.
   1. Asphyxia during labor: documented late decelerations, decreased variability, severe variable decelerations
   2. Apgar scores at 1 and 5 minutes
D. Review significant social history: mother with a sexually transmitted disease (STD), single parent, language barrier, substance abuse, and lack of support system.
E. Assess vital signs every 30 minutes for 2 hours, then every hour for 4 hours or until stabilized (Table 6-11).
F. Measure the neonate (Table 6-12).
G. Perform a physical examination of the newborn (Table 6-13).
H. Perform neuromuscular assessment. The absence of expected reflexes requires investigation into birth trauma and asphyxia or CNS anomaly (Table 6-14 and Fig. 6-19).
I. Perform a systematic gestational age assessment (Table 6-15; and see Fig. 6-18). Plot measurements on percentile scale to determine whether neonate is small, average, or large for gestational age.
J. Perform a behavioral assessment using the Brazelton Neonatal Behavioral Assessment Scale to evaluate newborn's behavioral uniqueness.
   1. Waiting 2 to 3 days to perform assessment gives neonate a chance to rid body of effects of analgesia, anesthesia, and trauma of birth.
   2. The scale measures six categories: habituation, orientation, motor activity, self-quieting ability, social behaviors, sleep and awake states.
   3. Performing test with the parents present familiarizes them with their newborn's uniqueness and may provide them with cues about the best ways to respond to the newborn.

Nursing Care of the Newborn

A. Aspiration
   1. Keep bulb syringe or suction immediately available: suction mouth, then nose.
   2. Turn neonate on side or stomach and pat firmly on the back, holding head 10 to 15 degrees lower than feet.

HESI Hint • Suction the mouth first and then the nose. Stimulating the nares can initiate inspiration, which could cause aspiration of mucus in oral pharynx.

B. Infection
   1. *Handwashing!* This is the most effective preventive measure.
   2. Scrupulous cord care: Swab cord with alcohol at each diaper change, or keep clean with mild soap and water (varies with hospital and provider).
   3. After circumcision a petrolatum gauze dressing or a generous amount of petrolatum may be applied with each diaper change for 1 or 2 days to prevent the diaper from adhering to the site.
   4. Do not allow visitors or personnel to attend to newborn if active infection is present or if newborn has diarrhea, open wounds, an infectious skin rash, or herpes virus.
   5. Encourage breastfeeding for immunologic factors.

HESI Hint • Circumcision has become controversial because there is no real medical indication for the procedure, and it does cause trauma and pain to the newborn. It was once thought to decrease the incidence of penile and cervical cancer, but some researchers say this is unfounded.

C. Hypothermia
   1. Keep newborn dry and warm.
   2. Place stockinette cap on head (greatest heat loss is through scalp).
   3. Take newborn's temperature at admission and every 4 to 6 hours.
   4. If newborn's temperature falls below 36.4° C, place in radiant warmer and apply skin temperature probe to regulate isolette temperature. May also double-wrap or put skin to skin (kangaroo) with mother.

HESI Hint • Hypothermia (heat loss) leads to depletion of glucose and, therefore, to the use of brown fat (special fat deposits fetus develops in last trimester; they are important to thermoregulation) for energy. This results in ketoacidosis and possible shock. Prevent by keeping neonate warm!

TABLE 6-11 Newborn Vital Sign Norms

Vital sign	Normal	Nursing Implications

Respirations	Rate: 30-60 breaths/min	• Remember the ABCs (airway, breathing, circulation)
		• Count 1 full minute by observing abdomen or auscultating breath sounds.
		• Note five symptoms of respiratory distress:
		  • Tachypnea
		  • Cyanosis
		  • Flaring nares
		  • Expiratory grunt
		  • Retractions

Heart rate	110-160 bpm; may decrease as low as 100 during sleep; may increase as high as 180 during crying	• Auscultate for 1 full minute at the PMI (point of maximal impulse): third to fourth intercostal space.
Temperature	Range: 36.5° C-37.5° C	• Rectal approach may perforate rectum; if taken rectally, insert only ¼ to ½ inch for 5 min and hold legs firmly to prevent trauma.
Blood pressure	Average 80/50 mm Hg	• Not usually measured unless problems in circulation have been assessed.

TABLE 6-12 Physical Measurements

Assessment	Normal	Nursing Implications
Weight	• Average: 3401.9 g • Majority weigh between 2700 and 4000 g (6-9 lb)	• Weigh at birth and daily, with neonate completely naked. • Normally lose 5%-15% (average 10%) of birth weight in first week of life; weight should be documented carefully.
Length	• Average range: 46-52.5 cm	• Measured from crown to rump and rump to heel, or from crown to heel at birth
Head circumference	• Average range: 33-35 cm (normally, 2 cm larger than chest circumference)	• Tape measure placed above eyebrows and stretched around fullest part of occiput, at posterior fontanel (FOC, frontal-occipital circumference)
Chest circumference	• Average range: 31-33 cm	• Tape measure is stretched around scapulae and over nipple line.

HESI Hint • *Physical Assessment*
A detailed physical assessment is performed by the nurse or physician. Regardless of who performs the physical assessment, the nurse must know normal versus abnormal variations in the newborn. Observations must be recorded and the physician notified regarding abnormalities.

TABLE 6-13 Physical Examination of the Newborn

Normal	Abnormal	Rationale
General Appearance		
• Awake • Flexed extremities • Moves all extremities • Strong, lusty cry • Obvious presence of subcutaneous fat • No obvious anomalies	• Little subcutaneous fat	• Intrauterine growth problems • Fetal stress
	• Frog position	• Prematurity
	• Flaccid	• Asphyxia • Prematurity
	• Hard to arouse	• Sepsis • CNS problems • Asphyxia
	• High-pitched cry	• CNS damage or anomalies • Hypoglycemia • Drug withdrawal

TABLE 6-13 Physical Examination of the Newborn—cont'd

Normal	Abnormal	Rationale
Integument		
• Smooth, elastic turgor and subcutaneous fat, superficial peeling after 24 hr; veins rarely visible • Milia, vernix increases • Lanugo, mottling • Harlequin sign (pink-red skin on one side of body) • Erythema toxicum (pink papular rash is normal) • Mongolian spots • Telangiectatic nevi (stork bites)	• Extreme desquamation	• Postmaturity
	• Many visible veins	• Prematurity
	• Meconium staining	• Fetal distress
	• Cyanosis	• Heart disease • Asphyxia
	• Jaundice (within 24 hr)	• Blood incompatibilities • Sepsis • Drug reactions
	• Vesicles	• Herpes, syphilis
	• Café-au-lait spots	• Neurofibromatosis
Head		
• Round or slightly molded • Caput succedaneum (edema over occiput) • Open, flat anterior and posterior fontanels, sutures slightly separated or overlapping due to molding	• Bulging fontanel	• Increased ICP
	• Sunken fontanel	• Dehydration
	• Widely separated sutures	• Hydrocephalus
	• Premature suture closure	• Genetic disorders
	• Cephalohematoma	• Blood under periosteum due to trauma

HESI Hint • It is difficult to differentiate between caput succedaneum (edema under the scalp) and cephalohematoma (blood under the periosteum). The caput crosses suture lines and is usually present at birth, whereas the cephalohematoma does not cross suture lines and manifests a few hours after birth. The danger of cephalohematoma is increased hyperbilirubinemia due to excess RBC breakdown.

Normal	Abnormal	Rationale
Eyes		
• Symmetrically placed • Pseudostrabismus • Chemical conjunctivitis (from eye prophylaxis) • Clear cornea • White-blue sclera • Subconjunctival hemorrhage from pressure • Absence of tears • Doll's eye movement (slight nystagmus)	• Purulent discharge	• Gonorrhea or chlamydia
	• Brushfield spots in iris	• Down syndrome
	• Absence of red reflex	• Congenital cataracts
	• Epicanthal folds	• Down syndrome
	• Setting-sun sign	• CNS disorders
	• Absent glabellar reflex (blink)	• CNS or neuromuscular problem
Ears		
• Pinna at or above level of line drawn from outer canthus of eye • Well formed and firm with instant recoil if folded against head	• Low-set	• Down syndrome
	• Unformed, soft	• Prematurity
	• Preauricular sinus	• Possible renal anomaly
Nose		
• In midline • Appears flattened • Is being used for breathing • Occasional sneezing	• Short, upturned, small philtrum (creases under nose)	• Fetal alcohol syndrome
	• Nasal flaring	• Respiratory distress
	• Grunting	• Respiratory distress • Choanal atresia (obstruction between nares and pharynx)
	• Snuffles	• Syphilis
	• Excessive sneezing	• Drug withdrawal

Continued

TABLE 6-13 Physical Examination of the Newborn—cont'd

Normal	Abnormal	Rationale
Mouth and Chin		
• Symmetrical movement • Intact lip and palate • Epstein pearls • Mobile tongue • Sucking pads in cheeks • Presence of rooting, sucking, swallowing, and gagging reflexes	• Asymmetry	• Facial nerve injury (Bell palsy)
	• Cleft lip	• Genetic disorder
	• White plaques on cheeks, tongue	• Monilia infection/thrush
	• Absence of protective reflexes	• Prematurity • CNS disorders
	• Excessive drooling	• Esophageal atresia
Neck		
• Short • Range of motion • Nonpalpable thyroid • Ability to lift head momentarily	• Limited range of motion	• Torticollis (wry neck)
	• Nuchal rigidity	• Meningitis
	• Enlarged thyroid	• Hyperthyroidism
	• Crepitus over clavicle	• Fractured clavicle
Chest		
• Symmetrical excursion • Breath sounds clear and equal • Transient rales at birth • Round • Breast engorgement (hormonal) • Transient murmurs	• Persistent murmur	• Patent ductus arteriosus
	• Visible activity over precordium	• Congenital heart anomaly • Heart failure
	• Retractions	• Respiratory distress
	• Asymmetrical chest	• Pneumothorax
Back, Hips, Buttocks, and Anus		
• Spine intact • Symmetrical gluteal folds • Equal limb lengths • Patent anus	• Pilonidal dimple or sinus (at base of sacrum)	• CNS anomaly • Covert spina bifida
	• Hip click • Unequal limb lengths • Asymmetrical gluteal folds	• Congenital hip dislocation
	• Absence of stools after 24 hours	• Imperforate anus • GI obstruction
Abdomen		
• Full, rounded, soft • Present bowel sounds • Palpable liver 1-2 cm below right costal margin • Two arteries, one vein in cord; white cord with Wharton jelly	• Scaphoid	• Diaphragmatic hernia
	• Distention	• Meconium ileus • GI obstruction • Hirschsprung disease
	• Hepatosplenomegaly	• Sepsis
	• Purulent discharge at base of cord, foul odor	• Omphalitis (cord infection)
	• One artery	• Renal or heart anomalies
	• Omphalocele	• Abdominal contents in umbilicus (anomaly)
	• Gastroschisis	• Abdominal contents outside of abdomen (anomaly)

TABLE 6-13 **Physical Examination of the Newborn—cont'd**

Normal	Abnormal	Rationale
Genitals		
Female	• Labia minora and clitoris visible	• Prematurity
• Slightly edematous labia covering clitoris and labia minora		
• Pseudomenstruation		
• Visible hymenal tag		
Male	• Undescended testes	• Prematurity
• Penis with foreskin intact	• Meatus on dorsal surface penis	• Epispadias
• Meatus in middle at tip of penis	• Meatus on ventral surface penis	• Hypospadias
• Descended testes	• Fluid in testes	• Hydrocele
• Slight edema of scrotum	• Intestine in inguinal canal	• Inguinal hernia
• Rugae on scrotum		
Extremities		
• Arms, hands, fingers, legs, feet, toes	• Incurving little finger	• Down syndrome
• Flexion	• Simian crease	• Down syndrome
• Symmetrical movement	• Flapping tremors	• Drug withdrawal
• Palpable brachial and radial pulses	• Polydactyly	• Extra digit (family trait)
• Palmar and plantar grasp reflex present	• Syndactyly	• Webbed digit (family trait)
• Strong grasp reflex	• Difference in pulses between upper and lower extremities	• Coarctation of aorta
• Multiple palmar and plantar creases		
• Slightly bowed legs	• Absence of plantar creases	• Prematurity
• Femoral pulses present	• Rigid fixation of ankle	• Club feet (talipes)
• Positive Babinski reflex	• Absent Babinski reflex	• CNS injury

HESI Hint • The umbilical cord should always be checked at birth. It should contain three vessels: one vein, which carries oxygenated blood to the fetus, and two arteries, which carry unoxygenated blood back to the placenta. This is the opposite of normal circulation in the adult. Cord abnormalities usually indicate cardiovascular or renal anomalies.

HESI Hint • Postnatally, the fetal structures of foramen ovale, ductus arteriosus, and ductus venosus should close. If they do not, cardiac and pulmonary compromise will develop.

D. Hypoglycemia
  1. Perform a heelstick blood glucose assessment on all small-for-gestational-age (SGA) or large-for-gestational-age (LGA) babies, on infants of diabetic mothers (IDMs), on jittery babies, and on babies with high-pitched cries (Box 6-3).
  2. Report any blood glucose levels under 40 mg/dL in the full-term infant, under 30 mg/dL in the preterm infant. Normal serum glucose is 40 to 80 mg/dL.
  3. Feed the baby early (breast milk or formula) if a low glucose level is detected.
  4. Prevent cold stress, which leads to hypoglycemia.

E. Hemorrhagic disorders: Administer vitamin K to prevent hemorrhagic disorders (Table 6-16).
F. Hyperbilirubinemia
  1. Evaluate for Rh isoimmunization (Rh+ newborn, Rh− mother; maternal Rh+ antibodies are passed to the fetus and cause RBC hemolysis) and for ABO incompatibility (mother blood type O, newborn blood type A or B; maternal anti-A or anti-B antibodies are passed to newborn and cause less severe hemolysis).
  2. Bilirubin (byproduct of RBC destruction) binds to protein for excretion or metabolism.

TABLE 6-14 Neuromuscular Assessment

Reflex	Normal Response	Lasts Until
Rooting	Baby turns toward stimulus when cheek or corner of lip is touched.	3-4 mo (possibly 1 yr)
Moro	When startled, baby symmetrically extends and abducts all extremities. Forefingers form a C shape.	3-4 mo
Tonic neck	When neck is turned to side, baby assumes fencing posture.	3-4 mo
Babinski	When sole of foot is stroked from heel to ball, toes hyperextend and fan apart from big toe.	1 yr to 18 mo
Palmar grasp	When examiner's finger is placed in the infant's palm, the newborn will curl his or her fingers around the examiner's finger.	Lessens by 3-4 mo
Plantar	A finger at base of toes causes them to curl downward	8 mo
Stepping	When infant is held in upright position with feet touching a hard surface, walking motions are made.	3-4 mo

HESI Hint • These neurologic reflexes are transient and, as such, disappear usually within the first year of life. In the pediatric client, prolonged presence of these reflexes can indicate CNS defects. Anticipate NCLEX-RN questions regarding normal newborn reflexes. Physical assessment questions focus on normal characteristics of the newborn and the differentiation of conditions such as caput succedaneum and cephalohematoma.

3. Promote stooling by early feedings of milk (protein binds bilirubin for excretion).
4. Assess at birth and daily for presence of jaundice:
   a. Yellowish skin color, sclera, and mucous membranes
   b. Proceeds cephalocaudally (relationship between the head and the base of the spine)
5. Give adequate fluids.
6. Monitor bilirubin levels.
7. Assist with phototherapy if needed.

HESI Hint • Physiologic jaundice occurs at 2 to 3 days of life. If it occurs before 24 hours or persists beyond 7 days, it becomes pathologic. Typically, NCLEX-RN questions ask about the normal problem of physiologic jaundice, which occurs 2 to 3 days after birth due to the immature liver's normal inability to keep up with RBC destruction and to bind bilirubin. Remember, unconjugated bilirubin is the culprit.

Nursing Plans and Interventions

A. The nurse is responsible for monitoring the newborn whether the infant is rooming-in or in the nursery!
B. Facilitate parent–infant attachment.
C. Document the infant's elimination pattern daily.
   1. Stool progression: meconium (black, tarry, sticky) stool within the first 24 hours to transitional (yellowish-green) to milk stool (yellow). Report if no stool within 24 hours.
   2. Infant should void within 4 to 6 hours of birth; then should use one diaper for each day of life, minimum, until day 6. On day 6 and beyond infant should use a minimum of six to eight diapers per day. Report if there is no urination within 24 hours. There may be brick-red "dust" in the first voidings (uric acid crystals).

HESI Hint • To evaluate exact urine output, weigh dry diaper before applying. Weigh the wet diaper after infant has voided. Calculate and record each gram of added weight as 1 mL urine.

D. Screen for phenylketonuria (PKU) after 24 hours of breast milk or formula ingestion. State laws differ regarding newborn screening. Many also screen for hypothyroidism, sickle cell, and galactosemia.
E. Document nutrition intake and calculate nutrition needs.

HESI Hint • Do *not* feed a newborn when the respiratory rate is over 60. Inform the physician and anticipate gavage feedings in order to prevent further energy utilization and possible aspiration.

NEUROMUSCULAR MATURITY

	−1	0	1	2	3	4	5
Posture							
Square Window (wrist)	>90°	90°	60°	45°	30°	0°	
Arm Recoil		180°	140° - 180°	110° - 140°	90° - 110°	<90°	
Popliteal Angle	180°	160°	140°	120°	100°	90°	<90°
Scarf Sign							
Heel to Ear							

PHYSICAL MATURITY

Skin	sticky friable transparent	gelatinous red, translucent	smooth pink, visible veins	superficial peeling or rash, few veins	cracking pale areas rare veins	parchment deep cracking no vessels	leathery cracked wrinkled
Lanugo	none	sparse	abundant	thinning	bald areas	mostly bald	
Plantar Surface	heel-toe 40-50 mm: -1 <40 mm: -2	>50 mm no crease	faint red marks	anterior transverse crease only	creases ant. 2/3	creases over entire sole	
Breast	imperceptible	barely perceptible	flat areola no bud	stippled areola 1-2 mm bud	raised areola 3-4 mm bud	full areola 5-10 mm bud	
Eye/Ear	lids fused loosely: -1 tightly: -2	lids open pinna flat stays folded	sl. curved pinna; soft; slow recoil	well-curved pinna; soft but ready recoil	formed & firm instant recoil	thick cartilage ear stiff	
Genitals (male)	scrotum flat, smooth	scrotum empty faint rugae	testes in upper canal rare rugae	testes descending few rugae	testes down good rugae	testes pendulous deep rugae	
Genitals (female)	clitoris prominent labia flat	prominent clitoris small labia minora	prominent clitoris enlarging minora	majora & minora equally prominent	majora large minora small	majora cover clitoris & minora	

MATURITY RATING

score	weeks
-10	20
-5	22
0	24
5	26
10	28
15	30
20	32
25	34
30	36
35	38
40	40
45	42
50	44

FIGURE 6-19 Estimation of gestational age. New Ballard scale for newborn maturity rating. Expanded scale includes extremely premature infants and has been refined to improve accuracy in more mature infants. (From Ballard J, et al: New Ballard score, expanded to include extremely premature infants, *J Pediatr* 119(3):4177, 1991.)

TABLE 6-15 Gestational Age Assessment

By Date	By Weight
Preterm: 20-37 wk gestation	Small for gestational age (SGA): Weight below the tenth percentile for estimated weeks of gestation
Term: 38-42 wk gestation	Average for gestational age (AGA): Weight between the tenth and ninetieth percentiles for estimated weeks of gestation
Postterm: >42 wk gestation	Large for gestational age (LGA): Weight above the ninetieth percentile for estimated weeks of gestation

BOX 6-3 *Heelstick Procedure for Newborns*

- Wash hands and put on gloves.
- Clean heel with alcohol and dry with a gauze pad.
- Choose a site for puncture that avoids the plantar artery in the middle of the heel.
- Use only the lateral surfaces of the heel.
- Puncture deep enough to trigger a free flow of blood. Wipe away first drop with sterile gauze pad.
- Collect blood in appropriate tube, on card, or on glucose "stick."

TABLE 6-16 Vitamin K

Drug	Indications	Adverse Reactions	Nursing Implications
Vitamin K (phytonadione)	• Prevention of hemorrhagic disorder in newborn • Infants are born with sterile gut; no enteric bacteria present for synthesis of vitamin K.	• Inflammation at the injection site	• Give IM in the first hour after birth. • Use the vastus lateralis muscle of the thigh. • Hold knee secure during procedure because neonate will try to move during injection.

1. Demand feeding (bottle or breast) is preferred.
2. Most bottlefed newborns eat every 3 to 4 hours; breastfed infants eat every 2 to 3 hours (the milk is digested more quickly).
3. After the initial weight loss period, the infant should gain approximately 1 oz (30 g) per day.
4. An infant needs about 50 calories/lb or 108 calories/kg of body weight, for the first 6 months.

HESI Hint • A 7 lb 8 oz (3.39 kg) baby would need 50 calories × 7 lb = 350 calories plus 25 calories (½ lb or 8 oz) = 375 calories per day. Most infant formulas contain 20 calories per oz. Dividing 375 by 20 = 18.75 oz of formula needed per day.

F. Monitor laboratory values for anemia, infection, and polycythemia (Appendix A).
   1. Hct
   2. Hgb
   3. Platelets
   4. WBC
   5. Provide parent and family with teaching plan for newborn care.
      a. *Bathing.* Teach *not* to submerge infant in water until cord falls off (7 to 10 days); continue cord care and keep diaper off cord.
      b. *Diapering.* Teach to use warm water to clean infant after voiding; use soap and water with stools. (Remember, cleanse female perineum front to back); may use A&D cream or ointment for rashes.
      c. *Crying.* Teach that infant may cry 2 hours per day when hungry, wet, or bored. Encourage picking the baby up. Teach to identify fussy periods and change environment when they occur.
      d. *Comfort.* Encourage parents to enjoy swaddling, to avoid startling infant when picking up; to try to burp when fussy or crying (may be a gas bubble).
G. Recognize signs and symptoms of a sick newborn who needs medical attention.
   1. Lethargy or difficulty waking
   2. Temperature above 37.8° C
   3. Vomiting (large emesis, not spitting up)
   4. Green, liquid stools
   5. Refusal of two feedings in a row

HESI Hint • Teach parents to take infant's temperature, both axillary and rectal. Axillary is recommended, but some pediatricians request a rectal (core) temperature.
• Axillary: Place thermometer under infant's arm and hold thermometer in place for 5 minutes.
• Rectal: Use thermometer with *blunt* end. Insert thermometer ¼ to ½ inch and hold in place for 5 minutes. Hold feet and legs firmly.

Review of the Normal Newborn

1. The newborn transitional period consists of the first _____ of life.
2. The nurse anticipates which newborns will be at greater risk for problems in the transitional period. State three factors that predispose to respiratory depression in the newborn.
3. What is the danger to the newborn of heat loss in the first few hours of life?
4. Normal newborn temperature is _____. Normal newborn heart rate is _____. Normal newborn respiratory rate is ____. Normal newborn blood pressure is ____.
5. The nurse records a temperature below 36.1° C on admission of the newborn. What nursing actions should be taken?
6. True or False: The newborn's head is usually smaller than the chest.
7. During the physical examination of the newborn, the nurse notes the cry is shrill, high-pitched, and weak. What are the possible causes?

Review of the Normal Newborn—cont'd

8. The nurse notes a swelling over the back part of the newborn's head. Is this a normal newborn variation?
9. What symptoms are common to most newborns with Down syndrome?
10. Identify three ways to determine the presence of congenital hip dislocation in the newborn.
11. Should the normal newborn have a positive or negative Babinski reflex?
12. A SGA newborn is identified as one who _____.
13. When suctioning the newborn with a bulb syringe, which should be suctioned first, the mouth or the nose?
14. A new mother asks the nurse whether circumcision is medically indicated in the newborn. How should the nurse respond?
15. Normal blood glucose in the term neonate is _____.
16. Why does the newborn need vitamin K in the first hour after birth?
17. Physiologic jaundice in the newborn occurs _____. It is caused by _____.
18. When is the screening test for PKU done?
19. A term newborn needs to take in _____ calories per pound per day. After the initial weight loss is sustained, the newborn should gain _____ per day.
20. List five signs and symptoms new parents should be taught to report immediately to a doctor or clinic.

Answers to Review

1. 6 to 8 hours
2. Cesarean section delivery; magnesium sulfate given to mother in labor; asphyxia or fetal distress during labor
3. It leads to depletion of glucose (there is very little glycogen storage in immature liver); body begins to use brown fat for energy, producing ketones and causing subsequent ketoacidosis and shock.
4. 36.5° to 37.4° C; 110 to 160 bpm; 30 to 60; 80/50
5. Place newborn in isolette or under radiant warmer, and attach a temperature skin probe to regulate temperature in isolette or radiant warmer. Double-wrap newborn if no isolette or warmer is available, and put cap on head. Watch for signs of hypothermia and hypoglycemia.
6. False: The head is usually 2 cm larger unless severe molding occurred.
7. CNS anomalies, brain damage, hypoglycemia, drug withdrawal
8. It depends on the finding. If it crosses suture lines and is a caput (edema), it is normal. If it does not cross suture lines, it is a cephalohematoma with bleeding between the skull and periosteum. This could cause hyperbilirubinemia. This is an abnormal variation.
9. Low-set ears, simian crease on palm, protruding tongue, Brushfield spots in iris, epicanthal folds
10. Hip click determination, asymmetric gluteal folds, unequal limb lengths
11. Positive; the transient reflex is present until 12 to 18 months of age.
12. Has a weight below the tenth percentile for estimated weeks of gestation.
13. The mouth; stimulating the nares can initiate inspiration, which could cause aspiration of mucus in oral pharynx.
14. There is controversy concerning this issue, but we do know it causes pain and trauma to the newborn, and the medical indications (prevention of penile and cervical cancer) may be unfounded.
15. 40 to 80 mg/dL
16. The sterile gut at delivery lacks intestinal bacteria necessary for the synthesis of vitamin K; vitamin K is needed in the clotting cascade to prevent hemorrhagic disorders.
17. Jaundice occurs at 2 to 3 days of life and is caused by immature liver's inability to keep up with the bilirubin production resulting from normal RBC destruction.
18. At 2 to 3 days of life, or after enough breast milk or formula, usually after 24 hours, is ingested to allow for determination of body's ability to metabolize amino acid phenylalanine.
19. 50; 1 oz, or 30 g
20. Lethargy, temperature > 37.7° C, vomiting, green stools, refusal of two feeds in a row

High-Risk Disorders

Antepartum Hemorrhage: Miscarriage (Spontaneous Abortion)

A. It is indicated by bleeding between conception and 20 weeks' gestation.
B. About 75% of spontaneous abortions occur between 8 and 13 weeks; they are usually related to chromosomal defects.
C. It is considered a medical emergency.

Nursing Assessment

A. Gestational age of 20 weeks or less; fetal viability absent
B. Uterine cramping, backache, and pelvic pressure
C. Bright-red vaginal bleeding
   1. Note number of perineal pads per hour.
   2. Note symptoms of shock:
      a. Rapid, thready pulse
      b. Pallor
      c. Hypotension
      d. Cool, clammy skin
   3. Assess client's and family's emotional status, needs, and support systems

Analysis (Nursing Diagnoses)

A. *Deficient fluid volume* related to …
B. *Anxiety* related to …

> **HESI Hint** • Spontaneous abortion may be the result of intimate partner violence. Intimate partner violence often begins or occurs more frequently during pregnancy.

Nursing Plans and Interventions

A. Identify type of abortion and subsequent management.
B. Monitor vital signs, level of consciousness every hour until stable.
C. Save all peripads, linens.
D. Start an IV with at least an 18-gauge over-the-needle catheter.
E. Give RhoGAM if indicated (Rh-negative mother).
F. Teach client to notify nurse if the following occur:
   1. Temperature above 38° C
   2. Foul-smelling vaginal discharge
   3. Bright-red bleeding accompanied by any tissue larger than a dime
G. Implement grief protocol if fetus loss occurs.
   1. Provide a memory packet (footprints, bracelet).
   2. Give client and family opportunity to see fetus (sex of fetus).
   3. Explain the grief process and refer to community resources for grief and loss. (RESOLVE and SHARE are examples of national bereavement support groups.)

Types and Treatments of Miscarriage

A. Threatened
   1. Description: spotting without cervical changes
   2. Treatment: bed rest for 24 to 48 hours; no sexual intercourse for 2 weeks
B. Inevitable or incomplete
   1. Description: moderate to heavy bleeding with tissue and products of conception present; open cervical os
   2. Treatment: hospitalization; D&C
C. Complete
   1. Description: all products of conception passed; cervix closed
   2. Treatment: no need for treatment
D. Septic
   1. Description: fever, abdominal pain and tenderness; foul-smelling vaginal discharge; bleeding from scant to heavy
   2. Treatment: termination of pregnancy; antibiotic therapy; monitoring for septic shock
E. Missed
   1. Description: fetus dead; placenta atrophied but passage of products of conception has *not* occurred; cervix closed
   2. Treatment: watchful waiting; check clotting factors and possibly terminate pregnancy to lessen the chances of developing disseminated intravascular coagulation (DIC).
F. Recurrent/habitual
   1. Description: loss of three or more previable pregnancies
   2. Treatment: varies based on cause; if premature cervical dilatation (incompetent cervix) is cause, prophylactic cerclage may be done.

> **HESI Hint** • Clients with prior traumatic delivery, history of D&C, and multiple abortions (spontaneous or induced) and daughters of diethylstilbestrol (DES) mothers may experience miscarriage or preterm labor related to incompetent cervix. The cervix may be surgically repaired before pregnancy or during gestation. A cerclage (a McDonald suture) is placed around the cervix to constrict the internal os. The cerclage may be removed before labor if labor is planned or left in place if cesarean birth is planned.

Gestational Trophoblastic Disease (Hydatidiform Mole)

A. Chorionic villi degenerate into a bunch of clear vesicles in grapelike clusters.
B. Hydatidiform mole is a developmental anomaly.
C. An embryo is rarely present.
D. It predisposes the client to choriocarcinoma.

B. ize and date discrepancy (uterus larger than expected for gestational age)

C. Other common findings
1. Anemia
2. Excessive nausea and vomiting
3. Abdominal cramping
4. Early symptoms of preeclampsia

Analysis (Nursing Diagnoses)

A. *Grieving* related to …
B. *Deficient knowledge* (specify) related to …
C. *Anxiety* related to …

Nursing Plans and Interventions

A. Provide preoperative and postoperative D&C care.
B. Assess the following:
1. Vital signs
2. Vaginal discharge
3. Uterine cramping
C. Provide discharge instructions.
1. Instruct to prevent pregnancy for 1 year.
2. Instruct to obtain monthly serum hCG levels for 1 year.
D. Teach signs of complications to be reported immediately to health care provider or clinic:
1. Bright-red, frank vaginal bleeding
2. Temperature spike over 100.4° F
3. Foul-smelling vaginal discharge

> **HESI Hint** • Pregnancy may mask the signs and symptoms of choriocarcinoma. If the client's hCG levels do not diminish, choriocarcinoma may develop.

E. Refer to community resource for grief and loss.

Ectopic Pregnancy

A. Fertilized ovum is implanted outside the uterine cavity, usually in a fallopian tube.
B. It occurs in 1 of 200 pregnancies.
C. It commonly occurs as the result of tubular obstruction or blockage that prevents normal transit of the fertilized ovum.
D. It is considered a medical emergency.

Nursing Assessment

A. Possible absence of early symptoms of pregnancy
B. Missed period; full feeling in lower abdomen, lower quadrant tenderness
C. Positive pregnancy test
D. Signs of acute rupture:
1. Vaginal bleeding
2. Adnexal or abdominal mass

5. Syncope; shock

Analysis (Nursing Diagnoses)

A. *Acute pain* related to …
B. *Grieving* related to …
C. *Risk for deficient fluid volume* related to …

Nursing Plans and Interventions

A. Provide admission care.
1. Assess vital signs stat.
2. Check for vaginal bleeding.
3. Start IV to administer fluids.
4. Notify health care provider immediately.
B. Perform gentle, moderate abdominal palpation and percussion.
C. Explain procedures as interventions continue; allow family member to be present if possible.
D. Prepare client for abdominal ultrasound.
E. Prepare client for possible laparotomy; give preoperative and postoperative surgical instructions.
F. Type and crossmatch for two units packed RBCs.

> **HESI Hint** • Suspect ectopic pregnancy in any woman of childbearing age who presents at an emergency room, clinic, or office with unilateral or bilateral abdominal pain. Most are misdiagnosed as appendicitis.

Abruptio Placentae and Placenta Previa

> **HESI Hint** • A client who is at 32 weeks' gestation calls the health care provider because she is experiencing dark-red vaginal bleeding. She is admitted to the emergency department, where the nurse determines the FHR to be 100 bpm. The client's abdomen is rigid and boardlike, and she is complaining of severe pain. What action should the nurse take first? First, the nurse must use her or his knowledge base to differentiate between abruptio placentae (this client) and placenta previa (painless bright-red bleeding occurring in the third trimester). The nurse should immediately notify the health care provider, and no abdominal or vaginal manipulation or examinations should be done. Administer O_2 by facemask. Monitor for bleeding at IV sites and gums because of the increased risk for DIC. Emergency cesarean section is required because uteroplacental perfusion to the fetus is being compromised by early separation of the placenta from the uterus.

Abruptio Placentae	Placenta Previa

A. Partial or complete premature detachment of the placenta from its site of implantation in the uterus
B. Occurs in 1 of 200 pregnancies
C. Usually occurs in late third trimester or in labor
D. Is the cause of 15% of maternal deaths
E. One-third of infants born to mothers with abruptio placentae die.
F. A medical emergency!
G. Cause unknown but is related to:
  1. Hypertensive disorders
  2. High gravidity
  3. Abdominal trauma (uncommon)
  4. Short umbilical cord
  5. Cocaine abuse
	A. Abnormal implantation of placenta in lower uterine segment
	B. Occurs in 1 of 250 pregnancies
	C. Bleeding usually begins in the third trimester
	D. Degrees of previas:
	  1. Partial: Placenta lies over part of cervical os.
	  2. Complete: Placenta lies over entire cervical os.
	  3. Marginal: Edge of placenta meets the rim of the cervical os.
	  4. Low-lying: Placenta implants in lower uterine segment with a placental edge lying near the cervical os.
	E. Associated with previous uterine scars, surgery, and fibroid tumors
	F. A medical emergency!

Nursing Assessment

Abruptio Placentae	Placenta Previa
A. Bleeding: concealed or overt (if overt, is dark red) B. Uterine tenderness C. Persistent abdominal pain D. Rigid, boardlike abdomen E. FHR abnormalities	A. Painless, bright-red vaginal bleeding in third trimester B. Soft uterus C. Possible signs of shock D. Placenta in lower uterine segment (indicated by ultrasound) E. FHR is usually normal

Nursing Plans and Interventions

Abruptio Placentae	Placenta Previa

A. Institute bed rest with *no* vaginal or rectal manipulation, and notify health care provider immediately.
B. Monitor BP and pulse every 15 minutes; apply electric BP monitor if available.
C. Apply external uterine and fetal monitor.
D. Place client in side-lying position to increase uterine perfusion.
E. Closely monitor contractions and FHR.
F. Begin IV infusion with 16- to 18-gauge catheter.
G. Review results for complete blood count (CBC), clotting studies, Rh factor, and type/crossmatch stat.
H. Watch for signs of developing DIC:
  1. Bleeding gums or nose
  2. Reduced laboratory values for platelets, fibrinogen, and prothrombin
  3. Bleeding from injection sites, IV sites
  4. Ecchymosis
I. Prepare for immediate emergency cesarean section.
J. Monitor blood loss; save pads and linens.
K. Provide constant nurse surveillance and allow presence of family if available.
L. Provide emotional support; teach regarding usual management and expected outcomes of abruption.
	A. Use bed rest to extend the period of gestation until fetal lung maturity is achieved (determined by an L/S ratio of at least 2:1); then delivery is accomplished.
	B. If determined during labor, institute bed rest immediately and notify physician.
	C. Monitor BP and pulse every 15 minutes.
	D. Start IV to administer fluids.
	E. Obtain blood specimen for CBC, clotting studies, Rh factor, and type/crossmatch.
	F. Monitor contractions and FHR; place external monitor on client immediately.
	G. Place in side-lying position.
	H. Continue monitoring blood loss; save pads and linen.
	I. Prepare client for ultrasound diagnosis.
	J. Prepare client and family for possible cesarean birth if placenta previa is complete.
	K. Provide emotional support and appropriate teaching regarding usual management and outcomes of placenta previa.

HESI Hint • DIC is a syndrome of abnormal clotting that is systematic and pathologic. Large amounts of clotting factors, especially fibrinogen, are depleted, causing widespread external and internal bleeding. DIC is related to fetal demise, infection and sepsis, pregnancy-induced hypertension (preeclampsia), and abruptio placentae. (DIC is discussed in greater detail in the Advanced Clinical Concepts section of Chapter 3.)

HESI Hint • Clients with abruptio placentae or placenta previa (actual or suspected) should undergo *no* abdominal or vaginal manipulation.
- No Leopold maneuvers
- No vaginal examination
- No rectal examinations, enemas, or suppositories
- No internal monitoring

Anemia

A. A decrease in the oxygen-carrying capacity of blood; often related to iron deficiency and reduced dietary intake
B. Occurs in 20% of pregnant women
C. Associated with increased incidence of miscarriage, preterm labor, preeclampsia, infection, postpartum hemorrhage, and intrauterine growth retardation

Nursing Assessment

A. Fatigue, pallor
B. Hgb and Hct signs of anemia:
    1. Hgb <11 g/dL, Hct <37% in first trimester
    2. Hgb <10.5 g/dL, Hct <35% in second trimester
    3. Hgb <10 g/dL, Hct <32% in third trimester
C. See Chapter 5, Sickle Cell Anemia.
D. Poor nutritional intake
E. Noncompliance with prenatal vitamin and iron supplementation

Analysis (Nursing Diagnoses)

A. *Ineffective peripheral tissue perfusion* related to ...
B. *Imbalanced nutrition: less than body requirements* related to ...

Nursing Plans and Interventions

A. Analyze 24-hour dietary recall.
B. Review and teach nutritional requirements for pregnancy (see Appendix B).
C. Teach about oral administration of iron (Table 6-17).

Infections

A. Includes STDs and general infections
B. Female circumcision
C. The antepartum period (Table 6-18)
D. Simple viral infections
E. STDs

HESI Hint • Female circumcision (aka *female genital mutilation [FGM]*) is a deeply entrenched cultural tradition that has no religious significance among some immigrants from Africa and the Middle East. It usually occurs to young girls between infancy and age 15. Often nonmedical personnel perform the procedure under nonsterile conditions that may lead to infections and other problems such as mechanical problems with urination or delivery of an infant. These procedures to the female genitals include pricking, piercing, scraping, cutting, and burning of the genital area.

Nursing Assessment

A. History of multiple sex partners
B. Previous history of STD or vaginal infections
C. Employment involving high exposure to infection (e.g., childcare worker, health care worker)
D. Nonspecific symptoms: fever, malaise

TABLE 6-17 Iron

Drug	Indications	Adverse Reactions	Nursing Implications
Ferrous sulfate	Iron deficiency anemia	• Constipation • Diarrhea • Gastric irritation • Nausea or vomiting	• Iron is best absorbed on an empty stomach. • To be taken with vitamin C source such as orange juice to increase absorption • Should not be taken with cereal, eggs, or milk, which decrease absorption • Should be taken in the evening if problem exists with morning sickness • Stools will turn dark green to black. • Laboratory values should be checked for increased reticulocytes and rising Hgb and Hct.

Continued

TABLE 6-18 Infections: Maternal and Fetal Effects

Infections	Maternal Effects	Fetal Effects	Treatment
• *Chlamydia trachomatis*	• Mucopurulent vaginal discharge • Dysuria • Acute salpingitis • Pelvic inflammatory disease (PID) • Sterility or infertility	• Stillbirth or neonatal death • Preterm birth • Ophthalmia neonatorum • Pneumonia	• Erythromycin • May need to treat partner: azithromycin (Zithromax)
HESI Hint • Tetracycline is contraindicated in pregnancy because it darkens the teeth of the newborn.			
• Human papillomavirus (HPV)	• Small or large, dry, wartlike growth on vulva, vagina, cervix, or rectum (condyloma acuminatum)	• Possible chronic respiratory papillomatosis	• Laser ablation or cryotherapy • In a pregnant woman, lesions usually left alone, unless mild laser treatment needed. • Explain need for possible abdominal delivery due to fetal effect.
HESI Hint • Podophyllin, which is usually used to treat HPV, is contraindicated in pregnancy because it is associated with fetal death, preterm labor, and cervical carcinoma. Quadrivalent human papillomavirus (types 6, 11, 16, 18) recombinant vaccine (Gardasil) is available to nonpregnant females 9 years and older to prevent HPV.			
• Gonorrhea (TORCH disease)	• Dysuria • Purulent vaginal discharge • PID	• Ophthalmia neonatorum • Sepsis	• Includes both partners • Penicillin and/or erythromycin and ceftriaxone used in pregnancy • Have partners use condoms until cultures negative two times
• Syphilis (TORCH disease)	• Chancre • Late abortion (syphilis is most common cause) • Positive antibody screen; will not show positive if tested too soon after exposure (usually positive 6 wk after exposure). • Positive tests for *Treponema pallidum* (FTA-ABS)	• Stillbirth • Congenital syphilis, characterized by snuffles (rhinitis) if mother has latent or tertiary syphilis • Hydrocephaly • Congenital cataracts • Copper-colored rash • Cracks around the mouth • Hypothermia (neonate may have difficulty with thermoregulation)	• Treatment before 16 weeks prevents placental transmission to fetus • Penicillin G • Erythromycin
• Toxoplasmosis (TORCH disease)	• Effects are absent or manifest as flulike symptoms.	• Stillbirth • Microcephaly • Hydrocephalus • Blindness • Deafness	• Treatment during pregnancy by sulfa drugs • May consider therapeutic abortion if discovered before 20 wk
HESI Hint • Toxoplasmosis is usually related to exposure to cats, gardening (where cat feces may be found), or eating raw meat.			

TABLE 6-18 Infections: Maternal and Fetal Effects—cont'd

Infections	Maternal Effects	Fetal Effects	Treatment
• Hepatitis (TORCH disease)	• May result in preterm birth	• Baby is HBsAg positive, IgM positive	• Carriers of hepatitis B are given a series of hepatitis immunizations that may prevent carrier status and chronic liver disease in newborn.
• Rubella (TORCH disease)	• Most severe if contracted in first trimester • Therapeutic abortion offered	• Congenital heart defects • IUGR • Congenital cataracts • Hearing or vision problems may arise in later childhood.	• No maternal treatment for the virus is available.
HESI Hint • Rubella is teratogenic to the fetus during the first trimester, causing congenital heart disease, congenital cataracts, or both. All women should have their titers checked during pregnancy. If a woman's titers are low, she should receive the vaccine after delivery and be instructed not to get pregnant within 3 months. Breastfeeding mothers may take the vaccine.			
• Cytomegalovirus (CMV) or cytomegalic inclusion disease (CID; TORCH disease)	• Maternal effects are absent or mononucleosislike	• Stillbirth • Congenital CMV • Microcephaly • IUGR • Cerebral palsy • Mental retardation • Rash • Jaundice • Hepatosplenomegaly	• No treatment is available for mother or infant.
• Herpes simplex virus (TORCH disease)	• A primary or recurrent infection • Painful vesicular genital lesions • Cesarean delivery recommended during active lesion breakout	• Disseminated or localized skin infection • CNS abnormalities	• Safety of systematic acyclovir (Zovirax) in pregnant clients has not been established; should be used in pregnant clients only when infection is life threatening.
HESI Hint • Acyclovir (used to treat herpes simplex) is not recommended during pregnancy.			
• Human immunodeficiency virus (HIV) • Acquired immune deficiency syndrome (AIDS) (TORCH disease)	• Usually asymptomatic • Chronic vaginitis • Susceptible to opportunistic diseases and immunologic suppression	• Affects fetus through transplacental transfer, exposure to maternal blood and body fluids, and through breast milk	• See Advanced Clinical Concepts, HIV Infection in Chapter 3.
• Bacterial vaginosis (vaginal infection)	• Milklike discharge with fishlike odor • Itching, burning pain • Can cause premature rupture of membranes • Postpartum endometritis	• Neonatal sepsis and death	• Treated with clindamycin or ampicillin or metronidazole (Flagyl)

Continued

TABLE 6-18 Infections: Maternal and Fetal Effects—cont'd

Infections	Maternal Effects	Fetal Effects	Treatment
• Monilial vaginitis (*Candida albicans*, yeast; vaginal infection)	• Common in diabetics and clients on long-term antibiotic therapy • Odorless thick, cheesy vaginal discharge • Severe vaginal itching • Dyspareunia	• Oral thrush or perineal rash	• Treated with miconazole nitrate cream or nystatin cream in pregnancy • Client to wear cotton undergarments and to abstain from intercourse until cured
• *Trichomoniasis vaginalis* (*Trichomonas protozoa*)	• Profuse, frothy, yellowish discharge • Irritation, itching • Dysuria • Dyspareunia	• Usually no fetal effects	• Treat with vaginal suppositories to reduce symptoms during the first and second trimesters of pregnancy

HESI Hint • Although metronidazole (Flagyl) is the treatment of choice for some vaginal infections, its use is contraindicated in the first trimester of pregnancy, and its use during the second trimester is controversial.

HESI Hint • Medications usually recommended for a nonpregnant client with an STD may be contraindicated for the pregnant client because of effects on the fetus.

E. General symptoms of STDs: vaginal discharge, genital lesions, dysuria, and dyspareunia
F. Specific symptoms (e.g., herpes simplex blisters)
G. Laboratory studies: antibody titers, TORCH, VDRL (may be negative if drawn too early), RPR, gonorrhea screen, vaginal wet-mount

Analysis (Nursing Diagnoses)

A. *Risk for injury (mother/fetus)* related to ...
B. *Deficient knowledge* (specify) related to ...

Nursing Plans and Interventions

A. See Nursing Plans and Interventions for STDs in Chapter 6.
B. Advise regarding immunity to rubella; if client lacks immunity, advise against working with children in terms of risk for exposure.
C. If diagnosed with infection, teach and counsel regarding maternal and fetal effects and how and why to follow the prescribed medical regimen.

Psychosocial Concerns: Teenage (Adolescent) Pregnancy

Definition: Pregnancy occurring at age 19 or younger
A. Teen pregnancy remains a problem and is addressed in Healthy People 2020.
B. Teen pregnancy is associated with anemia, preeclampsia, cephalopelvic disproportion (CPD), STDs, IUGR, and ineffective parenting.

Nursing Assessment

A. Determine that client's age is between 12 and 19.
B. Assess factors that influence the outcome of pregnancy.
   1. Previous history of menstrual or obstetric complications
   2. Nutritional status: 24-hour diet recall and analysis
   3. Attitude toward pregnancy and becoming a mother
   4. Access to prenatal care.
   5. Attitude toward pregnancy and becoming a mother
   6. Social support system (e.g., family, spouse, or boyfriend, friends, school)
   7. Cultural and spiritual beliefs
   8. Exposure to battering or force intercourse from boyfriend, spouse, father, or other male relative or other male
   9. Peer activities regarding smoking, drugs, and unsafe behaviors
   10. Client's activities regarding smoking, drugs, and unsafe behaviors
   11. Economic status
   12. Educational level, knowledge of pregnancy, childbearing, and childrearing

Analysis (Nursing Diagnoses)

A. *Deficient knowledge* (specify) related to ...
B. *Imbalanced nutrition: less than/more than body requirements* related to ...

Nursing Plans and Interventions

A. Establish trust and rapport through interview first, and then proceed to therapeutic relationship.
B. Avoid authoritative, punitive approach to counseling; use an information-sharing approach.
C. Provide information in private regarding options of pregnancy termination, adoption, and local agencies supporting pregnant adolescents.
D. Praise adolescent for all health-maintenance activities (e.g., coming for pregnancy testing, making prenatal visits, and well-thought-out questions).
E. Allow support person to attend prenatal visits.
F. Relate nutrition information to resumption of figure postpartum, skin health, hair integrity, and other normal adolescent concerns.
G. Teach dangers related to substance abuse during pregnancy.
  1. Smoking: low-birth-weight infant
  2. Alcohol: fetal alcohol syndrome
  3. Cocaine: preterm labor and abruptio placentae; subtle neurologic changes in the neonate
H. Teach that teratogenic fetal effects are highest in first trimester.
I. Encourage normal activities to achieve early developmental task of identity versus role confusion and late adolescent developmental task of intimacy versus isolation.
J. Encourage to stay in school, continue identity as student.
K. Prevent social isolation by encouraging adolescent to continue normal activities (e.g., attendance at school functions, games, and family activities).
L. Provide information regarding childbirth classes, peer support groups.
M. Teach major milestones in fetal development (major fetal growth in third trimester).
N. Monitor carefully for development of preeclampsia, nutritional disorders (anemia, IUGR).

> **HESI Hint** • The outcome of adolescent pregnancy depends on prenatal care. Nutrition is a key factor because the adolescent's physiologic needs for growth are already higher, and the additional stress of pregnancy only increases those needs.

Preterm Labor

Description

A. Onset of labor between 20 and 37 $^6/_7$ weeks' gestation
B. Predisposing factors to preterm labor include:
  1. Diabetes, cardiac disease, preeclampsia, and placenta previa
  2. Infection, especially UTI
  3. Overdistention of uterus due to multiple pregnancies, hydramnios, LGA baby
C. Psychosocial factors
  1. Working outside home, if stressful
  2. Two or more children under age 5
  3. Financial stress
  4. No social support system
  5. Smoking >10 cigarettes per day
D. Preterm labor is responsible for two of three neonatal deaths.
E. Neonates over 2000 g (4.5 lb) or 32 weeks' gestation have best chance of survival.

Nursing Assessment

A. True labor present: contractions with cervical changes occurring
B. FHR 110 to 160 bpm with no distress
C. No medical or obstetric disorder contraindicating continuance of pregnancy
D. Fetal fibronectin test obtained from a cervical swab indicating that preterm labor has begun

Analysis (Nursing Diagnoses)

A. *Anxiety* related to …
B. *Deficient knowledge* related to …
C. *Risk for injury (mother or fetus)* related to …

Nursing Plans and Interventions for Premature Labor

A. Antepartum
  1. Use fetal development chart to show client when baby has mature lungs (36 weeks).
  2. Teach warning signs of preterm labor.
    a. Uterine contractions every 10 minutes or more often
    b. Menstruallike cramps; low, dull backache; and pelvic pressure
    c. Increase or change in vaginal discharge
    d. ROM
  3. Teach self-assessment of uterine contractions.
    a. Instruct to lie on left side, place fingers on top of uterus.
    b. Teach to note a periodic hardening or tightening, with or without pain (contraction).
    c. Teach that more than five contractions in an hour should be reported immediately to health care provider or clinic.
  4. Use follow-up teaching with written instructions about signs of impending labor.
B. Intrapartum
  1. Home management
    a. Teach need for bed rest with fetus off of the cervix (e.g., no sitting or kneeling).
    b. Teach side-lying position and elevation of foot of bed to increase uterine perfusion and decrease uterine irritability.
    c. Teach side effects and warning signs of medications. (Client may be taking oral tocolytic drugs [terbutaline]; Table 6-19.)
    d. Teach to avoid sexual stimulation: no sexual intercourse, nipple stimulation, or orgasm.

TABLE 6-19 Medications for Intrapartal Complications

Drugs	Indications	Adverse Reactions	Nursing Implications

Terbutaline sulfate sympathomimetic agent, bronchodilator	• To stop preterm labor contractions	• CNS effects:
		  • Severe nervousness
		  • Tremulousness
		  • Headache
		• CV effects:
		  • Severe palpitations
		  • Tachycardia
		  • Chest pain
		  • Pulmonary edema
		• GI effects:
		  • Nausea
		  • Vomiting
		  • Diarrhea
		  • Epigastric pain
		• Laboratory value distortions:
		  • Low K^+
		  • Hyperglycemia
			• Administer IV.
			• Increase infusion rate every 15 min, depending on uterine response and maternal side effects.
			• Obtain maternal electrocardiogram (ECG) and laboratory values before beginning infusion.
			• Place mother on bedside cardiac monitor.
			• Monitor fetus continuously.
			• Monitor vital signs every 15 min.
			• Maternal pulse should not exceed 140 bpm.
			• FHR should not exceed 180 bpm.
			• I&O; weigh daily.
			• Prepare woman for side effects.
			• Notify health care provider of:
			  • High pulse, FHR changes, abnormal laboratory values
			  • Signs of heart failure: dyspnea, jugular vein distention, dry cough, rales in lung bases
			  • Have antidote available (e.g., a beta-blocking agent such as propranolol [Inderal])

Magnesium sulfate	• CNS depressant administered to a preeclamptic client to prevent seizures
	• May be used as a tocolytic to stop preterm labor contractions
		• CNS depression manifested by:
		  • Depressed respirations
		  • Depressed DTRs
		• Decreased urine output
		• Pulmonary edema
			• Hold if respiration <12/min, urine output <100 mL/4 hr.
			• DTRs absent
			• Monitor magnesium levels as prescribed and report values outside therapeutic range.
			• Remind client of warm, flushed feeling with IV administration.
			• Keep calcium gluconate (antidote) at bedside.

Nifedipine	• Calcium channel blocker
	• Relaxes smooth muscles of uterus by blocking calcium
	• Used as a first-line tocolytic or to continue treatment after stabilization with magnesium sulfate
		• Maternal
		  • Hypotension
		  • Fatigue
		  • Overdose produces nausea, drowsiness, confusion, slurred speech.
		  • Peripheral edema
		  • Facial flushing
		• Fetal/newborn (rare)
		  • Problems related to maternal hypotension, which would affect uteroplacental perfusion
			• Check BP for hypotension immediately before giving medication.
			• Avoid use with magnesium sulfate; can cause severe hypotension.
			• Rise slowly from lying to sitting position, then dangle feet at side of bed.
			• Do not use sublingual route of administration.

TABLE 6-19 Medications for Intrapartal Complications—cont'd

Drugs	Indications	Adverse Reactions	Nursing Implications

Indomethacin	• Prostaglandin synthetase inhibitor (NSAID)
	• Relaxes uterine smooth muscle by inhibiting prostaglandins
	• Used when other methods fail only if gestational age is less than 32 wk
		• Maternal
		  • Nausea and vomiting
		  • Dyspepsia, pyrosis
		  • Dizziness
		  • Oligohydramnios
		  • Reduced platelet aggregation, increasing risk for hemorrhage
		• Fetal
		  • Constriction of ductus arteriosus progressing to premature closure
		  • Decrease in renal function with oligohydramnios
		• Neonate
		  • Bronchopulmonary dysplasia, respiratory distress syndrome
		  • Intraventricular hemorrhage
		  • Necrotizing enterocolitis
		  • Hyperbilirubinemia
		  • Pulmonary hypertension
			• Administer for 48 hr or less.
			• Do not use for women with bleeding potential (coagulopathy, thrombocytopenia), NSAID-sensitive asthma, peptic ulcer disease, significant renal or hepatic impairment, oligohydramnios.
			• Determine amniotic fluid volume and function of fetal ductus arteriosus before initiating therapy and within 48 hr of discontinuing therapy; assessment is critical if therapy continues for more than 48 hr.
			• Administer with food or use rectal route to decrease GI distress.
			• Monitor for signs of postpartum hemorrhage.

HESI Hint • Although the toxic side effects of magnesium sulfate are well known and watched for, it is just as important to get serum blood levels of magnesium sulfate above 4 mg/dL in order to prevent convulsions and to reach therapeutic range.

HESI Hint • Hold next dose of magnesium sulfate and notify health care provider if any toxic symptoms occur (<12 respirations/min, urine output <100 mL/4 hr, absent DTRs, magnesium sulfate serum levels >8 mg/dL).

HESI Hint • When administering magnesium sulfate, always have antidote available (calcium gluconate).

HESI Hint • Tachycardia is the major side effect of tocolytic drugs, which are beta-adrenergic agents, such as terbutaline; they are used to stop preterm labor. Teach the client to take her pulse before administration and to withhold medication if pulse is not within the prescribed parameters (usually withheld if pulse is >120 to 140). If administration is via a continuous pump, teach client to monitor pulse periodically.

    e. Teach to increase oral fluid (2 to 3 L/day).
    f. Teach to empty bladder every 2 hours.
    g. Review what to do if membranes rupture or if signs of infection occur (fever, foul-smelling vaginal discharge).
  2. Hospital management
    a. Place on bed rest in side-lying position with continuous fetal monitoring (external).
    b. Notify health care provider *immediately*.
    c. Administer medications as prescribed:
      (1) Magnesium sulfate: decreases uterine activity through relaxation of smooth muscle secondary to magnesium's replacing calcium in the cells
      (2) Terbutaline and ritodrine: beta-adrenergic agent that acts on B_2 receptors, causing uterine muscle relaxation
      (3) Glucocorticoids (betamethasone): enhances fetal lung maturation or surfactant production if fetus is <35 weeks' gestation
    d. Prepare for birth or low-birth-weight infant if preterm labor is not arrested.
    e. Continuously monitor FHR.

Dystocia

A. Difficult birth resulting from any cause
B. Can result from any one or all of the 5 Ps:
1. Powers: primary uterine contractions and secondary abdominal bearing-down efforts
2. Passage: maternal pelvis, uterus, cervix, vagina, perineum
3. Passenger: fetus and placenta
4. Psyche: response to labor by woman
5. Position: position of the laboring woman
C. Dystocia is suspected when there is:
1. A lack of progress in cervical dilatation
2. A lack of fetal descent
3. A lack of change in uterine contraction characteristics (frequency, strength, and duration)
D. Dystocia, dysfunctional labor, and uterine inertia are terms used interchangeably.

Nursing Assessment

A. Hypertonic or hypotonic uterine contractions
B. Inability to bear down or push efficiently
C. Prolonged labor patterns (Table 6-20)

Analysis (Nursing Diagnoses)

A. *Acute pain* related to …
B. *Anxiety* related to …
C. *Risk for injury (mother/fetus)* related to …

Nursing Plans and Interventions

A. Notify health care provider if prolonged labor patterns occur according to the Friedman curve.
B. Assist with diagnostic procedures (ultrasound, pelvimetry, vaginal examination) to rule out CPD.
C. Assist with amniotomy performed by health care provider: Artificial rupture of membranes (AROM) may enhance labor forces.
1. Explain procedure (it is painless).
2. FHR is assessed *immediately* after rupture to determine whether there is a cord prolapse.
3. Assess fluid for color, odor, and consistency (blood, meconium, or vernix particles).
D. Initiate oxytocin infusion for induction (initiation) or augmentation (stimulation) of labor, and manage infusion delivery (Box 6-4).

HESI Hint • Dystocia frequently requires the use of oxytocin for augmentation or induction of labor. Uterine tetany is a harmful complication, and careful monitoring is required. The desired effect is contractions every 2 to 3 minutes, with duration of contractions no longer than 90 seconds. Continuously monitor FHR and uterine resting tone. If tetany occurs, turn off oxytocin, turn client to a side-lying position, and administer O_2 by facemask. Check output (should be at least 100 mL/4 hr). Oxytocin's

---

most important side effect is its antidiuretic (ADH) effect, which can cause water intoxication. Using IV fluids containing electrolytes decreases the risk for water intoxication.

Hypertensive Disorders of Pregnancy

A. Gestational hypertension
1. BP elevation occurs for the first time after midpregnancy.
2. There is no proteinuria.
B. Transient hypertension
1. Gestational hypertension, with no other signs of preeclampsia, is present at time of birth.
2. It resolves by 12 weeks after birth.
C. Preeclampsia
1. It is a pregnancy-specific syndrome that usually occurs after 20 weeks' gestation (except with gestational trophoblastic disease [hydatidiform mole]).
2. It involves gestational hypertension plus proteinuria.
D. Hemolysis, elevated liver enzymes, low platelets (HELLP) syndrome: Although not technically classified as a separate hypertensive disorder of pregnancy, HELLP syndrome is a variant of severe preeclampsia, and it can have a wide variety of risk factors and signs and symptoms.
E. Eclampsia: Seizures (with no known cause, like epilepsy) occur in a woman with preeclampsia.
F. Chronic hypertension: Hypertension has been observed before pregnancy or is diagnosed before the 20th week of gestation (with the exception of hydatidiform mole).
G. Preeclampsia superimposed on chronic hypertension: Chronic hypertension with new-onset proteinuria and a worsening of the already present hypertension, thrombocytopenia, or increased liver enzyme values.

Preeclampsia and Eclampsia

A. This is the most common hypertensive disorder; it develops during pregnancy and is characterized by elevated BP and proteinuria.
B. Preeclampsia is characterized by a BP of ≥140/90 mm with concomitant evidence of preeclampsia.
C. It usually develops during last 10 weeks of gestation or up to 48 hours postdelivery.
D. It occurs in 6% to 7% of all pregnancies.
E. It occurs predominantly in primigravida and in multigravida if experienced as a primigravida.
F. Preeclampsia is a major cause of maternal death and fetal hypoxia and death.
G. It is differentiated into three types:
1. Preeclampsia
2. Eclampsia: preeclampsia with seizures and coma
3. HELLP syndrome

TABLE 6-20 **Prolonged Labor Patterns**

Pattern	Nullipara	Multipara
Prolonged latent phase	>20 hr	>14 hr
Prolonged active phase	<1.2 cm/hr	<1.5 cm/hr
Secondary arrest	No change for >2 hr	No change for >2 hr
Prolonged deceleration phase	>3 hr	>1 hr
Protracted descent	Descent of fetus <1 cm/hr	Descent of fetus <2 cm/hr
Arrest of descent	>1 hr	>½ hr

BOX 6-4 *Nursing Protocol for Administration of Oxytocin*

- Determine any contraindications to use of oxytocin.
  - Known cephalopelvic disproportion (CPD)
  - Fetal stress
  - Placenta previa
  - Prior classical incision into uterus
  - Active genital herpes infection
  - Floating fetus
  - Unripe cervix
- Add oxytocin (Pitocin, Syntocinon) to IV fluid.
  - Piggyback at the lowest port on the primary IV line.
  - Using the lowest port ensures that very little oxytocin will be in the primary line if an emergency requires discontinuation of the drug.
  - Begin infusion slowly and increase at 20- to 30-minute increments until contractions occur every 2 to 3 minutes, are 40 to 60 seconds in duration, and are firm.
- The goal of oxytocin administration is to produce acceptable uterine contractions.
- Use external or internal fetal monitoring, continuously monitor the following:
  - FHR
  - Uterine resting tone
  - Contraction frequency, duration, and strength

HESI Hint • Women with previous uterine scars are prone to uterine rupture, especially if oxytocin or forceps are used. If a woman complains of a sharp pain accompanied by the abrupt cessation of contractions, suspect uterine rupture, which is a *medical emergency*. Immediate surgical delivery is indicated to save the fetus and the mother.

HESI Hint • The uterus is most sensitive to becoming tetanic at the beginning of the infusion. The client must *always* be attended and contractions monitored. Contractions should last no longer than 90 seconds to prevent fetal hypoxia.

H. There is no known cause of preeclampsia. Pathophysiology is characterized by:
1. Generalized vasospasm and vasoconstriction leading to vascular damage over time
2. Loss of plasma protein into the interstitial spaces (fluid is drawn into the extravascular spaces, which results in hypovolemia)
3. Hypovolemia, which results in decreased perfusion to major organs, including the uterus

Nursing Assessment

A. Baseline BP is obtained at first prenatal visit.
B. Risk factors associated with preeclampsia are:
1. Age under 17 years or above 35 years
2. Low socioeconomic status
3. Poor protein intake
4. Previous hypertension
5. Diabetes (gestational or preexisting)
6. Multiple gestations
7. Hydatidiform mole
8. Prior pregnancy with preeclampsia
9. Family history (mothers or sisters with preeclampsia)
C. Mild preeclampsia
1. BP rise to 30 mm Hg systolic and 15 mm Hg diastolic over previous baseline, or 140/90 or greater
2. Proteinuria of ≥0.3 g in a 24-hour specimen
3. Presence of associated conditions (outlined earlier)
4. Weight gain >2 lb/week
5. Proteinuria ≥1+
6. Edema, especially around eyes, face, and fingers
7. Reflexes may be normal or 2+
8. CNS symptoms: possible mild headache, slight irritability
9. IUGR, evidenced by size–date discrepancy
D. Severe preeclampsia: all of the earlier symptoms *plus* any two of the following:
1. BP of 160/110 mm Hg on two or more occasions
2. Proteinuria 2+ to 3+ (2 g in a 24-hour specimen)
3. Generalized edema (very puffy face and hands)
4. Deep tendon reflexes (DTR) 3+ or greater, plus clonus
5. Oliguria (less than 100 mL/4 hr)
6. CNS symptoms: severe headache, visual disturbances (blurred vision, photophobia, blind spots)
7. Elevated serum creatinine, thrombocytopenia, and marked liver enzyme elevation (aspartate aminotransferase [AST]) with epigastric pain related to liver spasms
E. Severe IUGR; late decelerations of the FHR
1. Eclampsia
2. Presence of seizure in a woman with preeclampsia
3. Tonic-clonic seizures
F. HELLP syndrome
1. It is characterized by hemolysis (H), elevated liver enzymes (EL), and low platelets (LP).

2. There is increased risk for abruption, acute renal failure, hepatic rupture, preterm birth, and fetal or maternal death or both.
3. Its causes arise from changes that occur with preeclampsia.
4. It is most commonly seen in older, white, multiparous women.
5. Signs and symptoms include history of malaise, epigastric or right-upper-quadrant pain, nausea, and vomiting.
6. Many women are normotensive and do not have proteinuria.
7. These women should still be treated prophylactically with magnesium sulfate (because of the increased CNS irritability that is part of the disease), even if hypertension is not present.
8. Women with HELLP are at high risk for developing the syndrome again in future pregnancies, as well as for developing preeclampsia in other pregnancies not complicated by HELLP.

Analysis (Nursing Diagnoses)

A. *Risk for injury (fetus/mother)* related to …
B. *Deficient knowledge* (specify) related to …

Nursing Care, in the Home, for the Client with Preeclampsia Antepartum

A. Home management
1. Inform client that absolute bed rest with bathroom privileges is necessary (except for regularly scheduled prenatal visits).
2. Have client weigh herself daily and report 907.18 g (2 lb)/week gain.
3. Teach client to test urine daily for protein.
4. Provide client with list of signs to report immediately to caregiver.
   a. CNS symptoms: visual disturbances, headache, nausea and vomiting, hyperreflexia, convulsions
   b. Hepatic sign: epigastric pain
   c. Renal signs: oliguria, proteinuria
   d. Fetal distress signs: decreased or absent fetal activity, unusual or extreme fetal activity
   e. Signs of abruptio placentae: vaginal bleeding, abdominal pain
5. Teach prescribed diet.
   a. High protein
   b. Limited salt intake (no longer completely restricted)
   c. Maintenance of minimum of 35 cal/kg of body weight
6. Teach that signs and symptoms include history of malaise, epigastric or right-upper-quadrant pain, nausea and vomiting.
7. Teach that many women are normotensive and do not have proteinuria.

8. Inform that the woman could be hospitalized to be treated prophylactically with magnesium sulfate (because of the increased CNS irritability that is part of the disease), even if hypertension is not present.
9. Teach that women with HELLP are at high risk for developing the syndrome again in future pregnancies, as well as for developing preeclampsia in other pregnancies not complicated by HELLP.

B. Hospital management
1. If mild eclampsia progresses to severe preeclampsia, hospitalization will be necessary.
2. Monitor level of consciousness, BP, and vital signs every 4 hours or more often if levels are elevated or abnormal.
3. Obtain fetal assessment continuously; apply external fetal monitor.
4. Assess for vaginal bleeding and abdominal pain.
5. Provide bed rest in left side-lying position.
6. Start IV infusion with 16- to 18-gauge venous catheter.
7. Insert indwelling urinary catheter with urine meter.
8. Monitor I&O hourly.
9. Maintain quiet, slightly darkened environment and limit visitors.
10. Administer magnesium sulfate and antihypertensive drugs (rare unless diastolic BP consistently over 100), and possibly oxytocin for initiation and augmentation of labor (see Table 6-19).
11. Assess daily for signs of coagulopathy.
    a. Petechiae under BP cuff
    b. Platelet decrease or increase
    c. Fibrinogen increase or decrease
12. Assess DTR and assess for clonus once each shift or more often if prescribed or abnormal.
13. Transfer to L&D department if necessary.
    a. Signs of pulmonary edema occur.
    b. HELLP syndrome occurs.
    c. Late decelerations of the FHR occur.
    d. Preterm labor begins.

Nursing Care for the Client with Preeclampsia Intrapartum

A. When a client with preeclampsia begins labor, control the amount of stimulation in the labor room.
1. Keep nurse-to-client ratio at 1:1.
2. If possible, put client in darkened, quiet private room.
3. Keep client on absolute bed rest, side-lying and with side rails up.
4. Disturb client as little as possible with nursing interventions.
B. Have client choose support person to stay with her and limit other visitors.
C. Constantly explain rationale for procedures and care.
D. Maintain IV line with 16- to 18-gauge catheter.

E. Monitor BP every 15 to 30 minutes, keeping BP cuff on or using electronic BP monitor if available.

F. Check urine for protein every hour and report any increase.

G. Determine DTR every hour and report any increase.

H. Administer magnesium sulfate (see Table 6-19).

1. It is usually given IV with a loading dose (specified by health care provider), administered over 15 to 30 minutes to get the blood level up to therapeutic serum levels.

2. Serum blood levels are usually maintained by infusing up to 2 g/hr after loading dose.

I. Monitor for toxicity during magnesium sulfate administration:

1. Urinary output <30 mL/hr
2. Respirations <12/min
3. DTR absent
4. Deceleration of the FHR, bradycardia

J. If convulsions or seizures do occur:

1. Stay with client and use call button to summon help. Have someone get health care provider stat!
2. Turn client onto side to prevent aspiration.
3. Do *not* attempt to force objects inside mouth or put fingers into woman's mouth.
4. Administer O$_2$ at 10 L/min by facemask and have suction available.
5. Give magnesium sulfate as prescribed (see Table 6-19).
6. Assess L&D status.

K. During the postdelivery period:

1. Assess BP, respirations, DTRs, and urine output every 4 hours for 48 hours (if still on magnesium sulfate, may assess every hour).
2. Carefully assess uterine tone and fundal height for uterine atony resulting from magnesium sulfate administration.
3. Monitor for blood loss: preexisting hypovolemia makes these women sensitive to even normal blood loss.
4. Instruct client to report headache, visual disturbances, or epigastric pain.
5. Check with the health care provider before administration of *any* ergot derivatives.

> **HESI Hint** • The major goal of nursing care for a client with preeclampsia is to maintain uteroplacental perfusion and prevent seizures. This requires the administration of magnesium sulfate. Withhold administration of magnesium sulfate if signs of toxicity exist: respirations <12/min, absence of DTRs, or urine output <30 mL/hr.

> **HESI Hint** • Rarely are antihypertensive drugs used in the preeclamptic client. They are given only in the event of diastolic BP above 110 mm Hg (danger of stroke). The drug of choice is hydralazine HCl.

> **HESI Hint** • Although delivery is often described as the "cure" for preeclampsia, the client can convulse up to 48 hours after delivery.

Maternal and Infant Cardiac Disease

A. Impaired cardiac function usually results from a congenital defect or history of rheumatic heart disease with valve prolapse or stenosis.

B. It is seen more commonly in women today because of surgical correction techniques in infancy that enable them to live to childbearing age.

C. Impaired cardiac function is dangerous because of the plasma volume increase that accompanies pregnancy.

D. Type and extent of disease

1. Class I: Unrestricted physical activity; ordinary physical activity does not cause cardiac symptomatology.
2. Class II: Ordinary activity causes fatigue, palpitations, dyspnea, and angina; physical activity is limited.
3. Class III: With less-than-ordinary activity, cardiac decompensation symptoms ensue; moderate to marked limitation of activity.
4. Class IV: Symptoms of cardiac insufficiency occur even at rest; no activity is allowed.

Nursing Assessment

A. History of preexisting cardiac disease

B. Cardiac decompensation

1. Subjective symptoms, determined by client
   a. Increasing fatigue
   b. Dyspnea
   c. Feeling of smothering
   d. Dry, hacking cough
   e. Racing heart
   f. Swelling of feet, legs, and fingers
2. Objective symptoms, determined by health professional
   a. Pulse >100 bpm
   b. Crackles at lung bases even after deep breathing
   c. Orthopnea and dyspnea
   d. Respirations >25/min
3. Anemia possible (Hct <32%, Hgb <10 mg/dL)

Analysis (Nursing Diagnoses)

A. *Deficient knowledge* (specify) related to ...

B. *Anxiety* related to ...

C. *Compromised family coping* related to ...

D. *Ineffective peripheral tissue perfusion* (specify) related to ...

Nursing Care for the Cardiac Maternity Client

A. Antepartum

1. Teach client to report any symptoms of cardiac decompensation (listed earlier).

2. Encourage 8 to 10 hours of sleep each night and daily rest periods.
3. Teach self-administration of heparin if prescribed.
   a. If self administration is prescribed teach client how to administer the medication.
   b. Prescribed for prevention of deep vein thrombolytic formation. Adverse reactions include: hemorrhage, GI irritation and bleeding, and thrombocytopenia
   c. Precautions: Monitor for unusual signs of bleeding; monitor CBC; give subcutaneously; caution client to use a soft toothbrush and to avoid cuts
   d. Cautions for client: Don't take aspirin or aspirin-containing medications; no salicylates; no NSAIDS, no cold, allergy products or pain relievers that contain any of these medications
   e. Follow HCP directions regarding monitoring laboratory blood work prior to administration of heparin; Be sure laboratory work is exactly what is ordered by HCP since there are two different types of laboratory tests and the therapeutic range is different for each of the laboratory tests.
   f. Report laboratory values to HCP to obtain correct dose
   g. Give client diet plan, which includes high iron, high protein, and adequate calorie intake.

5. Inform client of anticipated difficult period for control at 28 to 32 weeks, when plasma volume peaks in pregnancy.
6. Teach client to notify health care provider at first sign of infection.

B. Intrapartum
   1. Maintain a calm atmosphere, allowing presence of support persons, and keep family informed at all times.
   2. Maintain cardiac perfusion:
      a. Put client in semi-Fowler, side-lying position.
      b. Prevent Valsalva maneuvers, even during second stage (obstructs left ventricular outflow).
      c. Avoid hypotension if epidural anesthesia is used.
      d. Avoid use of stirrups in delivery room (can cause popliteal vein compression and decreased venous return).
   3. Provide pain relief and supportive measures because pain can contribute to cardiac distress.
   4. Monitor forceps delivery and episiotomy (will likely be performed to decrease the time of the second stage).

C. Postpartum
   1. Tailor care to the woman's functional classification.
   2. Continue semi- or high-Fowler position (head of bed raised), with side-lying maintained.
   3. Progress ambulation: dangling, sitting, standing, short to long ambulation according to tolerance and absence of symptoms of cardiac decompensation.
   4. Administer stool softeners as prescribed to prevent straining during bowel movement.
   5. Watch for symptoms of urinary infection: dysuria, white cells in urine, and pus in urine.
   6. Report *any* symptoms of cardiac decompensation to health care provider immediately:
      a. Tachycardia (pulse >100)
      b. Tachypnea (respirations >25)
      c. Dry cough
      d. Rales in the lung bases
   7. Report immediately any temperature spike over 38.0° C.
   8. Plan with the mother and family for support when returning home. If necessary, refer to community resources for homemaking services.

> **HESI Hint** • Nursing care during L&D for the client with cardiac disease is focused on prevention of cardiac embarrassment, maintenance of uterine perfusion, and alleviation of anxiety.

> **HESI Hint** • Because of the risk for myocardial ischemia, the use of a beta-adrenergic agent such as terbutaline and ritodrine HCL is contraindicated in treatment of preterm labor for clients who are diagnosed with cardiac disease.

> **HESI Hint** • Normal diuresis, which occurs in the postpartum period, can pose serious problems to the new mother with cardiac disease because of the increased cardiac output.

Congenital Heart Disease in the Newborn

Nursing Assessment

A. Weak cry, cyanosis worsening with crying
B. Lethargy, hypotonia, and flaccidity
C. Persistent bradycardia or tachycardia
D. Tachypnea or other signs of respiratory distress
E. Decreased or absent femoral or pedal pulses

Nursing Plans and Interventions

A. Decrease energy utilization immediately: no nippling (no pacifiers, no excessive stimulation).
B. Notify health care provider stat of findings.
C. Transfer neonate to neonatal intensive care unit (NICU) for diagnostic workup.

> **HESI Hint** • Heparin is the drug of choice during pregnancy; it does not cross the placental membrane. Warfarin (Coumadin) may *not* be taken during pregnancy due to its ability to cross the placenta and affect the fetus.

Hyperemesis Gravidarum

A. This is the inability to control nausea and vomiting during pregnancy.
B. Hyperemesis gravidarum is characterized by the inability to keep down fluids and solid foods for 24 hours.
C. It is linked to maternal hormones and possibly to psychological reactions to pregnancy.

Nursing Assessment

A. Weight loss during pregnancy
B. Signs of dehydration:
   1. Increased urine specific gravity
   2. Oliguria
C. Psychological distress (different from normal ambivalence in pregnancy)
D. Fluid and electrolyte imbalance; potential metabolic acidosis

Analysis (Nursing Diagnoses)

A. *Risk for fluid volume deficit* related to …
B. *Anxiety* related to …
C. *Imbalanced nutrition: less than body requirements* related to …

Nursing Plans and Interventions

A. Weigh daily at same time with like clothing.
B. Check urine three times daily for ketones.
C. Monitor electrolytes and hydration status. Report abnormal laboratory values to health care provider stat.
D. Progress diet from clear liquids to full liquids to bland diet to full diet.
E. Check FHR (if possible, auscultate by Doppler) every 8 hours.
F. Provide psychological support to offset client's concerns.

> **HESI Hint** • Research has found that infection by *Helicobacter pylori* (the bacterium that causes stomach ulcers) is another possible causative factor in hyperemesis. Other pregnancy and nonpregnancy risk factors for hyperemesis gravidarum include first pregnancy, multiple fetuses, age under 24, history of this condition in other pregnancies, obesity, and high-fat diets.

> **HESI Hint** • In severe cases of hyperemesis gravidarum, the health care provider may prescribe antihistamines, vitamin B$_6$, or phenothiazines to relieve nausea. The provider may also prescribe metoclopramide (Reglan) to increase the rate at which the stomach moves food into the intestines or antacids to absorb stomach acid and help prevent acid reflux.

> **HESI Hint** • Women diagnosed with hyperemesis gravidarum are often deficient in thiamin, riboflavin, vitamin B$_6$, vitamin A, and retinol-binding proteins.

Diabetes Mellitus

A. It may manifest for the first time in pregnancy as the diabetogenic effects of pregnancy increase.
B. Hormonal changes during pregnancy act to increase maternal cell resistance to insulin so that an abundant supply of glucose is available to the fetus.
C. A preexisting reduction in insulin and the glucose-sparing effects of pregnancy compromise the health of the mother and fetus.
D. If insulin cannot move glucose into maternal cells, the mother will begin to metabolize fat and protein for energy-producing ketones and fatty acids, which result in ketoacidosis.

Nursing Assessment

A. Predisposing factors include:
   1. Family history of diabetes
   2. History of more than two spontaneous abortions
   3. Hydramnios
   4. Previous baby with a weight over 4000 g (8 lb 13.5 oz)
   5. Previous baby with unexplained congenital anomalies
   6. High parity
   7. Obesity
   8. Recurrent monilial vaginitis
   9. Glycosuria
B. Abnormal glucose screen: A 1-hour glucose screen is routinely done on all pregnant women between 24 and 26 weeks' gestation.
C. Elevated glycosylated hemoglobin A$_{1c}$ used to evaluate diabetic control by reflecting blood glucose level during the previous 6 to 8 weeks indicates uncontrolled diabetes.
D. Types of diabetes mellitus include:
   1. Type 1 (insulin dependent). Client to be scheduled for hemoglobin A$_{1c}$ test (glycosylated hemoglobin reflects glucose control for the life span of the RBC, 120 days); prone to ketosis.
   2. Type 2 (non–insulin dependent). In pregnancy, insulin is required to control maternal blood glucose levels.
   3. Type 3 (gestational diabetes). Onset during pregnancy and return to normal glucose tolerance after delivery.
E. Symptoms include the three Ps: polyphagia, polydipsia, and polyuria.
F. Hypoglycemia (usually first trimester); insulin need may decrease.
G. Hyperglycemia (second and third trimesters); amount of insulin needed increases.
H. Increased incidence of preeclampsia, infection, and hydramnios

Analysis (Nursing Diagnoses)

A. *Deficient knowledge (diabetes mellitus during pregnancy)* related to …
B. *Risk for injury (fetus/mother)* related to …

Nursing Plans and Interventions

A. At diagnosis, implement the following:
   1. Review pathophysiology of disease.
   2. Teach home glucose monitoring (urine and blood).
   3. Demonstrate insulin administration.
   4. Identify signs of hypo- and hyperglycemia and the immediate actions to be taken if signs are noted (see Diabetes Mellitus in Medical-Surgical Nursing later in this chapter).
   5. Stress importance of regular prenatal visits.
   6. Encourage verbalization of concerns regarding diagnosis.
B. Refer client to dietitian for individualized diet management:
   1. Calories: 35 to 50 cal/kg of ideal body weight
   2. Complex carbohydrates: 50% of diet
   3. Proteins: 20% of diet
   4. Fat: less than 30% of diet
   5. Distribute calories among three meals and four snacks.
   6. Review relationship between exercise and diet. Hyperglycemia can be prevented by consistent utilization of calories through exercise.
C. Remind client of expected increased insulin needs in second and third trimesters, related to increasing diabetogenic effects of pregnancy.
D. Review situations that will complicate diabetic control: illness, diarrhea, and vomiting.
E. Teach client to drink orange juice followed by a glass of low-fat milk for hypoglycemic reaction or insulin reaction.
F. Teach client signs and symptoms of ketoacidosis (fruity odor to breath, nausea and vomiting, exaggerated respiratory effort, altered mental state) and that she should go to hospital immediately if any of these symptoms occur.
G. Remind client of need for the possibility of a scheduled induction between 38 and 40 weeks' gestation, when control of diabetes becomes more difficult.
H. See subsequent material: Nursing Care for the Maternity Client with Diabetes.
I. Provide care for the infant (see Nursing Care for Infant of a Mother with Diabetes later in this chapter)

HESI Hint • *Glucose Screen*
Client does not have to fast for this test; 50 g of glucose is given, and blood is drawn after 1 hour. If the blood glucose is greater than 140 mg/dL, a 3-hour glucose tolerance test (GTT) is done.

HESI Hint • A higher incidence of fetal anomalies occurs in pregnant women with diabetes. Therefore fetal surveillance is very important:
- Ultrasound examination
- Alpha-fetoprotein (to determine neural tube anomalies)
- Nonstress and contraction stress tests

HESI Hint • Oral hypoglycemics are not taken during pregnancy because of the potential teratogenic effects on the fetus. Insulin is used for therapeutic management.

HESI Hint • When a pregnant woman is admitted with a diagnosis of diabetes mellitus:
- She is more prone to preeclampsia, hemorrhage, and infection.
- Most diabetic pregnancies are allowed to progress to term (38 to 40 weeks' gestation) as long as metabolic control is maintained and fetal growth is within standards.

Nursing Care for the Maternity Client with Diabetes

A. Predelivery period
   1. Insert an IV line for infusion of insulin and a glucose-containing solution. Insulin does not cross the placental barrier.
   2. On the day of delivery, carefully assess client for insulin administration.
   3. Titrate regular insulin and glucose-containing solution to maintain blood glucose levels between 70 and 90 mg/dL during labor.
   4. Determine blood glucose hourly by fingerstick and maintain between 60 and 80 mg/dL.
   5. Position woman on left side to avoid pressure on vena cava by large fetus or hydramnios.
   6. Check urine for ketones hourly. Report any over 2+.
   7. Monitor fetus continuously, using electronic fetal monitoring system.
B. Postdelivery period
   1. Use a sliding-scale approach to insulin administration because of the precipitous fall in insulin requirements after delivery.
   2. Continue a 5% glucose infusion.
   3. Check urine each shift for ketones (sign of hyperglycemia, utilization of fat and protein for energy).
   4. Monitor for complications:
      a. Preeclampsia
      b. Postpartum uterine atony associated with uterine overdistention
      c. Infection
C. Encourage breastfeeding, which decreases insulin requirements. Insulin does not cross into breast milk.
D. Contraception: diaphragm with spermicide

HESI Hint • Insulin requirements are less during labor and drop precipitously after delivery; therefore it is useful to discontinue long-acting insulin administration on the day before delivery is planned.

Nursing Care for Infant of a Mother with Diabetes

A. Assessment
1. Macrosomia
2. IUGR
3. Hypoglycemia, hypocalcemia
4. Hyperbilirubinemia, polycythemia
5. Congenital anomalies
6. Infection
7. Prematurity
B. Nursing plans and interventions
1. Observe for birth trauma: clavicle fracture or cerebral trauma.
2. Perform heelsticks for glucose assessment at 30 minutes of age, 1 hour, and as prescribed.
3. Observe for hypoglycemia: jitteriness.
4. Observe for hypocalcemia: jitteriness.
5. Begin small, frequent feedings at 1 hour of age.

Emergency Delivery

Description: Emergency delivery (rapid, uncontrolled delivery) is a nonsterile or an unassisted delivery that can be managed without complications to mother or fetus.

Nursing Assessment

A. Bulging perineum
B. Woman screaming that the baby is coming
C. Presenting part visible at introitus

Analysis (Nursing Diagnoses)

A. *Risk for injury (mother or fetus)* related to …
B. *Anxiety* related to …

Nursing Plans and Interventions

A. Do not, at any time, leave the client alone. Have another nurse or staff member bring any equipment needed.
B. If possible, get precipitous delivery basin from emergency room or closet if birth is occurring in labor room (basin includes towels, scissors, cord clamps, bulb syringe, and placenta basin).
C. Place clean towel under mother's buttocks.
D. Have client use hee-blow or blow-blow breathing technique to slow expulsion of head over perineum.
E. If amnion is still present, rupture with fingers or clean implement when head crowns.
F. Apply gentle counterpressure against presenting part (vertex) to prevent the fetus from "popping" over the perineum, which can lacerate tissue and cause fetal cerebral trauma.

G. Check for cord around neck and remove if loose; cut if tight.
H. Deliver anterior shoulder first by gently pressing downward under symphysis.
I. Apply upward pressure over perineum to deliver posterior shoulder.
J. Deliver entire body, holding baby in slightly head-down position to facilitate mucus drainage.
K. Suction baby with bulb syringe quickly (mouth and nares).
L. Dry infant and cover with blanket or towel.
M. If equipment is available, clamp cord in two places and cut in between. If sterile supplies are not available, leave cord intact.
N. Do not milk the cord.
O. When signs of placental separation are seen (gush of blood, lengthening of cord), ask woman to gently push placenta out.
P. Put baby to mother's breast to contract uterus.

Cesarean Birth

A. Delivery of a fetus or fetuses through the abdomen
B. Whether planned (elective) or unplanned (emergency), such a client is prone to complications:
1. Anesthesia complications
2. Usual abdominal surgery complications
3. Sepsis
4. Thromboembolism
5. Injury to the urinary tract
C. The rate of cesarean-section births is more than 30% in the United States and is increasing.
D. Vaginal birth after cesarean (VBAC) rate is decreasing due to the complications associated with the procedure.

Nursing Assessment

A. Elective or repeat cesarean birth scheduled
B. Emergency cesarean birth performed to prevent harm to mother or fetus

Analysis (Nursing Diagnoses)

A. *Anxiety* related to …
B. *Risk for injury (mother)* related to …
C. *Impaired urinary elimination* related to …

Nursing Care for a Client with Cesarean Birth

A. Before cesarean birth
1. If surgery is planned, encourage couple to attend cesarean birth class.
   a. Tour of surgical area is usually provided.
   b. Film of cesarean birth is shown.
   c. Discussion is led by staff member.
2. If emergency cesarean is necessary, obtain informed consent, including health care provider's explanation of risks, benefits, and alternatives to surgery.
3. Inform anesthesiologist of need for preoperative assessment.

4. Assist with anesthesia, usually epidural.
5. Administer preoperative medications if prescribed.
   a. Usually, because fetus is in utero, no analgesia or sedative is prescribed preoperatively.
   b. Client may receive antacid to alkalize stomach contents (if aspiration occurs, less damage will be done to lung tissue) or a drug such as a histamine receptor antagonist, which is a gastric antisecretory drug that reduces the production of gastric secretions.
6. Shave abdomen from xiphoid to one quarter way down thigh, including pubic area (varies according to institution).
7. Insert Foley catheter.
8. Obtain laboratory studies: Type and crossmatch for two units packed RBCs, CBC, and chemistry.
9. Obtain catheterized or clean-catch urinalysis.
10. Have client remove dentures, contact lenses, rings, and fingernail polish and give to support person.
11. Notify nursery, neonatologist, and pediatrician of impending cesarean birth.
12. Allow presence of support person in operative suite unless hospital policy contraindicates it.
13. Maintain safety during transfer to operative suite.

B. Intraoperative care
   1. Before abdominal preparation:
      a. Place wedge under one hip to displace uterus laterally.
      b. Keep client warm with warm blankets.
      c. Monitor and document fetal heart tones continuously.
   2. Apply grounding pad to leg.
   3. Perform abdominal scrub (prep).
   4. Perform circulating nurse duties per institutional protocol.
   5. If client is awake, assess and meet psychosocial needs.

C. After cesarean birth
   1. Receive complete report, including the type of uterine incision performed.
   2. Fundal height and consistency assessment may be difficult due to abdominal bandage and pain. Note on chart if unable to determine, but gentle attempts should be made.

3. Assess temperature every hour in recovery room, then every 4 hours for 24 hours, and every 8 hours thereafter if temperature is within normal limits.
4. Assess heart rate, respirations, breath sounds, bowel sounds, and SaO_2 according to unit protocol.
5. Begin I&O assessment every 8 hours.
6. Administer pain medication as prescribed. The trend is toward patient-controlled analgesia (PCA pumps) and postoperative epidural analgesia with morphine sulfate (Duramorph), fentanyl citrate (Sublimaze) (Table 6-21).
7. Encourage participation in infant care as soon as possible, and take mother or couple to nursery often.
8. Demonstrate splinting of abdomen, coughing, deep breathing, and use of incentive spirometer to prevent respiratory complications due to stasis of lung secretions.
9. Maintain aseptic technique to prevent sepsis.
   a. Teach handwashing technique.
   b. Assess incisional healing every 8 hours.
   c. Perform scrupulous perineum care and pad changes.
   d. Assess lochia for foul odor (indicative of infection).

HESI Hint • If a woman is medicated, the responsible adult accompanying her must sign the necessary consent forms. State laws differ as to the acceptability of a friend signing the consent form rather than a relative.

HESI Hint • Babies delivered abdominally miss out on the vaginal squeeze and are born with more fluid in their lungs, predisposing them to transient tachypnea (TTN) and respiratory distress.

HESI Hint • The preferable low-transverse uterine incision usually results in less postoperative pain, less bleeding, and fewer incidents of ruptured uterus. The classical vertical incision of the uterus may involve part of the fundus, resulting in more postoperative pain, more bleeding, and an increased chance for uterine rupture.

TABLE 6-21 Narcotic Analgesics

Drugs	Indications	Adverse Reactions	Nursing Implications
Fentanyl citrate (Sublimaze)	Used as an adjunct to anesthesia	• Respiratory depression, apnea • Bradycardia, hypotension	• Have resuscitation equipment readily available. • Do not mix with IV barbiturates.
Morphine sulfate	Often first choice for severe pain	• Nausea, vomiting, constipation • Respiratory depression, depression of cough reflexes • Hypotension	• Check respirations and BP before administration; hold administration if respirations <12 or if hypotension exists. • Have antagonist, naloxone HCl (Narcan), available in case of respiratory depression.

HESI Hint • Cesarean birth clients have the same lochia changes, placental site healing, and aseptic needs as vaginal birth clients. The amount of lochia may be scant due to the exploration and cleansing of the uterus just after delivery of the placenta. However, pooling in the vagina and uterus while on bed rest may result in blood running down the client's leg when she first ambulates.

HESI Hint • A laparotomy of any kind, including cesarean birth, predisposes the client to postoperative paralytic ileus. When the bowel is manipulated during surgery, it ceases peristalsis, and this condition may persist. Symptoms include absent bowel sounds, abdominal distention, tympany on percussion, nausea and vomiting, and, of course, obstipation (intractable constipation). Early ambulation is an effective nursing intervention.

Review of High-Risk Disorders

1. What instructions should the nurse give the woman with a threatened abortion?
2. Identify the nursing plans and interventions for a woman hospitalized with hyperemesis gravidarum.
3. Describe discharge counseling for a woman after hydatidiform mole evacuation by D&C.
4. What condition should the nurse suspect if a woman of childbearing age presents to an emergency room with bilateral or unilateral abdominal pain, with or without bleeding?
5. List three symptoms of abruptio placentae and three symptoms of placenta previa.
6. What specific information should the nurse include when teaching about HPV detection and treatment?
7. State three principles pertinent to counseling and teaching a pregnant adolescent.
8. What complications are pregnant adolescents particularly prone to developing?
9. All pregnant women should be taught preterm labor recognition. Describe the warning symptoms of preterm labor.
10. List the factors predisposing a woman to preterm labor.
11. When is preterm labor able to be arrested?
12. What is the major side effect of beta-adrenergic tocolytic drugs (terbutaline)?
13. What special actions should the nurse take during the intrapartum period if preterm labor is unable to be arrested?
14. A prolonged latent phase for a multipara is _____ and for a nullipara is _____. Multiparas' average cervical dilatation is _____ cm/hr in the active phase, and nulliparas' average cervical dilatation is _____ cm/hr in the active phase.
15. What are the major goals of nursing care related to pregnancy-induced hypertension with preeclampsia?
16. Magnesium sulfate is used to treat preeclampsia.
    A. What is the purpose of administering magnesium sulfate?
    B. What is the main action of magnesium sulfate?
    C. What is the antidote for magnesium sulfate?
    D. List the three main assessment findings indicating toxic effects of magnesium sulfate.
17. What are the major symptoms of preeclampsia?
18. What is the priority nursing action after spontaneous or AROM?
19. What is the most common complication of oxytocin augmentation or induction of labor? List three actions the nurse should take if such a complication occurs.
20. List the symptoms of water intoxication resulting from the effect of oxytocin on the ADH.
21. State three nursing interventions during forceps delivery.
22. What is the cause of preeclampsia?
23. What interventions should the nurse implement to prevent further CNS irritability in the preeclampsia client?
24. A woman on the oral hypoglycemic tolbutamide asks the nurse if she can continue this medication during pregnancy. How should the nurse respond?
25. Name three maternal and three fetal complications of gestational diabetes.
26. When should the nurse hold the dose of magnesium sulfate and call the physician?
27. State three priority nursing actions in the postdelivery period for the client with preeclampsia.
28. What are the two most difficult times for control in the pregnant diabetic?
29. Why is regular insulin used in labor?
30. List three conditions clients with diabetes mellitus are more prone to developing.
31. When is cardiac disease in pregnancy most dangerous?
32. Does insulin cross the placenta–breast barrier?
33. The goal for diabetic management during labor is euglycemia. How is it defined?
34. What contraceptive technique is recommended for diabetic women?
35. List the symptoms of cardiac decompensation in a laboring client with cardiac disease.
36. What interventions can the nurse implement to maintain cardiac perfusion in a laboring cardiac client?
37. Gentle counterpressure against the perineum during an emergency delivery prevents _____ and _____.
38. When may a VBAC be considered by a woman with a previous cesarean section?
39. Before anesthesia for cesarean section delivery, the mother may be given an antacid or a gastric antisecretory drug (histamine receptor antagonist). State the reasons these drugs are given.
40. Clients who have had a cesarean section are prone to what postoperative complications?

Answers to Review

1. Maintain strict bed rest for 24 to 48 hours. Avoid sexual intercourse for 2 weeks.
2. Weigh daily; check urine ketone three times daily; give progressive diet; check FHR every 8 hours; monitor for electrolyte imbalances.
3. Prevent pregnancy for 1 year. Return to clinic or doctor for monthly hCG levels for 1 year. Postoperative D&C instructions: Call if bright-red vaginal bleeding or foul-smelling vaginal discharge occurs or temperature spikes over (38° C).
4. Ectopic pregnancy
5. Abruptio placentae: fetal distress; rigid, boardlike abdomen; pain; dark-red or absent bleeding. Previa: pain-free; bright-red vaginal bleeding; normal FHR; soft uterus
6. Detection of dry, wartlike growths on vulva or rectum. Need for Pap smear in the prenatal period. Treatment with laser ablation (cannot use podophyllin during pregnancy). Associated with cervical carcinoma in mother and respiratory papillomatosis in neonate. Teach about immunization for females age 9 to 30 with Gardasil.
7. Nurse must establish trust and rapport before counseling and teaching begin. Adolescents do not respond to an authoritarian approach. Consider the developmental tasks of identity and social and individual intimacy.
8. Preeclampsia, IUGR, CPD, STDs, anemia
9. More than five contractions per hour; cramps; low, dull backache; pelvic pressure; change in vaginal discharge
10. Urinary tract infection; overdistention of uterus; diabetes; preeclampsia; cardiac disease; placenta previa, psychosocial factors such as stress
11. Cervix is <4 cm dilated, <50% effacement, and membranes are intact and not bulging out of the cervical os.
12. Tachycardia
13. Monitor the FHR continuously and limit drugs that cross placental barriers so as to prevent fetal depression or further compromise.
14. >14 hours, >20 hours, 1.5, 1.2
15. Maintenance of uteroplacental perfusion; prevention of seizures; prevention of complications such as HELLP syndrome, DIC, and abruption
16. Answers are as follows:
    A. To prevent seizures by decreasing CNS irritability
    B. CNS depression (seizure prevention)
    C. Calcium gluconate
    D. Reduced urinary output, reduced respiratory rate, and decreased reflexes
17. Increase in BP of 30 mm Hg systolic and 15 mm Hg diastolic over previous baseline; proteinuria (albuminuria); CNS disturbances
18. Assessment of the FHR
19. Tetany. Turn off oxytocin. Turn pregnant woman onto side. Administer O_2 by facemask.
20. Nausea and vomiting, headache, and hypotension
21. Ensure empty bladder. Auscultate FHR before application, during process, and between traction periods. Observe for maternal lacerations and newborn cerebral or facial trauma.
22. The person who determines the exact cause will be our next Nobel Prize winner! However, the underlying pathophysiology appears to be generalized vasospasm with increased peripheral resistance and vascular damage. This decreased perfusion results in damage to numerous organs.
23. Darken room, limit visitors, maintain close 1:1 nurse-to-client ratio, place in private room, plan nursing interventions all at the same time so client is disturbed as little as possible.
24. No. Oral hypoglycemic medications are teratogenic to the fetus. Insulin will be used.
25. Maternal: hypoglycemia, hyperglycemia, ketoacidosis. Fetal: macrosomia, hypoglycemia at birth, fetal anomalies
26. When the client's respirations are <12/min, DTRs are absent, or urinary output is <100 mL/4 hr
27. Monitor for signs of blood loss. Continue to assess BP and DTRs every 4 hours. Monitor for uterine atony.
28. Late in the third trimester and in the postpartum period, when insulin needs drop sharply (the diabetogenic effects of pregnancy drop precipitously)
29. It is short acting, predictable, can be infused intravenously, and can be discontinued quickly if necessary.
30. Preeclampsia, hydramnios, infection
31. At peak plasma volume increase, between 28 and 32 weeks' gestation, and during stage II labor
32. No. Therefore insulin-dependent women may breastfeed.
33. 70 to 90 mg/dL
34. Diaphragm with spermicide; clients should avoid birth control pills, which contain estrogen, and intrauterine devices (IUDs), which are an infection risk.
35. Tachycardia, tachypnea, dry cough, rales in lung bases, dyspnea, and orthopnea
36. Position client in a semi- or high Fowler position. Prevent Valsalva maneuvers. Position client in a side-lying position for regional anesthesia. Avoid stirrups because of possible popliteal vein compression and decreased venous return.
37. Maternal lacerations, fetal cerebral trauma
38. If a low uterine transverse incision was performed and can be documented, and if the original complication does not recur, such as CPD
39. Antacid buffers alkalize the stomach secretions. If aspiration occurs, less lung damage ensues. An antisecretory drug reduces gastric acid, reducing the risk for gastric aspiration.
40. Paralytic ileus, infection, thromboembolism, respiratory complications, and impaired maternal–infant bonding

Postpartum High-Risk Disorders

Postpartum Infections

Description: Any clinical infection of the vaginal canal and perineum that occurs within 28 days of delivery

Nursing Assessment

A. Women predisposed to infection include those with:
1. ROM >24 hours
2. Any lacerations or operative incisions (forceps, episiotomy, or cesarean section)
3. Hemorrhage
4. Hematomas
5. Lapses in aseptic technique before or after delivery (e.g., faulty perineal care)
6. Anemia or poor physical health before delivery
7. Intrauterine manipulation, manual removal of placenta, retained placental fragments

B. Women predisposed to puerperal morbidity include those:
1. With a temperature of 38.0° C or higher
2. In whom morbidity occurs within the first 24 hours after delivery
3. In whom temperature elevation occurs on 2 successive days or in two successive 4-hour assessments

C. Signs of infection (see next section, Assessment Data for Puerperal Infection)

D. Most common organisms are streptococcal and anaerobic organisms; least common organism is staphylococcus.

Assessment Data for Puerperal Infection

A. Perineal infection
1. Temperature 38.3° C to 40° C
2. Red, swollen, very tender perineum (episiotomy site)
3. Purulent drainage, induration

B. Endometritis (infection of lining of uterus)
1. Temperature 38.3° C to 38.8° C
2. Pulse >100
3. Malaise, anorexia
4. Excess fundal tenderness long after it is expected
5. Uterine subinvolution
6. Lochia returning to rubra from serosa
7. Foul-smelling lochia

C. Parametritis (pelvic cellulitis)
1. Temperature 39.4° C to 40° C
2. Tachycardia, tachypnea
3. Severe uterine and cervical tenderness
4. WBC >25,000
5. Palpable pelvic abscess

D. Peritonitis
1. Chills and temperature to 105° F
2. Rapid, thready pulse to 140 bpm
3. Decreased urinary output
4. Paralytic ileus, abdominal distention, absence of bowel sounds

E. Thrombophlebitis (deep vein)
1. Minimal fever, if any
2. Positive Homan sign (if assessed)
3. Pain in calf or dull ache in leg
4. Swelling in extremity below pain

F. Urinary tract infection or cystitis (bladder)
1. Slight or no fever
2. Dysuria, frequency, urgency, suprapubic tenderness
3. Hematuria, bacteriuria
4. Cloudy urine

G. Pyelonephritis (kidney)
1. Temperature 38.8° C and higher, chills
2. Flank pain and costovertebral-angle tenderness
3. Nausea and vomiting
4. Dysuria, urgency, cloudy urine, hematuria, bacteriuria

H. Mastitis (breast)
1. Sore, cracked nipple
2. Flulike symptoms: malaise, chills, and fever
3. Red, warm lump in breast

Analysis (Nursing Diagnoses)

A. *Risk for injury* related to …
B. *Deficient knowledge* (specify) related to …
C. *Acute pain* related to …

Nursing Plans and Interventions

A. Implement general care pertinent to any client with a diagnosed infection:
1. Use and teach good handwashing technique.
2. Assess and record vital signs, especially temperature, every 4 hours or more often if indicated.
3. Manage fever by increasing fluids, providing cool cloths, administering acetaminophen (Tylenol) PO or by suppository.
4. Assess for signs of dehydration: inelastic skin turgor, dry mucous membranes, increased urine specific gravity.
5. Maintain hydration: Increase fluid intake to 2 to 3 L/day.
6. Promote nutrition: Teach to include four basic food groups and increase intake of foods containing vitamin C (for healing) and protein (for tissue repair).
7. Emphasize need for adherence to medication regimen (take entire antibiotic series).
8. Teach to maintain cleanliness, personal hygiene.
9. Implement medical and nursing interventions for specific diagnosed infections.

B. Perineal infection
1. Teach to stay warm, but not to use hot water bottle in bed if chilled.
2. Assess site daily for decrease in redness, pain, and discharge.
3. Assist with sitz bath and perineal lamp two to three times daily; encourage meticulous perineum care.
4. Administer antibiotics and analgesics as prescribed.

C. Endometritis
1. Usually maintain bed rest (Fowler or semi-Fowler position) with bathroom privileges.

2. Palpate fundus and abdomen every 8 hours to assess pain and involution.
3. Administer antibiotics, usually IV, commonly using a saline lock (Table 6-22).

D. Parametritis
1. Promote lochial and uterine drainage by instructing client to use semi-Fowler position.
2. Determine amount and odor of lochia (heavy, foul-smelling lochia usually indicates anaerobic bacteria).
3. Monitor for development of pelvic thrombophlebitis: Clot in ovarian vein will cause acute abdominal pain.
4. Administer IV antibiotics.

E. Peritonitis
1. Client is usually transferred to intensive care: *medical emergency.*
2. Give O$_2$ through mask.
3. Administer IV antibiotics.
4. Insert nasogastric tube for gastric decompression and prevention of vomiting caused by paralytic ileus.
5. Assess abdomen three times daily for tympany, distention, and bowel sounds.
6. Monitor and document I&O.

F. Mastitis
1. Obtain culture and sensitivity of breast milk.
2. Instruct client to breastfeed every 2 to 3 hours and to make sure breasts are emptied with each feed.
3. Do not let client cease breastfeeding abruptly unless health care provider so prescribes.
4. Tell client that she may have to discontinue breastfeeding if there is pus in breast milk or if antibiotic is contraindicated in breastfeeding. Mother should manually empty her breasts and discard the milk to maintain milk production and reduce congestion.

5. If the newborn develops diarrhea, contact health care provider regarding changing antibiotic.
6. Mastitis is usually treated at home by PO antibiotics.
7. Tell client to maintain bed rest for 48 hours.
8. Monitor client for abscess formation, need for incision, and drainage.

G. Deep vein thrombophlebitis
1. See Medical-Surgical Nursing for interventions in Chapter 4.
2. Administer anticoagulant therapy (heparin for 6 weeks; see Table 4-16).

H. Cystitis and pyelonephritis
1. Collect urine for analysis and culture.
2. Avoid catheterization if at all possible.

I. STDs
1. See Medical-Surgical Nursing in Chapter 6 for interventions.
2. Breastfeeding and rooming-in are affected when the mother has an STD (Table 6-23).

HESI Hint • A nurse must be especially supportive of a postpartum client with infection because it usually implies isolation from newborn until organism is identified and treatment begun. Arrange phone calls to nursery and window viewing. Involve family, spouse, and significant others in teaching, and encourage other family members to continue neonatal attachment activities.

HESI Hint • The most common iatrogenic cause of a UTI is urinary catheterization. Encourage clients to void frequently and not ignore the urge. IV antibiotics are usually administered to clients with pyelonephritis.

TABLE 6-22 Antibiotics

Drugs	Indications	Adverse Reactions	Nursing Implications
Clindamycin	Broad-spectrum antibiotic used to treat postpartum endometritis	• Nausea, vomiting • GI irritation • Diarrhea	• Must be used in combination with gentamicin
Ampicillin-sulbactam	Broad-spectrum antibiotic used to treat postpartum endometritis	• Rash, dermatitis • Nausea, vomiting • GI irritation	• Do not administer to clients with penicillin sensitivity. • Alternative to clindamycin and gentamicin combination
Gentamicin sulfate	Aminoglycoside antibiotic used for serious puerperal infections	• GI irritation • Nephrotoxicity • Ototoxicity • Neurotoxicity • Possible hypersensitivity	• Do not mix with any other drug. • Observe for ototoxicity: ataxia, tinnitus, headache. • Observe for nephrotoxicity: elevated BUN and creatinine levels. • Observe for neurotoxicity: paresthesia, muscle weakness. • Monitor I&O closely.
Cephalexin	Broad-spectrum antibiotic used to treat lactational mastitis	• Rash, dermatitis • Nausea, vomiting	• Do not administer to clients with penicillin allergy.

Postpartum Hemorrhage

A. It is a leading cause of maternal mortality that demands prompt recognition and intervention.
B. Hemorrhage can be caused by:
  1. Uterine atony (poor muscle tone)
  2. Lacerations of the vagina
  3. Hematoma development in the cervix, perineum, or labia
  4. Retained placental fragments
  5. Full bladder
C. Predisposing factors include:
  1. High parity
  2. Dystocia, prolonged labor

TABLE 6-23 Breastfeeding and Rooming-In Procedures for Mothers with Sexually Transmitted Diseases (STDs)

STDS	Rooming-In	Breastfeeding
AIDS/HIV positive	Yes	No
Cytomegalovirus (CMV)	Yes	No
Chlamydia	Yes	Yes
Gonorrhea (untreated)	No	No
Medication for 24 hr	Yes	Yes
Hepatitis	Yes	Yes
Herpes	Yes	Yes
Syphilis (untreated)	No	No
Medication × 24 hr	Yes	Yes
Trichomoniasis	Yes	Yes

3. Operative delivery: cesarean or forceps delivery; intrauterine manipulation
4. Overdistention of the uterus: polyhydramnios, multiple gestation, large neonate
5. Abruptio placentae
6. Previous history of postpartum hemorrhage
7. Infection
8. Placenta previa

Nursing Assessment

A. Excessive uterine bleeding during the first hour after delivery (hemorrhage, more than one saturated pad every 15 minutes)
B. Excessive uterine bleeding during the postpartum period (more than one saturated pad per hour)
C. Blood loss of more than 500 mL during vaginal delivery or loss of 1% or more of body weight (1 mL = 1 g)
D. Signs of hypovolemic shock:
  1. Decreased BP
  2. Weak, rapid pulse
  3. Cool, clammy skin, colored ashen or gray
E. Signs of hematomas developing in perineum:
  1. Intense perineal pain
  2. Swelling and blue-black discoloration on perineum
  3. Pallor, tachycardia, and hypotension (great blood loss); feeling of pressure in vagina, urethra, and bladder
  4. Possible urinary retention, uterine displacement
F. Signs of bleeding from unrepaired laceration:
  1. Continuous trickle from vagina
  2. Bleeding in spurts
  3. Bleeding in presence of contracted fundus
G. Signs of bleeding from uterine atony:
  1. Soft, boggy uterus usually above umbilicus
  2. Fundus that does not firm up with massage

Analysis (Nursing Diagnoses)

A. *Risk for deficient fluid volume* related to …
B. *Anxiety* related to …
C. *Risk for infection* related to …

Nursing Plans and Interventions

A. Early postpartum
  1. Review chart for predisposing factors.
  2. Monitor vital signs, fundus, lochia every 15 minutes for 1 hour; every 30 minutes for 1 hour; and every hour for the next 2 hours, or according to institution's policy.
  3. Monitor level of consciousness.
  4. Keep the bladder empty.
  5. Call physician if atony or bleeding continues despite massage.
  6. Anticipate increasing oxytocin IV infusion and administering ergot preparation IM.
  7. Count pads saturated and time required to saturate.
  8. Monitor I&O (at least 30 mL/hr output); be sure to maintain fluid replacement.

B. Late postpartum
   1. Anticipate quick hospitalization and determination of cause of bleeding.
   2. Type and crossmatch for possible blood transfusion.
   3. Administer oxytocic drugs and possibly ergot preparations as prescribed.
   4. Administer antibiotics as prescribed.
   5. Keep the client warm, and be alert for symptoms of shock.
   6. Prepare client for possible surgical repair of laceration, evacuation of hematomas, or curettage for removal of placental fragments (most common reason for late postpartum hemorrhage).
C. Hematoma development
   1. Apply ice pack to perineum to decrease swelling and pain.
   2. Prepare client for surgical incision if hematoma is large.
   3. Monitor vital signs closely. Because hemorrhage is covert, hypovolemia and anemia can occur without overt signs.
   4. Administer analgesics and antibiotics as prescribed.
   5. If severe hemorrhage and hypovolemic shock occur, notify physician immediately and:
      a. Increase IV infusion to wide open.
      b. Give O_2 at 10 L by facemask.
      c. Monitor vital signs every 5 to 15 minutes.

   d. Lower head of bed; position client supine.
   e. Assist with insertion of central venous pressure (CVP) line or hemodynamic catheter.
   f. Insert Foley catheter.

> **HESI Hint** • During medical emergencies such as bleeding episodes, clients need calm, direct explanations and assurance that all is being done that can be done. If possible, allow support person at bedside.

> **HESI Hint** • Risk factors for hemorrhage include dystocia, prolonged labor, overdistended uterus, abruptio placentae, and infection.

> **HESI Hint** • What immediate nursing actions should be taken when a postpartum hemorrhage is detected?
> • Perform fundal massage.
> • Notify the health care provider if the fundus does not become firm with massage.
> • Count pads to estimate blood loss.
> • Assess and record vital signs.
> • Increase IV fluids (additional IV line may be indicated).
> • Administer oxytocin infusion as prescribed.

Review of Postpartum High-Risk Disorders

1. May women with a positive HIV antibody try to breastfeed?
2. What are the common side effects of antibiotics used to treat puerperal infection?
3. How does the nurse differentiate the symptomatology of cystitis from that of pyelonephritis?
4. What are the signs of endometritis?
5. What are the nursing actions for endometritis and parametritis?
6. State four risk factors for or predisposing factors to postpartum infection.
7. State four risk factors for or predisposing factors to postpartum hemorrhage.
8. What immediate nursing actions should be taken when a postpartum hemorrhage is detected?
9. Must women diagnosed with mastitis stop breastfeeding?

Answers to Review

1. No, HIV has been found in breast milk.
2. GI adverse reactions: nausea, vomiting, diarrhea, and cramping. Hypersensitivity reactions: rashes, urticaria, and hives
3. Pyelonephritis has the same symptoms as cystitis (dysuria, frequency, and urgency) with the addition of flank pain, fever, and pain at costovertebral angle.
4. Subinvolution (boggy, high uterus); lochia returning to rubra with possible foul smell; temperature 38.0° C or higher; unusual fundal tenderness
5. Measures to promote lochial drainage; antipyretic measures (acetaminophen, cool cloths); administration of analgesics and antibiotics as prescribed; increase of fluids, with attention to high-protein and high-vitamin C diet
6. Operative delivery, intrauterine manipulation, anemia or poor physical health, traumatic delivery, and hemorrhage
7. Dystocia or prolonged labor, overdistention of the uterus, abruptio placentae, and infection
8. Fundal massage. Notify health care provider if massage does not firm fundus. Count pads to estimate blood loss. Assess and record vital signs. Increase IV fluids and administer oxytocin infusion as prescribed.
9. No, women who stop breastfeeding abruptly may make the situation worse by increasing congestion and engorgement and providing further media for bacterial growth. Client may have to discontinue breastfeeding if pus is present or if antibiotics are contraindicated for neonate.

Newborn High-Risk Disorders

Major Danger Signals in the Newborn

A. Of neonates requiring special care at birth, 60% can be identified through the prenatal history and another 20% through a review of intrapartal risk factors.

B. Infants with Apgar scores of 7 to 10 rarely need resuscitative efforts; scores of 4 to 6 indicate mild to moderate asphyxia, and scores of 0 to 3 indicate severe asphyxia.

C. The family experiences extreme challenges in adapting to the crisis of a sick baby.

Danger Signs by System

A. Central nervous system: lethargy, high-pitched cry, jitteriness, seizures, bulging fontanels

B. Respiratory system: apnea (lack of breathing for 15 seconds), tachypnea, flaring nares, retractions, seesaw breathing, grunting, abnormal blood gases

C. Cardiovascular system: abnormal rate and rhythm, persistent murmurs, differentials in pulse, dusky skin color, circumoral cyanosis

D. Gastrointestinal system: absent feeding reflexes, vomiting, abdominal distention, changes in stool patterns, no stool

E. Metabolic system: hypoglycemia, hypocalcemia, hyperbilirubinemia, labile temperature

F. Newborn weight is a major variable in determining survival
   1. Low birth weight (LBW): 2500 g or less
   2. Very low birth weight (VLBW): 1500 g or less

HESI Hint • "Jitteriness" is a clinical manifestation of hypoglycemia and hypocalcemia. Laboratory analysis is indicated to differentiate between the two causes.

HESI Hint • Cold stress leads to metabolic problems in the newborn. The number-one priority in managing the newborn is to prevent loss of body heat; that is followed by using ABCs. Prevent chilling (keep the neonate under radiant warmer or in the isolette).

If an infant is cold, the first signs exhibited are prolonged acrocyanosis, skin mottling, tachycardia, and tachypnea. Neonates produce heat by nonshivering thermogenesis, which involves the burning of brown fat. If an infant is cold-stressed warm slowly over 2 to 4 hours because rapid warming may produce apnea. A neonate needs glucose; he or she has little glycogen storage and needs to be fed.

Nursing Plans and Interventions for Management of Newborn Resuscitation

A. Ventilations are done over mouth and nose using a size 1 mask for a term neonate, a size 0 for a preterm.

B. With neonates, initial ventilation with peak inflating pressures of 30 to 40 cm H_2O at a rate of 40 to 60 per minute is usually successful in unresponsive term infants.

C. If the heart rate is under 60, compressions are done with thumbs side by side; hands encircle the thorax and cover the lower third of the sternum to a depth of one-third the anteroposterior chest diameter. The compression:ventilation ratio is 3:1 to achieve 120 events per minute (90 compressions plus 30 breaths).

D. Start IV fluids (usually in umbilical vein; may use peripheral vein).

E. Administer sodium bicarbonate or epinephrine as prescribed (Table 6-24).

F. Administer glucose as prescribed (stress rapidly causes hypoglycemia).

G. Assign someone to support parents during resuscitation.

H. Resuscitative efforts may be evaluated by the Silverman-Anderson Index of Respiratory Distress. Five criteria are graded:
   1. Upper chest synchronization
   2. Lower chest retractions
   3. Xiphoid retractions
   4. Nares dilation (flaring)
   5. Expiratory grunt

TABLE 6-24 **Newborn Resuscitation**

Drugs	Indications	Adverse Reactions	Nursing Implications
Sodium bicarbonate	Correction of severe metabolic acidosis in asphyxiated infants after adequate ventilation begun	• Fluid overload • Hypernatremia • Intracranial hemorrhage	• Do not mix with calcium solutions; causes precipitate. • Use *pediatric* concentration of the drug. • Infuse slowly and monitor I&O.
Epinephrine	Asystole or severe bradycardia	• Tachydysrhythmias	• Make sure ventilation of newborn is adequate. • Do not inject directly into artery. • Monitor apical pulse or connect to ECG before use.

> **HESI Hint** • A score of 10 on the Silverman-Anderson Index of Respiratory Distress indicates that a newborn is in severe respiratory distress. This is the exact *opposite* of the method used for Apgar scoring.

Oxygen Therapy for the Newborn

Nursing Plans and Interventions

A. Principle: Always administer O_2 at the lowest concentration possible when correcting hypoxia. Use an O_2 analyzer to determine the exact O_2 concentration because O_2 is a "drug." Hypoxia and hyperoxia are both dangerous.

B. O_2 toxicity results in:
  1. Retinopathy of prematurity (retrolental fibroplasias [RLF])
  2. Bronchopulmonary dysplasia (BPD)

C. O_2 is prescribed in percentages and represents the F_{IO_2} (fraction of inspired O_2 in the "air"). Room air has an F_{IO_2} of 21%. O_2 can be prescribed at between 21% and 199%.

D. Administration of O_2 to a newborn is done via:
  1. Oxy-Hood: for concentrations up to 100%
  2. Nasal prongs: for low concentrations
  3. Continuous positive airway pressure (CPAP), which:
     a. Reduces the work of breathing and keeps alveoli open to prevent atelectasis (works like the expiratory grunt)
     b. Is administered by nasal prongs or mechanical ventilator

E. Surfactant administration, with natural bovine lung extract, beractant (Survanta), or artificial surfactant, is administered via endotracheal tube as an adjunct to oxygen and ventilation therapy to prevent and treat respiratory distress syndrome (RDS) in premature infants.
  1. Prevention of RDS: Provided at birth to infants with clinical manifestations of surfactant deficiency or with a birth weight less than 1250 g
  2. Treatment of RDS: Administered to infants with confirmed diagnosis of RDS, preferably within 8 hours of birth
  3. Observe infant's condition for changes such as diuresis that may occur with improvement.
  4. Ventilator settings may need changing as the infant's ability to oxygenate increases.

F. Adverse effects may include respiratory distress immediately after administration, bradycardia, and oxygen desaturation. Extracorporeal membrane oxygenation (ECMO): Blood is oxygenated outside the body through a bypass procedure.

G. Monitor for problems associated with neonatal hypoxia:
  1. Respiratory acidosis
  2. Organ damage
     a. Necrotizing enterocolitis (NEC). Hypoxic-ischemic injury to the mucosa of the intestinal tract results in abdominal distention, sepsis, and nutritional impairment.
     b. Patent ductus arteriosus (PDA). There is a return to fetal circulation in an attempt to provide O_2 to brain and large organs; it results in worsening respiratory distress and pulmonary edema due to increased blood flow to lungs.
     c. Intraventricular hemorrhage (IVH). Hypoxia causes vessel damage in the tiny periventricular capillaries, resulting in symptoms of increased intracranial pressure (ICP) (e.g., seizures, decreased or absent reflexes, hypotonia, bulging fontanels, enlarged head circumference, setting-sun eyes, shrill cry, hypothermia, apnea, or bradycardia).

> **HESI Hint** • Watch a newborn's Hct. It is difficult to oxygenate either an anemic newborn (lack of oxygen-carrying capacity) or a newborn with polycythemia (Hct >80%, thick, sluggish circulation).

H. Closely monitor the partial pressure of O_2 in the newborn's arterial blood (i.e., P_{O_2}).

I. Monitor oxygenation status
  1. Monitor arterial oxygen saturation level using pulse oximetry. It has a direct relationship to the partial pressure of O_2 in the arterial blood. Oxygen saturation should not fall below 90.
  2. Monitor O_2 levels by placing a TcP_{O_2} (transcutaneous oxygen pressure monitor) on the newborn. TcP_{O_2} levels should range from 60 to 80 mm Hg.
  3. Draw blood gas determinations from an arterial line every 3 to 4 hours. *Always* correlate O_2 saturation (Sv_{O_2}) and TcP_{O_2} readings with blood gases.

J. Criteria for mechanical ventilation: Oxygen administration by other means does not reverse respiratory acidosis: pH <7.2, P_{O_2} <50, P_{CO_2} >60.

> **HESI Hint** • The P_{O_2} should be maintained between 50 and 90 mm Hg. P_{O_2} <50 signifies hypoxia; P_{O_2} >90 signifies oxygen toxicity problems.

Neonate with Sepsis

Infections, especially in a preterm infant, can be overwhelming because of the immaturity of the immune system.

Nursing Assessment

A. Lethargy
B. Temperature instability
C. Difficulty feeding
D. Subtle color changes: mottling, duskiness
E. "Just acts funny"; subtle changes in behavior
F. Respiratory distress, apnea
G. Hyperbilirubinemia

Analysis (Nursing Diagnoses)

A. *Ineffective thermoregulation* related to ...
B. *Risk for injury* related to ...

Nursing Plans and Interventions

A. Prevent infection in the high-risk newborn
   1. Meticulous handwashing: 3 minutes before day begins, 1 minute in between each baby
   2. Apply triple-dye antimicrobial to cord.
   3. Maintain sterile technique during procedures.
   4. Avoid wearing rings and other jewelry in nursery, and no artificial nails.
   5. During contact with body secretions, *use universal precautions! Wear gloves!*
   6. Document appearance of IV site every 30 to 60 minutes.
   7. Watch skin integrity: Use little tape; use sheepskin, waterbed, and range of motion.
   8. Be alert for any staff member who has a herpes lesion that has not reached the crusting stage; such a person should *not* be in the nursery.
   9. Maintain adequate nutrition: Calculate calorie, protein, and fluid needs according to weight.
B. If neonate develops signs of sepsis:
   1. Place in incubator or isolette and put in isolation room if possible.
   2. Assist health care provider with a sepsis workup: blood cultures, spinal tap (cerebrospinal fluid), urine collection, chest radiograph, chemistry, and CBC with differential.
   3. Administer antibiotics as prescribed.

> **HESI Hint** • Antibiotic dosage is based on the neonate's weight in kilograms. Peak and trough drug levels are drawn to evaluate whether therapeutic drug levels have been achieved. Closely monitor the neonate for adverse effects of all drugs.

Preterm Newborn Care

Definition: Supportive care for the neonate born at less than 38 weeks' gestation is based on the level of immaturity identified by gestational age and physical assessment.

Nursing Assessment

A. Respiratory distress due to:
   1. Lung immaturity
   2. Lack of surfactant lining alveoli (air sacs)
   3. Immaturity of respiratory center in brain causing apnea and bradycardia
   4. PDA, usually related to hypoxia
   5. Results in an RDS (hypoxia and hypercarbia)
B. Temperature instability related to:
   1. Insufficient subcutaneous fat
   2. Larger ratio of body surface area to body weight
   3. Extended, open body position
   4. Immature hypothalamus
C. Nutrition problems related to:
   1. Poorly developed suck
   2. Small stomach
   3. Immature digestion process: lacks some gastric and pancreatic enzymes (no bile salts)
   4. Hypoglycemia: decreased glycogen storage in liver
   5. Anemia: lack of fetal iron
   6. Hyperbilirubinemia: inability of immature liver to handle bilirubin metabolism
D. Fluid and electrolyte problems related to:
   1. Limited concentration/excretion ability of kidneys
   2. Metabolic acidosis: decreased buffering capacity
   3. Hypocalcemia (<7 mg/dL): inability to store and absorb calcium
E. Immunologic immaturity due to:
   1. No IgM antibodies
   2. No phagocytosis
   3. Thin skin barrier
   4. IVH: weak, fragile capillaries in ventricles of brain

> **HESI Hint** • Sepsis can be indicated by both a temperature increase and a temperature decrease.

Analysis (Nursing Diagnoses)

A. *Impaired gas exchange* related to ...
B. *Ineffective thermoregulation* related to ...
C. *Imbalanced nutrition: less than body requirements* related to ...
D. *Infection* related to ...

Nursing Plans and Interventions

A. Provide and monitor O_2 therapy.
B. Monitor thermoregulation.
   1. Place infant under radiant warmer.
   2. Cover infant with plastic wrap to reduce insensible water loss.
   3. Warm all things that touch newborn: hands, equipment, O_2, and surfaces.
   4. Maintain abdominal skin temperature at 36.6° C to 37.1° C (use skin temperature probe taped over liver), and report any temperature 36.1° C >37.2° C (both increase energy expenditure).
C. Monitor fluid and electrolytes. Observe for signs of:
   1. Hypoglycemia: jitteriness, tremors, lethargy, hypotonia, apnea, weak or high-pitched cry, eye rolling, and seizures
   2. Hypocalcemia: jitteriness, apnea, increased muscle tone, edema, abdominal distention, feeding intolerance, and Chvostek sign (twitching over tapped parotid gland)
   3. Excessive fluid volume: edema, tachycardia, bulging fontanels, and rales in lungs
   4. Deficient fluid volume: sunken fontanels, poor skin turgor, and dry mucous membranes

D. If infant weighs <1500 g, report weight loss >12% (180 g) in first few days of life.
E. Weigh diapers daily.
   1. Record diaper weight before putting it on infant.
   2. Weigh diaper after infant has voided (1 mL urine = 1 g of weight).
F. Maintain urine output of 1 mL/kg/hr and specific gravity of 1.005 to 1.012.
G. Prevent intracranial hemorrhage (increased risk in VLBW).
   1. Monitor vital signs, fontanels, muscle tone, and activity.
   2. Monitor Hct level.
   3. Follow minimal-stimulation protocol.
H. Maintain nutrition: Breast milk is best.
   1. Maintain 110 to 150 calories/kg/day; 140 to 160 mL/kg/day
   2. Give oral nipple feedings if neonate:
      a. Observe infant: can suck well, has gag reflex, and has a coordinated suck–swallow ability.
      b. Observe that infant >34 weeks' gestation is gaining 20 to 30 g/day.
      c. Observe that infant consumes feeding for 20 minutes or longer without signs of fatigue or tachycardia.
I. Use modified "preemie" formulas: provide 24 calories/oz (increase calories without increasing fluid).
J. Institute gavage feeding if necessary: indicated to avoid aspiration resulting from a weak suck, an uncoordinated suck, and respiratory distress (Box 6-5 and Fig. 6-20).
K. Provide total parenteral nutrition (TPN): for preterm or postsurgical neonate who cannot handle or cannot metabolize enteral feedings (Box 6-6).
   1. Monitor glucose, serum, and urine.
   2. Administer any IV fluid with a dextrose content above 12.5% through a central line.
   3. Monitor laboratory values daily; may include Hct and serum electrolytes.
   4. Administer calcium supplement and vitamin D to prevent rickets.
   5. Vitamin E (tocopherol) supplement is given as antioxidant to enhance cellular integrity (i.e., prevent oxygen toxicity and red cell destruction).
L. Prevent injury resulting from hyperbilirubinemia (see Nursing Care of Newborn with Hyperbilirubinemia later in this chapter).
M. Support family and parental adjustment.
   1. Refer to Box 6-7.
   2. Initiate early visitation, and accompany parents on first visit to intensive care unit (ICU).
   3. Provide information to parents daily.
   4. Teach caregiving skills
   5. Continue to enhance parent–infant bonding.
N. Plan for discharge using multidisciplinary approach.

HESI Hint • Drugs used to treat neonatal infections can be ototoxic and nephrotoxic. Close monitoring of therapeutic levels and observation for side effects are required.

HESI Hint • Closely monitor BUN and creatinine levels when administering the "-mycin" antibiotics to treat infections in a neonate. Renal immaturity in a preterm infant makes monitoring the administration of IV fluids and drugs crucial.

BOX 6-5 *Gavage Feeding*

Newborn Client

- Gather equipment: sterile feeding tube (5 to 8 Fr); calibrated syringe for formula; stethoscope; sterile syringe without needle; paper tape; formula; and medications, if prescribed.
- Position newborn with head slightly elevated and towel under shoulders.
- Measure distance from bridge of the infant's nose to the earlobe and then to a point halfway between the xiphoid process and the umbilicus.
- Pass tube along back of tongue, advancing as newborn swallows.
- Test placement:
  - Inject 0.5 mL air using a sterile syringe while simultaneously listening for air "bubble" into stomach with stethoscope over epigastrium.
  - Aspirate a small amount of stomach contents and check pH to verify gastric contents (<3).
- Aspirate and measure any residual stomach contents and reduce volume of feeding by amount of residual obtained (if health care provider so prescribes).
- Attach large feeding syringe to tube with plunger removed; pour in warmed formula or breast milk and allow to flow by gravity. Hold 6 to 8 inches above newborn's head for slow feeding: 20 minutes or 1 mL/min.
- Stop flow at neck of syringe by pinching tubing.
- Clear tubing with small amount of sterile water (1 to 2 mL).
- Pinch tubing and withdraw quickly to avoid administering the feeding nasopharyngeally.
- Infant may be burped.
- Position infant on right side to minimize possibility of regurgitation and aspiration.
- Postpone any treatments for 1 hour so feeding is retained.
- Record amount of residual, the type and amount of the feeding, the time the feeding was started and the time the feeding ended, and the newborn's response to the feeding.

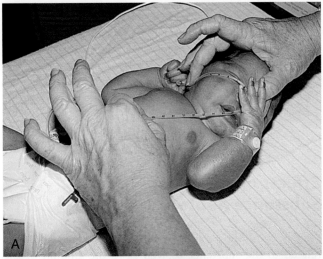

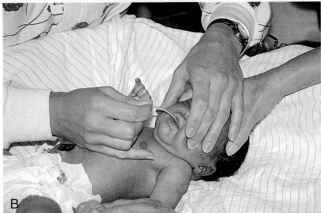

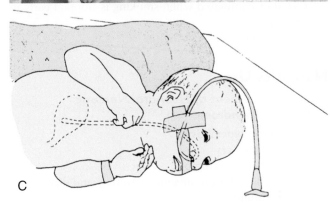

FIGURE 6-20 Gavage feeding. **A,** Measurement of gavage feeding tube from tip of nose to earlobe and then to midpoint between end of xiphoid process and umbilicus. Tape may be used to mark correct length on tube. **B,** Insertion of gavage tube using orogastric route. **C,** Indwelling gavage tube, nasogastric route. After feeding by orogastric or nasogastric tube, infant is propped on right side or placed prone (preterm infant) for 1 hour to facilitate emptying of stomach into small intestine. Note rolled towel for support. (**A** and **B,** courtesy Marjorie Pyle, RNC, Lifecircle, Costa Mesa, Calif. **C,** from Lowdermilk DL, Perry SE: *Maternity nursing,* ed 9, St. Louis, 2010, Mosby.)

Hyperbilirubinemia

Definition: Excessive accumulation of bilirubin (usually unconjugated) in the blood due to RBC hemolysis

Nursing Assessment

A. Predisposing risk factors
   1. Rh incompatibility
   2. ABO incompatibility
   3. Induction using oxytocin (Pitocin) because of IUGR
   4. Prematurity
   5. Sepsis
   6. Perinatal asphyxia
   7. Maternal diabetes mellitus or intrauterine infections
   8. Cephalohematoma
B. Jaundice: sclera, skin (if whole body is yellow or palms are yellow, there is danger of kernicterus [bilirubin encephalopathy] resulting from bilirubin deposition in brain)
C. Total bilirubin determinations
   1. Level increasing more than 5 mg/day
   2. Term: level >12 mg/dL
   3. LBW: level 10 to 12 mg/dL or greater
   4. Preterm: level >5 mg/dL (infant more sensitive to kernicterus at lower bilirubin concentrations)

D. Positive direct Coombs test. (This result indicates presence of maternal antibody in the fetal RBC, an indication of sensitization. If >1:64, an exchange transfusion is indicated.)
E. Increased reticulocyte count (usually indicates ABO incompatibility)
F. Anemia
G. Urine and stools may be dark.

Analysis (Nursing Diagnoses)

A. *Risk for injury* related to …
B. *Impaired gas exchange* related to …
C. *Anxiety (parental)* related to …

Nursing Plans and Interventions

A. Notify health care provider of any abnormal assessment factors present.
B. Implement orders for phototherapy. (Phototherapy decomposes bilirubin in the skin through oxidation.)
   1. Place unclothed neonate 18 inches below a bank of lights as prescribed until bilirubin levels fall to prescribed levels.
   2. Place opaque mask over eyes to prevent retinal damage.
   3. Monitor skin temperature.
   4. Cover genitals with a small diaper or mask to catch urine and stool while leaving skin surface open to light.
   5. Turn every 2 hours to avoid skin breakdown.
   6. Turn off the lights for 5 to 15 minutes every 8 hours to assess for conjunctivitis.
   7. Monitor for signs of dehydration.
C. Maintain hydration: nipple, gavage feedings, and IV fluids.
D. Assist with exchange transfusion.
E. Promote excretion of bilirubin by feeding in order to produce more stooling.
F. Provide a fiber-optic blanket for rooming-in or home phototherapy.

> **HESI Hint** • To assess for skin jaundice, apply pressure with thumb over bony prominences to blanch skin. After thumb is removed, the area will look yellow before normal skin color reappears. The best areas for assessment are the nose, forehead, and sternum. In dark-skinned infants, observe conjunctival sac and oral mucosa.

> **HESI Hint** • Unconjugated, indirect (fat-soluble) bilirubin is the dangerous bilirubin. It is measured by subtracting the direct from the total bilirubin. Laboratory tests measure total and direct bilirubin (conjugated, excretable, non–fat-soluble) levels.

> **HESI Hint** • Maintenance of hydration is crucial for all infants. Phototherapy treatment for hyperbilirubinemia increases the risk for dehydration. A preterm infant is already at risk for fluid and electrolyte imbalances caused by increased body surface area resulting from extended body positioning and larger body area in relation to body weight.

Effects on the Neonate of Substance Abuse

The effects on the neonate of maternal substance abuse are related to the substance as well as to the amount of the substance abused.

Cigarette Smoking

Nursing Assessment

A. Neonate is small.
B. IUGR; retardation increases with the number of cigarettes smoked.
C. Neonates of mothers who are exposed to smoke-filled environments are also at risk.

Nursing Plans and Interventions

A. Teach the antepartum client that IUGR can be minimized or eliminated when smoking is stopped early in pregnancy.
B. Treat infant as an SGA infant.

Narcotics Use

Nursing Assessment of Neonatal Narcotic Withdrawal Syndrome

A. Irritability, hyperactivity
B. High-pitched cry
C. Coarse, flapping tremors
D. Poor feeding, frantic sucking, vomiting, and diarrhea
E. Nasal stuffiness

Nursing Plans and Interventions

A. Swaddle and minimize handling.
B. Decrease environmental stimuli.
C. Provide pacifier.
D. Place in prone position with sheepskin.
E. Cover elbows and knees to prevent skin breakdown.
F. Keep bulb syringe close at hand.

Alcohol Intake

Nursing Assessment

A. Fetal alcohol syndrome (FAS):
   1. Microcephaly

2. Growth retardation
3. Short palpebral fissures
4. Maxillary hypoplasia
5. Strabismus
6. Abnormal palmar creases, irregular hair, whorls
7. Poor suck, cleft lip, cleft palate, small teeth
B. Long-term complications of FAS:
1. Mental retardation, hyperactivity, developmental delays, attention deficits
2. Poor coordination
3. Facial abnormalities
4. Behavioral deviations (irritability)
5. Cardiac and joint abnormalities

C. The combined effects of cigarette smoking and alcohol consumption during pregnancy cause greater fetal anomalies than the sum of their individual effects.

Nursing Plans and Interventions

A. Determine how much and how often the mother drank alcoholic beverages during pregnancy or while breast-feeding. (Alcohol intake has serious harmful effects on the fetus, especially when consumed during the sixteenth to eighteenth weeks of pregnancy.)
B. Decrease environmental stimuli.
C. Provide enteral feedings if neonate has incoordinate sucking and swallowing.

Review of Newborn High-Risk Disorders

1. List the major CNS danger signals that occur in the neonate.
2. A baby is delivered blue, limp, and with a heart rate <100. The nurse dries the infant, suctions the oropharynx, and gently stimulates the infant while blowing O_2 over the face. The infant still does not respond. What is the next nursing action?
3. What does the Silverman-Anderson Index measure?
4. What are the two major complications of O_2 toxicity?
5. NEC results from _____ and is manifested by _____. Ischemia/hypoxia result in _____.
6. IVH is more common in _____ and results in symptoms of _____.
7. What conditions make oxygenation of the newborn more difficult?
8. In order to prevent problems with oxygenating the newborn, what parameters can the nurse observe?
9. What are the cardinal symptoms of sepsis in a newborn?
10. A premature baby is born and develops hypothermia. State the major nursing interventions to treat hypothermia.
11. Nurses often weigh diapers in order to determine exact urine output in the high-risk neonate. Explain this procedure.
12. What factors does a nurse look for in determining a newborn's ability to take in nourishment by nipple and mouth?
13. What complications are associated with TPN?
14. In order to prevent rickets in the preterm newborn, what supplements are given?
15. List four nursing interventions to enhance family and parent adjustment to a high-risk newborn.
16. List the risk factors for hyperbilirubinemia.
17. List the symptoms of hyperbilirubinemia in the neonate.
18. Write one nursing diagnosis generated from the data pertinent to hyperbilirubinemia.
19. List three nursing interventions for the neonate undergoing phototherapy.
20. List the symptoms of neonatal narcotic withdrawal.
21. Neonates who are "sick" are prone to receiving too much stimulation in the form of invasive procedures and handling and too little developmentally appropriate stimulation and affection. How might such an infant respond?
22. How should a nurse determine the length of a tube needed for the oral gavage feeding of a newborn?
23. What are the two best ways to test for correct placement of the gavage tube in the infant's stomach?
24. What characteristics would the nurse expect to see in a neonate with fetal alcohol syndrome?

Answers to Review

1. Lethargy, high-pitched cry, jitteriness, seizures, and bulging fontanels
2. Begin oxygenation by bag and mask at 30 to 50 breaths per minute. If heart rate is <60, start cardiac massage at 120 events per minute (30 breaths and 90 compressions). Assist health care provider in setting up for intubation procedure.
3. Respiratory difficulty
4. RLF and BPD
5. Ischemic hypoxia, abdominal distention, sepsis, and a lack of absorption from intestines; injury to the intestinal mucosa
6. Premature neonates and VLBW babies; increased ICP
7. RDS: alveolar prematurity and lack of surfactant; anemia; and polycythemia
8. Po_2 50 to 90; Svo_2 60 to 80 mm Hg

9. Lethargy, temperature instability, difficulty feeding, subtle color changes, subtle behavioral changes, and hyperbilirubinemia

10. Place under radiant warmer or in incubator with temperature skin probe over liver. Warm all items touching newborn. Place plastic wrap over neonate.

11. Diaper is weighed in grams before being applied to infant. Diaper is weighed after infant has wet it. Each gram of added weight is calculated and recorded as 1 mL of urine.

12. Infant has good suck, has coordinated suck–swallow, takes less than 20 minutes to feed, gains 20 to 30 g/day.

13. Hyperglycemia, electrolyte imbalance, dehydration, and infection

14. Calcium and vitamin D

15. Initiate early visitation at ICU. Provide daily information to family. Encourage participation in support group for parents. Encourage all attempts at caregiving (enhances bonding).

16. Rh incompatibility, ABO incompatibility, prematurity, sepsis, perinatal asphyxia

17. Bilirubin levels rising 5 mg/day, jaundice, dark urine, anemia, high reticulocyte (RBC) count, and dark stools

18. Risk for injury related to predisposition of bilirubin for fat cells in brain

19. Apply opaque mask over eyes. Leave diaper loose so stools and urine can be monitored but cover genitalia. Turn every 2 hours. Watch for dehydration.

20. Irritability, hyperactivity, high-pitched cry, frantic sucking, coarse flapping tremors, and poor feeding

21. Failure to thrive, absence of crying

22. Measure from the bridge of the nose to the earlobe and then to a point halfway between the xiphoid and the umbilicus.

23. Aspiration of stomach contents and pH testing; auscultation of an air bubble injected into the stomach

24. Microcephaly, strabismus, growth retardation, short palpebral fissures, maxillary hypoplasia, abnormal palmar creases, irregular hair, whorls, poor suck, cleft lip, cleft palate, small teeth

For more review, go to http://evolve.elsevier.com/HESI/RN for HESI's online study examinations.

7 PSYCHIATRIC NURSING

Therapeutic Communication

Description: Includes both verbal and nonverbal interactions that include facial expressions, as well as body language, among the nurse, clients, colleagues, and health care providers. It is a reciprocal process that can create either a therapeutic interaction or communication barriers.

A. Communication is the primary tool used in the delivery of psychiatric nursing care and all nurse–client interactions (Table 7-1).
B. Face-to-face communication involves both the verbal and nonverbal expression of the sender's thoughts or feelings.
   1. Voice inflection, rate of speech, and words convey cognitive and affective messages.
   2. Nonverbal messages are communicated via body language, eye movements, facial expressions, and gestures (Fig. 7-1).
   3. Messages are conveyed by the sender to the recipient through sight, sound, touch, and smell. Nonverbal messages can be very powerful; for example, wrinkling your nose at a malodorous client conveys a negative and rejecting message (Fig. 7-2).
   4. The focus of therapeutic interaction is to establish a constructive relationship.
   5. It is the means through which nurses influence the behavior of others; therefore it is critical to the successful outcome of nursing interventions (Table 7-2).

Coping Styles (Defense Mechanisms)

Description: Coping styles are automatic psychological processes that protect the individual against anxiety and from awareness of internal and external dangers and stressors. The individual may or may not be aware of these processes (Table 7-3).

Treatment Modalities

Description: Psychiatric and mental health treatment modalities used to promote mental health

Types of Treatment Modalities

A. Milieu therapy
   1. The planned use of people, resources, and activities in the environment to assist in improving interpersonal skills, social functioning, and performing the activities of daily living (ADLs), as well as safety and protection for all clients.
   2. Occurs in inpatient and outpatient settings by providing clients an opportunity to actively participate in treatment, decrease social isolation, encourage appropriate social behaviors, and educate clients in basic living skills.
   3. Clients are provided a safe place to learn and adopt mature and responsible behavior through staff limit setting and client responses to maladaptive social responses.
   4. It uses limit setting; that requires consistent setting of appropriate limits by all staff, nurses, and physicians, and all health care workers to work with one another via shared communication to maintain and reestablish limit setting.
   5. It uses activities that support group sharing, cooperation, and compromise (e.g., unit-governing groups).
   6. Nursing interventions support client privacy and autonomy and provide clear expectations.
B. Behavior modification
   1. This process attempts to change ineffective or maladaptive behavioral patterns; it focuses on the consequences of actions rather than on peer pressure.
   2. Positive reinforcement is used to strengthen desired behavior (e.g., a client is praised or given a token that can be exchanged for a treat or desired activity).
   3. Negative reinforcement is used to decrease or eliminate inappropriate behavior (e.g., ignoring undesirable behavior, removing a token or privilege, giving a "time out").

TABLE 7-1 Helpful Techniques

Acknowledgment	Recognizing the client's opinions and statements without imposing your own values and judgment
Clarifying	The process of making sure you have understood the meaning of what was said
Confrontation	Should be used *judiciously*, Calling attention to inconsistent behavior
Focusing	Assisting the client to explore a specific topic, which may include sharing perceptions and theme identification
Information giving	Feedback about client's observed behavior
Open-ended questions	Questions that require more than a yes or no response
Reflecting/restating	Paraphrasing or repeating what the client has said (be careful not to overuse; client will feel as though you are not listening)
Silence	Can be therapeutic or can be used to control interaction; use carefully with paranoid client; may be misinterpreted or could be used to support paranoid ideation
Suggesting	Offering alternatives, for example, "Have you ever considered…?"

HESI Hint • The purpose of therapeutic interaction with clients is to allow them the autonomy to make choices when appropriate. Keep statements value free, advice free, and reassurance free. Remember, *just the facts! No opinions!*

HESI Hint • What action should the nurse take in a psychiatric situation when the client describes a physical problem? Assess, assess, assess! If a client in the psychiatric unit with paranoid schizophrenia complains of chest pain, take his or her blood pressure and pulse. If the obstetrical client who has delivered a dead fetus complains of perineal pain, look at the perineal area (she may have a hematoma). Just because the focus of the client's situation is on his or her psychological needs, it does not mean that the nurse can ignore physiologic needs.

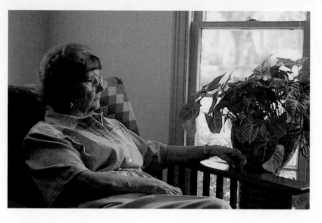

FIGURE 7-1 Body language is one important form of nonverbal communication. What might this woman's body language be saying? (From Harkreader H: *Fundamentals of nursing: caring and clinical judgment,* ed 3, Philadelphia, 2007, Saunders, p. 260, VitalBook file.)

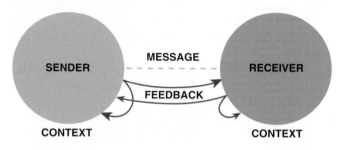

FIGURE 7-2 Communication (From Stuart G: *Principles and practice of psychiatric nursing,* ed 10, St. Louis, 2012, Mosby.

4. Role modeling and teaching new behaviors are important interventions.

C. Family therapy
 1. This form of group therapy identifies the entire family as the client.
 2. It is based on the concept of the family as a system of interrelated parts forming a whole.
 3. The focus is on the patterns of interaction within the family, not on any individual member.
 4. The therapist assists the family in identifying the roles assigned to each member based on family rules.
 5. Life scripts (living out parents' dreams) and self-fulfilling prophecies (unconsciously following what one thinks should happen, therefore setting it up to happen) are identified.
 6. Congruent and incongruent communication patterns and behaviors are identified.
 7. The goal is to decrease family conflict and anxiety and to develop appropriate role relationships.

D. Crisis intervention
 1. This form of therapy is directed at the resolution of an immediate crisis, which the individual is unable to handle alone.

TABLE 7-2 Useful and Forbidden Phrases

Description	Examples
Useful Phrases	
• These are phrases that are useful in therapeutic interaction. • Keep the interaction open, genuine, and client centered. • Keep the client as the focus. • Be aware of your own feelings and anxiety level.	• "Tell me about ..." • "Go on ..." • "I'd like to discuss what you're thinking ..." • "What are your thoughts ...?" • "Are you saying that ...?" • "What are you feeling?" • "It seems as if ..."
Forbidden Phrases	
• These are phrases that should *not* be used when interacting with clients. Avoid them at all costs (especially if they appear on an examination). • Avoid social interaction, clichés, and saying too much. • Avoid changing subjects. • Avoid words like *good, bad, right, wrong,* and *nice.*	• "You should ..." • "You'll have to ..." • "You can't ..." • "If it were me, I'd ..." • "Why don't you ..." • "I think you ..." • "It's the policy on this unit." • "Don't worry." • "Everyone ..." • "Why ...?" • "Just a second ..." • "I know ..."

HESI Hint • Basic communication principles can be applied to all clients:
• Establish trust.
• Demonstrate a nonjudgmental attitude.
• Offer self; be empathetic, not sympathetic.
• Use active listening.
• Accept and support client's feelings.
• Clarify and validate client's statements.
• Use matter-of-fact approach.

HESI Hint • Remember, a nurse's nonverbal communication may be more important than the verbal communication.

HESI Hint • A question concerning nurse–client confidentiality appears often on the NCLEX-RN®. For the nurse to tell a client that he or she will not tell anyone about their discussion puts the nurse in a difficult position. Some information must be shared with other team members for the client's safety (e.g., suicide plan) and optimal therapy.

2. A crisis may develop when previously learned coping mechanisms are ineffective in dealing with the current problem.
3. The individual is usually in a state of disequilibrium.
4. If a client is in a panic state as a result of the disorganization, be very directive.
5. Focus on the problem, not the cause.
6. Identify support systems.
7. Identify fast-coping patterns used in other stressful situations.
8. The goal is to return the individual to precrisis level of functioning.
9. Crisis intervention is usually limited to 6 weeks.

E. Cognitive therapy
1. It is directed at replacing a client's irrational beliefs and distorted attitudes.
2. It is focused, problem-solving therapy.
3. The therapist and client work together to identify and solve problems and overcome difficulties.
4. It is short-term therapy of 2 to 3 months' duration.
5. It involves cognitive restructuring.

F. Electroconvulsive therapy (ECT)
1. ECT involves the use of electrically induced seizures for psychiatric purposes. It is used with severely depressed clients who fail to respond to antidepressant medications and therapy. It may be used with extremely suicidal clients because 2 weeks are needed for antidepressants to take effect.
2. Nursing care before ECT
   a. Prepare client by teaching what the treatment involves.
   b. Avoid using the word "shock" when discussing the treatment with client and family.
   c. An anticholinergic (e.g., atropine sulfate) is usually given 30 minutes before treatment to dry oral secretions.
   d. A quick-acting muscle relaxant (e.g., succinylcholine [Anectine]) or a general anesthetic agent such as methohexital sodium is given to client before the ECT. This helps prevent bone or muscle damage.
   e. Have an emergency cart, suction equipment, and O_2 available in the room.
3. Nursing care after ECT
   a. Maintain patent airway; client is in an unconscious state immediately after ECT.
   b. Check vital signs every 15 minutes until client is alert.
   c. Reorient client after ECT (confusion is likely upon awakening, and short-term memory impairment may occur).

TABLE 7-3 Coping Styles (Defense Mechanisms)

Style	Description	Example
Denial	Unconscious failure to acknowledge an event, thought, or feeling that is too painful for conscious awareness	A woman diagnosed with cancer tells her family all the tests were negative.
Displacement	The transference of feelings to another person or object	After being scolded by his supervisor at work, a man comes home and kicks the dog for barking.
Identification	Attempt to be like someone or emulate the personality, traits, or behaviors of another person	A teenage boy dresses and behaves like his favorite singer.
Intellectualization	Using reason to avoid emotional conflicts	The wife of a substance abuser describes in detail the dynamics of enabling behavior yet continues to call her husband's workplace to report his Monday-morning absences as an illness.
Introjection	Incorporation of values or qualities of an admired person or group into one's own ego structure	A young man deals with a business client in the same fashion his father deals with business clients.
Isolation	Separation of an unacceptable feeling, idea, or impulse from one's thought process	A nurse working in an emergency room is able to care for the seriously injured by isolating or separating her feelings and emotions related to the clients' pain, injuries, or death.
Passive-aggression	Indirectly expressing aggression toward others; a facade of overt compliance masks covert resentment	An employee arrives late to a meeting and disrupts others after being reminded of the meeting earlier that day and promising to be on time.
Projection	Attributing one's own thoughts or impulses to another person	A student who has sexual feelings toward her teacher tells her friends the teacher is "coming on to her."
Rationalization	Offering an acceptable, logical explanation to make unacceptable feelings and behavior acceptable	A student who did not do well in a course says it was poorly taught and the course content was not important anyway.
Reaction formation	Development of conscious attitudes and behaviors that are the opposite of what is really felt	A person who dislikes animals does volunteer work for the Humane Society.
Regression	Reverting to an earlier level of development when anxious or highly stressed	After moving to a new home, a 6-year-old starts wetting the bed.
Repression	The *involuntary* exclusion of a painful thought or memory from awareness	A young man whose mother died when he was 12 years old cannot tell you how old he was or the year she died.
Sublimation	Substitution of an unacceptable feeling with a more socially acceptable one	A student who feels too small to play football becomes a champion marathon swimmer.
Suppression	The *intentional* exclusion of feelings and ideas	When about to lose Tara, Scarlet O'Hara says, "I'll think about it tomorrow."
Undoing	Communication or behavior done to negate a previously unacceptable act	A young man who used to hunt wild animals now chairs a committee for the protection of animals.

   d. Common complaints after ECT include:
     (1) Headache
     (2) Muscle soreness
     (3) Nausea
     (4) Retrograde amnesia

> **HESI Hint** • Vomiting by an unconscious client can lead to aspiration. Nausea is a common compliant after ECT. Because post-ECT clients are unconscious, the nurse must observe closely for the possibility of aspiration: *maintain a patent airway!*

G. Group intervention
   1. This process is used with two or more clients who develop interactive relationships and share at least one common goal or issue.
   2. The types of groups are as follows:
     a. The group may be closed (set group) or open (new members may join).
     b. The group may be small or large (>10 members).
     c. There are many types of groups (psychoeducation, supportive therapy, psychotherapy, self-help).
     d. Common nurse-led intervention groups include those that focus on medications, symptom management, anger management, and self-care.

   3. The phases in groups are as follows:
     a. The initial, or orientation, phase is characterized by:
      (1) High anxiety
      (2) Superficial interactions
      (3) Testing the therapist to see if he or she can be trusted
     b. The middle, or working, phase is characterized by:
      (1) Problem identification
      (2) The beginning of problem solving
      (3) The beginning of the group sense of "we"
     c. The termination phase is characterized by:
      (1) Evaluation of the experience
      (2) The expression of feelings ranging from anger to joy
   4. The advantages of groups are:
     a. The development of socializing techniques
     b. The opportunity to try new behaviors
     c. The promotion of a feeling of universality (i.e., not being alone with problems)
     d. The opportunity for feedback from the group, which may correct distorted perceptions
     e. The opportunity for clients to look at alternative ways of analyzing and dealing with problems

Review of Therapeutic Communication and Treatment Modalities

1. After the fourth group meeting, the informal leader makes the statement that she believes she can help the group more than the assigned facilitator and has better credentials. Identify the group dynamics and stage of development.
2. On an inpatient psychiatric unit, clients are expected to get up at a certain time, attend breakfast at a certain time, and arrive for their medications at the correct time. What form of therapy is incorporated into this unit?
3. The wife of a man killed in a motor vehicle accident has just arrived at the emergency department and is told of her husband's death. What nursing actions are appropriate for dealing with this crisis?
4. A 10-year-old is admitted to the children's unit of the psychiatric facility after stabbing his sister. His behavior is extremely aggressive with the other children on the unit. Using a behavior-modification approach with positive reinforcement, design a treatment plan for this child.
5. The 10-year-old, his sister, his mother, and the mother's live-in boyfriend are asked to attend a therapy meeting. Who is the "client" who will be treated during this session?
6. A 66-year-old woman is admitted to the psychiatric unit with agitated depression. She has not responded to antidepressants in the past. What would be the medical treatment of choice for this client?
7. Describe the nurse's role in preparing clients for ECT.
8. Describe the nursing interventions used to care for a client during and after ECT.

Answers to Review

1. The informal leader is "testing," which is a behavior indicative of a new group trying to establish trust. This group is still in the orientation phase of development.
2. Milieu
3. Take her to a quiet room, and ask her if there are family members, friends, or clergy you can call for her. Assess her need for medication and discuss it with the health care provider. Stay with her, be firm and directive, and assess previous successful coping strategies.
4. Assess what activities he enjoys. Set up a token system; when he displays nonaggressive behavior, he earns a token good toward participating in the activity selected. He loses a token when he becomes aggressive.
5. The entire family
6. ECT
7. Give accurate, nonjudgmental information about the treatment. Explore the client's concerns. Check emergency equipment. Be sure suction equipment and O_2 are available.
8. Maintain patent airway. Check vital signs every 15 minutes until client is alert. Remain with client after treatment until client is conscious. Reorient if client is confused.

Anxiety and Related Disorders

Anxiety

Description: Anxiety is unexplained discomfort, tension, apprehension, or uneasiness, which occurs when a person feels a threat to self. The threat may be real or imagined and is a very subjective experience.

Levels of Anxiety

A. Mild anxiety
   1. Is associated with daily life; motivates learning
   2. Produces increased levels of sensory awareness and alertness
   3. Allows for thoughts that are logical; client is able to concentrate and problem-solve
   4. Allows client to appear calm and in control
B. Moderate anxiety
   1. Continues to motivate learning with assistance from others
   2. Allows client to be attentive and able to focus and problem-solve but not at an optimal level
   3. Dulls perceptions of sensory stimuli; client becomes hesitant
   4. Causes client's speech rate and volume to increase; client becomes wordy
   5. Causes client to become restless (frequent body movements and gestures)
   6. May be converted into physical symptoms, such as headaches, nausea, diarrhea, and tachycardia
C. Severe anxiety
   1. Stimulates fight-or-flight response
   2. Causes sensory stimuli input to be disorganized
   3. May cause perceptions to be distorted
   4. Impairs concentration and problem-solving ability
   5. Results in selective attention, focusing on only one detail
   6. Results in the verbalization of emotional pain (e.g., "I need help, I can't stand this.")
   7. Causes tremors, increased motor activity (e.g., pacing, wringing hands)
D. Panic
   1. Causes perceptions to be grossly distorted; client is unable to differentiate real from unreal
   2. Causes client to be unable to concentrate or problem-solve; causes loss of rational, logical thinking. Client may have hallucinations.
   3. Causes client to feel overwhelmed, helpless
   4. Causes loss of control, inability to function
   5. Can elicit behavior that may be angry and aggressive or withdrawn, with clinging and crying
   6. Requires immediate intervention

HESI Hint • Common physiologic responses to anxiety include increased heart rate and blood pressure; rapid, shallow respirations; dry mouth and tight feeling in throat; tremors and muscle tension; anorexia; urinary frequency; and palmar sweating.

HESI Hint • When a nurse encounters a very anxious client, the nurse must first assess his or her own level of anxiety and remain calm. A calm nurse helps the client gain control, decrease anxiety, and increase feelings of security. Anxiety is very contagious and is easily transferred from client to nurse and from nurse to client.

Anxiety Disorders, Obsessive-Compulsive and Related Disorders, and Traumatic and Stressor Related Disorders

Generalized Anxiety Disorders

Description: Unrealistic, excessive, or persistent (lasting 6 months or longer) anxiety and worry about two or more life circumstances. Previously learned coping mechanisms are inadequate to deal with this level of anxiety. Anxiety must be out of proportion to the actual danger or threat in the situation (DSM-5).

Nursing Assessment

A. Severe anxiety
B. Motor tension
   1. Restlessness
   2. Quickly fatigued
   3. Feelings of "shakiness"
   4. Tension
C. Autonomic hyperactivity
   1. Shortness of breath
   2. Heart palpitations
   3. Dizziness
   4. Diaphoresis
   5. Frequent urination
D. Vigilance and scanning
   1. Difficulty concentrating
   2. Sleep disturbance
   3. Irritability, quick to become angry
E. On edge, appearance of being nervous
F. Low self-esteem

Analysis (Nursing Diagnoses)

A. *Anxiety* related to . . .
B. *Ineffective coping* related to . . .
C. *Disturbed sleep pattern* related to . . .

Nursing Plans and Interventions

A. Assess client so as to recognize anxiety and label the feeling (e.g., "What are you feeling now?").
B. Help client to identify the relationship between the stressor and the level of anxiety.
C. Provide opportunities to learn and test various adaptive coping responses.
D. Encourage exercise, deep-breathing techniques, visualization, relaxation techniques, and biofeedback.
E. Decrease environmental stimuli.

Panic Disorders and Phobias

A. Discrete periods of intense fear or discomfort that are unexpected and may be incapacitating.
B. It is characterized by an irrational fear of an external object, activity, situation, and feelings of impending doom.
C. It is a chronic condition that has exacerbations and remissions.
D. The client transfers anxiety or fear from its source to a symbolic object, idea, or situation.
E. The client recognizes that the fear is excessive and unrealistic but "can't help it."

Common Phobias

A. Acrophobia: fear of heights
B. Agoraphobia: fear of crowds or open places
C. Claustrophobia: fear of closed-in places
D. Hydrophobia: fear of water
E. Social anxiety disorder
F. Thanatophobia: fear of death

Nursing Assessment

A. Coping styles used (see Table 7-3):
   1. Displacement
   2. Projection
   3. Repression
   4. Sublimation
B. Autonomic hyperactivity
C. Panic attacks that usually peak at 10 minutes but can last up to 30 minutes, with a gradual return to normal functioning
D. Disruption in personal life as well as work life
E. Possible use of alcohol and drugs to decrease anxiety

Analysis (Nursing Diagnoses)

A. *Ineffective coping* related to …
B. *Social isolation* related to …

> **HESI Hint** • When a client describes a phobia or expresses an unreasonable fear, the nurse should acknowledge the feeling (fear) and refrain from exposing the client to the identified fear. After trust is established, a desensitization process may be prescribed. Desensitization is the nursing intervention for phobia disorders. The nurse should:

- Assist client to recognize the factors associated with feared stimuli that precipitate a phobic response.
- Teach and practice with client alternative adaptive coping strategies, such as the use of thought substitution (replacing a fearful thought with a pleasant thought) and relaxation techniques. (Role-playing is useful when the client is in a calm state.)
- Expose client progressively to feared stimuli, offering support with the nurse's presence.
- Provide positive reinforcement whenever a decrease in phobic reaction occurs.

Note: In all likelihood, the desensitization process will be overseen by a mental health practitioner (nurse practitioner) or psychologist.

> **HESI Hint** • The nurse should place an anxious client where there are reduced environmental stimuli (a quiet area of the unit, away from the nurses' station).

Nursing Plans and Interventions

A. Establish trust; listen, use a calm approach and direct, simple questions. Remain with client; do not leave alone.
B. Provide a safe environment.
C. Draw client's attention away from feared object or situation.
D. Discuss with the client alternative coping strategies and encourage use of such alternatives.
E. Suggest substitution of positive thoughts for negative ones.
F. Assist in desensitizing client.
G. Gradually and systematically introduce the client to the anxiety-producing stimuli.
H. Pair the anxiety-producing stimuli with another response such as relaxation or exercise.
I. Encourage the sharing of fears and feelings with others.
J. Administer antianxiety medications as prescribed (Table 7-4).
K. Administer selective serotonin reuptake inhibitors (SSRIs) or other medications as prescribed (Table 7-5).
L. Teach to decrease intake of caffeine and nicotine.

Obsessive-Compulsive and Related Disorders

Description: DSM-5 no longer considers Obsessive-Compulsive and Related Disorders a component of Anxiety Disorders; it is now a component of Personality Disorders. Anxiety associated with repetitive thoughts (obsession) or irresistible impulses (compulsion) to perform an action.

A. Fear of losing control is a major symptom of this disorder.
B. New disorders introduced in DSM-5 include:
   1. hoarding
   2. excoriation (skin-picking)

TABLE 7-4 Antianxiety Drugs

Drugs	Indications	Reactions	Nursing Implications
Benzodiazepines			
• Chlordiazepoxide HCl • Diazepam • Clorazepate dipotassium • Lorazepam	• Reduce anxiety • Induce sedation, relax muscles, inhibit convulsions • Treat alcohol and drug withdrawal symptoms • Safer than sedative-hypnotics	• Sedation • Drowsiness • Ataxia • Dizziness • Irritability • Blood dyscrasias • Habituation and increased tolerance	• Administer at bedtime to alleviate daytime sedation. • Greatest harm occurs when combined with alcohol or other central nervous system depressants. • Instruct to avoid driving or working around equipment. • Gradually taper drug therapy due to withdrawal effects; do not stop suddenly. • Used only as short-term drug and as supplement to other medications.
Nonbenzodiazepines			
• Buspirone	• Reduce anxiety • Help to control symptoms such as insomnia, sweating, and palpitations associated with anxiety	• Dizziness	• Takes several weeks for antianxiety effects to become apparent. • Intended for short-term use.
• Zolpidem	• Used for short-term treatment of insomnia	• Daytime drowsiness	• Give with food 1-1½ hr before bedtime.
• Ramelteon	• Approved for long-term treatment of insomnia • Selectively binds to melatonin receptors	• Dizziness	• Appropriate for clients with delayed sleep onset.

3. trichotillomania (hair-pulling disorder)
4. obsessive-compulsive and related disorder due to a medical condition
5. substance or medication induced obsessive-compulsive and related disorder

> **HESI Hint** • In addition, relevant obsessive-compulsive disorder may present with a range of insight into their disorder related beliefs including absent insight/delusion symptoms.

Nursing Assessment

A. Use of coping styles to control anxiety (see Table 7-3)
   1. Repression
   2. Isolation
   3. Undoing
B. Magical thinking (belief that one's thoughts or wishes can control other people or events)
C. Evidence of destructive, hostile, aggressive, and delusional thought content
D. Difficulty with interpersonal relationships
E. Interference with normal activities (e.g., a client who "must" wash her hands all morning and cannot take her children to school)

F. Safety issues involved in repetitive performance of the ritualistic activity (e.g., dermatitis occurring as a result of the continuous washing of hands)
G. Recurring intrusive thoughts
H. Recurring, repetitive behaviors that interfere with normal functioning

Analysis (Nursing Diagnoses)

A. *Social isolation* related to …
B. *Ineffective coping* related to …

Nursing Plans and Interventions

A. Provide for client's physical needs.
B. Allow performance of the compulsive activity with attention given to safety (e.g., skin integrity of a hand washer).
C. Explore meaning and purpose of the behavior with client.
D. Avoid punishing and criticizing.
E. Establish routine to avoid anxiety-producing changes.
F. Assist client with learning alternative methods of dealing with stress.
G. Avoid reinforcing compulsive behavior.
H. Limit the amount of time for performance of ritual, and encourage client to gradually decrease the time.

TABLE 7-5 **Antidepressant Drugs**

Drugs	Indications	Adverse Reactions	Nursing Implications
Tricyclics			
• Amitriptyline HCl • Desipramine HCl • Imipramine HCl • Nortriptyline HCl • Protriptyline HCl • Maprotiline	• Depression • Clients with morbid fantasies do not respond well to these drugs.	• Anticholinergic effects: dry mouth, blurred vision, constipation, and urinary retention • CNS effects: sedation, psychomotor slowing, and poor concentration • Cardiovascular effects: tachycardia, orthostatic, hypotension, quinidinelike effect on the heart (assess history of myocardial infarction), prolongation of QTc interval • GI effects: nausea and vomiting • Narrow therapeutic index (can be lethal in overdose)	• Administer at bedtime to minimize sedative effect. • Takes 2-6 wk to achieve therapeutic effects • 1-3 wk should elapse between discontinuing tricyclics and initiating MAO inhibitors. • Teach client to avoid alcohol. • Avoid concurrent use of antihypertensive drugs. • Carefully evaluate suicide risk. • Lethal in overdose.
MAO Inhibitors (Monoamine Oxidase Inhibitors)			
• Isocarboxazid • Phenelzine sulfate • Tranylcypromine sulfate • Selegiline	• Depression • Phobias • Anxiety	• Tachycardia • Urinary hesitancy, constipation • Impotence • Dizziness • Insomnia • Muscle twitching • Drowsiness • Dry mouth • Fluid retention • *Hypertensive crisis:* severe hypertension, severe headache, chest pain, fever, sweating, nausea and vomiting • Confusion	• Must *not* be used with tricyclics (cause *hypertensive crisis*) • Major concern is need for dietary restrictions—*certain drug and food interactions can cause hypertensive crisis.* • Instruct client *not* to eat foods with high tyramine content: aged cheese, red wine, beer, beef and chicken, liver, yeast, yogurt, soy sauce, chocolate, bananas. • May not be used with SSRIs • Teach client *not* to take over-the-counter drugs without physician approval. • Teach the warning signs of hypertensive crisis: headaches, palpitations, increased BP. • Teach client to use caution around machinery.
SSRIs (Selective Serotonin Reuptake Inhibitors)			
• Fluoxetine HCl • Paroxetine • Sertraline • Fluvoxamine • Citalopram	• Depression • Anxiety • Panic disorder • Aggression • Anorexia nervosa • OCD	• Drowsiness • Dizziness, lightheadedness • Headache • Insomnia • Depressed appetite	• Effective 2-4 wk after treatment is initiated. • Should *not* be used with MAO inhibitors: cause hypertensive crisis (violent reaction). • Should wait at least 14 days between discontinuing MAO inhibitor and starting fluoxetine (Prozac).

Continued

TABLE 7-5 Antidepressant Drugs—cont'd

Drugs	Indications	Adverse Reactions	Nursing Implications

• Escitalopram
• Vilazodone
	• Depression
	• Anxiety
	• Panic disorder
	• Aggression
	• Anorexia nervosa
	• OCD
		• Serotonin syndrome
		• Sexual dysfunction
		• Allergic reaction or rash; with-hold drug if occurs
		• Weight gain
			• At least 5 wk should lapse between discontinuing fluoxetine (Prozac) and initiating an MAO inhibitor.
			• May be given in evening if sedation occurs.
			• Monitor for serotonin syndrome (defined by at least three symptoms):
			  • Rapid onset of altered mental states
			  • Agitation
			  • Myoclonus
			  • Hyperreflexia
			  • Fever
			  • Shivering
			  • Diaphoresis
			  • Ataxia
			  • Diarrhea
			• Caution client about OTC use of St. John's wort.
			• Must be tapered slowly if discontinuing or changing from one SSRI to another.

Atypical Antidepressants			
• Trazodone	• Depression • With trazodone: insomnia, dementia with agitation	• Safer than tricyclics and MAO inhibitors in terms of side effects	• Effective 2-4 wk after treatment is initiated.
S/NRIs (Serotonin/Norepinephrine Reuptake Inhibitors)			
• Duloxetine • Venlafaxine • Desvenlafaxine	• Depression • Anxiety • Panic disorder • Aggression • Anorexia nervosa • OCD • Management of diabetic neuropathic pain	• Nausea • Dry mouth • Insomnia • Headache • Fatigue • Depressed appetite • Increased sweating • Sexual dysfunction • Withdrawal symptoms with abrupt cessation (agitation, tremors, headache, nightmares)	• Should not be used with MAO inhibitors: cause hypertensive crisis (violent reaction). • Should wait at least 14 days between discontinuing MAO inhibitor and starting S/NRIs. • Take baseline blood pressure and monitor periodically (can cause slight drop in BP). • Monitor for worsening of pretreatment symptoms and inform client of possibility. • See the previous section in this table on Nursing Implications for SSRIs.
Norepinephrine Dopamine Reuptake Inhibitors (NDRIs)			
• Bupropion • Mirtazapine	• Second line of antidepressant when SSRI and SNRI are not effective for depression and smoking cessation • Anxiety and sleep disturbances	• Insomnia, tremor, anorexia and weight loss, dry mouth • Sleep disturbances, poor appetite, pain, sexual dysfunction, sedation	• Lowers seizure threshold; should not be used for patients with seizure disorders or eating disorders because of increased seizure incidence in this group. • Herbal considerations: Ephedra may cause hypertensive crisis. • Inform client: exaggerated with alcohol use or other CNS depressants. Medication taken in evening due to sedative effects.

I. Administer antianxiety medications as prescribed (see Table 7-4).

J. Administer SSRIs and tricyclic antidepressants as prescribed (see Table 7-5).

> **HESI Hint** • Compulsive acts are used in response to anxiety, which may or may not be related to the obsession. It is the nurse's responsibility to help alleviate anxiety.
>
> Interfering will increase anxiety. The client's acts should be allowed as long as they are free of violence. The nurse should:
> - Actively listen to the client's obsessive themes.
> - Acknowledge the effects that ritualistic acts have on the client.
> - Demonstrate empathy.
> - Avoid being judgmental.

> **HESI Hint** • The best time for interaction with a client is at the completion of the performed ritual. The client's anxiety is lowest at this time; therefore it is an optimal time for learning.

Traumatic and Stressor Related Disorders

Description: DSM-5 no longer considers Posttraumatic Stress Disorder (PTSD) as a component of Anxiety Disorders. New nomenclature is Traumatic and Stressor Related Disorders. These disorders include severe anxiety, which results from experiencing or witnessing a traumatic event (e.g., war, earthquake, rape, incest) directly or indirectly and can include a persistent re-experiencing of the trauma. Symptoms include intrusion, negative mood, dissociation, and arousal.

Nursing Assessment

PTSD redefined in DSM-5 with four symptom clusters. They are:

A. Avoidance of events or situations that are reminders.

B. Persistent negative alterations in cognitions and mood.

C. Mood including numbing symptoms, as well as persistent negative emotional states.

D. Alterations in arousal and reactivity, including irritable or aggressive behavior and reckless or self-destructive behavior (suicidal ideation and substance abuse).

Other Stressor Related Disorders:

A. Anxiety level is proportional to the perceived degree of threat experienced by the client.

B. Anxiety is manifested in symptomatic behaviors:
1. Intrusive thoughts
2. Flashbacks of the experience
3. Nightmares
4. Emotional detachment

C. Responses to anxiety include: shock, anger, panic, or denial.

D. May manifest as self-destructive behavior such as suicidal ideation and substance abuse.

E. Visible reminders of the trauma (e.g., scars, physical disabilities) may trigger reactions.

Analysis (Nursing Diagnoses)

A. *Posttrauma syndrome* related to …

B. *Ineffective coping* related to …

C. *Risk for other-directed/self-directed violence* related to …

Nursing Plans and Interventions

A. Provide consistent, nonthreatening environment.

B. Implement suicidal and homicidal precautions if assessment indicates risk.

C. Listen to client's details of events to identify the most troubling aspect of events.

D. Assist client to develop objectivity in perceiving event and identify areas of no control.

E. Assist client to regain control by identifying past situations that have been handled successfully.

F. Administer antianxiety and antipsychotic medications as prescribed so as to decrease anxiety, manage behavior, and provide rest (Table 7-6; and see Table 7-3).

> **HESI Hint** • For clients diagnosed with traumatic and stressor related disorders, the nurse should:
> - Actively listen to client's stories of experiences surrounding the traumatic event.
> - Assess suicide risk.
> - Assist client to develop objectivity about the event and problem-solve regarding possible means of controlling anxiety related to the event.
> - Encourage group therapy with other clients who have experienced the same or related traumatic events.

TABLE 7-6 **Antipsychotic Drugs**

Traditional Drugs	Indications	Adverse Reactions	Nursing Implications
Phenothiazines			

• Chlorpromazine HCl
• Trifluoperazine HCl
• Thioridazine HCl
• Perphenazine
• Triflupromazine
• Loxapine
	• To control psychotic behavior: hallucinations, delusions, and bizarre behavior	• Drowsiness
		• Orthostatic hypotension
		• Weight gain
		• Anticholinergic effects
		• Extrapyramidal effects
		  • Pseudoparkinsonism
		  • Akathisia
		  • Dystonia
		  • Tardive dyskinesia
		• Photosensitivity
		• Blood dyscrasias: granulocytosis, leukopenia
		• Neuroleptic malignant syndrome
			• Extrapyramidal effects are *major* concern.
			• Monitor older clients closely.
			• Takes 2-3 wk to achieve therapeutic effect
			• Keep client supine for 1 hr after administration and advise to change positions slowly because of effects of orthostatic hypotension.
			• Teach client to avoid:
			  • Alcohol
			  • Sedatives (potentiate effect of CNS depressants)
			  • Antacids (reduce absorption of drug)

• Fluphenazine HCl	• To control psychotic behavior • Useful in treatment of psychomotor agitation associated with thought disorders	• Same as other phenothiazines	• Absorbed slowly • Used with noncompliant clients because it can be administered IM once every 14 days.
Nonphenothiazines			
• Haloperidol • Thiothixene HCl • Pimozide	• To control psychotic behavior • Less sedative than phenothiazines	• Severe extrapyramidal reactions • Leukocytosis • Blurred vision • Dry mouth • Urinary retention	• Teach client to avoid alcohol. • Pimozide (Orap) is used only for Tourette syndrome.
Long-Acting Drugs			
• Fluphenazine decanoate • Haloperidol decanoate	• Clients who require supervision with medication regimens	• Similar to fluphenazine (Prolixin) and haloperidol (Haldol)	• Similar to Haldol and Prolixin • Prolixin can be given every 7-28 days. • Haldol can be given every 4 wk. • Requires several months to reach steady-state drug levels
Atypical Antipsychotic Drugs			
• Risperidone • Olanzapine • Quetiapine • Aripiprazole • Ziprasidone • Clozapine	• Treat positive and negative symptoms of schizophrenia without significant EPS. • Clients who have not responded well to typical antipsychotics or have side effects with typical antipsychotics • Fewer side effects • Clozapine has superior efficacy in clients who have been treatment resistant.	• Risperdal: neuroleptic malignant syndrome (NMS), EPS, dizziness, GI symptoms (nausea, constipation), anxiety • Zyprexa: drowsiness, dizziness, EPS, agitation • Seroquel: drowsiness, dizziness, headache, EPS, weight gain, anticholinergic effects • Clozaril: agranulocytosis, drowsiness, dizziness, GI symptoms, NMS	• Monitor WBC weekly for first 6 mo, then biweekly. • Baseline vital signs (VS) and ECG; report abnormal VS. • Monitor for symptoms of NMS and EPS. • Teach to change positions slowly. • Abilify is a new class of antipsychotic drugs, dopamine system stabilizers (DSSs) for schizophrenia and acute bipolar mania. • Seroquel: monitor lipids, especially for obese, diabetic, or hypertensive clients.

Review of Anxiety Disorders, Obsessive-Compulsive and Related Disorders, and Traumatic and Stressor Related Disorders

1. State five autonomic responses to anxiety.
2. Identify the coping style used by a person who feels guilty about masturbating as a child and develops a handwashing compulsion as an adult.
3. Identify anxiety-reducing strategies the nurse can teach.
4. Which levels of anxiety facilitate learning?
5. A veteran of the wars in Afghanistan and Iraq is plagued by nightmares and is found trying to strangle his roommate one night. List in order of priority the appropriate nursing interventions.
6. A client displays a phobic response to flying. Describe the desensitization process that would probably be implemented.
7. A client is in the middle of an extensive ritual that focuses on food during lunch. However, the client is scheduled for group therapy, which is about to start. What action should the nurse take?

Answers to Review

1. Shortness of breath, heart palpitations, dizziness, diaphoresis, frequent urination
2. Undoing
3. Deep-breathing techniques, visualization, relaxation techniques, exercise, biofeedback
4. Mild to moderate
5. Protect roommate from harm. Stay with client. If the client is agitated, administer antianxiety medications as prescribed. Arrange for private room. Place client on homicidal precautions at night.
6. Talk about planes. Look at pictures of planes. Make plans to accompany client during a visit to airport. Accompany client onto a plane. Allow the client to board a plane alone. Accompany the client on a short flight while listening to a relaxation tape.
7. Allow client to complete the ritual. Discuss with the group leader the possibility of allowing the client to enter the group late. Arrange for client to begin lunch earlier so that the ritual can be completed before scheduled activities.

Somatic Symptom Disorder and Related Disorders

A. Clients diagnosed with somatic symptoms plus abnormal thoughts, feelings, and behaviors *may or may not* have a diagnosed medical condition.
B. Clients diagnosed with somatic symptom disorders are persistently preoccupied with their perceived health issues and frequently demand unnecessary tests
C. May not comply with health care provider recommendations.
D. These clients incur large care costs due to the significant distress and dysfunction related to their symptoms.
E. These clients often seek treatment from several health care providers (referred to as *doctor shopping*) because a health care provider may not provide the answer to the client's distress.

Types of Somatic Symptom Disorders

A. The client with somatic symptom disorder has a long history of visits to health care providers for multiple somatic complaints. Most frequent symptoms are pain (back, chest, head, pelvic), palpitations, or dizziness.
B. Psychological factors affecting other medical conditions comprise a new mental disorder in DSM-5. This disorder and factitious disorder are placed among the somatic symptom and related disorders because somatic symptoms are predominant in both disorders, and both are most often encountered in medical settings.
C. Factitious disorder is a deliberate exaggeration; induce or fabricate symptoms or self-injury without obvious gains such as a financial incentive (for example, use medication incorrectly or inappropriately).
D. Munchausen syndrome is a severe and chronic form of factitious disorder that may result in severe self-harm that requires treatment in the hospital (e.g., surgery or other invasive procedures).
E. Factitious disorder by proxy occurs when a person foists deliberate fabricated symptoms onto another person.
F. Munchausen syndrome by proxy occurs when a caregiver (usually the mother) causes a child to require treatment for an illness or injury stimulated by the mother.
G. Malingering occurs when a client creates complaints for secondary gain (e.g., to obtain a disability check).

Nursing Assessment

A. Preoccupation with pain or bodily function for at least 6 months' duration
B. History of frequent "doctor shopping"
C. Absence of emotional concern regarding the physical impairment
D. Women may report excessive dysmenorrhea

E. Vital signs may be elevated, as in a panic attack
F. Fear of having a serious disease
G. Excessive use of analgesics
H. Rumination about physical symptoms
I. Drug abuse; drug screening needed to determine presence of abuse and, if present, the level of abuse
J. Depression and presence of suicidal ideation
K. Social or occupational impairment
L. Presence of blindness, deafness, paralysis, or seizures suggestive of a neurologic disease

Analysis (Nursing Diagnoses)

A. *Chronic pain* related to ...
B. *Ineffective coping* related to ...
C. *Disturbed personal identity* related to ...

Nursing Plans and Interventions

A. Convey a nonjudgmental attitude.
B. Record duration and intensity of pain with attention to factors that precipitate onset.
C. Encourage expression of angry feelings.
D. Implement suicide precautions if indicated.
E. No one medication is particularly recommended. Comorbid disorders such as anxiety and depression are treated with disorder-specific medications.
F. Focus interactions and activities away from self and pain.
G. Help client identify connection between pain and anxiety.
H. Increase time and attention given to client as reward for not focusing on self or physical symptoms.

TABLE 7-7 Terms Associated with Somatic Symptom Disorders

Term	Definition
La belle indifference	Term used to describe the lack of concern over physical illness; seen in conversion reactions
Primary gain	A decrease in anxiety resulting from the ability to deal with a stressful situation
Secondary gain	The rewards obtained from the sick role, such as freedom from certain responsibilities, sympathy

I. Help client identify needs met by the sick role (e.g., attention and freedom from responsibility) (Table 7-7).
J. Encourage use of anxiety-reducing techniques such as deep breathing, visualization, meditation, exercise, and relaxation.

> **HESI Hint** • Be aware of your own feelings when working with these clients. It is a challenge to be nonjudgmental. The pain is real to the person experiencing it. These disorders cannot be explained medically; they result from internal conflict. The nurse should:
> • Acknowledge the symptom or complaint.
> • Reaffirm that diagnostic test results reveal no organic pathology.
> • Determine the secondary gains acquired by the client.

Review of Somatic Symptom Disorder and Related Disorders

1. Describe the difference between primary and secondary gains.
2. An air traffic controller suddenly develops blindness. All physical findings are negative. The client's history reveals increased anxiety about job performance and fear about job security. What type of disorder is this? What purpose is the blindness serving? What nursing interventions are indicated?
3. A 29-year-old secretary, who is obese, has visited seven different doctors in the past year with a complaint of chest pain and shortness of breath. This individual is certain she is having a heart attack in spite of the health care provider's reassurance that all tests are normal. What type of disorder is this? What nursing actions are indicated?
4. Five years ago, a man was involved in a motor vehicle accident that killed the friend who was a passenger in the car he was driving. Since that time, he has been unable to work because of severe back pain. The pain is unrelieved by prescribed medications. What type of disorder is this? What are the contributing causes? Describe the nursing care.

Answers to Review

1. The primary gain is a decrease in anxiety that results from some effort made to deal with stress. The secondary gain is the advantage, other than reduced anxiety, that occurs as a result of the sick role.

2. Conversion reaction; decreases the anxiety about job; assist with ADLs, encourage expression of anger, teach relaxation techniques, and assist with the identification of anxiety related to job security and performance.

Continued

Answers to Review—cont'd

3. Functional neurologic symptom disorder (formerly conversion reaction or disorder) is a condition by which clients display psychological stress in physical ways. That is, an emotional crisis, a very stressful incident, converts to a physical problem. One example is the air traffic controller reading about a near-miss airline crash. The client develops blindness even though neurological and physical evaluation cannot determine any underlying cause for the client's signs and symptoms. Interventions may focus on ways to decrease the anxiety, for example, about the job; assist with ADLs; encourage expression of anger; teach relaxation techniques; and assist with the identification of anxiety related to job security and performance.

4. Somatization disorder; unresolved grief, anxiety; evaluate pain medication use or abuse; document duration and intensity of pain; assist client to identify precipitating factors related to request for medication.

Dissociative Disorders

A. These disorders involve alteration in the function of consciousness, personality, memory, or identity.
B. Dissociative disorders may be sudden and temporary or gradual and chronic.
C. Clients diagnosed with these types of disorders handle stressful situations by "splitting" from the situation and going into a fantasy state.
D. The disorders are an unconscious defense mechanism that protects one against overwhelming anxiety.

Types of Dissociative Disorders

A. Dissociative amnesia
1. Is the sudden temporary inability to recall extensive personal events.
2. The memory loss includes gaps in memory for extended periods of time or memories of the precipitating event.
3. It usually occurs after a traumatic event, such as a threat of death or injury, an intolerable life situation, or a natural disaster.
4. It is the most common dissociative disorder.
5. Dissociative amnesia with fugue.
   a. It is characterized by a person suddenly leaving home or work with the inability to recall his or her identity, so this involves flight as well as loss of memory.
   b. The person may even assume a new identity.
   c. This disorder rarely occurs.
B. Dissociative identity disorder (formerly called *multiple personality disorder*)
1. The person assumes two or more identities simultaneously.
2. The dissociative aspect emerges during stress.
3. It is a severe form of dissociation thought to be a coping mechanism.
4. It is characterized by the client's dissociation from events that occur in everyday life or a traumatic experience such as severe child abuse or sexual, physical, or psychological abuse.
C. Depersonalization disorder
1. It is characterized by a temporary loss of one's reality and the ability to feel and express emotions.
2. Expresses detachment with regard to surroundings (e.g., objects or individuals). The client experiences others as unreal or visually distorted.

Nursing Assessment

A. Depression, mood swings, insomnia, potential for suicide
B. Varying degrees of orientation
C. Varying levels of anxiety
D. Impairment of social and occupational functioning
E. Alcohol or drug abuse (Drug screening is necessary to determine presence and level of abuse.)

Analysis (Nursing Diagnoses)

A. *Ineffective coping* related to …
B. *Potential for self-directed/other-directed violence* related to …
C. *Disturbed personal identity* related to …

Nursing Plans and Interventions

A. Reduce environmental stimulation to decrease anxiety.
B. Stay with client during periods of depersonalization. (The client is often fearful, and the nurse's presence assists in providing support and comfort during fearful episode.)
C. Demonstrate acceptance of client's behavior during various experiences and personalities.
D. Document emergence of different personalities, if present.
E. Implement suicide precautions if assessment indicates risk.
F. Encourage client to identify stressful situations that cause a transition from one personality to another.
G. Help client to identify effective coping patterns used in other stressful situations.
H. Assist client in using new alternative coping methods.

HESI Hint • The nurse should be aware that all behavior has meaning.

HESI Hint • Avoid giving clients diagnosed with dissociative disorders too much information about past events at one time. The various types of amnesia that accompany dissociative disorders provide protection from pain. Too much, too soon may cause decompensation.

Review of Dissociative Disorders

1. Describe the relationship between dissociative amnesia and dissociative amnesia with fugue state.

2. What is dissociative identity disorder?
3. List three possible causes of dissociative amnesia.

Answers to Review

1. Dissociative amnesia is characterized by the sudden onset of the client's temporary inability to remember extensive information about the client's personal life. It usually occurs after a traumatic event (e.g., death or natural disaster). A dissociative fugue is a rare occurrence that is also a subcategory of dissociative amnesia. It is characterized by the client's sudden flight from home or work with an inability to recall his or her own identity.
2. Dissociative identity disorder involves the development of two or more distinct personalities within one individual. The assumption of multiple identities may or may not occur in response to severe stress such as sexual assault.
3. Everyday events as well as traumatic events such as a threat of death or injury may trigger dissociative amnesia; examples of triggers are an intolerable life situation; a natural disaster; or any ordinary event occurring in the home or at work

Personality Disorders (DSM-5 Criteria)

Personality Disorders
Schizotypal
Antisocial
Borderline
Narcissistic
Avoidant
Obsessive-compulsive

Description: Individuals with personality disorders display inappropriate emotional responses to stresss and in interpersonal relationships. These individuals have vast disability in personal and work relationships. Often their perception and interpretation of the world and other people around them is inaccurate. Impulse control is often difficult for these individuals to maintain.

The following is a list of reasons individuals with personality disorders have difficulty in work and personal relations:
- Insensitivity to the needs of others
- Demanding and fault finding
- Inability to trust others
- Passive-aggressive traits
- Blurs boundaries between self and others
- Lack of individual accountability
- Tendency to evoke intense interpersonal conflict (relationships are often marked by hostility that leads to serious interpersonal conflict and in some cases violence directed at others).
- Often people with personality disorders have the ability to "get under the skin" of others.
- Most people with personality disorders have problematic relationships with others; they are often socially isolated because of their maladaptive coping skills and their rigidity, including the need to control others, which complicates their interactions with others.

A. Schizotypal personality
  1. Has interpersonal deficits
  2. Has eccentricities and odd beliefs
  3. Is socially isolated
  4. Example: a person who spends hours walking the streets dressed in all sorts of mismatched clothing while wearing a hat with all kinds of things hanging from it.
B. Antisocial personality
  1. Shows aggressive acting-out behavior pattern without any remorse
  2. Is clever and manipulative in order to meet own self-centered needs
  3. Lacks social conscience and ability to feel remorse; is emotionally immature and impulsive
  4. Has ineffective interpersonal skills that impair the forming of close and lasting relationships
  5. Verbally: is disparaging, humiliating, and belligerent toward those perceived as a threat

6. Nonverbally: is cold, callous, and insensitive to others; can display socially gracious behaviors in order to meet own needs
7. Example: a prison inmate who tries to get special privileges by bribing the guards (e.g., acting out the role of a con artist)

C. Borderline personality
1. Has disturbances regarding self-image and sexual, social, and occupational roles
2. Shows impulsive, self-damaging behavior; makes suicidal gestures
3. Is other-directed, overly dependent on others
4. Is unable to problem-solve or learn from experience
5. Tends to view others as either all good or all bad (e.g., "splitting" behavior)
6. Verbally: is self-critical, demanding, whiny, manipulative, and argumentative and can become verbally abusive
7. Nonverbally: has highly changeable and intense affect, impulsive behaviors
8. Shows inappropriate intense anger or difficulty controlling anger
9. Example: a teenage girl who threatens to commit suicide when her boyfriend leaves, but in 6 weeks has new boyfriend and is clinging to him

D. Narcissistic personality
1. Perceives self as all-powerful and important, is critical of others, arrogant
2. Has exaggerated feeling of self-importance and self-love
3. Needs attention and admiration
4. Is preoccupied with power and appearance
5. Exploits others
6. Verbally: talks about self incessantly and does whatever necessary to draw attention to self
7. Nonverbally: is inattentive and indifferent to others, appears concerned only with self
8. Lacks empathy
9. Example: a star football player whose success has gone to his head

E. Avoidant personality
1. Is socially inhibited
2. Feels inadequate
3. Is hypersensitive to negative criticism, rejection
4. Longs for relationships
5. Example: a man who refuses to play on the employees' softball team because he is afraid his teammates will make fun of him

F. Dependent personality
1. Has unreasonable wishes and wants, and expresses needs in a demanding, whining manner while professing independence and denying dependent behavior
2. Is passive, without accepting responsibility for consequences of his or her own behavior
3. Has low self-esteem, sees self as stupid, unable to make decisions
4. Is dependent on others to meet his or her needs
5. Verbally: is self-deprecating, demanding others to meet needs
6. Nonverbally: appears dull, uninterested in others, dissatisfied with self
7. Example: an adult who exhibits adolescent-type behavior, wants others to take care of him or her while at the same time declaring independence

G. Obsessive-compulsive personality
1. Attempts to control self through the control of others or the environment
2. Shows inattention to new facts or different viewpoints
3. Is cold and rigid toward others
4. Is a perfectionist, inflexible, and stubborn
5. Acts with blind conformity and obedience to rules
6. Is excessively neat and clean, preoccupied with lists, rules, details, and orders
7. Is preoccupied with work efficiency and productivity
8. Verbally and nonverbally: expresses disapproval of those whose behaviors and standards are different from own
9. Example: a nurse who insists that all staff on the unit wear a freshly starched uniform every day and has no tolerance for staff that do not dress as professionally as this individual

Nursing Assessment

A. Assess degree of social impairment.
B. Determine degree of manipulative behavior.
C. Assess degree of anxiety.
D. Determine the risk for self- or other-directed violence.

Analysis (Nursing Diagnoses)

A. *Disturbed personal identity* related to …
B. *Ineffective coping* related to …
C. *Social isolation* related to …
D. *Risk for self-directed/other-directed violence* related to …

Nursing Plans and Interventions

A. Establish trust; use straightforward approach.
B. Protect client from injury to self and others.
C. Assist client to recognize manipulative behavior.
D. Focus on client's strengths and accomplishments.
E. Set limits on manipulative behaviors when necessary.
F. Reinforce independent, responsible behaviors.
G. Assist client to recognize the need to respect the needs and rights of others.
H. Encourage socialization with others to improve skills.

HESI Hint • Personality disorders are characterized by anxious and fearful behaviors.

HESI Hint • Personality disorders are long-standing behavioral traits that are maladaptive responses to anxiety and that cause difficulty in relating to and working with other individuals. NCLEX-RN® questions sometimes test personality disorder content by describing management situations.

HESI Hint • Persons with personality disorders are usually comfortable with their interactions with others and believe that they are right and the world is wrong. These individuals usually have very little motivation to change.

Review of Personality Disorders

State the diagnosis that should be made based on the following behaviors or symptoms:

1. Orderly, rigid
2. Unable to conform to social norms
3. Needy, always in a crisis, self-mutilating, unable to sustain relationships, splitting behavior
4. Unable to make decisions for self, allows others to assume responsibility for his or her life
5. Feelings of self-importance and entitlement; may exploit others to get own needs met
6. Dramatic, flamboyant, needs to be the center of attention

Answers to Review

1. Borderline personality disorder
2. Obsessive-compulsive personality disorder
3. Avoidant personality disorder
4. Schizotypal personality disorder
5. Antisocial personality disorder
6. Narcissistic personality disorder

Eating Disorders

HESI Hint • Clients diagnosed with eating disorders are often concurrently diagnosed with psychiatric disorders.

Anorexia Nervosa

A. There are two subtypes in anorexia:
1. The client who restricts her or his intake of food and consequently does not maintain minimal weight for height and age.
2. The client who employs binge eating and/or purging as a mechanism to control body weight.
B. A distorted body image and intense fear of becoming obese drive excessive dieting and exercise.
C. A reported 15% to 20% of those diagnosed die.
D. Anorexia is more prevalent in females. (Females often experience amenorrhea.)
E. It occurs in adolescence and may continue across the lifespan.
F. Male and female athletes exhibit a greater incidence of eating disorders.
G. Eating disorders are frequently comorbid with other mental health illnesses (i.e., depression, bipolar disorder, obsessive-compulsive disorders, and social phobia)
H. Possible causes
1. Neurobiological and neuroendocrine abnormalities are associated with both anorexia and bulimia; how-

ever, there is currently no consensus on whether the abnormalities caused the eating disorder or the eating disorder contributed to the abnormality.
2. Genetic factors contribute to the risk of developing an eating disorder.
a. There is a 70% concordance rate for identical twins.
b. For fraternal twins, there is a 20% concordance rate.
3. Psychological determinants of eating disorders are thought to be:
a. Low self-esteem and harsh self-judgment focused primarily on the subject of weight
b. Results of anorexic clients living in families that are controlling and emphasize perfection
c. Results of bulimic clients living among chaotic and emotionally expressive families
4. Eating disorders occur globally; these disorders occur among ethnic minorities in the United States as well as in non-Western countries.

Nursing Assessment

A. Weight loss of at least 15% of ideal or original body weight
B. Excessive exercise
C. Apathy about physical condition and inordinate pleasure in weight loss
D. Skeletal appearance (usually hidden by baggy clothes)
E. Distorted body image (usually sees self as fat)
F. Low self-esteem
G. Hair loss and dry skin
H. Irregular heartbeat, decreased pulse and blood pressure (BP) resulting from decreased fluid volume

I. Delayed psychosexual development (adolescents) or disinterest in sex (adults)
J. Dehydration and electrolyte imbalance (decreased potassium, sodium, and chloride) resulting from:
1. Diet pill abuse
2. Enema and laxative abuse
3. Diuretic abuse
4. Self-induced vomiting

Analysis (Nursing Diagnoses)

A. *Imbalanced nutrition: less than body requirements* related to …
B. *Disturbed personal identity* related to …
C. *Interrupted family process* related to …

Nursing Plans and Interventions

A. Monitor weight, vital signs, and electrolytes (especially potassium, thyroid levels, and calcium/phosphorus for osteoporosis).
B. Provide a structured, supportive environment, especially during mealtimes.
C. Set a time limit for eating.
D. Carefully monitor food and fluid intake.
E. Be alert to client's choosing low-calorie foods.
F. Be alert to possible discarding of food through others or in pockets, wastebaskets, or drawers.
G. Monitor client after meals for possible vomiting.
H. Monitor activity level to prevent excessive exercise.
I. Use positive reinforcement to build self-esteem and develop a realistic body image.
J. Devise a behavior-modification program if indicated.
1. Include an established weight goal and weigh on a regular schedule.
2. Weigh in same clothes, with back to scale; this prevents manipulation and arguing about exact weight.
3. Praise weight gain rather than food intake.
K. Focus interactions away from food and eating.
L. Administer antidepressant medications as indicated.
M. Teach client that sudden withdrawal from medications may cause seizures.
N. Encourage family therapy.
O. Provide snacks between meals.
P. Monitor activity and assess for weakness, fatigue, and pathologic fractures.
Q. Provide safe environment and assess for suicide ideation. Implement suicide precautions if necessary.
R. Assess for water loading before weighing.

HESI Hint • Do not allow clients diagnosed with anorexia to plan or prepare food for unit-based activities. Clients diagnosed with anorexia gain pleasure from providing others with food and watching them eat. These behaviors reinforce the client's perception of self-control.

Bulimia Nervosa

A. An eating disorder characterized by eating excessive amounts of food followed by self-induced purging by vomiting, misuse of laxatives, diuretics or other medications, fasting, and/or excessive exercise
B. Bulimic clients usually report a loss of control over eating during the bingeing

Nursing Assessment

A. Refer to Nursing Assessment described in Anorexia Nervosa.
B. Diarrhea or constipation, abdominal pain, and bloating
C. Dental damage due to excessive vomiting (gastric hydrochloric acid erodes dental enamel)
D. Sore throat and chronic inflammation of the esophageal lining, with possible ulceration
E. Financial stressors related to food budget
F. Concerns with body shape and weight; bulimics usually are not underweight.

Analysis (Nursing Diagnoses)

A. *Disturbed personal identity* related to …
B. *Interrupted family process* related to …
C. *Ineffective coping* related to …
D. *Risk for self-directed violence* related to …

Nursing Plans and Interventions

A. Monitor weight, vital signs, and electrolytes (especially potassium).
B. Provide a structured, supportive environment, especially around mealtime.
C. Monitor client after meals for possible vomiting.
D. Assist client to learn strategies other than eating for dealing with feelings.
E. Encourage client to express feelings of anger.
F. Discuss strategies to stop vomiting and laxative use.
G. Use positive reinforcement to build self-esteem and develop a realistic body image.
H. Administer antidepressant medications as indicated.
I. Promote family therapy.

HESI Hint • Binge eating disorder is a new diagnosis introduced in DSM-5. These individuals report recurrent episodes of eating large amounts of food in a short period and describe feeling guilty or shameful after overindulging. They do not purge, nor are they obese. Binge eating often coexists with other psychiatric disorders (e.g., bipolar disorder, depressive disorder and anxiety disorder).

HESI Hint • Individuals with bulimia often use syrup of ipecac to induce vomiting. If ipecac is not vomited and is absorbed, cardiotoxicity may occur and can cause conduction disturbances, cardiac dysrhythmias, fatal myocarditis, and circulatory failure. Because heart failure is not usually seen in this age group, it is often overlooked. Assess for edema and listen to breath sounds.

HESI Hint • Physical assessment and nutritional support are priorities; the physiologic implications are great. Nursing interventions should increase self-esteem and develop a positive body image. Behavior modification is useful and effective. Family therapy is most effective because issues of control are common in these disorders. (Therapy is usually long term.)

Review of Eating Disorders

1. Describe the clinical symptoms of anorexia nervosa.
2. A client with anorexia has her friend bring her several cookbooks so she can plan a party when she is discharged. What nursing intervention is appropriate in addressing this behavior?

3. What might the initial treatment include for a client admitted to the hospital with a diagnosis of bulimia nervosa?

Answers to Review

1. Weight loss of at least 15% of ideal or original body weight; hair loss; dry skin; irregular heart rate; decreased pulse; decreased BP; amenorrhea; dehydration; electrolyte imbalance
2. Discuss activities that don't involve food that can take place after discharge. Discuss the cookbooks with the

treatment team, and if the treatment plan so indicates, take the books from the client.
3. Blood work to evaluate electrolyte status; replenishment of electrolytes and fluids as indicated; careful monitoring for evidence of vomiting

Mood Disorders

Definition: Disturbances in mood manifested by extreme sadness or extreme elation

Depressive Disorders

Definition: Pathologic grief reactions ranging from mild to severe states

Symptoms of Varying Degrees of Depression
A. Mild
   1. Feelings of sadness
   2. Difficulty concentrating and performing usual activities
   3. Difficulty maintaining usual activity level
B. Moderate
   1. Feelings of helplessness and powerlessness
   2. Decreased energy
   3. Sleep pattern disturbances
   4. Appetite and weight changes
   5. Slowed speech, thought, movement (may also be agitated and hyperactive)
   6. Rumination on negative feelings
C. Severe
   1. Feelings of hopelessness, worthlessness, guilt, shame

   2. Despair
   3. Flat affect
   4. Indecisiveness
   5. Lack of motivation, anergia, and decreased concentration
   6. Change in physical appearance (slumped posture, unkempt)
   7. Suicidal thoughts
   8. Possible delusions and hallucinations
   9. Sleep and appetite disturbances
   10. Loss of interest in sexual activity
   11. Constipation

HESI Hint • The most important signs and symptoms of depression are a depressed mood with a loss of interest in the pleasures in life. The client has sustained a loss. Other symptoms include:
• Significant change in appetite, often accompanied by a change in weight, either weight loss or gain
• Insomnia or hypersomnia (usually sleeping during the day, often because the client is not sleeping at night due to anxiety)
• Fatigue or lack of energy
• Feelings of hopelessness, worthlessness, guilt, or overresponsibility
• Loss of ability to concentrate or think clearly
• Preoccupation with death or suicide

Nursing Assessment

A. Determine degree of depression.
B. Determine current suicide risk.
C. Laboratory tests:
   1. Decreased serotonin level is indicative of depression.
   2. Decreased norepinephrine level is indicative of depression.

Analysis (Nursing Diagnoses)

A. *Risk for self-directed violence* related to …
B. *Self-care deficit* (specify) related to …
C. *Disturbed sleep pattern* related to …
D. *Ineffective coping* related to …

Nursing Plans and Interventions

A. Directly ask client about feelings and plans to harm self.
B. Implement suicide precautions if assessment indicates risk (see Care of the Suicidal Client later in this chapter).
C. Monitor sleep, nutrition, and elimination patterns.
D. Assist client with ADLs.
E. Initiate interaction with client (use a nonthreatening and nonchallenging approach).
F. Strongly encourage participation in activities. Do not give the client a choice about participating in activities (e.g., "It's time to go to the gym for basketball").
G. Observe for sudden elevation in mood; may indicate increased risk for suicide.
H. Assist client in identifying a support system.
I. Encourage discussion of feelings of helplessness, hopelessness, loneliness, and anger.
J. Ask about medications and complementary and alternative medications (CAM) and treatments.
K. Sit in silence if client is nontalkative.
L. Spend time with client and return when promised.

HESI Hint • Depressed clients have difficulty hearing and accepting compliments because of their lowered self-concept. Comment on signs of improvement by noting the behavior (e.g., "I notice you combed your hair today" not, "You look nice today").

HESI Hint • *Complementary and Alternative Medicine.* Clients are reluctant to share information regarding CAM. St. John's wort is available over the counter for effective self-treatment of depression. However, it may induce mania in bipolar clients and enhance photosensitivity. It may also reduce the plasma concentrations of other medications such as oral contraceptives, statins, and warfarin. If combined with SSRI or tricyclic antidepressants, St. John's wort may trigger serotonin syndrome.

Kava kava is a herb. It is believed to relieve anxiety, elevate mood and induce feelings of relaxation and contentment. Research studies indicate kava kava may be dangerous because it may induce psychiatric symptoms. There is a potential risk of liver failure associated with the use of kava kava. Multiple drug interactions and potentiation of medications such as anticonvulsants and antianxiety agents have been reported with the concomitant use of kava kava.

Valerian is often effectively used to alleviate insomnia. Others use it to alleviate anxiety and psychological stress. When used in medical amounts for a short time frame it is considered safe for most people. However there are side effects associated with valerian: uneasiness, excitability, headaches, and insomnia.

HESI Hint • The nurse knows depressed clients are improving when they begin to take an interest in their appearance or begin to perform self-care activities that were previously of little or no interest to them.

HESI Hint • The nurse should suspect an imminent suicide attempt if a depressed client becomes "better" (i.e., happy or even elated). Be aware: a happy affect may signify that the client feels relieved that a plan has been made and is prepared for the suicide attempt.

Care of the Suicidal Client

Suicide Precautions

A. Obtain history:
   1. A previous suicide attempt is a most significant risk factor. Other risk groups include those with biologic and organic causes of depression, such as substance abuse, organic brain disorders, or other medical problems.
   2. Clients with a history of a family member's suicide are at heightened risk for suicide.
B. Be aware of the major warning signs of an impending suicide attempt:
   1. A client begins giving away his or her possessions.
   2. When a previously depressed client becomes happy, frequently he or she may have made the decision to commit suicide and is no longer debating the possibility. The client may have regained the energy to act on suicidal feelings and has figured out how to accomplish the suicide.

Evaluation of Intent

A. Directly ask the client about his or her intent. Example: "Have you thought about harming yourself?"
B. Offer the client hope. Example: "We have medication and treatments that can help you through the bad times."

C. Identify the method chosen; the more lethal the method, the higher the probability that an attempt is imminent. "What is your plan for harming yourself?" Example: A client mentions a shotgun and plans to put it to his head and pull the trigger.

D. Determine the availability of the method chosen. If the method is readily available, the attempt is more likely. Example: The client has a loaded shotgun in his room, so it is readily available.

Nursing Interventions

A. Express concern for the client. Example: "I am very concerned that you are feeling so bad that you want to harm yourself."

B. Tell the client that you will share this information with the staff. Example: "I need to share this with the staff so that we can provide for your safety until you are feeling better."

C. Offer the client hope. Example: "You're feeling bad at this moment, but these feelings will pass. We have medications and treatments that can help you through the bad times."

D. Stay with the client. Never leave a suicidal client alone. Legally, the nurse should follow the policy of the institution regarding suicidal clients and should be able to demonstrate that these policies were carried out. Follow the agency policy regarding the removal of potentially hazardous objects such as razors, etc.

> **HESI Hint** • When dealing with a depressed client, encourage independence. If needed, assist with personal hygiene and urge the client to initiate grooming activities even when he or she does not feel like doing so. This helps promote self-esteem and a sense of control.

> **HESI Hint** • An important nursing intervention for the depressed client is to sit quietly with the client. When answering NCLEX-RN questions, remember that you are working at Utopia General and there is plenty of time and staff to provide ideal nursing care. Do not let the realities of clinical situations deter you from choosing the best nursing intervention. The best intervention is to sit quietly with the client, offering support with your presence.

> **HESI Hint** • There are always questions about drugs on the NCLEX-RN. Here are some tips:
> Know the common side effects of drug groups. For example:
> • Antianxiety drugs: sedation, drowsiness

• Kava (CAM), an effective over-the-counter herbal remedy used for the treatment of anxiety that modulates the GABA receptors. It is hepatotoxic, potentiates benzodiazepines, and inhibits the effects of levodopa in patients with Parkinson disease
• Parsley and St. John's wort is an effective CAM used for the treatment of mild depression. However, it may increase the client's risk for serotonin syndrome. In addition it should not be used in conjunction with MAOI inhibitors.
• Antidepressant drugs: anticholinergic effects, postural hypotension
• Monoamine oxidase (MAO) inhibitors: hypertensive crisis when mixed with SSRIs, tyramines, or medications with pseudoephedrine

Know specific problems and concerns in drug therapy. For example:
• Lithium requires serum lithium levels and renal function assessment and monitoring (especially for signs of toxicity).
• Phenothiazines cause extrapyramidal symptoms (EPS); in long-term treatment, tardive dyskinesia can be permanent if client is not assessed regularly for possible signs!

Know specific client teachings about drug therapy. For example:
• Phenothiazines cause photosensitivity, so client must wear protective clothing and sunglasses.
• MAO inhibitors require dietary restrictions (no food with tyramines, such as raisins, red wine, or aged cheese) to prevent hypertensive crisis.
• -SSRI and MAO inhibitors require two weeks time lapse from the previous MAO inhibitor or SSRI before switching from one of those medications to the other.

Bipolar Disorder, or Manic-Depressive Illness

A. It is an affective disorder that is manifested by mood swings involving euphoria, grandiosity, and an inflated sense of self-worth. This disorder may or may not include sudden swings to depression.

B. In order to be diagnosed with a bipolar disorder, according to the DSM-5 classification, a client must have at least one episode of major depression. A client may cycle, going from elevation to depression, with periods of normal activity in between.

Characteristics of Varying Degrees of Mania

A. Mild
   1. Feeling of being on a high
   2. Feelings of well-being
   3. Minor alterations in habits
   4. Usually does not seek treatment because of pleasurable effect

B. Moderate
1. Grandiosity
2. Talkativeness
3. Pressured speech
4. Impulsiveness
5. Excessive spending
6. Bizarre dress and grooming

C. Severe
1. Extreme hyperactivity
2. Flight of ideas
3. Nonstop activity (e.g., running, pacing)
4. Sexual acting out; explicit language
5. Talkativeness
6. Overresponsiveness to external stimuli
7. Easily distracted
8. Agitation and possibly explosiveness
9. Severe sleep disturbance
10. Delusions of grandeur or persecution

Nursing Assessment

A. Determine level of depression exhibited (see previous section on Symptoms of Varying Degrees of Depression).
B. Determine level of mania exhibited (see previous section on Characteristics of Varying Degrees of Mania).
C. Assess nutrition and hydration status.
D. Assess level of fatigue.
E. Assess danger to self and others in relation to level of impulse impairment present.

Analysis (Nursing Diagnoses)

A. *Risk for self-directed/other-directed violence* related to …
B. *Self-care deficit* (specify) related to …
C. *Ineffective denial* related to …
D. *Disturbed sleep patterns* related to …

Nursing Plans and Interventions

A. Maintain client's physical health: Provide nutrition, rest, and hygiene.
B. Provide safe environment (grandiose thinking and poor impulse control can result in accidents and/or altercations with other clients).
C. Decrease environmental stimulation (e.g., place in private room or seclusion room).
D. Implement suicide precautions if assessment indicates risk.
E. Use consistent approach to minimize manipulative behavior.
F. Use frequent, brief contacts to decrease anxiety.
G. Implement constructive limit setting.
H. Avoid giving attention to bizarre behavior (e.g., dress and language).
I. Try to meet needs as soon as possible to keep client from becoming aggressive.
J. Provide small, frequent feedings of food that can be carried (e.g., small finger sandwiches).
K. Engage in simple, active, noncompetitive activities.
L. Avoid distracting or stimulating activities in the evening to help promote sleep and rest.
M. Praise self-control, acceptable behavior.
N. Promote family involvement in therapy, teaching, and medication compliance.
O. Administer lithium, sedatives, and antipsychotics as prescribed (Table 7-8).

HESI Hint • Monitor serum lithium levels carefully. The therapeutic and toxic levels are very close to each other on the readings. Signs of toxicity are evident when lithium levels are more than 1.5 mEq/L. Blood levels should be drawn 12 hours after *last* dose.

HESI Hint • Clients who are experiencing mania can be very caustic toward authority figures. Be prepared for personal putdowns. Avoid arguing or becoming defensive.

HESI Hint • What activities are appropriate for a manic client? Noncompetitive physical activities that require the use of large muscle groups.

HESI Hint • Where should a manic client be placed on the unit?
Make every attempt to reduce stimuli in the environment. Place the client in a quiet part of the unit.

HESI Hint • What interventions should the nurse use if a client becomes abusive?
• Redirect negative behavior or verbal abuse in a calm, firm, nonjudgmental, nondefensive manner.
• Suggest a walk or other physical activity.
• Set limits on intrusive behavior. For example, "When you interrupt, I cannot explain the procedure to the others; please wait your turn."
• If a client becomes totally out of control, administer medication or use seclusion if the client is a danger to self or others. Always remember to use compassion with clients.

TABLE 7-8 Mood-Stabilizing Drugs

Drugs	Indications	Adverse Reactions	Nursing Implications
Lithium carbonate	• Bipolar disorders, especially the manic phase	• Nausea, fatigue, thirst, polyuria, and fine hand tremors • Weight gain • Hypothyroidism • Early signs of toxicity: diarrhea, vomiting, drowsiness, muscle weakness, lack of coordination • Possible renal impairment	• Lithium is excreted by the kidney. Maintain adequate serum levels. • Assess electrolytes, especially sodium. • Baseline studies of renal, cardiac, and thyroid status must be obtained before lithium therapy is begun. • Teach client *early* symptoms of lithium toxicity. If drug is continued, coma, convulsions, and death may occur. • Instruct client to keep salt usage consistent. • Use with diuretics is contraindicated. Diuretic-induced sodium depletion can increase lithium levels, causing toxicity.
Anticonvulsant Mood Stabilizers			
Valproic acid	• Used in bipolar disorder alone or with lithium	• GI distress: nausea, anorexia, vomiting • Hepatotoxicity • Neurologic symptoms: tremor, sedation, headache, dizziness	• Administer with food. • Monitor blood levels. • Maintain serum levels 50-125 µg/mL.
Carbamazepine	• Used in bipolar disorders • Used as alternative to lithium	• Dizziness • Ataxia • Blood dyscrasias	• Maintain serum levels at 8-12 g/mL. • Stop drug if WBC drops below 3000/mm³ or neutrophil count goes below 1500/mm³. • Monitor hepatic and renal function.
Lamotrigine	• Used in bipolar disorder alone or with other mood stabilizers	• Headache • Dizziness • Double vision • Rash (Stevens-Johnson syndrome)	• To minimize risk of severe rash, give low dose, 25-50 mg/day initially, then gradually increase to maintenance dose of 200 mg/day (used alone) or 100 mg/day (with valproate) or 400 mg/day (with carbamazepine).

Review of Mood Disorders

1. Identify the physiologic changes that commonly occur with depression.
2. A client who has been withdrawn and tearful comes to breakfast one morning smiling and interacting with her peers. Before breakfast she gave her roommate her favorite necklace. What actions should the nurse take and why?
3. Name the components of a suicide assessment.
4. A client on your unit refuses to go to group therapy. What is the most appropriate nursing intervention?
5. A client is standing on a table loudly singing "The Star-Spangled Banner" and is encircled by sheets, which have been set afire. In order of priority, describe appropriate nursing actions.

Answers to Review

1. Weight change (loss or gain), constipation, fatigue, lack of sexual interest, somatic complaints, and sleep disturbances
2. Assess for suicidal ideation, plan, and means of carrying out plan. Place on precautions as indicated. A sudden change in mood and giving away possessions are two possible signs that a suicide plan has been developed.
3. Existence of a plan, existence of a method, availability of method chosen, lethality of method chosen, identified support system, and history of previous attempts
4. Accompany client to the group; do not give client option. Client needs to be mobilized.
5. Remove client and other persons in the vicinity to a safe area and have someone activate the hospital fire plan. When area is safe, place client in quiet environment with low stimulation and medicate as indicated.

Schizophrenia Spectrum and Other Psychotic Disorders

Schizophrenia

Description: Psychiatric disorder characterized by thought disturbance, altered affect, withdrawal from reality, regressive behavior, difficulty with communication, and impaired interpersonal relationships, as well as an impaired ability to perceive reality.

A. Key symptoms of schizophrenia
1. Delusions
2. Hallucinations
3. Disorganized speech
4. Disorganized behavior
5. Negative symptoms

> **HESI Hint** • Positive symptoms: Hallucinations, delusions
> Negative symptoms: Movement disorders, flat affect, anhedonia (lack of pleasure), inability to begin or sustain planned activities, poverty of speech
> Cognitive symptoms: Difficulty understanding information, trouble paying attention, inability to use information after learning it

> **HESI Hint** • Catatonia occurs across several categories of disorders and can be used with depressive, bipolar, or psychotic disorders. In addition, catatonia occurs in the context of other medical conditions.

B. Catatonia
1. Stupor (decrease in reaction to the environment) or mutism
2. Rigidity (maintenance of a posture against efforts to be moved)
3. Posturing (waxy flexibility)
4. Negativism (resistance to instructions)
5. Excitement (severely agitated, out of control)
6. Potential for violence to self or others during stupor or excitement

C. Schizoaffective disorder diagnosis must include presence of a major mood episode for the majority of the disorder's total duration.

> **HESI Hint** • When evaluating client behaviors, consider the medications the client is receiving. Exhibited behaviors may be manifestations of schizophrenia or a drug reaction.

Nursing Assessment

A. Assess for disturbance in thought process.
1. Interpret content of internal and external stimuli.
   a. Symbolism: meaning given to words by client to screen thoughts and feelings that would be difficult to handle if stated directly
   b. Delusions: fixed false beliefs that may be persecutory, grandiose, religious, or somatic in nature
   c. Ideas of reference: belief that conversations or actions of others have reference to the client
2. Note form: construction of verbal communication.
   a. Looseness of association: lack of clear connection from one thought to the next
   b. Tangential or circumstantial speech: failing to address the original point, giving many nonessential details
   c. Echolalia: constantly repeating what is heard
   d. Neologism: creating new words
   e. Preseveration repeating same word or phrase in response to different questions
   f. Word salad: speaking a jumbled mixture of real and made-up words
3. Note process: flow of thoughts.
   a. Blocking: gap or interruption in speech due to absent thoughts
   b. Concrete thinking: thinking based on fact versus abstract and intellectual points
B. Assess for disturbance in perception.
1. Hallucinations: false sensory perception, usually auditory or visual in nature
2. Illusions: misinterpretation of external environment
3. Depersonalization: perceives self as alienated or detached from real body
4. Delusions: false, fixed beliefs that cannot be changed by reason
C. Assess for disturbance in affect (feelings or mood).
1. Blunted or flat
2. Inappropriate
3. Incongruent with context of situation or event
D. Assess for disturbance in behavior.
1. Incoherent and disorganized
2. Impulsive, uninhibited
3. Posturing, unusual mannerisms
4. Social withdrawal, neglect of personal hygiene
5. Exhibiting echopraxia: repetition of another person's movements
E. Assess for disturbance in interpersonal relationships.
1. Difficulty establishing trust
2. Difficulty with intimacy
3. Fear and ambivalence toward others

Analysis (Nursing Diagnoses)

A. *Disturbed sensory perception* related to …
B. *Disturbed personal identity* related to …
C. *Risk for self-directed/other-directed violence* related to …

Nursing Plans and Interventions

A. Establish trust.
B. Sit with mute clients.
C. Provide safe and secure environment.
D. Assist with physical hygiene and ADLs.
E. Use matter-of-fact, nonjudgmental approach.
F. Use clear, simple, concrete terms when talking with client.
G. Accept and support client's feelings; use clarification.
H. Reinforce congruent thinking. Stress reality.
I. Avoid arguing and avoid agreeing with inaccurate communications.
J. Set limits on behavior.
K. Avoid stressful situations.
L. Structure time for activities so as to limit time for withdrawal.
M. Encourage client to identify positive characteristics related to self.
N. Praise socially acceptable behavior.
O. Avoid fostering a dependent relationship.
P. Promote family involvement in therapy, teaching, and medication compliance.

> **HESI Hint** • Use Bleuler's four As to help remember the important characteristics of schizophrenia:
> - Autism (loss of connection with reality; client's thoughts are odd and internally stimulated)
> - Affect (flat or blunted, for example, lack of emotional expression)
> - Associations (loose, for example, rapidly changes from one subject to an unrelated subject)
> - Ambivalence (for example, simultaneously holding two different attitudes about a situation)

Delusional Disorders

Description: Characterized by suspicious, strange behavior, which can be precipitated by a stressful event and can manifest as an intense hypochondriasis

Nursing Assessment

A. Determine degree of suspiciousness and mistrust of others.
B. Assess degree of anxiety.
C. Determine whether delusions are present.
  1. Reference or control
  2. Persecution
  3. Grandeur
  4. Somatic
  5. Jealousy
D. Assess degree of insecurity.

Analysis (Nursing Diagnoses)

A. *Risk for self-directed/other-directed violence* related to …
B. *Social isolation* related to …

Nursing Interventions for Delusional and Hallucinating Clients

Client Is Delusional	Client Is Hallucinating
A. Encourage recognition of distorted reality. B. Divert focus from delusional thought to reality; do not permit rumination on false ideas.	A. Protect client from injury that might result from responding to commands of the voices; pay attention to the content.
C. Do not agree with or support delusions. D. Avoid arguing about the delusion. Be very matter of fact. E. Avoid physically touching client, especially if delusions are persecutional. F. Administer antipsychotic drugs (see Table 7-6). G. Monitor and treat side effects of psychotropic drugs (Table 7-9). H. Administer anticholinergic drugs (Table 7-10).	B. Avoid denying or arguing with client about the hallucination. C. Discuss your observations with client (e.g., "You appear to be listening to something."). D. Make frequent but brief remarks to interrupt the hallucinations. E. Administer antipsychotic drugs (see Table 7-6). F. Monitor and treat side effects of psychotropic drugs (see Table 7-9). G. Administer anticholinergic drugs (see Table 7-10).

> **HESI Hint** • Observe for increased motor activity and/or erratic response to staff and other clients. The client may be experiencing an increase in command hallucinations. When this occurs, there is an increased potential for aggressive behavior.

> **HESI Hint** • Do not argue with a client about the delusions. Logic does not work; it only increases the client's anxiety. Be matter of fact and divert delusional thought to reality. Trust is the basis for all interactions with any clients. Be supportive and nonjudgmental. Stress increases anxiety and the need for delusions and hallucinations. Do not agree that you hear voices (you should be the client's contact with reality), but acknowledge your observation of the client; for example, "You look like you're listening to something," or, "I understand you are hearing voices that I can't hear."

TABLE 7-9 Side Effects of Psychotropic Drugs and Nursing Interventions

Side Effects	Characteristics	Nursing Interventions
Blood Dyscrasias		
• Agranulocytosis: occurs in first weeks of treatment • Thrombocytopenia: decreased platelets	• Sore throat, fever, chills (most often seen with clozapine)	• Protect from infections. • Provide comfort measures: gargle for sore throat, use lozenges and analgesics.
	• Bruises easily, petechia	• Teach client safety measures.
Extrapyramidal Effects		
• Parkinsonism: occurs within 1-4 wk after initiation of treatment • Akathisia: occurs within 1-6 wk after initiation of treatment • Dystonia: occurs within 1-2 days after initiation of treatment • Tardive dyskinesia: develops late in treatment	• Rigidity, shuffling gait, pill-rolling hand movements, tremors, dyskinesia, masklike face • Restlessness, agitation, and pacing; sudden difficulty sitting still (can be confused with tardive dyskinesia) • Limb and neck spasms; uncoordinated, jerky movements; difficulty speaking and swallowing; rigidity and muscle spasms • Involuntary tongue and lip movements; blinking, choreiform movements of limbs and trunk	• Administer anticholinergic drugs (i.e., Cogentin, Artane). Other drugs for EPS include Benadryl, Symmetrel, Ativan, Klonopin; Inderal for akathisia and vitamin E for tardive dyskinesia. • Rule out anxiety. Can ask client, "Are you feeling so restless that you can't sit still?" • Emergency treatment is with IM anticholinergics. *Have respiratory emergency equipment available.* • Permanent side effect; anticholinergic drugs are of no help in decreasing symptoms. • Teach client and family to report side effects *early.*
• Photosensitivity	• Sunlight: exposed skin turns blue and color changes occur in eyes, but does not cause vision impairment.	• Teach client to stay out of sun, wear protective clothing and sunglasses. • Skin discoloration will disappear within 6 mo after drug is discontinued.
• Neuroleptic malignant syndrome	• Life-threatening emergency: high fever, tachycardia, stupor, increased respirations, severe muscle rigidity	• Increased risk with phenothiazines • Early recognition is important; transfer to medical facility for hydration, nutritional support, and treatment of possible respiratory failure and renal failure.
• Serotonin syndrome	• Confusion, disorientation, autonomic dysfunction	• Notify health care provider immediately. • Provide systems support.
• Anticholinergic effects	• Dry mouth, blurred vision, tachycardia, nasal congestion, constipation, urinary retention, orthostatic hypotension	• Encourage sips of water, chewing sugarless gum or sucking hard candy. • Increase fiber in diet. • Change positions slowly to avoid dizziness. • Report urinary retention to physician. • Tolerance to these side effects will usually occur.

HESI Hint • Know the side effects of drugs commonly used to treat schizophrenia because client behavioral changes may be due to drug reactions instead of schizophrenia.

TABLE 7-10 Anticholinergic Drugs

Drugs	Indications	Adverse Reactions	Nursing Implications
• Trihexyphenidyl HCl (Artane) • Benztropine mesylate (Cogentin) • Amantadine (Symmetrel)	• Acts on the extrapyramidal system to reduce disturbing symptoms	• Anticholinergic effects • Drowsiness • Headaches • Urinary hesitancy • Memory impairment	• Usually given in conjunction with antipsychotic drugs

Review of Thought Disorders

1. A client is sitting alone talking quietly. There is no one around. What nursing action should be taken?
2. A client has been sitting in the same position for 2 hours. He is mute. What type of illness is this client experiencing? Describe appropriate nursing interventions for this client.
3. A client is very agitated. He believes that the Central Intelligence Agency (CIA) has tapped the phone and is sending messages through the television and that you are an agent who has been planted by the agency. In order of priority, list the appropriate nursing actions when intervening in this situation. What type of delusion is this client experiencing?
4. The nurse asks the client, "What brought you to the hospital?" The client's response is, "The bus." What type of thinking is this client exhibiting?
5. What CAM herb is used to relieve insomnia? List two potential side effects of that herb.

Answers to Review

1. Quietly approach the client and note the behavior. Assess the content of the hallucinations (e.g., "I noticed you talking. Are you hearing voices? Can you tell me about the voices you are hearing?") Schizophrenia; spend time with client; assist with ADLs; be alert to potential for violence toward self or others; be aware of fluid and nutrition needs.
2. Delusion of grandeur; approach client and offer solitary activity as distraction. Assess need for medication. Encourage verbalization of feelings and promote outlet for expression. The delusion is paranoid disorder with delusions of reference.
3. Approach client and offer solitary activity as distraction. Assess need for medication. Encourage verbalization of feelings and promote outlet for expression. The delusion is paranoid disorder with delusions of reference (CIA).
4. Concrete
5. Valerian is used to alleviate insomnia. Potential side effects include: headaches, uneasiness, and insomnia.

Substance Abuse Disorder

Description: Regular use of psychoactive substances that affect the central nervous system (CNS), resulting in significant impairment or distress occurring in a 12-month time frame. Clients diagnosed with substance abuse disorder demonstrate a problematic pattern of behaviors. The DSM-5 lists nine known classes of psychoactive substances: alcohol; caffeine; cannabis; hallucinogens (phencyclidine or other hallucinogens); inhalants; opioids; sedatives; hypnotics; and anxiolytics, stimulants, and tobacco.

Nursing Assessment

A. Patterns indicative of alcoholism:
1. Episodic drinking (binges)
2. Continuous drinking
3. Morning drinking
4. Increase in family fighting about drinking
5. Increase in absences from work or school, especially Mondays
6. Blackouts
7. Hiding drinking pattern
8. Legal problems, such as drinking under the influence (DUI)
9. Health problems such as gastritis
10. Defense mechanisms: denial, projection, and rationalization
B. Family history of alcoholism or substance abuse
C. Dependency, yet resentfulness of authority
D. Impulsive, abusive behavior
E. Impaired judgment, memory loss
F. Incoordination, slurred speech
G. Mood varying between euphoria and depression
H. Intoxication as determined by blood alcohol level (BAL; 0.10% or greater is considered intoxication)
I. Previous experience with treatment centers or Alcoholics Anonymous (AA)
J. Alcohol withdrawal symptoms:
1. Begin shortly after drinking stops, as early as 4 to 6 hours after
2. Peaks in 48 to 72 hours and decreases within 4 to 5 days
3. Sudden or gradual increase in all vital signs (autonomic hyperactivity)
4. Delirium tremens (DTs); may appear 12 to 36 hours after last drink:
   a. Tachycardia (>100 bpm), tachypnea, diaphoresis
   b. Marked hand tremors, insomnia, and/or psychomotor agitation
   c. Transient visual, auditory, or tactile hallucinations or illusions (with alcohol-induced psychotic disorder, the client may describe feeling bugs crawling on the skin)
   d. Nausea and vomiting may be present
   e. Paranoia
5. Grand mal seizures and death (possible)
K. Chronic alcohol-related illnesses:
1. Chronic gastritis
2. Cirrhosis and hepatitis
3. Korsakoff syndrome: organic syndrome that frequently follows DTs; associated with chronic alcoholism
4. Wernicke syndrome: a severe disorder (encephalopathy) occurring in chronic alcoholics; probably due to a

deficiency of vitamin B_1 (thiamine); may escalate Korsakoff syndrome; is treated with thiamine chloride

5. Malnutrition and dehydration
6. Pancreatitis
7. Peripheral neuropathy

Analysis (Nursing Diagnoses)

A. *Risk for injury* related to …
B. *Ineffective family coping* related to …
C. *Imbalanced nutrition: less than body requirements* related to …
D. *Situational low self-esteem* related to …

Nursing Plans and Interventions

A. Maintain safety, nutrition, hygiene, and rest.
B. Obtain a BAL on admission or when a client appears intoxicated after admission.
C. Implement suicide precautions if assessment indicates risk.
   1. Monitor vital signs, I&O, electrolytes.
   2. Observe for impending DTs.
   3. Prevent aspiration; implement seizure precautions.
   4. Reduce environmental stimuli.
   5. Medicate with antianxiety medication, usually chlordiazepoxide (Librium) or lorazepam (Ativan) (see Table 7-4).
   6. Provide high-protein diet and adequate fluid intake (limit caffeine).
   7. Provide vitamin supplements, especially vitamins B_1 and B complex.
   8. Provide emotional support.
D. Provide care during withdrawal.
   1. Use direct, matter-of-fact, nonjudgmental attitude.
   2. Confront denial and rationalization (main coping styles used by alcoholics).
   3. Confront manipulations; set firm limits on behavior.
   4. Set short-term, realistic goals.
   5. Help increase self-esteem.
   6. Explore ways to increase frustration tolerance without alcohol.
   7. Identify ways to decrease loneliness.
   8. Encourage client to accept responsibility for own behavior.
   9. Identify availability of support systems (family, friends, church, AA).
   10. Identify activities and friendships not related to drinking.
   11. Provide group and family therapy; refer family to AA family groups or Alateen.
E. Provide client and family teaching regarding the side effects of disulfiram (Antabuse) if it is used as a deterrent to drinking (Table 7-11).
F. Provide client and family teaching regarding the side effects of disulfiram, acamprosate (Campral), or naltrexone if it is used to promote recovery (see Table 7-11).

Substance Use Disorder

Description: Abuse refers to the habitual use of psychoactive substances that is not socially acceptable nor a medical necessity. The substance is purposely used to alter the client's emotion, mood, or state of consciousness.

Addiction refers to behavior that is focused on drug use and drug-seeking behaviors. Drug cravings stimulate drug-seeking behavior. Substance abuse addiction is a chronic, potentially relapsing brain disorder. One client may remain abstinent for a lifetime, whereas another client may remain substance free for a long time, followed by a relapse into substance use and abuse.

The most commonly used illicit psychoactive substance is marijuana. Club drugs usage is on the rise; those substances include ecstasy, gamma-hydroxybutyric (GHB) acid, lysergic acid diethylamide (LSD), and methamphetamine.

Nonmedical use of prescription drugs is also a form of substance abuse. Painkillers (oxycodone [OxyContin]), sedatives, and stimulants may necessitate withdrawal precautions when a client is in the hospital. Sometimes abuse of prescription drugs leads to unintentional overdose and death.

Anabolic-androgenic steroids are also abused.

Nursing Assessment

Dual diagnosis: Although a large percentage of individuals with mood disorders or schizophrenia abuse psychoactive substances, research studies are seeking to determine whether there is a link between the neurotransmitter dopamine and schizophrenia and mood disorders, as well as between dopamine and addictive substances. Other researchers are studying gene disorders and their link to mental health disorders.

People who abuse alcohol or psychoactive substances are at high risk for suicide.
A. Pattern of psychoactive substance use
   1. What psychoactive substances are used?
   2. What is the psychoactive substance of choice?
   3. How much is used and how often?
   4. How long have the psychoactive substances been used?
B. Physical evidence of psychoactive substance usage
   1. Needle track marks
   2. Cellulitis at puncture site
   3. Poor nutritional status
   4. Inflammation of nasal passages
C. Possible causes of psychoactive substance use
   1. Desire to escape reality and problems
   2. Low self-esteem and lack of success in life
   3. Peer or culture pressure
   4. Lack of meaningful relationships
   5. Intolerance to pain and frustration
D. Symptoms of withdrawal and overdose are specific for the drug used (Table 7-12).

TABLE 7-11 Alcohol Deterrents

Drugs	Indications	Adverse Reactions	Nursing Implications
Disulfiram	• Treatment of alcoholism; aversion therapy • Interferes with breakdown of alcohol, causing an accumulation of acetaldehyde (a byproduct of alcohol in the body)	• *Severe side effects* occur if alcohol is consumed: ○ Nausea and vomiting ○ Hypotension, headaches ○ Rapid pulse and respirations ○ Flushed face and bloodshot eyes ○ Confusion ○ Chest pain ○ Weakness, dizziness	• Teach client what to expect if alcohol is consumed while taking the drug. • Be aware that some alcoholic clients use the side effects as a means of "punishing" themselves or as a form of masochism, and if a client repeatedly consumes alcohol while taking the drug, the health care provider should be notified. • Persons with serious heart disease, diabetes, epilepsy, liver impairment, or mental illness should not take Antabuse. • Use in motivated clients who have shown the ability to stay sober.
Acamprosate	• Treatment of alcohol dependence by reducing anxiety and unpleasant effects that trigger resuming drinking • Balances GABA and glutamate neurotransmitters	• Headache • Nausea and diarrhea	• Helps reduce cravings • Does not reduce or eliminate withdrawal symptoms

HESI Hint • What medications can the nurse expect to administer to chemically dependent clients? In treating alcohol withdrawal, chlordiazepoxide (Librium) or lorazepam (Ativan) is commonly used. Disulfiram (Antabuse) is often used as a deterrent to drinking alcohol. Client teaching should include the effects of consuming any alcohol while on Antabuse. Encourage client to read all labels of over-the-counter medications and food products that may contain small amounts of alcohol (e.g., cough medicine, shaving lotion).

Analysis (Nursing Diagnoses)

A. *Risk for injury* related to …
B. *Risk for infection* related to …
C. *Disturbed personal identity* related to …

Nursing Plans and Interventions

A. Assess level of consciousness and vital signs. (Rapid withdrawal can be fatal for persons addicted to barbiturates, antianxiety medications, and hypnotics.)
B. Monitor I&O and electrolytes.
C. Implement suicide precautions if assessment indicates risk.
D. Provide adequate nutrition, hydration, and rest.
E. Administer medications according to detoxification protocol of medical unit.
F. Phenothiazines may be used to decrease the discomfort of withdrawal.
G. Confront denial (main coping style used by substance abusers).
  1. Focus on substance abuse problem.
  2. Confront the placing of blame on external problems.
H. Reinforce reality in simple, concrete terms.
I. Encourage verbal expression of anger and depression.
J. Assist with identification of stressors and areas of conflict.
K. Encourage exploration of alternative coping strategies.
L. Positively reinforce insight into behavior patterns.
M. Help identify an appropriate support system.
N. Provide support to significant others.
O. Teach danger of acquired immune deficiency syndrome (AIDS) and other blood-related diseases.

HESI Hint • Know what defense mechanisms are used by chemically dependent clients. Denial and rationalization are the two most common coping styles used. Their use must be confronted so the client's accountability for his or her own behavior can be developed.

HESI Hint • What basic needs take priority when working with chemically dependent clients? Alcohol and psychoactive substance intake has superseded the intake of food for these clients. Nutrition is a priority. Poor nutrition with an alcoholic client results in inadequate intake of thiamine and niacin, leading to confabulation (falsification of memory), peripheral neuropathy, and amnesia (symptoms of Wernicke-Korsakoff syndrome). Therefore thiamine is part of the protocol for treating alcoholic clients.

HESI Hint • What behaviors are expected during withdrawal? In the alcoholic, DTs occur 12 to 48 hours after the last intake of alcohol. Know the symptoms. In drug abuse, withdrawal symptoms are specific to the type of drug.

HESI Hint • Fetal alcohol syndrome (FAS) and fetal alcohol spectrum disorders (FASDs) resulting in mental retardation, delayed growth and development, and distinctive facial abnormalities are the result of alcohol use during pregnancy. Lifelong permanent physical disabilities (hearing, eyesight, heart and kidney defects) and behavioral problems (hyperactivity and poor impulse control) are also associated with FAS and FASDs.

TABLE 7-12 Drug Withdrawal and Overdose Symptoms

Drugs	Withdrawal	Overdose	Effect
Opiates			
• Heroin • Morphine • Codeine • Opium • Methadone	• Watery eyes, runny nose, dilated pupils • Anxiety • Diaphoresis, fever • Nausea, vomiting, and diarrhea • Achiness • Abdominal cramps • Insomnia • Tachycardia	• Constricted pupils • Respiratory depression leading to respiratory arrest • Circulatory depression leading to cardiac arrest • Unconsciousness leading to coma • Death	• General physical and mental deterioration • Rapid tolerance • Impaired judgment
• Cocaine	• Depression • Fatigue • Disturbed sleep • Anxiety • Psychomotor agitation	• Tachycardia • Pupillary dilatation • Increased BP • Cardiac arrhythmias • Perspiration, chills • Nausea, vomiting	• Psychological dependence • Tolerance within hours or days
• Amphetamines	• Depression • Fatigue • Disturbed sleep	• Restlessness • Tremors • Rapid respiration • Confusion • Assaultive behavior • Hallucinations • Panic	• Paranoid delusions
• Hallucinogenics	• No withdrawal	• Panic • Psychosis	• Flashbacks • Impaired judgment
Antianxiety Drugs			

• Benzodiazepines:
  ○ Valium
  ○ Serax
  ○ Ativan
	• Tremors
	• Agitation
	• Anxiety
	• Abdominal cramps
	• Nausea and vomiting
	• Grand mal seizures
		• Drowsiness
		• Confusion
		• Hypotension
		• Convulsion
		• Shock
		• Coma → death
			• Withdrawal occurs if there is abrupt cessation
			• Temporary psychosis

HESI Hint • What type of therapy is used with chemically dependent clients? Group therapy is effective, as are support groups such as Alcoholics Anonymous and Narcotics Anonymous.

HESI Hint • Harm reduction is a community health strategy designed to reduce the harm of substance abuse to families, individuals, community, and society. Examples: More compassionate drug treatment options, including abstinence and drug-substitution models; HIV-related interventions such as needle exchanges; directed drug-use management should the client wish to continue use; changes in laws concerning possession of paraphernalia and drug use.

Review of Substance Abuse Disorder

1. Three days ago, a client was admitted to the medical unit for a gastrointestinal (GI) bleed. His BP and pulse rate gradually increased, and he developed a low-grade fever. What assessment data should the nurse obtain? What kind of anticipatory planning should the nurse develop?
2. What physical signs might indicate that a client is abusing intravenous medications?
3. What behaviors would indicate to the nurse manager that an employee has a possible substance abuse problem?

4. A client becomes extremely agitated, abusive, and very suspicious. He is currently undergoing detoxification from alcohol with chlordiazepoxide (Librium) 15 mg every 6 hours. What nursing actions are indicated?
5. A client in the third week of a cocaine rehabilitation program returns from an unsupervised pass. The nurse notices that he is euphoric and is socializing with the other clients more than he has in the past. What nursing actions are indicated?

Answers to Review

1. Obtain a drug and alcohol consumption assessment, including type, frequency, and time of last dose or drink. Call the health care provider and report findings. Anticipate withdrawal and DTs. Provide a quiet, safe environment. Place on seizure precautions. Anticipate giving a medication such as chlordiazepoxide (Librium). Call the health care provider and report findings.
2. Needle track marks; cellulitis at puncture site; poor nutritional status

3. Change in work performance, withdrawal, increase in absences (especially Mondays and Fridays), increase in number of times tardy, long breaks, lateness returning from lunch
4. Notify the health care provider immediately and anticipate an increase in dose or frequency of Librium to 50 mg. Provide a quiet, safe environment. Approach in a quiet, calm manner. Avoid touching client.
5. Notify health care provider of observed behavior change. Get a urine drug screen as prescribed. Confront client with observed behavior change.

Abuse

Intimate-Partner Violence

A. It is a criminal act of physical, emotional, economic, or sexual abuse between an assailant and a victim who most commonly are, or were, in an intimate relationship (may be married or dating).
B. Abuse is usually a tension-releasing action, as well as a lack of impulse control.
C. Assailant may come from a family in which battering and physical violence were present.
D. Persons act more violently when drinking alcohol or using psychoactive substances.
E. The relationship is usually characterized by issues of power and control.
F. Women in a battering relationship may lack self-confidence and feel trapped. They may be embarrassed about their situation, which results in isolation and dependency on the abuser.
G. Abuse often begins during pregnancy or occurs more frequently during pregnancy.
H. See Figure 7-3.

Nursing Assessment

A. Delay between time of injury and time of treatment
B. Anxious when answering questions about injury
C. Abdominal injuries during pregnancy
D. Looks to abuser for answers to questions related to injuries
E. Depression or suicidal ideation
F. Feeling of responsibility for "provoking" partner
G. Low self-esteem
H. Abrasions, cuts, lacerations, sprains, black eyes
I. Psychosomatic (somatoform) complaints
J. Concurrent use of alcohol or psychoactive substances

Analysis (Nursing Diagnoses)

A. *Fear* related to …
B. *Risk for injury* related to …
C. *Powerlessness* related to …

Nursing Plans and Interventions

A. Establish trust; use nonjudgmental approach.
B. Treat physical wounds and injuries. Remember, clients of the same gender also are survivors of family violence.
C. Interview the survivor when the spouse/partner is not present; send her/him out of the room to admissions, etc., thus allowing the survivor to tell what happened.

1. Tension-building phase

The man engages in increasingly hostile behaviors such as throwing objects, pushing, swearing, and threatening. He often consumes increased amounts of alcohol or drugs.

The woman tries to stay out of the way or to placate the man during this phase and thus avoid the next phase.

2. Battering incident

The man explodes in violence. He may hit, burn, beat, or rape the woman, often causing substantial physical injury.

The woman feels powerless and simply endures the abuse until the episode runs its course, usually 2 to 24 hours.

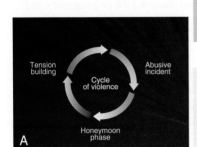

3. Honeymoon phase

The batterer will do anything to make up with his partner. He is contrite and remorseful and promises never to do it again. He may insist on having intercourse to confirm that he is forgiven.

The battered woman wants to believe the promise that the abuse will never happen again, but this is seldom the case.

A   B

FIGURE 7-3 The cycle of violence.

D. Treat physical wounds and injuries.

E. Document factual, objective statements about client's physical condition, injuries (take photos that become part of the medical record; use body chart to indicate location of injuries), and interaction with partner or family.

F. Determine potential for further violence.

G. Ask the survivor if there is a safe place to go to; offer to contact a safe place.

H. Provide crisis intervention.

I. Assist with referral to shelter if necessary or desired, with adult's consent.

J. Assist client with contacting authorities if charges are to be pressed.

HESI Hint • Women who are abused may rationalize the spouse's behavior and unnecessarily accept blame for his actions. The woman may or may not choose to press charges. Be sure to give her the number of a shelter or help line for future occurrences, and help her to develop a safety plan.

HESI Hint • Survivors of intimate partner violence may have been raped by the partner. Survivors of rape are at high risk for posttraumatic stress disorder (PTSD). Intervention to diminish distress is vital. The nurse should assess and intervene for sequelae such as unwanted pregnancy, sexually transmitted diseases, and HIV risk.

HESI Hint • Questions on the NCLEX-RN examination regarding physical and sexual abuse usually focus on three aspects:

1. Physical manifestations of abuse.
2. Client safety.
3. Legal responsibilities of the nurse.

For children, the nurse is legally responsible for reporting all suspected cases of abuse. In intimate-partner abuse, it is the adult's decision; the nurse should be supportive of the decision. Remember to document objective factual assessment data and the client's exact words in cases of sexual abuse and rape.

Review of Abuse

1. When does battering of women often begin or escalate?
2. What dynamics prevent a battered spouse from leaving the battering situation?
3. Identify nursing interventions for working with a rape survivor.

Answers to Review

1. During pregnancy
2. A woman in a relationship of intimate-partner violence may lack self-confidence and feel trapped because she lacks financial support for herself and her children. She is often embarrassed to tell friends and family, so she becomes isolated and dependent on the abuser.
3. Communicate nonjudgmental acceptance. Provide physical care to treat injuries. Give clear, concise explanations

of all procedures to be performed. Notify police; encourage victim to prosecute. Collect and label evidence carefully in the presence of a witness. Document factual, objective statements about physical condition. Record client's exact words in describing the assault. Notify rape crisis team or counselor if available in the community. Allow discussion of feelings about the assault. Advise of potential for venereal disease, HIV, or pregnancy, and describe medical care available.

Neurocognitive Disorder (DSM-5)

Description: Abnormal psychological or behavioral signs and symptoms that occur as a result of cerebral disease, systemic dysfunction, or use of or exposure to exogenous substances. These disorders go beyond normal aging, and there must be significant impairment in cognitive functioning.

Neurocognitive Disorder (Delirium and Dementia)

Delirium	Dementia
Description: Acute process that, if treated, is usually reversible. It is recognized by its sudden onset. A. It occurs in response to a specific stressor, such as: 1. Infection 2. Drug reaction 3. Substance intoxication or withdrawal 4. Electrolyte imbalance 5. Head trauma 6. Sleep deprivation B. The treatment of choice is the correction of the causative disorder.	Description: Cognitive impairments characterized by gradual, progressive onset; it is irreversible. Judgment, memory, abstract thinking, and social behavior are affected. Some examples of symptoms are aphasia, apraxia, and agnosia. A. It is most commonly seen in: 1. Alzheimer's disease (see Table 8-2) 2. Multiinfarctions (brain) B. It also occurs in: 1. Huntington chorea 2. Parkinson disease 3. Multiple sclerosis and brain tumors 4. Wernicke-Korsakoff syndrome (chronic alcoholics)

HESI Hint • The basic difference between delirium and dementia is that delirium is acute and reversible, whereas dementia is gradual and permanent.

Nursing Assessment

A. Limited attention span, easily distracted
B. Confusion and disorientation, impaired judgment
C. Delusions, visual hallucinations, or sensory illusions
D. Labile affect; sudden anger
E. Anxiety and depression
F. Loss of recent and remote memory
G. Confabulation (making up responses, stories to fill in lost memory)
H. Impaired coordination
I. Increased psychomotor activity
J. Slurring of speech
K. Decreased personal hygiene
L. Sleep deprivation, day–night reversal
M. Incontinence and constipation

Analysis (Nursing Diagnosis)

A. *Dressing/grooming self-care deficit* related to …

Nursing Plans and Interventions

A. Provide safe, consistent environment.
B. Maintain health, nutrition, safety, hygiene, and rest.
C. Assist with ADLs.
D. Provide support to client and family.
E. Provide routine in daily activities.
F. Mark the bathroom clearly.
G. Reorient the client as needed.
H. Use simple, direct statements.
I. See Medical-Surgical in Chapter 4; Psychiatric Nursing Neurocognitive Disorders in this chapter; and Neurological System in this chapter.

HESI Hint • Think "sudden change" when obtaining a history. Such changes are usually due to a specific stressor, and treatment of the causative stressor will usually result in correcting the confusion. Confusion in older adults is often accepted as being part of growing old. However, the confusion may be due to dehydration with resulting electrolyte imbalance.

HESI Hint • Confabulation is a false memory created by the client that is accepted as truth to fill in gaps when real experience cannot be recalled. It is a plausible but imagined memory.

HESI Hint • Nursing interventions for the confused older adult should focus on:
- Maintaining the client's health and safety
- Encouraging self-care
- Reinforcing reality orientation (e.g., saying, "Today is Monday," and calling the client by name)
- Providing a consistent, safe environment; engaging the client in simple tasks and activities to build self-esteem

HESI Hint • Providing a consistent caregiver is a priority in planning nursing care for the confused older client. Change increases anxiety and confusion.

Review of Neurocognitive Disorders

1. List six causes of delirium.
2. Describe the nursing care for a client with Alzheimer disease.
3. Identify three or more causes of dementia.

Answers to Review

1. Infection, medication interaction, alcohol withdrawal, electrolyte imbalance, sleep deprivation, brain injury (e.g., subdural hematoma).
2. Provide a safe, consistent environment. (Do not make changes, if possible. Change increases anxiety and confu-
sion.) Stick to routines. If client wanders, make sure he or she has a name tag. Provide assistance as needed with ADLs. Make sure bathroom is clearly labeled.
3. Alzheimer disease, multiinfarcts (brain), Huntington chorea, multiple sclerosis, Parkinson disease

Childhood and Adolescent Disorders

Attention-Deficit (Hyperactivity) Disorder (ADD/ADHD)

Description: Developmentally inappropriate attention, impulsiveness, and hyperactivity

Nursing Assessment

A. Physical assessment
B. More prevalent in boys
C. Failure to listen to and follow instructions
D. Difficulty playing quietly and sitting still
E. Disruptive, impulsive behavior
F. Distractibility to external stimuli
G. Excessive talking
H. Shifting from one unfinished task to another
I. Underachievement in school performance

Analysis (Nursing Diagnoses)

A. *Risk for injury: trauma* related to ….
B. *Social isolation* related to …
C. *Interrupted family process* related to …

Nursing Plans and Interventions

A. Decrease environmental stimuli.
B. Set limits on behavior when indicated.
C. Provide a safe, comfortable environment.
D. Administer medications as prescribed (Table 7-13).

Autism Spectrum Disorder (ASD)

Description: This is a new DSM-5 name that reflects a single condition with different levels of symptoms. Autism, Asperger disorder, childhood disintegrative disorder, and pervasive developmental disorder not otherwise specified are now combined. ASD is characterized by two components that must be met for the diagnosis of ASD. Deficits in social communication and restrictive repetitive behaviors, interests, and activities (RRBs) must be present.

ASD is essentially a group of developmental disabilities that cause problems with the following:
- Social skills (avoids eye contact, avoids or resists physical contact, and prefers to play alone). Maintains flat or inappropriate facial expressions. At age 12 months does not respond to being called by name.
- Communication is characterized by delayed language and speech skills; talks in a singsong or a flat, robotic voice
- Repetitive behaviors and routines
- Emotional attachment

Communication: Delayed speech and language skills; echolalia (repeats words or phrases over and over); talks in a flat, robotlike, or singsong voice; does not understand jokes, sarcasm, or teasing; gives unrelated answers to questions; uses few or no gestures

Repeated behaviors and routines: Repetitive motions repeated over and over (flaps hands, rocks body, or spins self in circles; repeatedly turns light on and off), plays with toys the same way every time, gets upset by minor changes

TABLE 7-13 Stimulants

Drugs	Indications	Adverse Reactions	Nursing Implications
• Dextroamphetamine sulfate • Methylphenidate HCl • Pemoline • Lisdexamfetamine • Amphetamine/dextroamphetamine • Dexmethylphenidate	• Treat ADD/ADHD • Methylphenidate is also used to treat narcolepsy.	• May interact with MAO inhibitors, producing fever and hypertensive crisis • Nervousness and insomnia; dizziness • Tourette syndrome • Tachycardia, palpitations, angina, dysrhythmias • Anorexia, weight loss, nausea, and abdominal pain	• Short-acting, 2-4 hr. • Teach to take last dose at least 6 hr before bedtime if insomnia occurs. • Administer 1-3 doses daily. • Administer with or after meals to avoid appetite suppression. • Monitor heart rate, rhythm, and BP. • Monitor height and weight to detect growth suppression.

(changes furniture around, changes route going someplace familiar), has obsessive interest. When behaviors or routines are changed usually has temper tantrum or severe frustration

Other symptoms: Unusual eating habits; aggression; cause self-injury; impulsive; hyperactivity; unusual reactions to the way things sound, smell, taste, look, or feel

In some children, ASD can be detected by age 18 months or younger. At age 2 an experienced health care provider can diagnose ASD.

There are two steps to diagnosing ASD:
• Developmental screening
• Comprehensive diagnostic evaluation

Developmental screening is a short test to tell if children are learning basic skills when they should, or if they might have delays. The health care provider might talk to or play with the child during examination to assess how the child learns, behaves, moves, and speaks. Delays in any of these areas could be indicative of a developmental problem. All children should be screened for developmental delays and disabilities during regular well-child doctor visits.

Children at high risk for developmental problems are those who were preterm birth, low birth weight, or other reasons. Additional risk factors are relatives who were diagnosed with ASD.

Disruptive, Impulse-Control, and Conduct Disorders

Definition: Conduct disorder characterized by callous and unemotional interpersonal relationships. Symptoms cause significant impairment in social, educational, or occupational functioning.

Definition: Oppositional defiant disorder is characterized by behavior that causes significant problems at school, work, or home. Criteria for diagnosis must not meet criteria for conduct disorder or antisocial personality disorder.

Nursing Assessment: Conduct Disorder

A. Physical fighting
B. Running away from home
C. Lying, stealing
D. Cruelty to animals
E. Frequent truancy
F. Vandalism, arson
G. Use of alcohol, drugs

Nursing Assessment: Oppositional Defiant Disorder

A. Argumentativeness
B. Blaming others for own problems
C. Defying rules and authority
D. Using obscene language
E. Acting resentful, vindictive

Analysis (Nursing Diagnoses): Conduct and Defiant Disorders

A. *Risk for other-directed violence* related to …
B. *Chronic low self-esteem* related to …
C. *Ineffective family coping* related to …

Nursing Plans and Interventions: Conduct and Defiant Disorders

A. Assess verbal and nonverbal cues for escalating behavior so as to decrease outbursts.
B. Use a nonauthoritarian approach.
C. Avoid asking "why" questions.
D. Initiate a "show of force" with a child who is out of control.
E. Use a "quiet room" when external control is needed.
F. Clarify expressions or jargon if meanings are unclear.
G. Teach to redirect angry feelings to safe alternative, such as a pillow or punching bag.
H. Implement behavior modification therapy if indicated.
I. Role-play new coping strategies with client.

HESI Hint • In depression, children often present with complaints of headache, stomachaches, and other somatic complaints.

HESI Hint • Adolescents are at increased risk for suicide. Monitor frequently and alert parents.

HESI Hint • Important points to remember when answering NCLEX-RN questions:
- A child in this situation may be involved in a self-fulfilling prophecy (e.g., "Mom says that I'm a troublemaker; therefore I must live up to Mom's expectations").
- Confront the client with his or her behavior (e.g., lying). This gives the client a sense of security.
- Provide consistent interventions; this helps prevent manipulation. Inconsistency does not help the client develop self-control.

Review of Childhood and Adolescent Disorders

1. A 7-year-old boy is disruptive in the classroom and is described by his parents as being hyperactive. What is the most probable psychiatric disorder? What are the signs and symptoms of this disorder? What drug is usually prescribed for this disorder?
2. A 15-year-old boy is threatening to drop out of school.

His parents, both alcoholics, say they can't stop him. He has just been arrested for stealing a car and breaking into a house. What is the most probable disorder? Develop nursing diagnoses and interventions for this disorder.

Answers to Review

1. Attention-deficit (hyperactivity) disorder (ADD/ADHD). More prevalent in boys; failure to listen to or follow instructions; difficulty playing quietly; disruptive behavior; impulsive behavior; difficulty sitting still; distractibility to external stimuli; excessive talking; shifting from one unfinished task to another; and underachievement in school performance. Methylphenidate (Ritalin).
2. Conduct disorder
   A. Risk for violence related to ..., depending on client.
   B. Disturbed self-esteem related to ..., depending on client.
   C. Ineffective family coping related to ..., depending on client.
   D. Assess verbal and nonverbal cues for escalating behavior so as to decrease outbursts. Use a nonauthoritarian approach. Avoid asking "why" questions. Initiate a show of force with a child who is out of control. Initiate suicide precautions when assessment indicates risk. Use a quiet room when external control is needed. Clarify expressions or jargon if meanings are unclear. Teach to redirect angry feelings to a safe alternative, such as a pillow or punching bag. Implement behavior modification therapy if indicated. Role-play new coping strategies.

Healthy aging is now an achievable goal for many. Aging and disease are separate entities. Aging is an individual process that affects each person differently. The chronologic age of 65 is the standard in the United States for being considered an older adult (elderly). By 2050, one in five Americans will be over the age of 65.

The concept of aging is further defined as young-old (65 to 74), middle-old (75 to 84), old-old (over 85), elite-old (over 90), and centenarian (100+).

Eighty percent of people over the age of 70 have at least one chronic condition, and 50% have multiple health problems.

Theories of Aging

Psychosocial Theories

A. Disengagement theory: Progressive social disengagement occurs naturally with aging and is accepted by the older adult. Variation in disengagement across older populations is related to cultural style and behaviors in different geographic regions.
B. Activity theory: Successful aging requires a high level of activity and involvement to maintain life satisfaction and positive self-esteem.

Biologic Theories

A. Pacemaker theory: A programmed decline or cessation of many components occurs in the nervous and endocrine systems.
B. Immunity theory: A programmed accumulation of damage and decline of the immune system's function (immunosenescence) takes place due to oxidative stress.
C. Wear-and-tear theory: After repeated use, damaged cells in the body structures wear out from the harmful effects of internal and external stressors, now known as *free radicals*.

> **HESI Hint** • The concept of aging is shifting from frail and dependent to healthy living. The majority of those aged 65 and older regard their health as good or excellent. The ability to perform activities of daily living (ADLs) is a more accurate measure of age than chronologic age.

Developmental Theories

A. Erik Erikson's theory: Theory identifies eight stages of developmental tasks throughout the life span; the eighth stage is integrity versus despair.
B. Maslow's theory: Maslow's hierarchy of needs ranks an individual's needs from the most basic to the most complex. Maslow uses the terms *physiologic, safety and security, belonging, self-esteem,* and *self-actualization* needs to describe the process that generally motivates individuals to move through life.

Physiologic Changes

A. Aging affects every cell in every organ of the body, but not at the same rate.
B. Three physiologic changes are clinically significant in making older adults vulnerable to injury and disease:
   1. Loss in compensatory reserve
   2. Progressive loss in efficiency of the body to repair damaged tissue
   3. Decreased functioning of the immune system processes
C. Diseases in older adults do not always present with classic signs and symptoms.
D. Physiologic changes increase more rapidly with increasing age.
E. Aging changes are influenced by genetic makeup and environment.

> **HESI Hint** • Changes in the heart and lungs result in less efficient utilization of O_2, which reduces an individual's capacity to maintain physical activity for long periods. Physical training for older people can significantly reduce blood pressure (BP) and increase aerobic capacity. NCLEX-RN® questions may ask about teaching and designing rehabilitation programs for older adults. The answers should contain something about exercise and nutrition.

> **HESI Hint** • Older people often complain that they cannot get to sleep at night and do not sleep soundly even after they fall asleep. This is because they have shorter stages of sleep, particularly shorter cycles

Continued

between stages 1 and 4 and REM sleep (stage 4 is deep sleep). They are easily awakened by environmental stimuli. They often compensate by napping during the day, which leads to further disruptions of night sleep. A common response is the use of prescription sleeping pills, which can create still further problems of disorientation, etc.

Integumentary System

Description: Skin, hair, and nail changes occur with aging and can cause problems concerning discomfort and self-esteem.

A. Thin skin provides a less effective barrier to trauma due to a loss of subcutaneous tissue.
   1. Increased risk for dehydration due to decline in lean mass and loss of body water
   2. Decreased ability of the skin to detect and regulate temperature
   3. Dry skin resulting from a decrease in endocrine secretion
   4. Loss of elastin and increased vascular fragility
B. Keratinocytes become smaller and regeneration slows; wound healing is slower.
C. Hair loss occurs; women have increased facial hair.
D. Vascular hyperplasia causes more varicosities (brown or blue discolorations).
E. Increased appearance of "age spots" and/or "liver spots" and raised lesions (seborrheic keratosis).
F. Nails become brittle and thick.

Nursing Assessment

A. Skin dryness and tears
B. Nails for changes in shape, color, and brittleness
C. Lesions to differentiate normal from abnormal
D. Bony prominences for signs of pressure ulcers

Analysis (Nursing Diagnoses)

A. *Impaired skin integrity* related to …
B. *Risk for injury* related to …
C. *Risk for infection* related to …

Nursing Plans and Interventions

A. Encourage the use of oils or lubricants on the skin at least twice a day.
B. Discourage the use of powder, which can be drying.
C. Teach to avoid overexposure to sunlight.
D. Encourage balanced nutrition and increased fluid intake.
E. Teach to maintain adequate humidity in the environment.
F. Teach to avoid temperature extremes.
G. Teach good foot care.
H. Observe bony prominences for signs of pressure.
I. Teach that poor peripheral circulation may slow the healing of foot and hand lesions.

HESI Hint • Peripheral circulation decreases as one ages. Regular assessment of the feet is very important because it increases the opportunity to discover and treat skin care problems early. These problems could become more serious because of decreased circulation.

HESI Hint • Differentiation of normal and pathologic causes for skin and hair conditions is essential; for example, seborrheic keratosis from melanomas.

Musculoskeletal System

Description: Age-related changes in the musculoskeletal system are gradual but have a significant impact on levels of mobility, which puts older adults at risk for falls and fractures.

A. The musculoskeletal system is composed of bones, joints, tendons, ligaments, and muscles.
B. Age-related changes are not life threatening but can affect function and quality of life.
C. Bone loss begins around age 40 and is more common in women than in men; thus, osteoporosis occurs more often in women. (See Medical-Surgical Nursing in Chapter 4)
D. This is a shortening of the trunk due to thinning of vertebral disks.
E. Loss of bone calcium, atrophic cartilage, and muscle occurs.
F. Bone mineral density (BMD) decreases, resulting in osteopenia and osteoporosis.
G. Range of motion (ROM) of joints decreases.
H. Progressive loss of cartilage occurs, resulting in osteoarthritis.
I. Muscle cells are lost and not replaced.
J. Lean body mass decreases with increased body fat.

Nursing Assessment

A. Dietary intake of calcium and vitamin D
B. Weight; underweight or overweight
C. Lifestyle habits; inappropriate nutrition, smoking, and inadequate exercise
D. History of fractures
E. ROM
F. Pain and chronic pain management strategies

Analysis (Nursing Diagnoses)

A. *Acute/chronic pain* related to …
B. *Risk for disuse syndrome* related to …
C. *Risk for injury* related to …
D. *Impaired physical mobility* related to …

Nursing Plans and Interventions

A. See Medical-Surgical Nursing, Osteoporosis in Chapter 4.
B. Teach that adequate calcium intake may help lessen osteoporotic changes.

C. Establish muscle-strengthening program (small weights, aquatic therapy).

D. Prevent accidents by ensuring a clutter-free, safe environment.

E. Provide adequate lighting day and night to prevent falls.

F. Teach clients not to back up but to turn around to move in the direction they wish to go.

G. Teach clients to walk looking straight ahead instead of looking down at their feet to optimize balance.

H. Encourage regular exercise inclusive of balance, weight-bearing, and low-resistance training.

I. Teach to avoid excessive joint strain.

J. Teach that medications (diuretics and sedatives) may contribute to falls.

K. Discourage excessive alcohol intake and encourage smoking cessation.

L. Encourage older people to change positions slowly to prevent orthostatic hypotension.

HESI Hint • Impaired mobility, impaired skin integrity, decreased peripheral circulation, and a lack of physical activity place older adults at risk for the development of pressure ulcers.

HESI Hint • The following are ways to help prevent or decrease the occurrence of falls:
- Install adequate lighting
- Wear proper footwear that supports the foot and contributes to balance; shoes should be made of non-slippery materials.
- Place a bell on any resident cats; cats move quickly and can get underfoot.
- Paint the edges of stairs a bright color.

Cardiovascular System

A. Age-related changes in the cardiovascular system predispose the older person to the development of dysrhythmias and other cardiac problems.

B. Cardiac output decreases as a result of a decrease in heart rate and stroke volume.

C. Cardiac output decreases because vessels lose elasticity. The heart's contractility decreases in response to increased demands.

D. Diastolic murmurs are present in more than one half of older adults because the mitral and aortic valves become thick and rigid.

E. Dysrhythmias (bradycardia, tachycardia, atrial fibrillation, and heart block) become more common as one ages, in part because of higher systolic BP and increased size of the atria.

F. Significant increases in systolic BP occur as a result of altered distribution of blood flow and increased peripheral resistance.

G. Arteriosclerosis increases with age and can cause cardiovascular problems:
1. Peripheral vascular disease
2. Edema
3. Coronary artery disease: acute coronary insufficiency, myocardial infarction (MI), dysrhythmias, heart failure (HF)

H. Much heart disease is preventable.

HESI Hint • Both systolic and diastolic BPs tend to increase with normal aging, but the elevation of systolic is greater. Remember the physiology of blood pressure, which is expressed as a ratio of systolic to diastolic pressure. Systolic refers to the level of BP during the contraction phase, and diastolic refers to the stage when the chambers of the heart are filling with blood.

Nursing Assessment

A. BP and vital signs

B. History of dizziness or blackouts with sudden position change (orthostatic hypotension)

C. Diuresis after lying down

D. Feelings of heart palpitations

E. Swelling in hands and feet (rings and shoes have become tight)

F. Weight gain without changes in eating pattern

G. Difficulty breathing at night (without elevation of the head of the bed). Confusion, personality changes can result from oxygen deficit.

Analysis (Nursing Diagnoses)

A. *Activity intolerance* related to …

B. *Ineffective tissue perfusion* (specify) related to …

C. *Decreased cardiac output* related to …

D. *Risk for injury* related to …

Nursing Plans and Interventions

A. Monitor BP in lying, sitting, and standing positions.

B. Encourage frequent rest periods to avoid fatigue.

C. Encourage regular, low-impact exercise.

D. Teach to change positions slowly to avoid falls and injuries.

E. Take apical and radial pulse; note deficits or rhythm abnormalities.

F. Teach to avoid extreme hot and cold because of decreased peripheral sensation.

G. Teach to avoid sitting with feet in a dependent position.

H. Assess edema: Weigh daily if indicated.

I. Encourage strict adherence to medication regimen.

J. Teach not to stop medications without prior approval from health care provider.

K. Determine support system for follow-up.

> **HESI Hint** • Dysrhythmias in older adults are particularly serious because older people cannot tolerate decreased cardiac output, which can result in syncope, falls, and transient ischemic attacks (TIAs). Pulse may be rapid, slow, or irregular.

> **HESI Hint** • Angina symptoms may be absent in older adults, or they may be confused with gastrointestinal symptoms.

Respiratory System

A. Older adults have increased demands for oxygen. The life span of an older adult increases the chance for exposure to toxic or infectious agents. Due to the aging process, multiple exposures over time can be damaging to the lungs and even life threatening.
B. Major age-related changes to the respiratory system:
   1. Breathing mechanics: Lungs lose elasticity; muscles become rigid and lose muscle mass and strength.
   2. Oxygenation: Increased ventilation and perfusion are imbalanced; increased dead space in the lungs and a decrease of alveolar surface area
   3. Ventilation control: Decreased reaction of peripheral and central chemoreceptors to hypoxia and hypercapnia
   4. Immune response: Decrease of cilia; decreased ability to clear mucus secretions, decreased ability to cough and deep-breathe, and a decreased immune response
   5. Exercise capability: Decrease of strength and muscle mass in the body
   6. Breathing ability: Decreased reaction to hypoxemia and hypercapnia

> **HESI Hint** • With aging, the muscles that operate the lungs lose elasticity so that respiratory efficiency is reduced. Vital capacity (the amount of air brought into the lungs at one time) decreases. Breathing may become more difficult after strenuous exercise. The rate of decline has been found to be slower in more active people. The nurse should encourage older people to remain physically active for as long as possible.
> Declining muscle strength may impair cough efficiency. This fact makes older people more susceptible to chronic bronchitis, emphysema, and pneumonia.

Nursing Assessment

A. Confusion (may be the first sign of respiratory infection)
B. Vital signs for elevated temperature, BP
C. Lungs for congestion or atelectasis
D. Vital capacity
E. Dyspnea and fatigue
F. Cough reflex and sputum production

Analysis (Nursing Diagnoses)

A. *Ineffective breathing pattern* related to …
B. *Impaired gas exchange* related to …
C. *Ineffective airway clearance* related to …
D. *Activity intolerance* related to …

> **HESI Hint** • Chronic obstructive pulmonary disease (COPD) is the major cause of respiratory disability in older adults. Aspiration pneumonia is a major cause of death in older adults.

Nursing Plans and Interventions

A. Encourage clients to receive an influenza vaccine yearly and the pneumonia vaccine after age 65 (a second dose may be given one additional time after about 5 years).
B. Remember that hypoxia can manifest as confusion.
C. If the client is a smoker, encourage him or her to stop. (Regardless of age, cardiovascular and respiratory status improves with smoking cessation and exercise.)
D. For older postoperative clients, turning, deep breathing, and use of incentive spirometer are imperative to prevent complications.
E. Encourage deep breathing. Teach breathing techniques such as pursed-lip breathing to facilitate respirations.

Gastrointestinal (GI) System

A. Age-related changes are bothersome and can affect comfort, function, and quality of life, but are rarely a direct cause of death.
B. Decreased saliva and dry mouth (xerostomia) are common.
C. Dental caries (tooth decay) and loss of teeth increase, resulting in decreased ability to chew food.
D. Hunger sensations decrease due to diminishing taste buds.
E. Relaxation of the lower esophageal sphincter or a sliding hiatal hernia increases the risk for gastroesophageal reflux disease (GERD) and aspiration.
F. The production of pepsin and hydrochloric acid decreases.
G. Delayed gastric emptying makes digestion of large amounts of food difficult.
H. Decreased peristalsis and decreased absorption in the small intestine of protein, fats, minerals (calcium), vitamins B_1 and B_2, and carbohydrates contribute to constipation problems.

I. Decreased enzyme production in the liver affects drug metabolism and detoxification processes.
J. Weight changes, especially weight loss, can be early indicators of health problems.

HESI Hint • The following are changes that contribute to chronic constipation with age:
- The number of enzymes in the small intestine is reduced, and simple sugars are absorbed more slowly, resulting in decreased efficiency of the digestive process.
- The smooth-muscle content and the muscle tone of the wall of the colon decrease. Anatomic changes in the large intestine result in decreased intestinal motility.
- Psychological factors, as well as abuse of over-the-counter laxatives, are factors.
- Decreases in fluid intake and mobility contribute to constipation.

Nursing Assessment

A. Brittle teeth due to thinning enamel
B. Receding gums resulting from periodontal disease (the major cause of tooth loss after the age of 30)
C. Decrease in taste sensation and appetite
D. Dry mouth due to a decrease in saliva production
E. Elimination pattern for evidence of constipation or diarrhea
F. Poor tolerance of high-fat meals and poor absorption of fat-soluble vitamins
G. Decreased glucose tolerance
H. Fluid intake

HESI Hint • Tooth loss is not a normal aging process. Good dental hygiene, good nutrition, and dental care can prevent tooth loss.

Analysis (Nursing Diagnoses)

A. *Constipation* related to …
B. *Risk for deficient/imbalanced fluid volume* related to …
C. *Impaired oral mucous membrane* related to …
D. *Imbalanced nutrition: less than/more than body requirements* related to …

Nursing Plans and Interventions

A. Encourage good oral hygiene (the use of a soft toothbrush, dental floss, and regular dental visits).
B. Assess dentures for proper fit.
C. Educate older clients about hidden sodium (canned soups, antacids, over-the-counter medications).
D. Promote adequate bowel functioning:
 1. Determine what is normal GI functioning for each individual.
 2. Encourage client to increase fiber and bulk in the diet.

3. Provide adequate hydration.
4. Encourage regular exercise.
5. Encourage eating small, frequent meals.
6. Discourage the use of laxatives and enemas.
7. Document bowel movements: frequency and consistency.

HESI Hint • Older people may appear to eat small quantities of food at mealtimes. This is because the digestive system of older people features a decrease in the contraction time of the muscles, and more time is needed for the cardiac sphincter to open. Therefore it takes more time for the food to be transmitted to the stomach. Thus the sensation of fullness may occur before the entire meal is consumed.

HESI Hint • Poor nutrition and malnutrition are significant concerns in the older adult. Some reasons for poor nutrition include chronic illness, which suppresses appetite; hospitalization and surgery; difficulty chewing; alcohol use; cognitive changes; depression; grief; loneliness; social isolation; and problems with food procurement. An early sign of malnutrition may be changes in weight.

Genitourinary System

Description: There are functional and structural changes, as well as psychosocial changes, in the older adult pertaining to the urinary system.

Kidney

A. Size and weight of the kidney decrease due to reduced renal tissue growth.
B. Glomerular filtration rate decreases due to a decrease in renal blood flow resulting from lower cardiac output. Decreased renal clearance of drugs is the result.
C. Tubular function diminishes.
D. Increased risk for reflux of urine into the ureters.
E. Chronic diseases such as atherosclerosis and hypertension also decrease renal functioning in older adults.

Nursing Assessment

A. Signs of dehydration or electrolyte imbalance:
 1. Skin turgor
 2. Intake/output
 3. Confusion
 4. Concentrated urine
 5. Medications such as diuretics
B. Laboratory values
 1. Proteinuria
 2. Increased blood urea nitrogen (BUN) and creatinine
 3. Presence of blood in urine

Analysis (Nursing Diagnoses)

A. *Risk for electrolyte imbalance* related to …
B. *Risk for imbalanced fluid volume* related to …
C. *Impaired urinary elimination* related to …
D. *Risk for ineffective renal perfusion* related to …

Nursing Plans and Interventions

A. Encourage an intake of at least 2 to 3 liters of fluid daily, if not contraindicated.
B. Instruct client about signs and symptoms of dehydration and to contact health care provider immediately.
C. Instruct client about the importance of completing antibiotics until the entire prescription is gone, even if symptoms go away.
D. Write out antibiotic schedule, including any special instructions. Print in large letters.

Bladder

A. The capacity of the bladder decreases by one half, resulting in urinary frequency and nocturia.
B. Emptying the bladder may become difficult because of a weakening of the bladder and perineal muscles and because of a decrease in sensation of urge to void. (This sets up a propensity for urinary tract infections [UTIs] due to residual urine in the bladder.)
C. Increased frequency and dribbling may occur in men because of a weakened bladder and an enlarged prostate.
D. Prostatic enlargement may cause urinary retention and bladder infection in men.
E. Women may experience stress incontinence.

Analysis (Nursing Diagnoses)

A. *Disturbed personal identity* related to …
B. *Sexual dysfunction* related to …
C. *Risk for impaired skin integrity* related to …
D. *Disturbed sleep pattern* related to …

Nursing Plans and Interventions

A. Initiate a bladder-training program if indicated.
B. Encourage older women to void at first urge when possible.
C. Initiate a skin-care program if incontinence is present.
D. Provide methods of dealing with incontinence. Kegel exercises can help.
E. Teach to avoid sleeping pills and sedation, which may cause nocturnal incontinence.
F. Teach to avoid caffeine because it promotes diuresis.

HESI Hint • The nurse should pay careful attention to urinary output in older clients because it is the first sign of loss of renal integrity. Older people have a higher risk for the development of renal failure because normal age-related changes result in compromised renal functioning.

HESI Hint • Kegel exercises consist of tightening and relaxing the vaginal and urinary meatus muscles. (They can be done unobtrusively at home.) When performed consistently, these exercises have been very successful in reducing the incidence of incontinence.

HESI Hint • Older adults may be embarrassed because they are incontinent. They may seek isolation, thereby predisposing themselves to loneliness.

HESI Hint • An assessment of sensitivity to bladder problems is essential when planning nursing care. Older people may be more sensitive to alcohol and caffeine because these substances inhibit the production of antidiuretic hormone (ADH). From 15% to 30% of community-based older adults and almost 50% of older adults living in nursing homes suffer from difficulties with bladder control.

HESI Hint • *MEDICATION ALERT!*
A decrease in the filtration efficiency of the kidneys has grave implications for people who are taking medication, particularly penicillin, tetracycline, and digoxin, which are cleared from the bloodstream primarily by the kidneys. These drugs remain active longer in an older person's system. As people age, the total number of functioning glomeruli decreases until renal function has been reduced by nearly 50%. Therefore they may be more potent, indicating a need to adjust the dose and frequency of administration.

Reproductive System

HESI Hint • Many older adults are sexually active or maintain an interest in sexual activities; therefore nurses should obtain a sexual assessment among older women and men in the acute care, community, and long-term care settings.

A. Age-related changes are related to hormonal and nervous system control.
B. Unless there is a medical condition, women do not have difficulty maintaining sexual function as they age.
  1. Women's ovarian function decreases; breast tissue involutes.
  2. Ovaries and the uterus slowly atrophy, and neither may be palpable.

    3. Perineal muscle weakness and atrophy of the vulva occur with age.

    4. Vaginal mucous membrane becomes dry, elasticity of tissue decreases, surface becomes smooth, and secretions become reduced and more alkaline. May lead to dyspareunia (painful intercourse).

    5. Libido may or may not decline.

C. Age-related changes:

    1. Testes atrophy, lose weight, and soften.

    2. Erection changes are seen.

    3. Prostate enlargement due to changes in testosterone levels

    4. Libido may or may not decline.

D. Older men may still experience orgasmic pleasure. For older men, the most common physiologic changes are:

    1. An erection that is less firm

    2. Shorter duration of erection

    3. Diminished force of ejaculation

E. The term for male menopause is *andropause*. Diminished testosterone is believed to be the cause of androgen decline in the aging male (ADAM).

Nursing Assessment: Women

A. Vital signs (temperature), discharge, or labial or vulvar redness and pruritus for possible infections (vaginitis)

B. Complaints of hot flashes, mood swings, or night sweat

C. Dyspareunia (painful intercourse)

Nursing Assessment: Men

A. Assess for complaints of urinary problems; prostate enlargement.

B. Assess testosterone hormone levels.

Analysis (Nursing Diagnoses)

A. *Disturbed body image* related to …

B. *Anxiety* related to …

C. *Sexual dysfunction* related to …

D. *Impaired urinary elimination* related to …

Nursing Plans and Interventions: Women

A. Teach client signs of vaginitis; report and treat if present.

B. Promote perineal care as needed.

C. Prescription creams can help with vaginal dryness.

D. Encourage client to obtain mammogram per guidelines.

Nursing Plans and Interventions: Men

A. Encourage annual digital examination for early identification of prostate cancer.

> **HESI Hint** • Sexually active older adults are at risk for sexually transmitted diseases if they seek sexual relations with different partners.

Neurologic System

Description: Neurocognitive disorders (DSM-5) are the major cause of disability in older adults. Dementia, cerebrovascular disorders, and movement disorders (e.g., Parkinson disease) are the major disorders in this category (see Medical-Surgical Nursing in Chapter 4).

A. The nervous system is the most complex of all systems and functions alone and in conjunction with many systems.

B. There is a decrease of neurons and neurotransmitters in the brain, which do not regenerate.

C. The neurologic system consists of two main components: the central nervous system (CNS) and the peripheral nervous system (PNS): decrease in both CNS and PNS functioning.

D. Intelligence remains constant in the healthy older adult.

E. Central processing decreases; performance of tasks is slower.

F. PNS changes in aging people may include the following:

    1. Significantly lower or nonexistent vibratory senses in the lower extremities

    2. Decrease of tactile sensitivity

    3. Loss of connection in nerve endings in the skin

    4. Loss of proprioception, affecting balance

Nursing Assessment

A. Comprehensive functional assessment; weaknesses, tremors, and gait disturbances

B. History of falls

C. Pain, headaches, ROM, and neuropathies in extremities

D. Sudden changes in vision, cognition, and muscle weakness

E. Depression

Analysis (Nursing Diagnoses)

A. *Risk for ineffective cerebral tissue perfusion* related to …

B. *Impaired verbal communication* related to …

C. *Risk for injury* related to …

D. *Risk for falls* related to …

Nursing Plans and Interventions

A. Perform a complete mental status examination, including depression.

B. Screen for cognitive impairment.

C. Monitor BP and hydration status.

D. Request physical and occupational service evaluations, if indicated.

E. Provide assistive devices as needed for ambulation.

F. Encourage walking, ROM, and balance exercises.

G. Teach individual relaxation techniques, stress management, and adaptive self-care management.

H. Minimize potential sources of injury in the environment.

I. Educate family and caregivers about support groups and other resources (agencies).

Nursing Plans and Interventions: Older Adults

A. Address client with respect: "Good Morning Mrs. Jones."
B. Orient the client to the purpose and length of the interview
C. Give the older adult time to respond because verbal response slows with age.
D. Choose words based on the clients sociocultural background and formal education; don't use slang or jargon (Fig. 8-1).
E. Keep questions short and to the point.
F. Give nonverbal cues and responses such as nodding, direct eye contact; avoid patting or stroking the client.
G. Active listening validates the older person. Reminiscence is an excellent way to obtain data about the client's current health problems and support systems (Fig. 8-2).

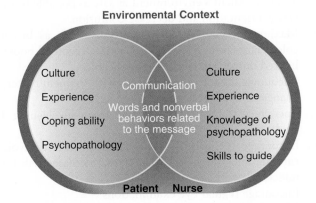

Environmental Context

Culture
Experience
Coping ability
Psychopathology

Communication
Words and nonverbal behaviors related to the message

Culture
Experience
Knowledge of psychopathology
Skills to guide

Patient   Nurse

FIGURE 8-1 Variables in the therapeutic communication environment. (From Keltner N, Steele D: *Psychiatric nursing*, ed 7. St. Louis, 2014, Mosby, pp 77-78.)

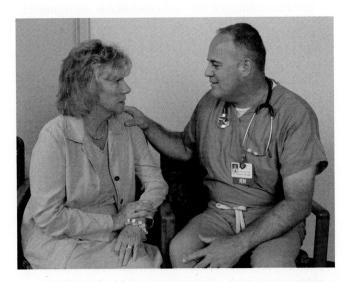

FIGURE 8-2 Body language and communication. (From Potter P, Perry AG, Stockert P, Hall A: *Basic nursing, multimedia enhanced version*, 7 ed. St. Louis, 2013, Mosby, p. 529.)

HESI Hint • Normal loss of brain cells is compounded by alcohol, smoking, and breathing polluted air. As a result, cognitive and safety issues can develop in the older adult. To help accommodate such losses, the nurse should teach older clients to shop during less crowded times in stores that are familiar to them, slow down well in advance of traffic signals, stay in the slower lane of the freeway, avoid freeways during rush hours, and leave for appointments well ahead of time.

HESI Hint • Alzheimer disease is the most common irreversible neurocognitive disorder of old age. It is characterized by deficits in attention, learning, memory, and language skills. Discuss the problems family members have in dealing with clients with Alzheimer disease in relation to the following disease manifestations:
• Depression
• Night wandering
• Aggressiveness or passiveness
• Inability to recognize family members

Endocrine System

Description: In the older adult, glands atrophy and decrease the rate of secretion. The impact is unclear, except it is more prevalent in women than in men due to the decline of estrogen, which causes menopause.

A. Consists of the thyroid, parathyroid, pituitary, adrenal, and pineal glands; the thymus; and the endocrine pancreas
B. Thyroid activity decreases (see Medical-Surgical Nursing, Hypothyroidism in Chapter 4). Symptoms are commonly undiagnosed in the older adult because they are attributed to being "normal for age."
C. Metabolic rate slows.
D. Estrogen production ceases with menopause; ovaries, uterus, and vaginal tissue atrophy.
E. Gonadal secretion of progesterone and testosterone decreases.
F. Insulin production decreases or insulin resistance increases.
G. T_4 (thyroxine) and T_3 (triiodothyronine) secreted by the thyroid gland remain unchanged with aging; however, their metabolic clearance rate is decreased. Production of parathyroid hormone decreases, which is made evident by osteoporosis.
H. Adrenal changes may affect circadian patterns of adrenocorticotropic hormone (ACTH).

Nursing Assessment

A. Signs and symptoms of diabetes in older adults; dehydration and confusion
B. History of recurrent infections, fatigue, and nausea; delayed wound healing; and paresthesias

C. Weight loss or gain without change in eating pattern
D. Laboratory values; hemoglobin A$_{1c}$, aldosterone, and cortisol levels
E. Bone density testing
F. Sleeping pattern
G. Depression

Analysis (Nursing Diagnoses)

A. *Risk for imbalance in body temperature* related to ...
B. *Risk for electrolyte imbalance* related to ...
C. *Imbalanced nutrition* related to ...
D. *Disturbed sleep pattern* related to ...
E. *Risk for unstable glucose levels* related to ...

Nursing Plans and Interventions

A. Encourage thyroid testing for older clients who seem depressed. Hypothyroidism is often dismissed as depression.
B. Refer to Medical-Surgical Nursing, Hypothyroidism in Chapter 4.
C. Older clients may have difficulty with lifelong medication regimens. Develop memory cues for medications and caution against abrupt withdrawal.
D. See Medical-Surgical Nursing, Diabetes in Chapter 4.
E. Encourage annual physical examination with routine laboratory tests.
F. Encourage annual eye examinations.
G. Teach daily foot care and monthly toenail care.

> **HESI Hint** • The most common endocrine disorders in the older adult are thyroid dysfunction and type 2 diabetes.

Sensory System

Description: The sensory system consists of vision, hearing, taste, touch, and smell. Changes in the sensory system, including balance, occur gradually and are often unnoticed.

A. A loss of cells in the olfactory bulb of the brain and a decrease in sensory cells in the nasal lining occur.
B. Sensitivity to smells declines.
C. Taste perception decreases due to loss of taste buds on the tongue.
D. Tear production decreases.
E. Abnormal, progressive clouding or opacity of the lens in the eyes occurs (cataracts).
F. A partial or complete white ring encircles the periphery of the cornea (arcus senilis).
G. Increased intraocular pressure (IOP), usually bilaterally, leads to optic nerve damage (glaucoma).
H. Hearing of high pitches diminishes first; the ability to discriminate tones is lost (presbycusis).

Nursing Assessment

A. Assess visual and hearing acuity, as well as glasses and/or hearing aids used
B. Eyes for cloudiness or opacity
C. Ears for wax and hearing loss
D. Evaluate dietary intake for unplanned weight loss and salt and sugar intake

Analysis (Nursing Diagnoses)

A. *Risk for falls* related to ...
B. *Risk for injury* related to ...
C. *Social isolation* related to ...
D. *Imbalanced nutrition: less than body requirements* related to ...

Nursing Plans and Interventions

A. Provide interventions to supplement loss of sensory input.
B. Encourage social interaction.
C. Make the client's environment as safe as possible to increase orientation and decrease confusion.
D. Maximize visual and nonvisual aids, such as bright colors, large print for written material, recorded books, lighted mirror, and glasses, if applicable.
E. Encourage the use of hearing aids with frequent battery changes if applicable.
F. Encourage the use of glasses and frequent cleaning if applicable.
G. Encourage the use of artificial tears; teach to avoid rubbing and touching of the eyes (increases risk for infection).
H. Encourage regular eye examinations.
I. Directly face hearing-impaired clients so they may read lips and view facial expressions.
J. Adapt ethnic favorites to dietary and taste limitations.
K. Educate the client's support system about interventions to maintain a safe and comfortable environment.

> **HESI Hint** • Diminished eyesight results in the following:
> - A loss of independence (driving and the ability to perform ADLs)
> - A lack of stimulation
> - The inability to read (recommend audiotapes)
> - The fear of blindness

> **HESI Hint** • Lower the tone of your voice when talking to an older person who is hearing impaired. High-pitched tones (e.g., women's voices) are the first to become difficult to hear; therefore lowering the pitch of your voice increases the likelihood that an older person with a hearing loss will be able to hear you speak.

Neurocognitive Disorder (NCD): Dementia

Description: Dementia is the permanent, progressive impairment in cognitive functioning manifested by memory loss (both long term and short term) and accompanied by impairment in judgment, abstract thinking, and social behavior.

A. Characterized by the following:
1. Personality changes
2. Confusion
3. Disorientation
4. Deterioration of intellectual functioning, loss of memory
5. Decline of appropriate judgment and ADLs
B. The four As of cognitive impairment are agnosia, amnesia, apraxia, and aphasia.
C. Types of dementia:
1. Alzheimer disease: The brains of individuals with Alzheimer disease have an abundance of beta amyloid plaques, neurofibrillary tangles, and atrophic brain cells and tissue. Alzheimer disease is the most common brain disorder and is one of the leading causes of death in the older adult.
2. Vascular or multifocal dementia: Ischemic brain lesions develop as a result of a history of hyperlipidemia, hypertension, smoking, or obesity.
3. Dementia with Lewy bodies (DLB): Microscopic deposits develop in the brain that damage nerve cells.
4. Frontotemporal dementia (Pick disease): The frontal and temporal lobes of the brain degenerate.

Nursing Assessment

A. Memory complaints: short term/long term; recognition of family, friends, or environment
B. Impaired physical functioning: shuffling, difficulty swallowing, and inability to perform ADLs
C. Conditions that mimic dementia

D. Unrecognized medical conditions
E. History of medications and changes

Analysis (Nursing Diagnoses)

A. *Chronic confusion* related to …
B. *Self-neglect* related to …
C. *Readiness for enhanced family coping* related to …
D. *Impaired memory* related to …

Nursing Plans and Interventions

A. Administer screening tools for depression and cognitive impairment.
B. Keep the client functioning and actively involved in social and family activities for as long as possible.
C. Maintain an orderly, almost ritualistic, schedule to promote a sense of security.
D. Maintain a regularly scheduled reality orientation on a daily basis.
1. Keep the client oriented as to time, place, and person (repeatedly).
2. Keep a calendar and clock within sight at all times.
    a. Display a calendar and clock that can be read by the older person (i.e., a clock with large numbers and a calendar that can be read by those with deteriorating vision).
    b. Be sure the date and time are accurate (i.e., keep the calendar current and the clock in working order).
E. Keep familiar objects, such as family pictures, in the older adult's environment to promote a sense of continuity and security.
F. Administer prescribed drugs to reduce emotional lability, agitation, and irritability or prescribed antidepressant, as indicated.
G. Speak in a slow, calm voice; avoid excitement.
H. Provide support and education to family and long-term caregivers.
I. Encourage end-of-life planning, including a will, do not resuscitate (DNR) status, power of attorney, and funeral arrangements.

TABLE 8-1 Alzheimer Medications

Drugs	Adverse Reactions	Nursing Implications
Acetylcholinesterase Inhibitors		
• Tacrine HCl • Donepezil HCl • Rivastigmine • Galantamine	• Overall—nausea and diarrhea • Cognex: considerable GI distress, elevated liver enzymes	• Teach clients that they should take *no* anticholinergic medication. • Medications should not be used in cases of severe liver impairment. • Take with meals to avoid GI upset. • Do not discontinue abruptly.
N-Methyl-D-Aspartate (NMDA) Antagonist		
• Memantine	• Headaches, dizziness, and constipation	• Add to acetylcholinesterase inhibitors in moderate to severe Alzheimer disease.

Psychosocial Changes

Loss

A. Loss includes loss of functional ability, decreased self-image, and death of significant others (family members, friends, or pets).
B. Loss is a universal, incontestable event of the human experience.
C. Regardless of the loss, each event has the potential to cause grief and the process called *bereavement* or *mourning*.
D. Grief is an individual response and is different depending on social and cultural norms.
E. Losses may be compounded (e.g., relocation, loss of support network, economic changes, and/or role changes), causing bereavement overload.

> **HESI Hint** • Older people undergo a great many changes, which are usually associated with loss (loss of spouse, friends, career, home, health, etc.). Therefore some older people are extremely vulnerable to emotional and mental stress, depression, and substance abuse.

Nursing Assessment

A. Any loss or losses
B. The older adult's day-to-day functioning (e.g., eating and sleeping and work or social patterns)
C. Level of depression and suicide risk
D. The support system in place to assist with loss
E. Ability to express emotions related to the loss or losses
F. Any feelings of uselessness and nonparticipation in social events
G. Any loss of income that affects health care needs and quality of life
H. New or increased alcohol consumption on a daily or weekly basis
I. Past coping styles used with past losses

Analysis (Nursing Diagnoses)

A. *Powerlessness* related to …
B. *Risk for social isolation* related to …
C. *Anxiety* related to …
D. *Grieving* related to …

Nursing Plans and Interventions

A. If needed, refer to grief counseling or a support group.
B. Encourage activities that allow the individual to use past coping strategies that will promote a feeling of self-worth and increased self-esteem.
C. Encourage the individual to share his or her feelings.
D. Encourage socialization with family peers and reminiscing about significant life experiences.

> **HESI Hint** • Integrity versus despair is Erikson's final stage of growth and development. Reminiscing is a means of setting one's life in order (accepting life and self), which is the task of this stage. The goal of this stage is to feel a sense of the meaning of one's life, rather than to feel despair or bitterness that one's life has been wasted. The major task of older adults is to redefine self in relation to a changed role.

> **HESI Hint** • Think about the following situations and discuss the nursing care for each:
> • A nursing supervisor who has had a stroke and is sent to a long-term facility for rehabilitation
> • An oil company executive who retires after 42 years with the company to travel in his recreational vehicle with his wife and dog
> • Shortly after their sixtieth wedding anniversary a man's wife has a cerebrovascular accident (CVA) and is paralyzed.

Health Maintenance and Preventive Care

Nursing Plans and Interventions

A. Encourage periodic health appraisal and counseling to prevent illness.
   1. Electrocardiogram (ECG) to detect subtle heart abnormalities
   2. Chest radiograph to detect tuberculosis or lung cancer
   3. Pulmonary function tests to detect chronic bronchitis and emphysema
   4. Tonometer test to measure IOP as a test for glaucoma
   5. Blood glucose to detect diabetes mellitus
   6. Pap smear to detect cancer of the cervix; digital rectal examination to detect cancer of the prostate
   7. Hearing and vision testing to detect sensory deprivation
   8. Breast self-examination and mammogram, if indicated
   9. Serum cholesterol as indicated by health status
   10. Screen at-risk older adults for bone density, thyroid functioning, and abdominal aneurysm (in males).
   11. Screen for depression and cognitive impairment.
   12. Screen for BP as indicated by health status.
   13. Screen for obesity.
   14. Screen for substance abuse.
   15. Screen for physical or emotional abuse.
B. Promote accident prevention.
   1. Educate about safety measures to take to prevent falls.
   2. Encourage physical and mental activities to promote mobility and confidence.
   3. Encourage regular muscle-strengthening and balance-training exercises.
   4. Encourage the use of assistive devices when needed (e.g., cane, walker, glasses, hearing aids).
   5. Monitor driving skills; encourage American Association of Retired Persons (AARP) driving evaluation and training.
C. Protect against infectious diseases.
   1. Encourage handwashing.
   2. Educate older adults to avoid individuals who are ill.
   3. Encourage immunization for influenza, pneumonia, and Td/Tdap.
   4. Recommend herpes zoster (shingles); hepatitis A and B; and measles, mumps, rubella, and varicella immunizations if risk factors are present.
D. Avoid temperature extremes; prevent hypothermia.
E. Encourage the older person to stop smoking, and discourage excessive alcohol intake.
F. Educate clients about proper foot care.

G. Encourage proper nutrition and weight control.
H. Encourage social interaction and use of support services (e.g., Meals On Wheels) and support groups (e.g., church).
I. Discourage the use of over-the-counter medications.
J. Review all medications yearly and encourage the client to throw away outdated drugs and prescriptions.
K. Diseases and conditions that affect older adults are the same as those that affect younger adults. However, in older adults, the signs and symptoms of pathology may be subtle, slow to develop, and quite different from those seen in younger people (Table 8-2).

End-of-Life Care

End-of-life care shifts care from invasive interventions aimed at prolonging life to supportive interventions that focus on control of symptoms. Insurance and hospice entities view the end-of-life stage as 6 months before death. However, a major problem with this definition is the difficulty in predicting the period of client survival. Health care providers may overestimate or underestimate survival time. Care includes:

A. Pain management is a priority in end-of-life care because untreated or undertreated pain consumes energy; interferes with function; affects quality of life and social interactions; and contributes to sleep disturbances, hopelessness, and loss of control.
B. Alleviating dyspnea can contribute to the client's comfort and decrease the family's anxiety. Dyspnea (distressing shortness of breath) may be related to pulmonary, cardiac, neuromuscular, or metabolic disorders; obesity; anxiety; and spiritual distress. Families need support, in particular when the gurgling sound ("death rattle") occurs close to the end of life.
C. Listening, reassuring, and reinforcing nonpharmacologic interventions to help manage anxiety (a mild to severe subjective feeling of apprehension, tension, insecurity, and uneasiness) may need to be followed by pharmacologic agents.
D. Managing GI symptoms of nausea, vomiting, gastritis, constipation, and diarrhea ensures comfort and quality of life.
E. Assessing for psychiatric symptoms of depression and delirium common at the end of life and providing care as needed. If unrecognized, they can rob clients of quality of life and quality of care.
F. Recognizing the spiritual needs of older adults can help them come to terms with their illness and the end of their life. *Spirituality* is a broad concept that encompasses the search for meaning in life experiences, relationships with others, and a sense of connectedness to a personal deity. Recognition of spiritual distress is important to help the dying client come to terms with the end of life.

TABLE 8-2 Diseases and Conditions in Older Adults

Disease or Condition	Description in Terms of the Older Adult	Nursing Implications
Delirium	• Acute confused state with rapid onset, usually the result of systemic illness or medication. • Decreased level of consciousness.	• Establish a meaningful environment. • Help maintain body awareness. • Help client cope with confusion, delusions, and illusions. • Review medications for syngestic effects
Dementia	• Slow onset of symptoms. • Level of consciousness may be intact.	• See Nursing Interventions for NCD.
Cardiac dysrhythmias	• Incidence increases with age. • More serious in older adults because of lower tolerance of decreased cardiac output (can result in syncope, falls, TIAs, and confusion). • Symptoms result from compromised circulation and O_2 deficit.	• Assess, prevent, and manage dysrhythmias. • Advise smoking cessation. • Encourage exercise and weight control.
Cataracts	• Often a result of normal aging changes. • Most common pathologic problem affecting the eyesight of older adults. • Treatment is surgical removal.	• Teach instillation of eye drops. • Reduce glare in environment. • Assistance is required postoperatively because affected eye is covered, and disorientation may occur.
Glaucoma	• Risk of acquiring increases with age.	• Loss of sensory input can result in confusion.
Macular degeneration	• Principal cause of blindness.	• Loss of sensory input can result in confusion. • Yearly examination important.
Cerebrovascular accident (CVA)	• Interruption of cerebral circulation, caused by occlusion or hemorrhage in the brain. • Risk increases with age.	• Prevent deterioration of client's condition. • Maximize functional abilities (occupational therapy). • Assist client in accepting physical deficits. • Check gag reflex before client receives food or fluids. • Prevent injuries to paralyzed limbs.
Pressure ulcer	• Immobility puts older adults at risk.	• Reposition frequently. • Massage bony prominences. • Provide adequate nutrition.
Hypothyroidism	• Usually occurs after age 50. • Symptoms are often similar to normal aging changes and have an insidious onset, making it difficult to detect in older adults. • Older adults are at greater risk for development of myxedema coma, which is life threatening.	• Often diagnosed as depression; with treatment, signs of depression disappear. • Caution against abruptly discontinuing medication.
Thyrotoxicosis (Graves disease)	• Symptoms may be absent or attributed to other, more common diseases in older adults. • Weight loss and HF may be predominant symptoms.	• It is precipitated by stressful events such as trauma, surgery, or infection. Be alert for signs and symptoms. • Can be fatal if untreated.

Continued

TABLE 8-2 Diseases and Conditions in Older Adults—cont'd

Disease or Condition	Description in Terms of the Older Adult	Nursing Implications
Chronic obstructive pulmonary disease (COPD)	• A major cause of respiratory disability in older adults • Most older people exhibit both chronic bronchitis and chronic emphysema. • Fatigue is a common result because of the increased work required to breathe (dyspnea).	• Encourage to stop smoking. • Keep in mind older person's state of confusion when teaching about treatment regimen. • Plan rest periods to allow patient to maintain oxygen levels.
Urinary tract infections (UTIs)	• Their incidence increases with age. • Older people are often asymptomatic or exhibit vague, ill-defined symptoms. • With infections, older people often become confused.	• Suspect UTI when client's voiding habits change.

G. Supporting family caregivers is important because family caregivers may do everything for the client, from assisting with ADLs to giving medications and managing medical equipment and treatments. Often they are the ones who serve as go-betweens for the client and health care providers. Although caregivers may find great satisfaction in their role, they often experience stress and diminished physical health.

H. Family bereavement support is essential because survivors are at an increased risk for illness or death. Normal responses to grief can be physical, psychological, cognitive, and/or spiritual. Uncomplicated grief is a dynamic, pervasive, and highly individualized process. Individuals who are overwhelmed or remain interminably in the state of grief without progression through the mourning process to completion may be experiencing complicated grief. When the nurse identifies complicated grief, it should be reported so that a referral for help can be made to the correct provider, such as a bereavement counselor.

Review of Gerontologic Nursing

1. What are the normal memory changes that occur as one ages?
2. What three physiologic changes are clinically significant in older adults?
3. Why can the BP of older adults be expected to increase?
4. What is the major cause of respiratory disability in older adults?
5. List five nursing interventions to promote adequate bowel functioning for older people.
6. What lifestyle factors negatively affect nearly every system in the older adult's body?
7. What visual problem most commonly occurs in older adults?
8. What are the three most common disorders that result from changes in the neurologic system?
9. What is the difference between delirium and NCD?
10. Falls are the result of what physiologic changes?
11. What are two factors that cause a decrease in the excretion of drugs by the kidneys?
12. What areas are important for end-of-life care?

Answers to Review

1. Short-term memory declines, whereas long-term memory stays the same.
2. Loss in compensatory reserve, progressive loss in efficiency of the body to repair damaged tissue, and decreased functioning of the immune system processes
3. The heart's work increases in response to increased peripheral resistance.
4. COPD
5. Determine what is "normal" GI functioning for each individual, increase fiber and bulk in the diet, provide adequate hydration, encourage regular exercise, and encourage eating small meals frequently.
6. Smoking, excessive alcohol intake, sedentary lifestyle (inactivity), and excessive dietary intake versus energy output
7. Cataracts
8. Dementia disorders, cerebrovascular disorders, and movement disorders (e.g., Parkinson disease)
9. Delirium has a sudden onset and is reversible; NCD is a slowly progressive, irreversible disease.
10. Falls are the result of cardiovascular changes, musculoskeletal system changes, and neurologic system changes.
11. Decrease in glomerular filtration and slowed organ functioning
12. Pain, dyspnea, anxiety, GI symptoms, psychiatric symptoms, spirituality, support for family caregivers, and family support during the bereavement period are important for end-of-life care.

NORMAL VALUES

Test	Adult	Child	Infant/Newborn	Older Adult	Nursing Implications
Hematologic					
Hgb Hemoglobin: g/dL	Male: 14-18 Female: 12-16 Pregnant: >11	1-6 yr: 9.5-14 6-18 yr: 10-15.5	Newborn: 14-24 0-2 wk: 12-20 2-6 mo: 10-17 mo-1 yr: 9.5-14	Values slightly decreased	High-altitude living increases values. Drug therapy can alter values. Slight Hgb decreases normally occur during pregnancy.
Hct Hematocrit: %	Male: 42-52 Female: 37-47 Pregnant: >33	1-6 yr: 30-40 6-18 yr: 32-44	Newborn: 44-64 2-8 wk: 39-59 2-6 mo: 35-50 mo-1 yr: 29-43	Values slightly decreased	Abnormalities in RBC size may alter Hct values.
RBC Red blood cell count: million/mm³	Male: 4.7-6.1 Female: 4.2-5.4	1-6 yr: 4-5.5 6-18 yr: 4.5-5	Newborn: 4.8-7.1 2-8 wk: 4-6 2-6 mo: 3.5-5.5 mo-1 yr: 3.5-5.2	Same as adult	Exercise and high altitudes can cause an increase in values. Pregnancy values are usually lower. Drug therapy can alter values.
WBC White blood cell count: 1000/mm³	Both sexes: 5-10	≤2 yr: 6.2-17 ≥2 yr: 5-10	Newborn, term: 9-30	Same as adult	Anesthetics, stress, exercise, and convulsions can cause increased values. Drug therapy can decrease values for 24-48 hr. Pregnancy (final month) and labor may cause increased WBC levels.
Platelet count: 1000/mm³	Both sexes: 150-400	150-400	Premature infant: 100-300 Newborn: 150-300 Infant: 200-475	Same as adult	Values may increase if living at high altitudes, exercising strenuously, or taking oral contraceptives. Values may decrease due to hemorrhage, disseminated intravascular coagulation (DIC), reduced production of platelets, infections, prosthetic heart valves, and drugs (acetaminophen, aspirin, chemotherapy, H2 blockers, INH, levofloxacin (Levaquin), streptomycin, sulfonamides, thiazide diuretics).

Test	Adult	Child	Infant/ Newborn	Older Adult	Nursing Implications
HESI Hint • The laboratory values that are most important to know for the NCLEX-RN® examination are Hgb, Hct, WBCs, Na, K, blood urea nitrogen (BUN), blood glucose, arterial blood gases (ABGs), bilirubin for newborn, and therapeutic ranges for prothrombin time/international; normalized ratio (PT/INR) and partial thromboplastin time (PTT).					
SED rate, ESR-Erythrocyte sedimentation rate: mm/hr	Male: up to 15 Female: up to 20 Pregnant: ↑ all trimesters	Up to 10	Newborn: 0-2	Same as adult	Rate is elevated during second and third trimesters of pregnancy.
PT Prothrombin time: seconds	Both sexes: 11-12.5 Pregnant: Slight ↓	Same as adult	Same as adult	Same as adult	Used in regulating warfarin (Coumadin) therapy. Therapeutic range is 1.5-2 times normal/control.
INR International Normalized Ratio	Both sexes 0.8-1.1	Same as adult	Same as adult	Same as adult	Used to monitor anticoagulation therapy. INR must be individualized.
PTT Partial thromboplastin time: seconds (see aPTT)	Both sexes: 60-70 Pregnant: Slight ↓	Same as adult	Same as adult	Same as adult	It is used in regulating heparin therapy. Therapeutic range is 1.5-2.5 times normal or control.
aPTT Activated partial thromboplastin time: seconds	Both sexes: 30-40	Same as adult	Same as adult	Same as adult	It is used in regulating heparin therapy. Therapeutic range is 1.5-2.5 times normal or control.
Blood Chemistry					
Alkaline phosphatase: IU/L	Both sexes: 30-120	2-8 yr: 65-210 9-15 yr: 60-300 16-21 yr: 30-200	<2 yr: 85-235	Slightly higher than adults	Hemolysis of specimen can cause a false elevation in values.
Albumin: g/dL	Both sexes: 3.5 -5 Pregnant: slight	4-5.9	Premature infant: 3-4.2 Newborn: 3.5-5.4 Infant 4.4-5.4	Same as adult	No special preparation is needed.
Bilirubin total: mg/dL	Total: 0.3-1 Indirect: 0.2-0.8 Direct: 0.1-0.3	Same as adult	Newborn: 1-12	Same as adult	Client is to be NPO except for water for 8-12 hr before testing. Prevent hemolysis of blood during venipuncture. Do *not* shake tube; it can cause inaccurate values. Protect blood sample from bright light.
Total calcium: mg/dL	Both sexes: 9-10.5	8.8-10.8	<10 days: 7.6-10.4 Umbilical: 9-11.5 days-2 yr: 9-10.6	Values tend to decrease	No special preparation is needed. Use of thiazide diuretics can cause increased calcium values.

Continued

Test	Adult	Child	Infant/ Newborn	Older Adult	Nursing Implications
Chloride: mEq/L	Both sexes: 98-106	90-110	Newborn: 96-106 Premature infant: 95-110	Same as adult	
Cholesterol: mg/dL	Both sexes: <200	120-200	Infant: 70-175 Newborn: 53-135	Same as adult	Instruct client to fast 12-14 hr after eating a low-fat meal.
High-density lipo-protein (HDL; alpha lipopro-teins), which are predominantly protein with a small amount of cholesterol	Male: >45 Female: >55	1-9 yr: 53-56 10-14 yr: 52-55 15-19 yr: 46-52	Newborn: 35	Same as adult	
Low-density lipoprotein (LDL; beta lipopro-teins), which are primarily cholesterol	<130	1-9 yr: 93-100 10-14 yr: 97 15-19 yr: 94-96	Newborn: 29	Same as adult	Target LDL is ≤70 for client with high risk for coronary heart disease (CHD).
CPK Creatine phospho-kinase: IU/L	Male: 55-170 Female: 30-135	Same as adult	Newborn: 65-580	Same as adult	Specimen must not be stored before running test.
Creatinine: mg/dL	Male: 0.6-1.2 Female: 0.5-1.1	Child: 0.3-0.7 Adolescent: 0.5-1	Newborn: 0.2-0.4 Infant: 0.3-1.2	Decrease in muscle mass may cause de-creased values.	It is preferred but not neces-sary to be NPO 8 hr before testing. A ratio of 20:1, BUN to creatine, indicates adequate kidney functioning.
Glucose: mg/dL	Both sexes: 70-110	≤2 yr: 60-100 >2 yr: 70-110	Cord: 45-96 Premature infant: 20-60 Newborn: 30-60 Infant: 40-90	Increase in nor-mal range after age 50	Client to be NPO except for water 8 hr before testing. Caffeine can cause increased values. Stress (e.g., myocardial infarc-tion [MI], infection, general anesthesia) can cause iatro-genic hyperglycemia.
CO_2 Total CO_2, Carbon dioxide content	Both sexes: 23-30	Same as adult: 20-28	Infant: 20-28 Newborn: 13-22	Same as adult	None Included in assessments of electrolytes and acid-base status
Iron: mcg/dL	Male: 80-180 Female: 60-160	50-120	Newborn: 100-250	Same as adult	Client to be NPO 8 hr before testing.
TIBC Total iron-binding capacity: mcg/dL	Both sexes: 250-460	Same as adult	Same as adult	Same as adult	None

Test	Adult	Child	Infant/ Newborn	Older Adult	Nursing Implications
LDH Lactic dehydroge- nase: IU/L	Both sexes: 100-190	60-170	Infant: 100-250 Newborn: 160-450	Same as adult	No intramuscular (IM) injec- tions are to be given 8-12 hr before testing. Hemolysis of blood will cause false positive.
Potassium: mEq/L	Both sexes: 3.5-5	3.4-4.7	Infant: 4.1-5.3 Newborn: 3-5.9	Same as adult	Hemolysis of specimen can result in falsely elevated values. Exercise of the forearm with tourniquet in place may cause increased potassium levels.
Protein total: g/dL	Both sexes: 6.4-8.3	6.2-8	Premature infant: 4.2-7.6 Newborn: 4.6-7.4 Infant: 6-6.7	Same as adult	It is preferred but not neces- sary to be NPO 8 hr before testing.
AST/SGOT Aspar- tate aminotrans- ferase: IU/L	0-35 Female slightly lower than adult males	3-6 yr: 15-50 6-12 yr: 10-50 12-18 yr: 10-40	0-5 days: 35-140 <3 yr: 15-60	Slightly higher than adult	Hemolysis of specimen can result in falsely elevated values. Exercise may cause an in- creased value.
ALT/SGPT Alanine amino- transferase: IU/ mL	Both sexes: 4-36	Same as adult	Infant may be twice as high as an adult.	Slightly higher than adult	Hemolysis of specimen can result in falsely elevated values. Exercise may cause an in- creased value.
Sodium: mEq/L	Both sexes: 136-145	136-145	Infant: 134-150 Newborn: 134-144	Same as adult	Do not collect from an arm with an infusing intravenous (IV) solution.
Triglycerides: mg/dL	Male: 40-160 Female: 35-135	Male 6-11 yr: 31-108 12-15 yr: 36-138 16-19 yr: 40-163 Female 6-11 yr: 35-114 12-15 yr: 41-138 16-19 yr: 40-128	Male 0-5 yr: 30-86 Female 32-99	Same as adult	Client is to be NPO 12 hr before testing. No alcohol for 24 hr before test.
Urea nitrogen: mg/ dL	Both sexes: 10-20	5-18	Infant: 5-18 Newborn: 3-12 Cord: 21-40	Slightly higher	None

Continued

Test	Adult	Child	Infant/ Newborn	Older Adult	Nursing Implications
Thyroid-stimulating hormone (TSH, thyrotropin)	Both sexes: 2-10	Same as adult	Newborn: 3-18 Cord: 3-12	Same as adult	The TSH test is used to differentiate primary and secondary hypothyroidism. TSH levels are subject to a diurnal variation. Some drugs may cause increased levels (antithyroid medications, lithium, potassium iodide, and TSH injection). Some drugs may cause decreased levels (aspirin, nonsteroidal antiarthritics, dopamine, heparin, steroids, and T_3). No food or drink restrictions are necessary.
Triiodothyronine (T_3), ng/dL	Both sexes: 70-205	1-5 yr: 105-270 6-10 yr: 95-240 ng/dL 11-15 yr: 80-215 ng/dL 16-20 yr: 80-210 ng/dL	Newborn: 100-740 Infant: 105-245	>50 yr: 40-180	Primarily to diagnose hyperthyroidism. Total T_3 values are increased in pregnancy because serum proteins are increased at that time.
Total thyroxine (T_4), mcg/dL	Male: 4-12 Female: 5-12	1-5 yr: 7-15 5-10 yr: 6-13 10-15 yr: 5-12	Newborn: 1-3 days: 11-22 1-2 wk: 10-16 Infant: 8-16	>60 yr: 5-11	Newborns are screened to detect hypothyroidism, so mental retardation can be prevented with early diagnosis. A heelstick is used to collect the blood. Slight increase in T_4 levels during pregnancy. Stop taking exogenous T_4 medication 1 month before testing.
Arterial Blood Chemistry					
pH	Both sexes: 7.35-7.45	Same as adult	2 mo-2 yr: 7.34-7.46 Newborn: 7.32-7.49	Same as adult	Specimen must be heparinized. Specimen must be iced for transport. All air bubbles must be expelled from sample. Direct pressure to puncture site must be maintained.

Test	Adult	Child	Infant/ Newborn	Older Adult	Nursing Implications
Pco_2: mm Hg	Both sexes: 35-45	Same as adult	<2 yr: 26-41	Same as adult	Specimen must be heparinized. Specimen must be iced for transport. All air bubbles must be expelled from sample. Direct pressure to puncture site must be maintained.
Po_2: mm Hg	Both sexes: 80-100	Same as adult	Newborn: 60-70	Same as adult	Specimen must be heparinized. Specimen must be iced for transport. All air bubbles must be expelled from sample. Direct pressure to puncture site must be maintained.
Hco_3: mEq/L	Both sexes: 21-28	Same as adult	Infant/newborn: 16-24	Same as adult	Specimen must be heparinized. Specimen must be iced for transport. All air bubbles must be expelled from sample. Direct pressure to puncture site must be maintained.
O_2 saturation: %	Both sexes: 95-100	Same as adult	Newborn: 40-90	95	Specimen must be heparinized. Specimen must be iced for transport. All air bubbles must be expelled from sample. Direct pressure to puncture site must be maintained.

Urinalysis (UA)

Characteristic	Normal	Nursing Implications
Appearance	Clear	May be a midstream, clean-catch specimen. Cloudy urine may be caused by the presence of pus (necrotic WBCs), RBCs, or bacteria or ingestion of certain foods. Urine that has been refrigerated for longer than 1 hr can become cloudy.
Color	Yellow to amber	Pale yellow to amber color because of the pigment urochrome (product of bilirubin metabolism). The color indicates the concentration of the urine (dilute urine: straw-colored; concentrated urine: deep amber and varies with specific gravity). Color can change with ingestion of certain foods or medications. Urine darkens with prolonged standing.
Odor	Aromatic	Diabetic ketoacidosis has the strong, sweet smell of acetone. Urinary tract infection (UTI): the urine may have a foul odor. When urine stands for a long time and starts to decompose, it has an ammonialike smell.

Continued

Characteristic	Normal	Nursing Implications
pH	4.6-8.0 (average, 6.0)	Bacteria, UTI, or a diet high in citrus fruits or vegetables may cause increased urine pH. Urine pH becomes alkaline on standing. The urine pH of an uncovered specimen will become alkaline. A first-voided specimen is best for testing urine specific gravity.
Protein	0-8 mg/dL 50-80 mg/24 hr (at rest) <250 mg/24 hr (during exercise)	Proteinuria indicator of renal disease Test the urine of all pregnant women for proteinuria, an indicator of preeclampsia. If significant protein is noted at urinalysis, a 24-hr urine specimen should be collected so that the quantity of protein can be measured. Transient proteinuria may be associated with severe emotional stress, excessive exercise, and cold baths. A first-voided specimen is best to test for protein.
Specific gravity	Adult: 1.005-1.030 (usually, 1.010-1.025) Older adult: values decrease with age Newborn: 1.001-1.020	Renal disease tends to diminish concentrating capability. Specific gravity is a measurement of hydration status: with overhydration the urine is more dilute; with dehydration the urine is more concentrated. Drugs that may cause increased specific gravity include dextran and sucrose.
Leukocyte esterase	Negative	Positive results indicate UTI. False-positive results may occur in specimens contaminated by vaginal secretions (heavy menstrual discharge, *Trichomonas* infection, parasites) that contain WBCs. False-negative results may occur in specimens containing high levels of protein or ascorbic acid.
Nitrites	None	Chemical testing is done with a dipstick containing a reagent that reacts with nitrites to produce a pink color. A positive test result indicates the need for a urine culture.
Ketones	None	Ketones spill over into the urine when blood glucose levels in diabetic patients are elevated. Ketonuria is associated with poorly controlled diabetes. Ketonuria may occur with acute febrile illnesses, especially in infants and children. Special diets (carbohydrate-free, high-protein, high-fat) and some drugs may cause ketonuria. Testing for ketones can be performed immediately after urine collection. Dip a reagent stick (Ketostix) into the urine specimen. Read the strip in 15 seconds by comparing it with the color chart.
Bilirubin	None	Obstruction of the bile duct by a gallstone causes conjugated hyperbilirubinemia, and unlike the unconjugated form, conjugated bilirubin is water soluble and can be excreted into the urine. Bilirubin is not stable in urine, especially when exposed to light.
Crystals	None	Crystals found on microscopic examination indicate that renal stone formation is imminent, if not already present. Radiographic contrast media may cause precipitation of urinary crystals.

Characteristic	Normal	Nursing Implications
Casts	None	For casts to form, the pH must be acidic and the urine concentrated. Two types of casts: Hyaline casts are conglomerations of protein, and cellular casts are conglomerations of degenerated cells.
Glucose	Fresh specimen: none 24-hr specimen: 50-300 mg/24 hr	Glucose is not excreted by the kidney unless blood levels exceed approximately 180 mg/dL, so can reflect the degree of glucose elevation in the blood. Collect a fresh double-voided specimen. In pregnancy glycosuria is common, but persistent and significantly high levels may indicate gestational diabetes.
White blood cells (WBCs)	0-4 per low-power field	The presence of five or more WBCs in the urine indicates a UTI involving the bladder or kidneys or both. A clean-catch urine culture should be done for further evaluation. Vaginal discharge may contaminate the urine specimen and factitiously cause WBCs in the urine.
WBC casts	None	WBC casts are most frequently found in infections of the kidney, poststreptococcal glomerulonephritis, or inflammatory nephritis.
Red blood cells (RBCs)	≤ 2	Hematuria can be microscopic or gross. Bladder, ureteral, and urethral diseases are the most common causes of RBCs in the urine. The most common cause of RBCs in the urine is from contamination of menses, so before collection of the sample, determine whether the patient is having a period. Traumatic urethral catheterization may cause RBCs in the urine.
RBC casts	None	RBC casts suggest glomerulonephritis interstitial nephritis, acute necrosis, pyelonephritis, renal trauma, or renal tumor. Strenuous physical exercise may cause RBC casts.
Volume		A 24-hr specimen is required. If a 24-hr urine collection is needed, refrigerate urine during the collection period.

Source: Pagana KD, Pagana TJ: *Mosby's diagnostic and laboratory test reference*, ed 10, St. Louis, 2011, Mosby.

Fat-Soluble Vitamins

Vitamin	Food Source
A	Liver Egg yolks, fortified margarine, and butter Dark green and deep orange fruits and vegetables (e.g., apricots, broccoli, cantaloupe, carrots, pumpkin, winter squash, sweet potatoes, and spinach)
D	Fortified and full-fat dairy products Fish oil Can be synthesized in the skin when exposed to sunlight
E	Vegetable oils and their products such as salad oils, margarine, nuts, seeds, avocado, and mango
K	Green leafy vegetables (e.g., lettuce, cabbage, spinach), peas, asparagus, meat, milk, and soybean oil

Water-Soluble Vitamins

Vitamin	Food Sources
C	Citrus fruits, cantaloupes, strawberries, tomatoes, potatoes, broccoli, green peppers, and spinach
B$_1$ (thiamine)	Pork, beef, liver, whole grains, legumes, and wheat germ
B$_2$ (riboflavin)	Liver, milk, milk products, soybeans, and enriched cereals
B$_3$ (nicotinic acid)	Meat, poultry, fish, peanuts, and enriched grains
B$_6$ (pyridoxine)	Meat, poultry, grains, seeds, and seafood
Folic acid	Liver, beans, peas, spinach, and yeast
B$_{12}$	Shellfish, liver, fish, and lean meat

Minerals

Mineral	Food Sources
Calcium	Milk, cheese, dark green vegetables, dried figs, soy, and legumes
Phosphorus	Milk, liver, legumes, fish, and soy
Magnesium	Whole grains, green leafy vegetables, tea, nuts, and fruit
Iron	Meats, eggs, legumes, whole grains, green leafy vegetables, and dried fruits
Iodine	Marine fish, shellfish, dairy products, iodized salt, and some breads
Potassium	Citrus fruits and dried fruits, bananas, watermelon, potatoes, legumes, tea, and peanut butter
Zinc	Meats, seafood, and whole grains

Foods High in Sodium

Vegetables	Condiments	Miscellaneous
Canned vegetables Carrots, particularly canned Tomatoes, particularly canned Tomato catsup Tomato juice	Bouillon cubes Mustard, prepared Olives, pickled, canned, or bottled Pickles, cucumber, dill Salad dressings, commercially prepared Soy sauce	Bacon Cheeses Ready-to-eat breakfast cereals Peanut butter Soups, commercially prepared, canned Corned beef

Important website for nutrition teaching: www.mypyramid.gov/

COMMON LABORATORY TESTS

Test	Purpose	Significance
Blood grouping with Rh factor and antibody screen	To determine blood type screen for possible maternal-fetal blood incompatibility	Identifies possible causes of maternal-fetal blood incompatibility. If father is Rh positive and mother is Rh negative and unsensitized, $Rh_o(D)$ immune globulin will be given during pregnancy and after birth
Complete blood count (CBC)	To identify infection, anemia, or cell abnormalities	More than $15,000/mm^3$ white blood cells or decreased platelets require follow-up
Hemoglobin (Hgb) or hematocrit (Hct)	To detect anemia Often checked several times during pregnancy	Low Hgb or Hct may indicate a need for added iron supplementation
Venereal Disease Research Laboratory (VDRL) or rapid plasma reagin (RPR)	To screen for syphilis	Treat if positive. Retest if indicated.
Rubella titer	To determine immunity	If titer is 1:8 or less, mother is not immune Immunize postpartum if not immune
Tuberculin skin test	To screen for tuberculosis	If positive, refer for additional testing or therapy
Genetic testing (for sickle cell anemia, cystic fibrosis, Tay-Sachs disease, and other genetic conditions)	Offered if there is an increased risk for certain genetic conditions	If mother is positive, check partner Counseling appropriate to the results of testing
Hepatitis B	To detect presence of antigens in maternal blood	If present, infants should be given hepatitis immune globulin and vaccine soon after birth
Human immunodeficiency virus (HIV) screen	Voluntary test encouraged at first visit to detect HIV antibodies	Positive results require retesting, counseling, and treatment to lower infant infection
Urinalysis	To detect renal disease or infection	Requires further assessment if positive for more than trace protein (renal damage, preeclampsia), ketones (fasting or dehydration), or bacteria (infection)
Papanicolaou (Pap) test	To screen for cervical neoplasia	Treat and refer if abnormal cells are present
Cervical culture	To detect group B streptococci and sexually transmitted diseases	Treat and retest as necessary, treat group B streptococci during labor

Continued

Test	Purpose	Significance
Multiple marker screen: Maternal serum alpha-fetoprotein, human chorionic gonadotropin, and estriol. Inhibin A may also be measured. May be combined with ultrasound.	To screen for fetal anomalies	Abnormal results may indicate chromosomal abnormality (such as trisomy 18 or 21) or structural defects (such as neural tube defects)
Glucose challenge test	To screen for gestational diabetes	If elevated, a glucose tolerance test is recommended

From McKinney E, James S, Murray S, Nelson K, Ashwill J: *Maternal-child nursing,* ed 4. Philadelphia, W.B. Saunders Company, 2012.

INDEX

Page numbers followed by *b*, *t*, and *f* indicate boxes, tables, and figures, respectively.

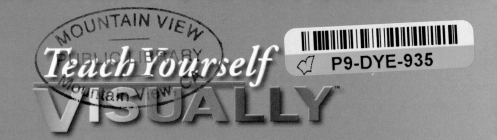

macOS™ Sierra

Paul McFedries

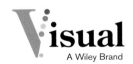

V·isual
A Wiley Brand

Teach Yourself VISUALLY™ macOS™ Sierra

Published by
John Wiley & Sons, Inc.
10475 Crosspoint Boulevard
Indianapolis, IN 46256

www.wiley.com

Published simultaneously in Canada

Wiley publishes in a variety of print and electronic formats and by print-on-demand. Some material included with standard print versions of this book may not be included in e-books or in print-on-demand. If this book refers to media such as a CD or DVD that is not included in the version you purchased, you may download this material at http://booksupport.wiley.com. For more information about Wiley products, visit www.wiley.com.

Library of Congress Control Number: 2016953459

ISBN: 978-1-119-30061-8 (pbk); ISBN: 978-1-119-30063-2 (ebk); ISBN: 978-1-119-30062-5 (ebk)

Manufactured in the United States of America

10 9 8 7 6 5 4 3 2 1

Trademark Acknowledgments

Contact Us

For general information on our other products and services, please contact our Customer Care Department within the U.S. at 877-762-2974, outside the U.S. at 317-572-3993 or fax 317-572-4002.

For technical support, please visit www.wiley.com and select the Contact Us link to reach Customer Care.

Credits

Executive Editor
Jody Lefevere

Project Editor
Sarah Hellert

Technical Editor
Galen Gruman

Copy Editor
Scott Tullis

Production Editor
Barath Kumar Rajasekaran

Manager, Content Development & Assembly
Mary Beth Wakefield

Vice President, Professional Technology Strategy
Barry Pruett

About the Author

Paul McFedries is a full-time technical writer. Paul has been authoring computer books since 1991, and he has more than 90 books to his credit. Paul's books have sold more than four million copies worldwide. These books include the Wiley titles *Teach Yourself VISUALLY Windows 10 Anniversary Update, Teach Yourself VISUALLY Excel 2016, The Facebook Guide for People Over 50*, and *iPhone 6 Portable Genius*. Paul is also the proprietor of Word Spy (www.wordspy.com), a website that tracks new words and phrases as they enter the language, and Word Spy Press (https://wordspy.com/index.php?page=press), books for people who love words. Paul invites you to drop by his personal website at www.mcfedries.com or follow him on Twitter @paulmcf or @wordspy.

Author's Acknowledgments

It goes without saying that writers focus on text, and I certainly enjoyed focusing on the text that you'll read in this book. However, this book is more than just the usual collection of words and phrases. A quick thumb-through the pages will show you that this book is also chock full of images, from sharp screenshots to fun and informative illustrations. Those colorful images sure make for a beautiful book, and that beauty comes from a lot of hard work by Wiley's immensely talented group of designers and layout artists. I thank them for creating another gem. Of course, what you read in this book must also be accurate, logically presented, and free of errors. Ensuring all of this was an excellent group of editors that included project editor Sarah Hellert, copy editor Scott Tullis, and technical editor Galen Gruman. Thanks to all of you for your exceptional competence and hard work. Thanks, as well, to Wiley executive editor Jody Lefevere for asking me to write this book.

How to Use This Book

Who This Book Is For

This book is for the reader who has never used this particular technology or software application. It is also for readers who want to expand their knowledge.

The Conventions in This Book

❶ Steps

This book uses a step-by-step format to guide you easily through each task. Numbered steps are actions you must do; bulleted steps clarify a point, step, or optional feature; and indented steps give you the result.

❷ Notes

Notes give additional information — special conditions that may occur during an operation, a situation that you want to avoid, or a cross reference to a related area of the book.

❸ Icons and Buttons

Icons and buttons show you exactly what you need to click to perform a step.

❹ Tips

Tips offer additional information, including warnings and shortcuts.

❺ Bold

Bold type shows command names, options, and text or numbers you must type.

❻ Italics

Italic type introduces and defines a new term.

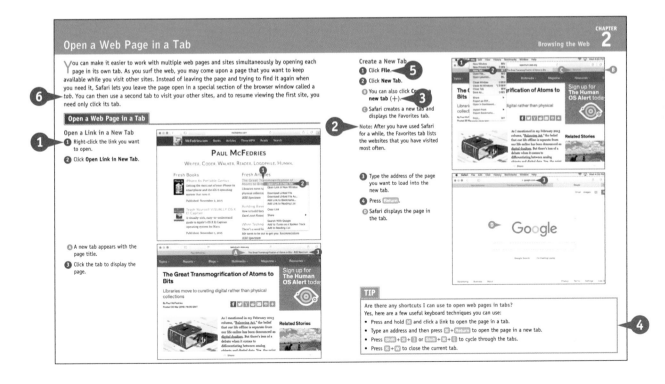

Table of Contents

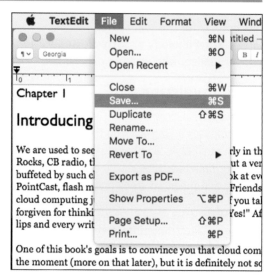

Chapter 2 Browsing the Web

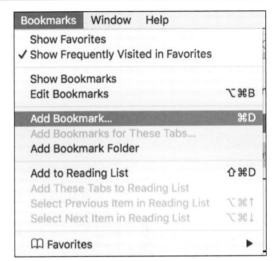

Chapter 3 Communicating via Email

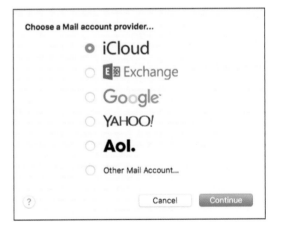

Table of Contents

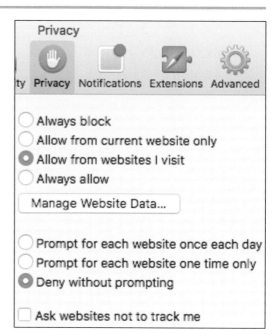

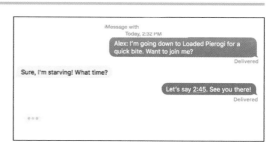

Chapter 6 | Tracking Contacts and Events

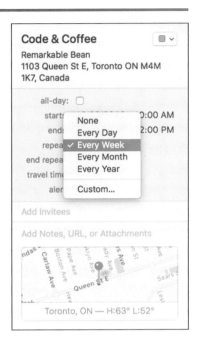

Chapter 7 | Playing and Organizing Music

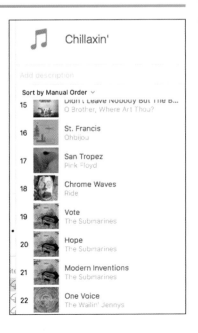

Table of Contents

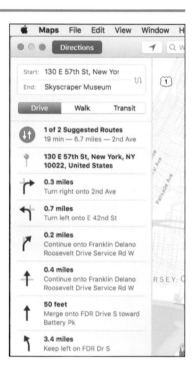

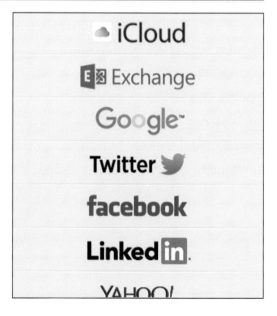

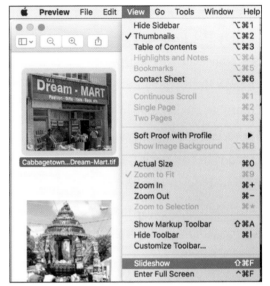

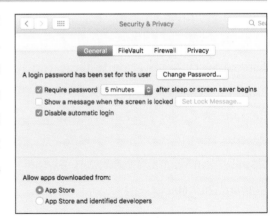

Table of Contents

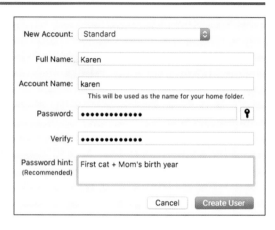

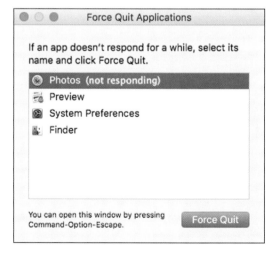

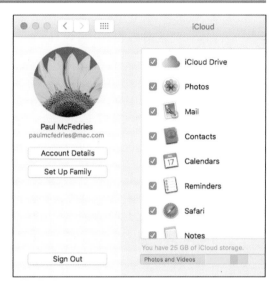

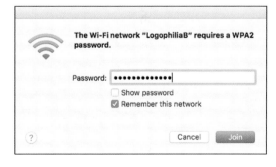

Learning Basic macOS Tasks

macOS (formerly OS X) has a few basic tasks that you need to know to make the rest of Mac chores faster and easier. These chores include starting and managing applications, searching your Mac for documents and data, saving your work, and fundamental file operations such as opening, printing, and copying.

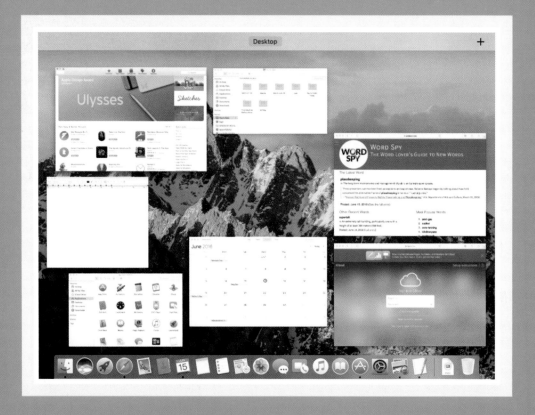

Start an Application

To perform tasks of any kind in macOS, you use one of the applications installed on your Mac. The application you use depends on the task you want to perform. For example, if you want to surf the World Wide Web, you use a web browser application, such as the Safari program that comes with macOS. Before you can use an application, however, you must first tell macOS what application you want to run. macOS launches the application and displays it on the desktop. You can then use the application's tools to perform your tasks.

Start an Application

Using the Dock

1 If the application that you want to start has an icon in the Dock, click the icon to start the application.

A You can position the mouse pointer (▶) over a Dock icon to see the name of the application.

Using Spotlight

1 Click **Spotlight** (🔍).

2 Start typing the name of the application you want to start.

B macOS displays a list of matching items.

3 When the application appears in the results, click it to start the program.

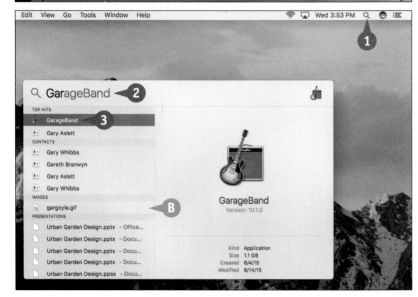

Using Finder

1 Click **Finder** ( ).

The Finder window appears.

2 Click **Applications**.

Note: You can also open Applications in any Finder window by pressing Shift + ⌘ + A or by clicking **Go** and then clicking **Applications**.

3 Double-click the application you want to start.

Note: In some cases, double-clicking the icon just displays the contents of a folder. In this case, you then double-click the application icon.

C The application appears on the desktop.

D macOS temporarily adds a button for the application to the Dock.

E The menu bar displays the menus associated with the application.

Note: Another common way you can launch an application is to use Finder to locate a document you want to work with and then double-click that document.

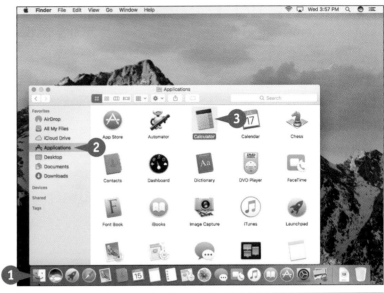

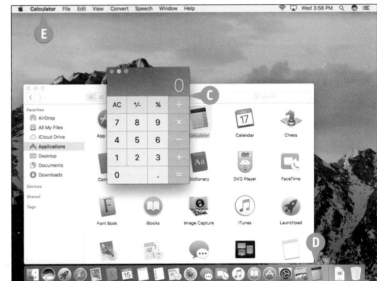

TIPS

How do I add an icon to the Dock for an application I use frequently?

To add an icon to the Dock, repeat steps **1** to **3** in the subsection "Using Finder." Right-click the application's Dock icon, click **Options**, and then click **Keep in Dock**.

How do I shut down a running application?

To shut down a running application, right-click the application's Dock icon and then click **Quit**. Alternatively, you can switch to the application and press ⌘ + Q.

Start an Application Using Launchpad

You can start an application using the Launchpad feature. This is often faster than using the Applications folder, particularly for applications that do not have a Dock icon.

Launchpad is designed to mimic the Home screens of the iPhone, iPad, and iPod touch. So if you own one or more of these devices, then you are already familiar with how Launchpad works.

Start an Application Using Launchpad

1 Click **Launchpad** ().

The Launchpad screen appears.

2 If the application you want to start resides in a different Launchpad screen, click the dot that corresponds to the screen.

Launchpad switches to the screen and displays the applications.

3 If the application you want to start resides within a folder, click the folder.

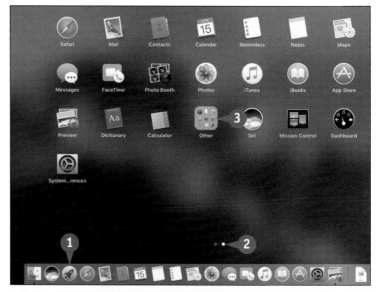

Launchpad opens the folder.

4 Click the icon of the application you want to start.

macOS starts the application.

Note: To exit Launchpad without starting an application, you can press Esc.

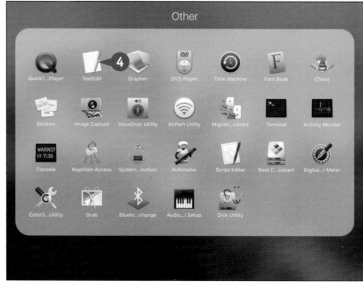

6

Locate the Mouse Pointer

macOS includes a feature that helps you locate the mouse pointer. This is useful because although you can control certain features of macOS using the keyboard or by using gestures on a trackpad or similar device, most macOS tasks require the mouse or trackpad. Clicking, double-clicking, dragging, and other standard mouse techniques make using macOS easy and efficient, but not if you have trouble locating the mouse pointer. This can happen very easily if your screen is crowded with windows.

Locate the Mouse Pointer

1 Jiggle the pointer several times:

If you have a mouse, move the mouse back and forth.

If you have a trackpad or a Magic Mouse, slide your finger back and forth on the surface of the trackpad or the top of the Magic Mouse.

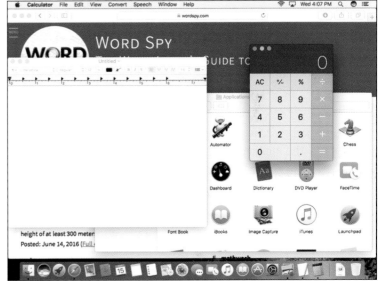

A macOS temporarily increases the size of the mouse pointer (🔍).

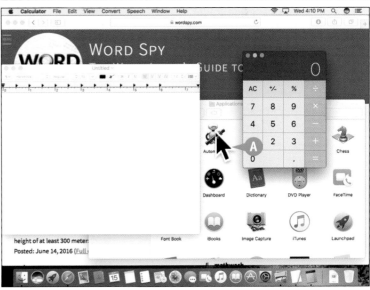

Switch Between Applications

If you plan on running multiple applications at the same time, you need to know how to easily switch from one application to another. In macOS, after you start one application, you do not need to close that application before you open another one. macOS supports a feature called *multitasking*, which means running two or more applications simultaneously. This is handy if you need to use several applications throughout the day.

Switch Between Applications

1 Click the Dock icon of the application you want to switch to.

Note: If you can see part of the application's window, you can also switch to the application by clicking its window.

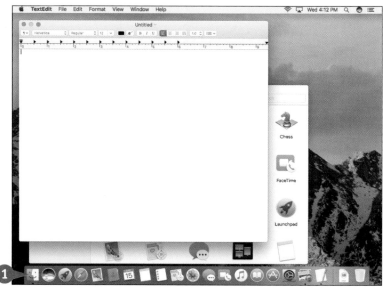

A macOS brings the application window(s) to the foreground.

B The menu bar displays the menus associated with the application.

Note: To switch between applications from the keyboard, press and hold ⌘ and repeatedly press Tab until the application that you want is highlighted in the list of running applications. Release ⌘ to switch to the application.

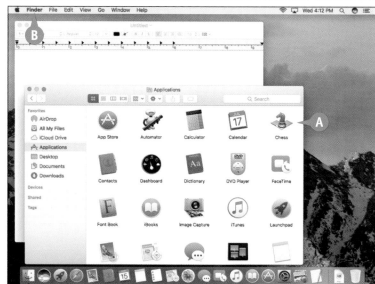

8

View Running Applications with Mission Control

The Mission Control feature makes it easier for you to navigate and locate your running applications. macOS allows you to open multiple applications simultaneously, and the only real limit to the number of open applications you can have is the amount of memory contained in your Mac. In practical terms, this means you can easily open several applications, some of which may have multiple open windows. To help locate and navigate to the window you need, use the Mission Control feature.

View Running Applications with Mission Control

1 Click **Launchpad** (🚀).

2 Click **Mission Control.**

Note: You can also invoke Mission Control by pressing ⒡⒊ or by placing four fingers on the trackpad of your Mac and then swiping up.

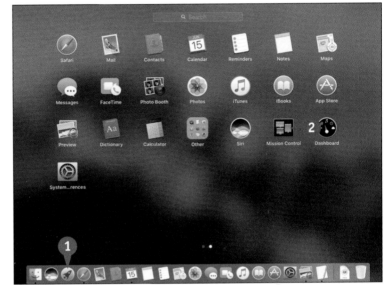

Ⓐ Mission Control displays each open window.

To switch to a particular window, click it.

Ⓑ To close Mission Control without selecting a window, you can click **Desktop** or press ⒠⒮⒞.

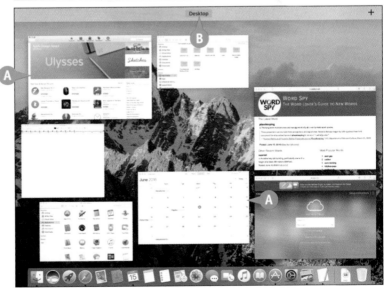

Run an Application Full Screen

You can maximize the viewing and working areas of an application by running that application in full-screen mode. When you switch to full-screen mode, macOS hides the menu bar, the application's status bar, the Dock, and the top section of the application window (the section that includes the Close, Minimize, and Zoom buttons). macOS then expands the rest of the application window so that it takes up the entire screen. Note that not all programs are capable of switching to full-screen mode.

Run an Application Full Screen

1 Click **View**.

2 Click **Enter Full Screen**.

You can also press **Control** + **⌘** + **F**.

A In applications that support Full Screen, you can also click **Zoom** (●).

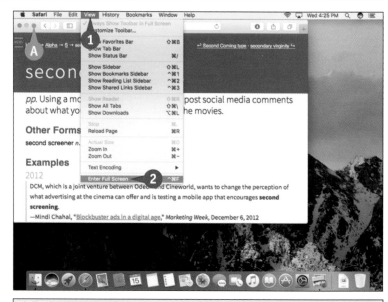

macOS expands the application window to take up the entire screen.

Note: To exit full-screen mode, move the mouse pointer (🡕) up to the top of the screen to reveal the menu bar, click **View**, and then click **Exit Full Screen**. You can also click **Zoom** (●), press **Esc**, or press **Control** + **⌘** + **F**.

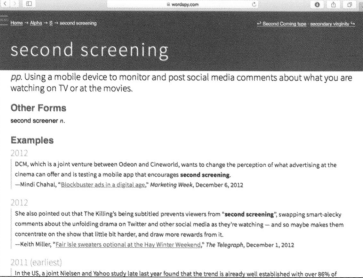

Split the Screen with Two Applications

Y ou can make your macOS desktop more convenient and more efficient by splitting the screen with two application windows. Splitting the screen means that macOS switches to full-screen mode, where one application window takes up the left side of the desktop, and a second application window takes up the right side of the desktop. With these windows arranged side by side, the content of both windows remains visible at all times, so you can easily refer to one window while working in the other.

Split the Screen with Two Applications

1 Click and hold **Zoom** (⬤).

2 Drag the mouse pointer (➤) to either the left or the right side of the screen.

Ⓐ macOS displays a blue background to show you where the application window will reside.

3 Release the mouse.

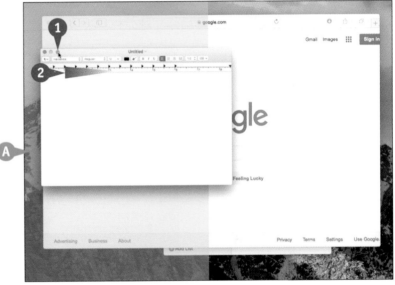

Ⓑ macOS switches to full-screen mode and displays the application in the half of the screen you selected.

Ⓒ macOS displays thumbnail versions of the other open windows.

4 Click a window.

macOS displays the window in the other half of the screen.

Note: To exit split-screen mode, move the mouse pointer (➤) to the top of the screen, click **View**, and then click **Exit Full Screen**. You can also click **Zoom** (⬤), press `Esc`, or press `Control`+`⌘`+`F`.

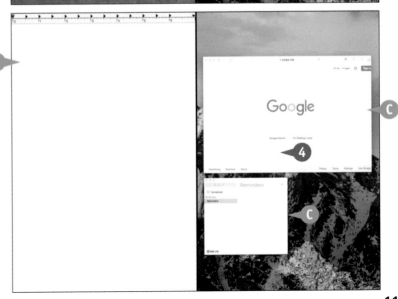

Search Your Mac

You can save time and make your Mac easier to use by learning how to search for the apps, settings, or files that you need.

After you have used your Mac for a while and have created many documents, you might have trouble locating a specific file. You can save a great deal of time by using the macOS Spotlight search feature to search for your document. You can also use Spotlight to search for apps as well as information from the Internet, the iTunes Store, the App Store, and more. Alternatively, you can use Finder's Search box to search just your Mac.

Search Your Mac

Search with Spotlight

1 Click **Spotlight** (🔍).

You can also press ⌘+**Spacebar**.

A The Spotlight window appears.

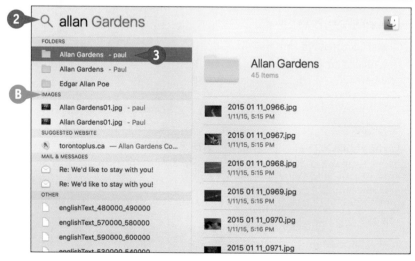

2 Type a word or short phrase that represents the item or information you want to locate.

B As you type, Spotlight displays the Mac and online items that match your search text.

3 Click the item you want to view or work with.

macOS opens the item.

Search Your Mac

1. Click **Finder** ( ).

2. If you want to search within a specific folder, open that folder.

3. Click inside the Search box.

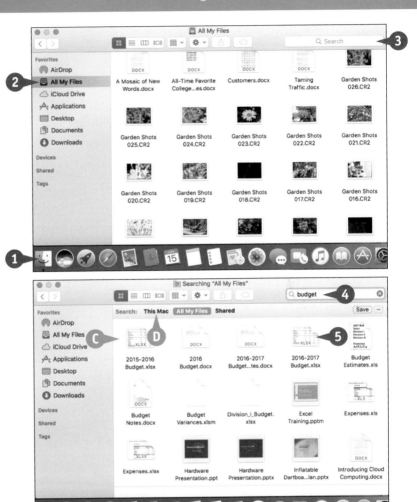

4. Type a word or short phrase that represents the item you want to locate.

C. As you type, Spotlight displays the items that match your search text.

D. If you are searching a specific folder, you can click **This Mac** to switch to searching your entire Mac.

5. Click the item you want to work with.

   macOS opens the item.

TIP

Can I remove item types from the Spotlight search results?

Yes. Spotlight supports a number of different *categories*, such as Applications, Documents, and Contacts. If there are categories that you never search for, such as system preferences or movies, you should remove them to make it easier to navigate the Spotlight search results.

To remove one or more categories from the Spotlight results, click **System Preferences** ( ) in the Dock and then click **Spotlight**. In the Search Results pane, click the check box beside each category you want to remove (changes to).

Voice-Operate Your Mac with Siri

I f your Mac comes with a built-in microphone or if you have connected a headset or microphone to your Mac, you can use the Siri voice-activated assistant to control macOS. You can use Siri to search your Mac, search the web, and start apps. You can also use Siri to run commands within certain apps. For example, you can use Siri to schedule appointments, start an email, or display a contact.

Before you can use Siri, you must have a microphone — either one that comes with your Mac or one that you connect to your Mac — and you must enable Siri in System Preferences.

Voice-Operate Your Mac with Siri

Enable Siri

1 Click **System Preferences** (⚙).

2 Click **Siri**.

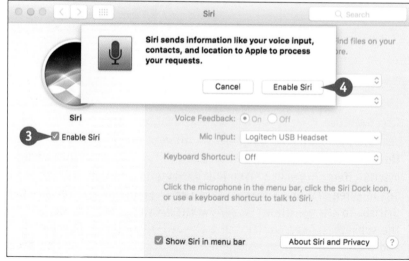

The Siri preferences appear.

3 Click the **Enable Siri** check box (☐ changes to ☑).

System Preferences asks you to confirm.

4 Click **Enable Siri**.

You can now use Siri to operate your Mac with voice commands.

Access Siri

1 Click **Siri** (⬤) in the Dock.

Note: See the second Tip to learn how to access Siri using a keyboard shortcut.

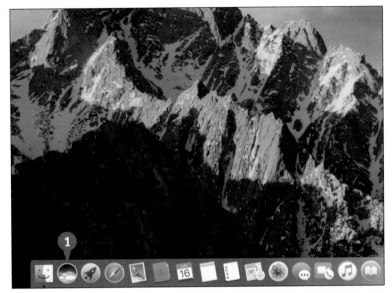

The Siri window appears and prompts you to ask something.

A You can also click **Siri** (⬤) in the menu bar.

2 Use your microphone to ask a question.

B The Siri window runs through several screens that show you the types of questions you can ask.

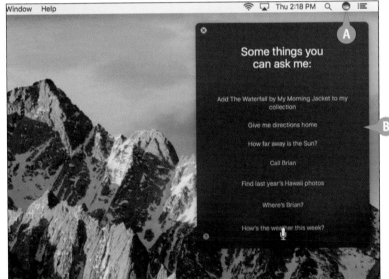

TIPS

How do I change the voice that Siri uses?
macOS offers six English male and female voices for Siri in three accents: American, Australian, and British. To change the voice, follow steps **1** and **2** in the subsection "Enable Siri," click the **Siri Voice** ⬦, and then click the voice you prefer.

Can I access Siri using the keyboard?
Yes, although this feature is turned off by default. To enable this feature, follow steps **1** and **2** in the subsection "Enable Siri," click the **Keyboard Shortcut** ⬦, and then click **Function Space**. You can now access Siri by pressing **Fn** + **Spacebar**.

Save a Document

After you create a document and make changes to it, you can save the document to preserve your work. When you work on a document, macOS stores the changes in your computer's memory. However, macOS erases the contents of the Mac's memory each time you shut down or restart the computer. This means that, unless the app you are using saves changes automatically, as many now do, the changes you make to your document are lost when you turn off or restart your Mac. Saving the document preserves your changes on your Mac's hard drive.

Save a Document

1 Click **File**.

2 Click **Save**.

In most applications, you can also press ⌘+⑤.

If you have saved the document previously, your changes are now preserved, and you do not need to follow the rest of the steps in this section.

If this is a new document that you have never saved before, the Save As dialog appears.

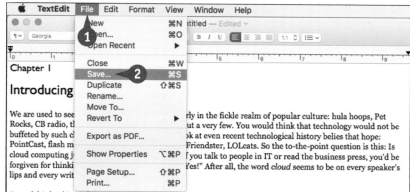

3 Type the filename you want to use in the Save As text box.

A To store the file in a different folder, you can click the **Where** ◌ and then select the location that you prefer from the pop-up menu.

4 Click **Save**.

The application saves the file.

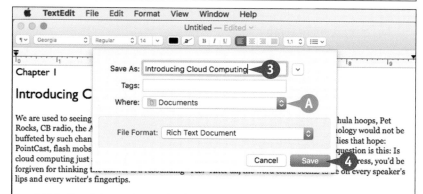

Open a Document

To work with a document that you have saved in the past, you can open it in the application that you used to create it. When you save a document, you save its contents to your Mac's hard drive, and those contents are stored in a separate file. When you open the document using the same application that you used to save it, macOS loads the file's contents into memory and displays the document in the application. You can then view or edit the document as needed.

Open a Document

1 Start the application you want to work with.

2 Click **File**.

3 Click **Open**.

In most applications, you can also press ⌘+O.

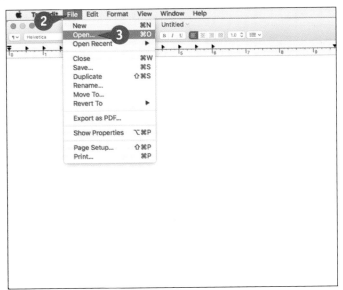

The Open dialog appears.

A To select a different folder from which to open a file, you can click ⊙ and then click the location that you prefer.

4 Click the document.

5 Click **Open**.

The document appears in a window on the desktop.

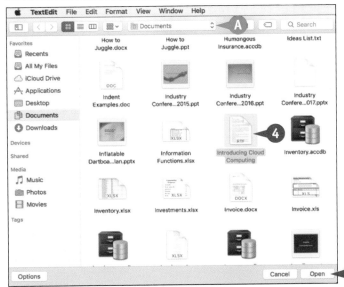

Print a Document

When you need a hard copy of your document, either for your files or to distribute to someone else, you can send the document to your printer. Most applications that deal with documents also come with a Print command. When you run this command, the Print dialog appears. You use the Print dialog to choose the printer you want, as well as to specify how many copies you want to print. Many Print dialogs also enable you to see a preview of your document before printing it.

Print a Document

1 Turn on your printer.

2 Open the document that you want to print.

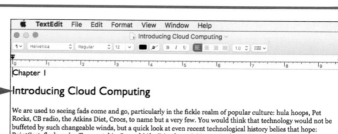

3 Click **File**.

4 Click **Print**.

In many applications, you can select the Print command by pressing ⌘+P.

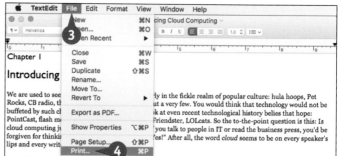

The Print dialog appears.

The layout of the Print dialog varies from application to application. The version shown here is a typical example.

5 If you have more than one printer, click the **Printer** ⬍ to select the printer that you want to use.

6 To print more than one copy, type the number of copies to print in the Copies text box.

7 Click **Print**.

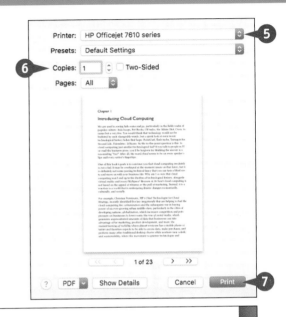

A macOS prints the document. The printer's icon appears in the Dock while the document prints.

Introducing Cloud Computing

We are used to seeing fads come and go, particularly in the fickle realm of popular culture: hula hoops, Pet Rocks, CB radio, the Atkins Diet, Crocs, to name but a very few. You would think that technology would not be buffeted by such changeable winds, but a quick look at even recent technological history belies that hope: PointCast, flash mobs, Tamagotchis, Second Life, Friendster, LOLcats. So the to-the-point question is this: Is cloud computing just another technological fad? If you talk to people in IT or read the business press, you'd be forgiven for thinking the answer is a resounding "Yes!" After all, the word *cloud* seems to be on every speaker's lips and every writer's fingertips.

One of this book's goals is to convince you that cloud computing resolutely is *not* a fad. It may be overhyped at the moment (more on that later), but it is definitely not some passing technical fancy that you can turn a blind eye to and move on with your business life. Why am I so sure that cloud computing won't end up in the dustbin of technological history, alongside virtual reality and (soon) MySpace? Because at its heart cloud computing is not based on the appeal of whimsy or the pull of marketing. Instead, it is a reaction to a world that is undergoing drastic changes economically, culturally, and socially.

For example, Christian Verstraete, HP's Chief Technologist for Cloud Strategy, recently identified five key megatrends that are helping to fuel the cloud computing fire: *urbanization* and the subsequent rise in buying power of an ever-growing urban middle class, particularly in the cities of developing nations; *globalization*, which increases competition and puts pressure on businesses to lower costs; the *rise of social media*, which generates unprecedented amounts of data that businesses can take advantage of for marketing, product development, and more; the *mainstreaming of mobility* where almost everyone has a mobile phone or tablet and therefore expects to be able to access data, make purchases, and perform many other **A** ional desktop chores while nowhere near a desk; and *sustainability*, where the movement to greener tech. logies and smaller

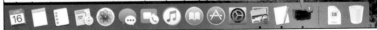

TIP

Can I print only part of my document?

Yes, you can print either a single page or a range of pages, although the steps you use to specify what you want to print vary from one application to another. In the Pages word-processing application, for example, you use the Pages pop-up menu to select what you want to print: All, Single, or Range.

If you select the Single option, use the text box (or the stepper, ⬍) to specify the number of the page you want to print.

If you select the Range option, use the two text boxes (or their associated steppers, ⬍) to specify the numbers of the first and last pages you want to print.

Copy a File

You can use macOS to make an exact copy of a file. This is useful when you want to make an extra copy of an important file to use as a backup. Similarly, you might require a copy of a file if you want to send the copy on a disc to another person. Finally, copying a file is also a real timesaver if you need a new file very similar to an existing file: You copy the original file and then make the required changes to the copy. You can copy either a single file or multiple files. You can also use this technique to copy a folder.

Copy a File

1 Locate the file that you want to copy.

2 Open the folder to which you want to copy the file.

To open a second folder window, click **File** and then click **New Finder Window**, or press ⌘+N.

3 Press and hold **Option**, and then click and drag the file and drop it inside the destination folder.

Ⓐ The original file remains in its folder.

Ⓑ A copy of the original file appears in the destination folder.

You can also make a copy of a file in the same folder, which is useful if you want to make major changes to the file and you would like to preserve a copy of the original. Click the file, click **File**, and then click **Duplicate**, or press ⌘+D. macOS creates a copy with the word "copy" added to the filename.

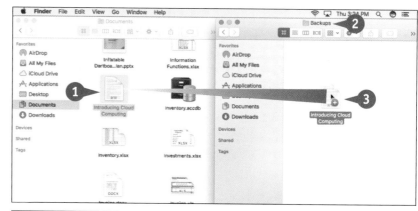

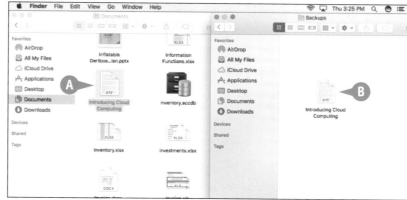

Move a File

When you need to store a file in a new location, the easiest way is to move the file from its current folder to another folder on your Mac. When you save a file for the first time, you specify a folder on your Mac's hard drive. This original location is not permanent, however. Using the technique in this section, you can move the file to another location on your Mac's hard drive. You can use this technique to move a single file, multiple files, and even a folder.

Move a File

1 Locate the file that you want to move.

2 Open the folder to which you want to move the file.

To create a new destination folder in the current folder, click **File** and then click **New Folder**, or press `Shift`+`⌘`+`N`.

3 Click and drag the file and drop it inside the destination folder.

Note: If you are moving the file to another drive, you must press and hold `⌘` while you click and drag the file. Otherwise a copy is made.

A The file disappears from its original folder.

B The file moves to the destination folder.

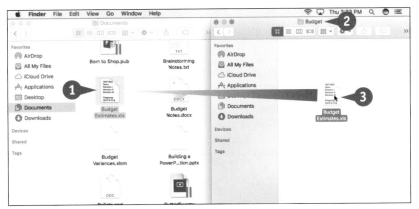

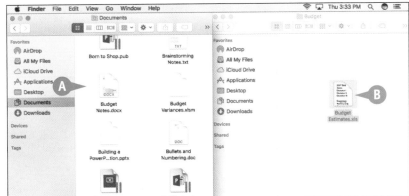

Rename a File

You can change the name of a file, which is useful if the current filename does not accurately describe the contents of the file. Giving your document a descriptive name makes it easier to find the file later. You should rename only those documents that you have created or that have been given to you by someone else. Do not try to rename any of the macOS system files or any files associated with your applications, or your computer may behave erratically or even crash.

Rename a File

1 Open the folder containing the file that you want to rename.

2 Click the file.

3 Press Return.

A A text box appears around the filename.

You can also rename any folders that you have created.

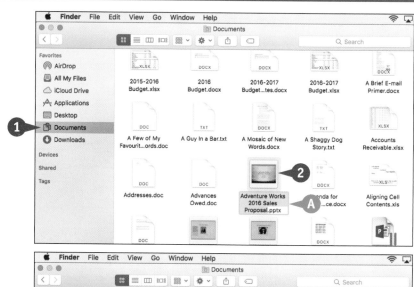

4 Edit the existing name or type a new name that you want to use for the file.

If you decide that you do not want to rename the file after all, you can press Esc to cancel the operation.

5 Press Return or click an empty section of the folder.

The new name appears under the file icon.

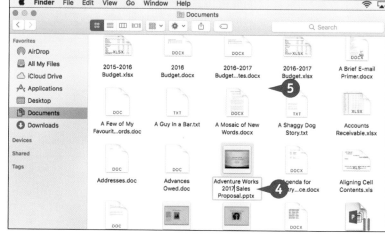

Delete a File

When you no longer need a file, you can delete it. This helps to prevent your hard drive from becoming cluttered with unnecessary files. You should ensure that you delete only those documents that you have created or that have been given to you by someone else. Do not delete any of the macOS system files or any files associated with your applications, or your computer may behave erratically or even crash.

Delete a File

1 Locate the file that you want to delete.

2 Click and drag the file and drop it on the **Trash** icon ( ) in the Dock.

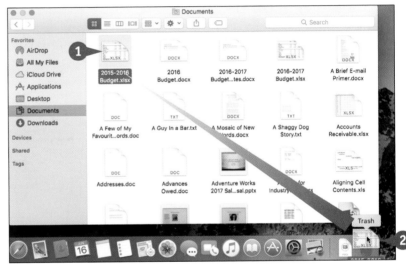

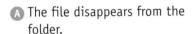

A The file disappears from the folder.

You can also delete a file by clicking it and then pressing ⌘ + Delete .

If you delete a file accidentally, you can restore it. Click the Dock's **Trash** icon ( ) to open the Trash window. Right-click the file and then click **Put Back**.

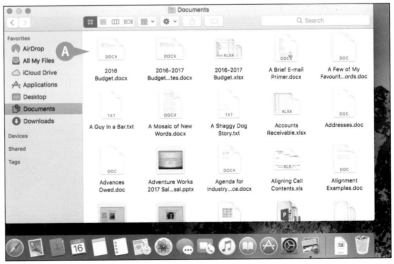

Open a Folder in a Tab

You can make it easier to work with multiple folders simultaneously by opening each folder in its own tab within a single Finder window. As you work with your documents, you may come upon one or more folders that you want to keep available while you work with other folders. Instead of cluttering the desktop with multiple Finder windows, macOS enables you to use a single Finder window that displays each open folder in a special section of the window called a *tab*. To view the contents of any open folder, you need only click its tab.

Open a Folder in a Tab

1 Right-click the folder you want to open.

2 Click **Open in New Tab**.

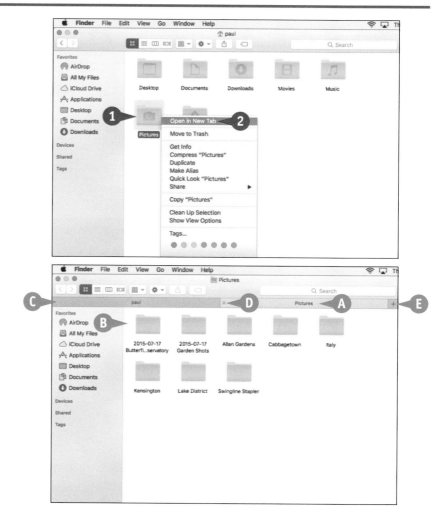

Ⓐ A new tab appears for the folder.

Ⓑ The folder's contents appear here.

Ⓒ You can click any tab to display its contents in the Finder window.

Ⓓ To close a tab, you can position the mouse pointer (►) over the tab and then click **Close Tab** (✕).

Ⓔ If you already have two or more tabs open, you can also click **Create a new tab** (+).

Note: You can also create a new tab by clicking **File** and then clicking **New Tab**.

Open a Document in a Tab

You can make it easier to work with multiple documents at the same time by opening each document in its own tab within a single application window. This is a new feature in macOS Sierra and is supported by a number of macOS apps as well as some third-party apps. Now, instead of cluttering the desktop with multiple app windows, you can use a single app window that displays each open document in a special section of the window called a tab. To view the contents of any open document, you click its tab.

Open a Document in a Tab

1 In an app that supports tabs, click **File**.

2 Click **New Tab**.

You can also press ⌘+T.

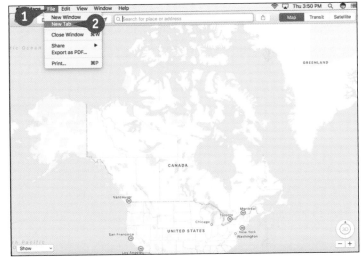

A A new tab appears.

B The tab's contents appear here.

C You can click any tab to display its contents in the app window.

D To close a tab, you can position the mouse pointer (🔺) over the tab and then click **Close Tab** (✕).

E If you already have two or more tabs open, you can also click **Create a new tab** (+).

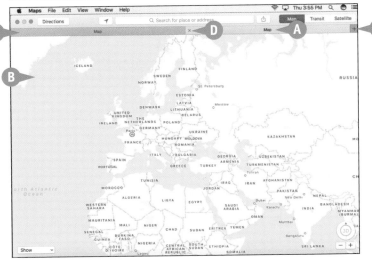

CHAPTER 2

Browsing the Web

If your Mac is connected to the Internet, you can use the Safari browser to navigate, or *surf*, websites. Safari offers features that make it easier to browse the web. For example, you can open multiple pages in a single Safari window, and you can save your favorite sites for easier access.

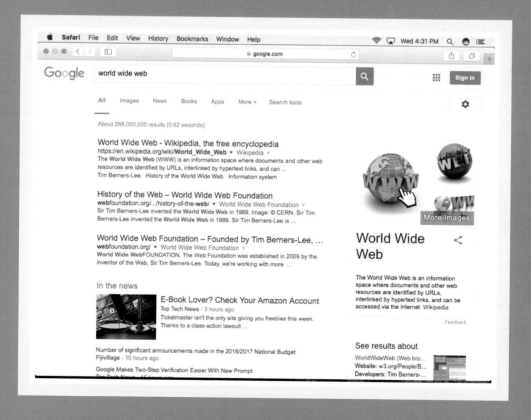

Open a Web Page in a Tab

You can make it easier to work with multiple web pages and sites simultaneously by opening each page in its own tab. As you surf the web, you may come upon a page that you want to keep available while you visit other sites. Instead of leaving the page and trying to find it again when you need it, Safari lets you leave the page open in a special section of the browser window called a *tab*. You can then use a second tab to visit your other sites, and to resume viewing the first site, you need only click its tab.

Open a Web Page in a Tab

Open a Link in a New Tab

1 Right-click the link you want to open.

2 Click **Open Link in New Tab**.

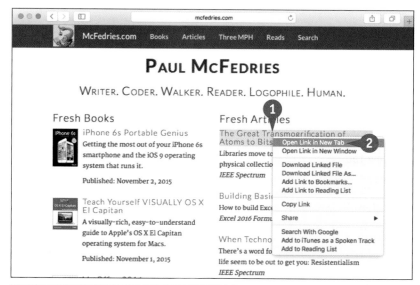

A A new tab appears with the page title.

3 Click the tab to display the page.

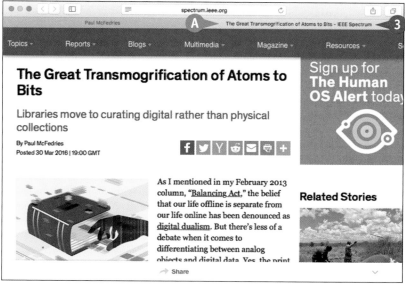

Create a New Tab

1 Click **File**.

2 Click **New Tab**.

Ⓑ You can also click **Create a new tab** (+).

Ⓒ Safari creates a new tab and displays the Favorites tab.

Note: After you have used Safari for a while, the Favorites tab lists the websites that you have visited most often.

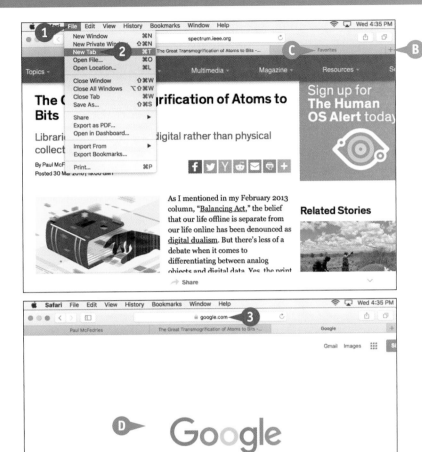

3 Type the address of the page you want to load into the new tab.

4 Press **Return**.

Ⓓ Safari displays the page in the tab.

Google

TIP

Are there any shortcuts I can use to open web pages in tabs?

Yes, here are a few useful keyboard techniques you can use:

- Press and hold ⌘ and click a link to open the page in a tab.
- Type an address and then press ⌘+**Return** to open the page in a new tab.
- Press **Shift**+⌘+**]** or **Shift**+⌘+**[** to cycle through the tabs.
- Press ⌘+**W** to close the current tab.

Navigate Web Pages

After you have visited several pages, you can return to a page you visited earlier. Instead of retyping the address or looking for the link, Safari gives you some easier methods. When you navigate from page to page, you create a kind of path through the web. Safari keeps track of this path by maintaining a list of the pages you visit. You can use that list to go back to a page you have visited. After you go back to a page you have visited, you can use the same list to go forward through the pages again.

Navigate Web Pages

Go Back One Page

1 Click **Previous Page** (<).

The previous page you visited appears.

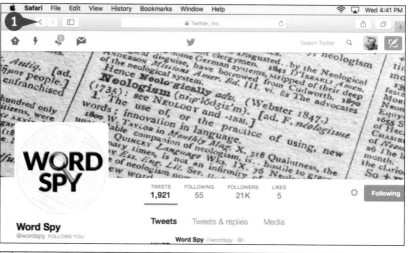

Go Back Several Pages

1 Click and hold down the mouse pointer (▶) on **Previous Page** (<).

A list of the pages you have visited appears.

Note: The list of visited pages is different for each tab that you have open. If you do not see the page you want, you may need to click a different tab.

2 Click the page you want to revisit.

The page appears.

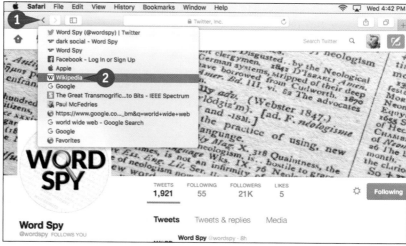

Go Forward One Page

1 Click **Next Page** (>).

The next page appears.

Note: If you are at the last page viewed up to that point, the Next Page icon (>) is not active.

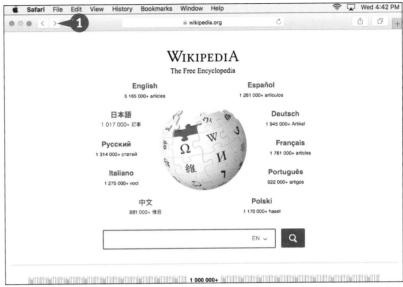

Go Forward Several Pages

1 Click and hold down the mouse pointer (**k**) on **Next Page** (>).

A list of the pages you have visited appears.

Note: The list of visited pages is different for each tab that you have open. If you do not see the page you want, you may need to click a different tab.

2 Click the page you want to revisit.

The page appears.

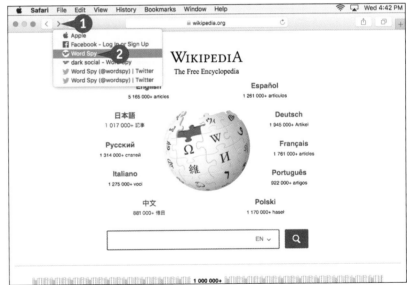

TIP

Are there any shortcuts I can use to navigate web pages?
Yes, a few useful keyboard shortcuts you can use follows:

- Press ⌘+[to go back one page.
- Press ⌘+] to go forward one page.
- Press Shift+⌘+H to return to the Safari home page (the first page you see when you open Safari).

Navigate with the History List

The Previous Page and Next Page icons (< and >) enable you to navigate pages in the current browser session. To redisplay sites that you have visited in the past few days or weeks, you need to use the History list, which is a collection of the websites and pages you have visited over the past month.

If you visit sensitive places such as an Internet banking site or your corporate site, you can increase security by clearing the History list so that other people cannot see where you have been.

Navigate with the History List

Load a Page from the Recent History List

1 Click **History**.

Safari displays a menu of recent dates that you used the program.

2 Click the date when you visited the page.

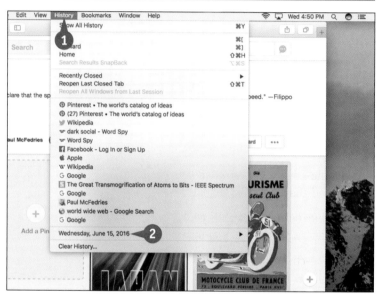

A A submenu of pages that you visited during that day appears.

3 Click the page you want to revisit.

Safari opens the page.

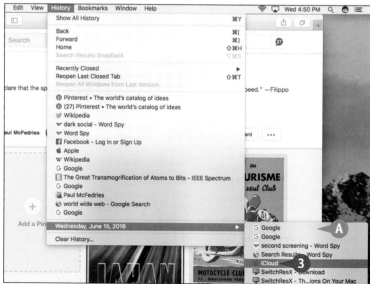

Load a Page from the Full History List

1 Click **History**.

2 Click **Show All History**.

Note: You can also run the Show All History command by pressing ⌘+Y.

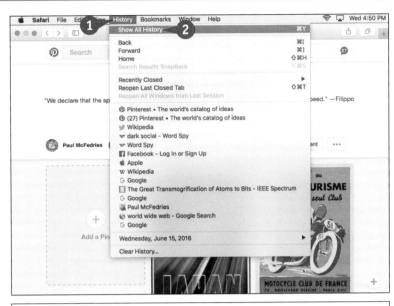

Safari displays the full History list.

3 Double-click the date when you visited the page.

B A submenu of pages that you visited during that day appears.

4 Double-click the page you want to revisit.

Safari opens the page.

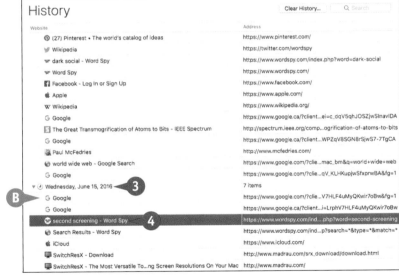

How can I control the length of time that Safari keeps track of the pages I visit?

In the menu bar, click **Safari** and then **Preferences**. The Safari preferences appear. Click the **General** tab. Click the **Remove history items** ⊘ and then select the amount of time you want Safari to track your history. Click **Close** (⬤).

Is there an easier way to find the page I am looking for?

If you know some or all of the page's title or address, you can search for the page. Press ⌘+Y to open History, click the Search box in the lower-right corner, and then type what you can remember of the page title or address.

Change Your Home Page

Your home page is the web page that appears when you first start Safari. The default home page is usually the Apple.com Start page, but you can change that to any other page you want, or even to an empty page. This is useful if you do not use the Apple.com Start page, or if there is another page that you always visit at the start of your browsing session. For example, if you have your own website, it might make sense to always begin there. Safari also comes with a command that enables you to view the home page at any time during your browsing session.

Change Your Home Page

Change the Home Page

1. Display the web page that you want to use as your home page.

2. Click **Safari**.

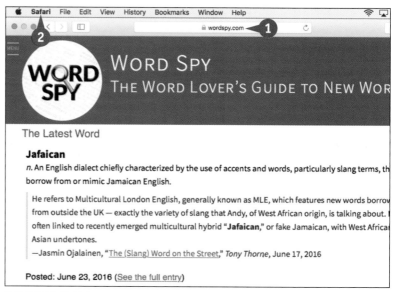

3. Click **Preferences**.

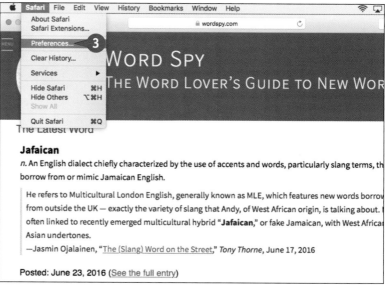

④ Click **General**.

⑤ Click **Set to Current Page**.

Ⓐ Safari inserts the address of the current page into the Homepage text box.

Note: If your Mac is not currently connected to the Internet, you can also type the new home page address manually using the Homepage text box.

⑥ Click **Close** (●).

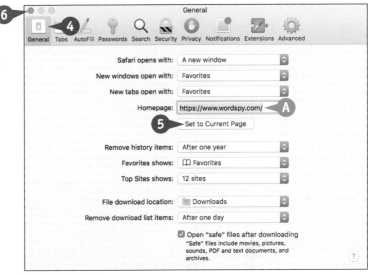

View the Home Page

① Click **History**.

② Click **Home**.

Note: You can also display the home page by pressing Shift + ⌘ + H.

Safari displays the home page.

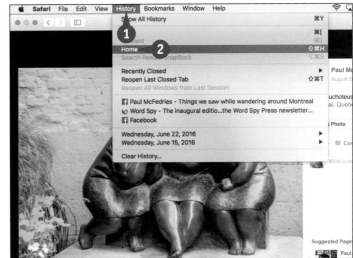

How can I get Safari to open a new tab without displaying the home page?

In the menu bar, click **Safari** and then **Preferences**. The Safari preferences appear. Click the **General** tab. Click the **New tabs open with** ⬍ and then select **Empty Page** from the pop-up menu. Click **Close** (●) to close the Safari preferences.

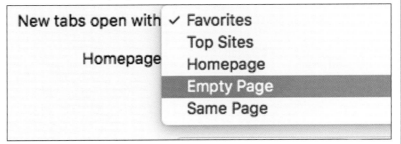

Bookmark Web Pages

I f you have web pages that you visit frequently, you can save yourself time by storing those pages as bookmarks — also called favorites — within Safari. This enables you to display the pages with just a couple of clicks.

The bookmark stores the name as well as the address of the page. Most bookmarks are stored on the Safari Bookmarks menu. However, Safari also offers the Favorites bar, which appears just below the address bar. You can put your favorite sites on the Favorites bar for easiest access.

Bookmark Web Pages

Bookmark a Web Page

1 Display the web page you want to save as a bookmark.

2 Click **Bookmarks**.

3 Click **Add Bookmark**.

Ⓐ You can also run the Add Bookmark command by clicking **Share** (⬆) and then clicking **Add Bookmark**.

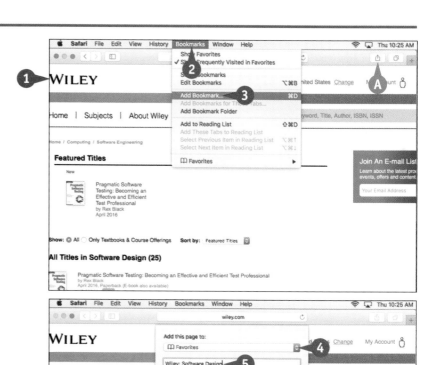

The Add Bookmark dialog appears.

Note: You can also display the Add Bookmark dialog by pressing ⌘+D.

4 Click ⬦ and then click the location where you want to store the bookmark.

5 Edit the page name, if necessary.

6 Click **Add**.

Safari adds a bookmark for the page.

Display a Bookmarked Web Page

1 Click **Show sidebar** (□).

2 Click **Bookmarks** (📖).

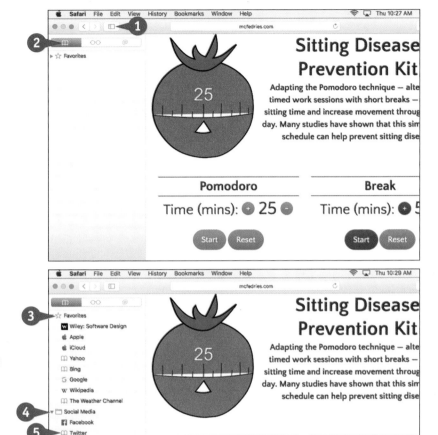

The sidebar appears with the Bookmarks tab displayed.

3 Click the location of the bookmark, such as **Favorites**.

4 Click the folder that contains the bookmark you want to display.

5 Click the bookmark.

The web page appears.

TIPS

Is there an easier way to display favorite pages?

Yes. Click **View** and then click **Show Favorites Bar**. Safari assigns keyboard shortcuts to the first nine bookmarks, counting from left to right and excluding folders. Display the leftmost bookmark by pressing ⌘+1. Moving to the right, the shortcuts are ⌘+2, ⌘+3, and so on.

How do I delete a bookmark?

If the site is on the Favorites bar, right-click the bookmark and then click **Delete**, or press and hold ⌘ and drag it off the bar. For all other bookmarks, click **Show sidebar** (□) and then **Bookmarks** (📖) to display the sidebar's Bookmarks tab. Locate the bookmark to remove, right-click the bookmark, and then click **Delete**.

Pin a Web Page Tab

If you have one or more web pages that you visit frequently, you might want even easier access to those pages than you get when you bookmark them. For example, you might want the web page to be available every time you launch Safari and every time you open a new Safari window. You can have that convenience and efficiency by using Safari to pin a web page's tab. This places a small icon for the tab to the left of the current tabs in every open Safari window. The pinned tabs also stay in place when you close and reopen Safari.

Pin a Web Page Tab

1 Open the web page you want to pin.

2 Click **Window**.

3 Click **Pin Tab**.

A You can also pin a tab by dragging the tab to the left of the existing tabs.

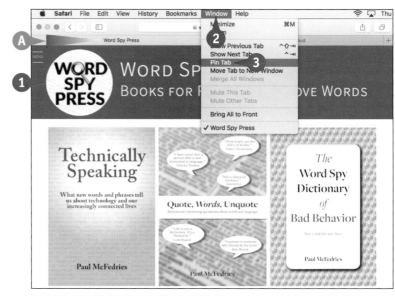

B Safari pins the tab.

C To open the tab, you can either right-click the pinned tab and then click **Unpin Tab**, or drag the pinned tab to the right.

Note: To remove the pinned tab, you can right-click it and then click **Close Tab**.

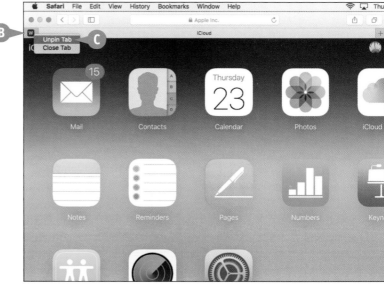

Mute a Web Page Tab

If a web page tab is playing sound, but you are not sure which tab is the source of the audio, you can have Safari mute all the open tabs. Having many web pages open in tabs is convenient, but a tab might suddenly begin playing sound, likely an ad or video that had a delayed start. The more tabs you have open, the less likely you are to know which tab is playing the sound. To avoid this frustration, tell Safari to mute all the tabs.

Mute a Web Page Tab

1 On the tab that is playing sound, click **Mute This Tab** (◁›)).

A If multiple tabs are playing sound, you can mute them all by switching to a tab that is not playing audio and then clicking **Mute Other Tabs** (◁›)) in the address bar.

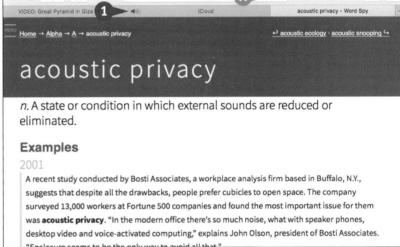

Safari mutes the sound (◁›)) changes to ◁).

2 To resume playing the sound, click **Unmute This Tab** (◁).

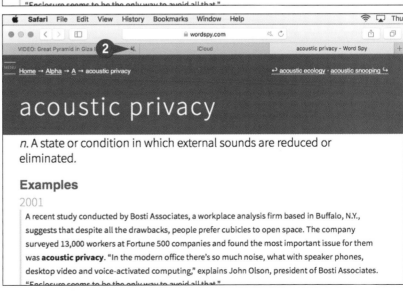

Display a Web Page Video as Picture-in-Picture

I f you want to watch an online video while performing other tasks, you can display the video as a picture-in-picture screen that stays visible while you work in other windows. This is useful for those times when you want to watch an online video, but you do not need to give the video your full attention. When you display the video as picture-in-picture, the video window stays visible even when you switch to another app. This enables you to read or work with that app while still being able to view the video playback.

Display a Web Page Video as Picture-in-Picture

1 Open the web page that contains the video you want to watch.

2 Right-click the video.

A menu of the video's built-in commands appears.

3 Right-click the video a second time.

A A menu of Safari's video commands appears.

4 Click **Enter Picture-in-Picture**.

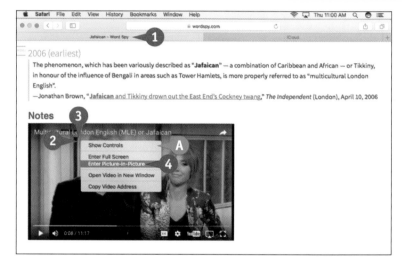

B Safari displays the video in a separate picture-in-picture window.

C When you switch to another app, the video remains visible.

D To close the video window, you can position the mouse pointer (⟍) over the video and click **Close** (⊗).

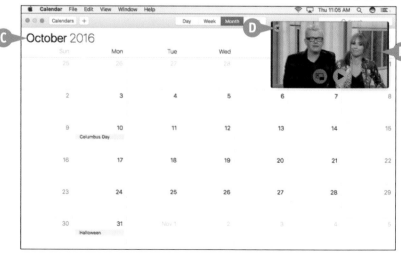

Search for Sites

If you need information on a specific topic, Safari has a built-in feature that enables you to quickly search the web for sites that have the information you require. The web has a number of sites called *search engines* that enable you to find what you are looking for. By default, Safari uses the Google search site (www.google.com). Simple, one-word searches often return tens of thousands of *hits*, or matching sites. To improve your searching, type multiple search terms that define what you are looking for. To search for a phrase, enclose the words in quotation marks.

Search for Sites

1 Click in the address bar and then type a word, phrase, or question that represents the information you want to find.

A If you see the search text you want to use in the list of suggested searches, you can click the text and skip step **2**.

2 Press **Return**.

B A list of pages that matches your search text appears.

3 Click a web page.

The page appears.

Note: To rerun a recent search, click **History** and then click **Search Results SnapBack** (or press **Option** + **⌘** + **S**).

Note: To change the search engine, click **Safari**, click **Preferences**, click the **Search** tab, click the **Search engine** ◊, and then click the search engine you prefer: Google, Yahoo!, Bing, or DuckDuckGo.

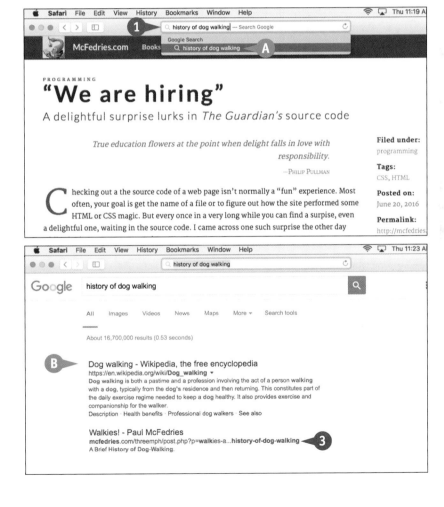

Download a File

Some websites make files available for you to open on your Mac. To use these files, you can download them to your Mac using Safari. Saving data from the Internet to your computer is called *downloading*. For certain types of files, Safari may display the content right away instead of letting you download it. This happens for files such as text documents and PDF files. In any case, to use a file from a website, you must have an application designed to work with that particular file type. For example, if the file is an Excel workbook, you need either Excel for the Mac or a compatible program.

Download a File

1. Navigate to the page that contains the link to the file.

2. Scroll down and click the link to the file.

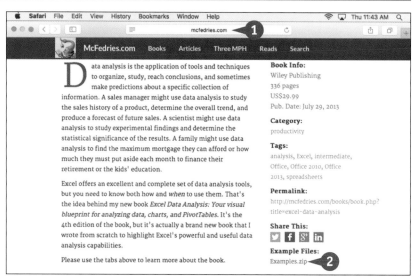

Safari downloads the file to your Mac.

Ⓐ The Show Downloads button shows the progress of the download.

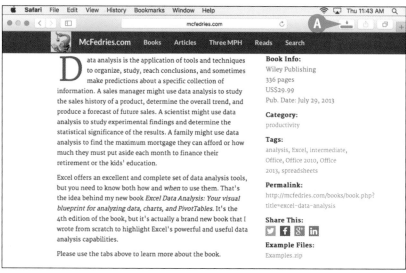

3 When the download is complete, click **Show Downloads** (⬇).

4 Right-click the file.

B You can also double-click the icon to the left of the file.

C You can click **Show in Finder** (🔍) to view the file in the Downloads folder.

5 Click **Open**.

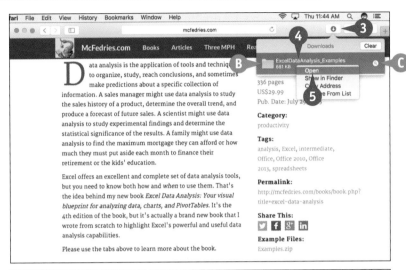

The file opens in Finder (in the case of a compressed Zip file, as shown here) or in the corresponding application.

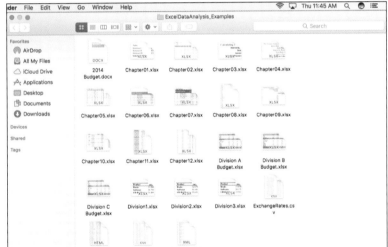

TIPS

If Safari displays the file instead of downloading it, how do I save the file to my Mac?
Click **File** and then click **Save As**. Type a name for the new file, choose a folder, and then click **Save**.

Is it safe to download files from the web?
Yes, but download files only from sites you trust. If you notice that Safari is attempting to download a file without your permission, cancel the download immediately; the file likely contains a virus or other malware. Fortunately, macOS has built-in safeguards against installing malware, so even if you download a malware program by accident, macOS will not allow it to be installed.

View Links Shared on Social Networks

You can make your web surfing more interesting and your social networking more efficient by using Safari to directly access links shared by the people you follow. Social networks are about connecting with people, but a big part of that experience is sharing information, particularly links to interesting, useful, or entertaining web pages. You normally have to log in to the social network to see these links, but if you have used macOS to sign in to your accounts, you can use Safari to directly access links shared by your Twitter and LinkedIn connections.

View Links Shared on Social Networks

Note: For more information on signing in to your social networking accounts, see Chapter 9.

1 Click **Show sidebar** (▢).

The Bookmarks sidebar appears.

2 Click **Shared Links** (@).

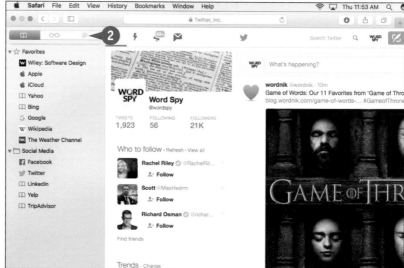

Safari displays the Shared Links sidebar, which lists the most recent links shared by the people you follow on Twitter and LinkedIn.

Note: If you do not see any links, it means you have not set up any social media accounts in macOS. See Chapter 9.

③ Click the shared link you want to view.

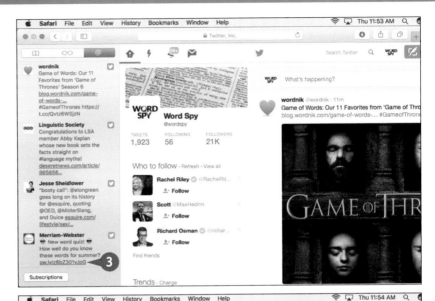

Ⓐ Safari displays the linked web page.

Ⓑ For a Twitter link, if you want to retweet the link to your followers, you can click **Retweet**.

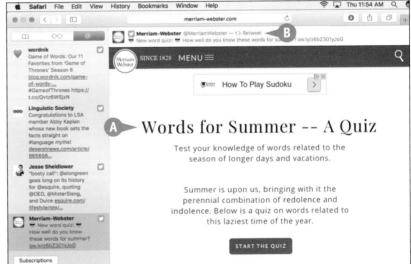

How can I be sure that I am seeing the most recent shared links?

Safari usually updates the Shared Links list each time you open it. However, to be sure that you are seeing the most recent links shared by people you follow on Twitter or are connected to on LinkedIn, click the **View** menu and then click **Update Shared Links**.

How do I hide the Shared Links sidebar when I do not need it?

To give yourself more horizontal screen area for viewing pages, hide the sidebar by clicking **Show sidebar** (▭) again. You can also toggle the Shared Links sidebar on and off by pressing Control + ⌘ + 3.

Create a Web Page Reading List

If you do not have time to read a web page now, you can add the page to your Reading List and then read the page later when you have time. You will often come upon a page with fascinating content that you want to read, but lack the time. You could bookmark the article, but bookmarks are really for pages you want to revisit often, not for those you might read only once. A better solution is to add the page to the Reading List, which is a simple list of pages you save to read later.

Create a Web Page Reading List

Add a Page to the Reading List

1 Navigate to the page you want to read later.

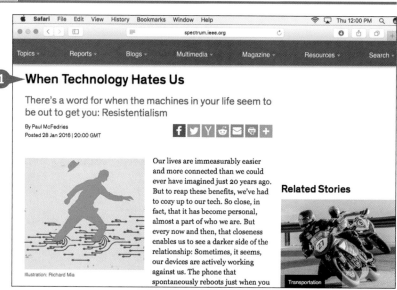

2 Click **Bookmarks**.

3 Click **Add to Reading List**.

Safari adds the page to the Reading List.

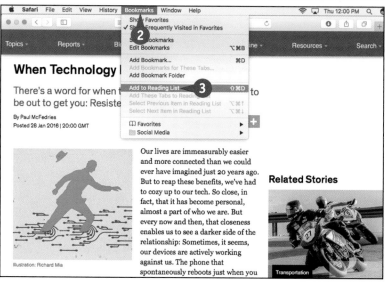

Select a Page from the Reading List

1 Click **Show sidebar** (□).

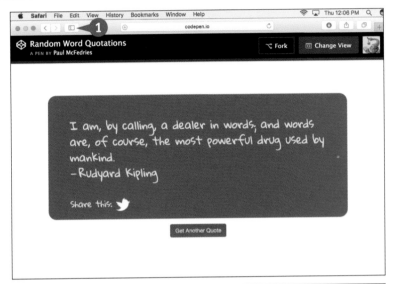

The Bookmarks sidebar appears.

2 Click **Reading List** (∞).

3 Drag the list down slightly to see the controls.

4 Click **Unread**.

A If you want to reread a page you have read previously, you can click **All** instead.

5 Click the page.

B Safari displays the page.

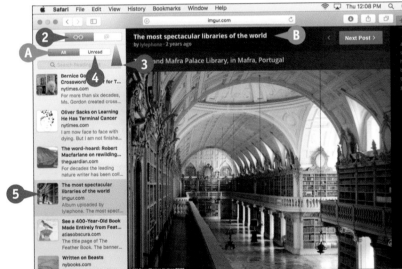

TIP

Are there easier ways to add a web page to my Reading List?

Yes, Safari offers several shortcut methods you can use. The easiest is to navigate to the page and then click **Add to Reading List** (⊕) to the left of the address bar. You can also add the current page to the Reading List by pressing Shift + ⌘ + D. To add all open tabs to the Reading List, click **Bookmarks** and then click **Add These Tabs to Reading List**. To add a link to the Reading List, press and hold Shift and click the link.

CHAPTER 3

Communicating via Email

macOS comes with the Apple Mail application that you can use to exchange email messages. After you type your account details into Mail, you can send email to friends, family, colleagues, and even total strangers almost anywhere in the world.

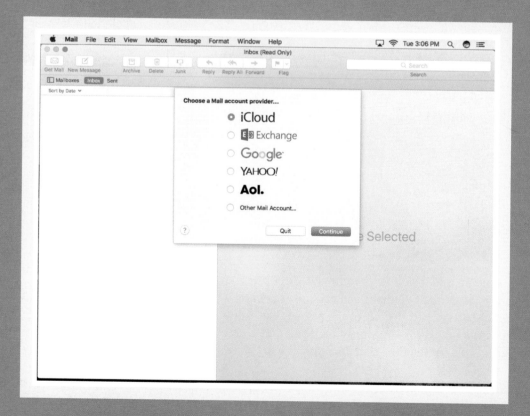

Add an Email Account

To send and receive email messages, you must add your email account to Mail. This is usually a POP (Post Office Protocol) or IMAP (Internet Message Access Protocol) account supplied by your Internet service provider (ISP), which should have sent you the account details. You can also use services such as Yahoo! and Gmail to set up a web-based email account, which enables you to exchange messages from any computer. If you have an Apple ID — that is, an account on the Apple iCloud service (www.icloud.com) — you can also set up Mail with your Apple account details.

Add an Email Account

Get Started Adding an Account

1 In the Dock, click **Mail** (📧).

2 Click **Mail**.

3 Click **Add Account**.

Note: If you are just starting Mail and the Welcome to Mail dialog is on-screen, you can skip steps **2** and **3**.

4 Click the type of account you are adding (⚪ changes to 🔘).

A For a POP or IMAP account, you can click **Other Mail Account**.

5 Click **Continue**.

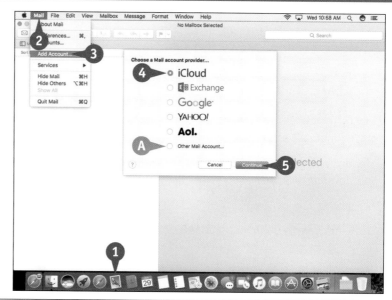

Add an iCloud Account

1 Type your Apple account address.

2 Type your Apple account password.

3 Click **Sign In**.

Mail signs in to your Apple account.

Note: Mail prompts you to choose which services you want to use with iCloud. See Chapter 14 to learn more.

4 Click **Add Account** (not shown).

Mail adds your Apple account.

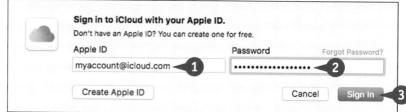

Add a POP or IMAP Account

1 Type your name.

2 Type your account address.

3 Type your account password.

4 Click **Sign In**.

Note: If the sign-in is successful, you can skip the rest of the steps in this section.

5 Edit the User Name text as required.

6 Click the **Account Type** ◘ and then click **POP** or **IMAP**.

7 Type the address of the account's incoming mail server.

8 Type the address of the account's outgoing mail server.

9 Click **Sign In**.

Mail signs in to your POP or IMAP account.

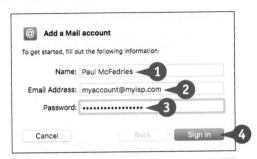

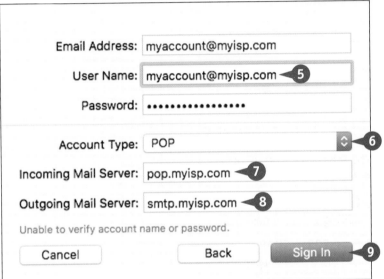

TIP

My email account requires me to use a nonstandard outgoing mail port. How do I set this up?
In the menu bar, click **Mail** and then click **Preferences**. The Mail preferences appear. Click the **Accounts** tab. Click the **Outgoing Mail Server (SMTP)** ◘ and then click **Edit SMTP Server List**. Click the outgoing mail server. Click the **Advanced** tab. Use the Port text box to type the nonstandard port number. Click **OK**. Click **Close** (●) and then click **Save**.

Send an Email Message

I̲f you know the recipient's email address, you can send a message to that address. An email address is a set of characters that uniquely identifies the location of an Internet mailbox. Each address takes the form *username@domain*, where *username* is the name of the person's account with the ISP or with an organization, and *domain* is the Internet name of the company that provides the person's account. When you send a message, it travels through your ISP's outgoing mail server, which routes the messages to the recipient's incoming mail server, which then stores the message in the recipient's mailbox.

Send an Email Message

1 Click **New Message** (☑).

Note: You can also start a new message by pressing ⌘+Ⓝ.

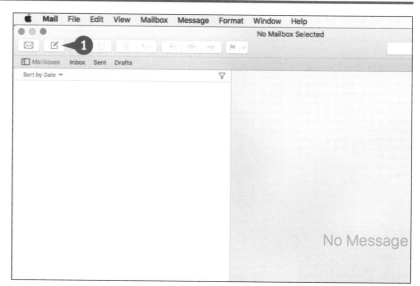

A message window appears.

2 Type the email address of the person to whom you are sending the message in the To field.

3 Type the email address of the person to whom you are sending a copy of the message in the Cc field.

Note: You can add multiple email addresses in both the To field and the Cc field by separating each address with a comma (,).

4 Type a brief description of the message in the Subject field.

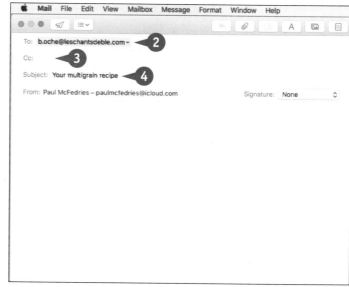

5 Type the message.

Ⓐ To change the message font, you can click **Fonts** (A) to display the Font panel.

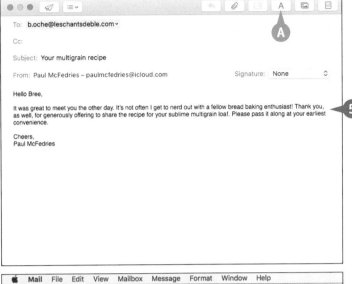

6 Click **Send** (✈).

Mail sends your message.

Note: Mail stores a copy of your message in the Sent folder.

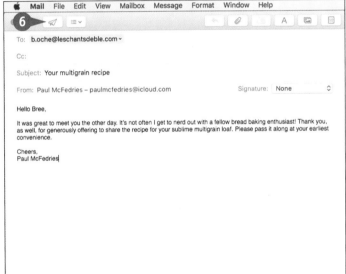

How can I compose a large number of messages offline?
You can compose your messages offline by following these steps: While disconnected from the Internet, click **Mail** (📧) in the Dock to start Mail. To ensure you are working offline, click **Mailbox**. If the Take All Accounts Offline command is enabled, click that command. Compose and send the message. Each time you click **Send** (✈), your message is stored temporarily in the Outbox folder. When you are done, connect to the Internet. After a few moments, Mail automatically sends all the messages in the Outbox folder.

Add a File Attachment

I f you have a file you want to send to another person, you can attach it to an email message. A typical message is fine for short notes, but you may have something more complex to communicate, such as budget numbers or a slideshow, or some form of media that you want to share, such as an image.

These more complex types of data come in a separate file — such as a spreadsheet, presentation file, or picture file — so you need to send that file to your recipient. You do this by attaching the file to an email message.

Add a File Attachment

① Click **New Message** (☑).

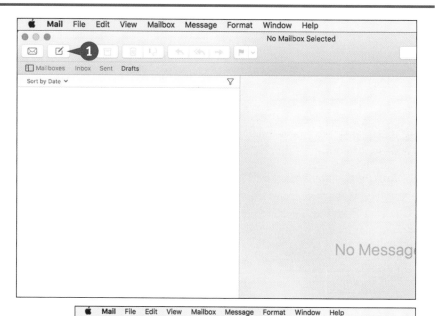

A message window appears.

② Fill in the recipients, subject, and message text as described in the previous section, "Send an Email Message."

③ Press `Return` two or three times to move the cursor a few lines below your message.

④ Click **Attach** (⬭).

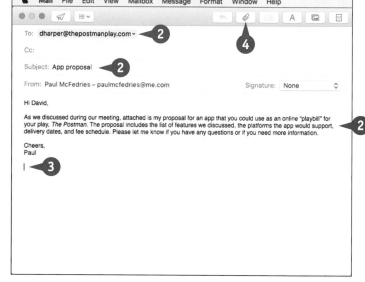

A file selection dialog appears.

5 Click the file you want to attach.

6 Click **Choose File**.

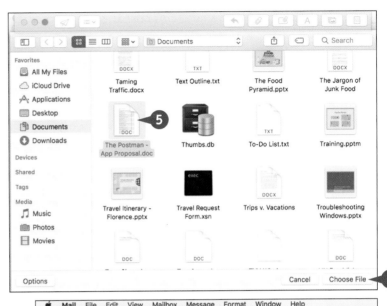

A Mail attaches the file to the message.

Note: Another way to attach a file to a message is to click and drag the file from Finder and drop it inside the message.

7 Repeat steps **4** to **6** to attach additional files to the message.

8 Click **Send** (✈).

Mail sends your message.

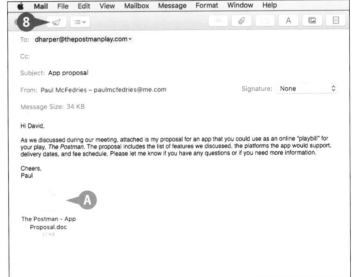

TIP

Is there a limit to the number of files I can attach to a message?

The number of files you can attach to the message has no practical limit. However, you should be careful with the total *size* of the files you send to someone. Many ISPs place a limit on the size of a message's attachments, which is usually between 2MB and 10MB. If you have an iCloud account, when you send a large attachment Mail asks if you want to use the Mail Drop feature, which stores the attachment in iCloud. Click **Use Mail Drop** to enable your recipient to download the attachment from iCloud.

Add a Signature Block

Asignature block is a small amount of text that appears at the bottom of an email message. Instead of typing this information manually, you can save the signature in your Mail preferences. When you compose a new message, reply to a message, or forward a message, you can click a button to have Mail add the signature block to your outgoing message.

Signature blocks usually contain personal contact information, such as your phone numbers, business address, and email and website addresses. Mail supports multiple signature blocks, which is useful if you use multiple accounts or if you use Mail for different purposes such as business and personal.

Add a Signature Block

Create a Signature Block

1 Click **Mail**.

2 Click **Preferences**.

The Mail preferences appear.

3 Click **Signatures**.

4 Click the account for which you want to use the signature.

5 Click **Create a signature** (**+**).

Mail adds a new signature.

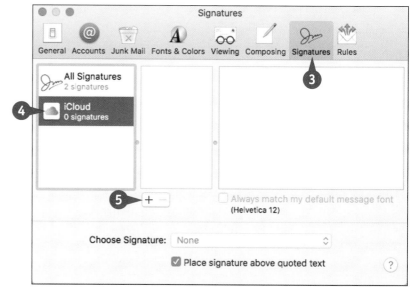

6 Type a name for the signature.

7 Type the signature text.

8 Repeat steps **4** to **7** to add other signatures, if required.

Note: You can add as many signatures as you want. For example, you may want to have one signature for business use and another for personal use.

9 Click **Close** (●).

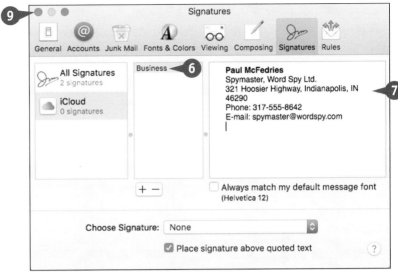

Insert the Signature

1 Click **New Message** (✎) (not shown) to start a new message.

Note: To start a new message, see the section "Send an Email Message."

2 In the message text area, move the insertion point to the location where you want the signature to appear.

3 Click the **Signature** ◊ and then click the signature you want to insert.

A The signature appears in the message.

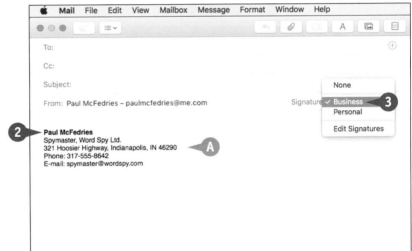

TIPS

I have multiple signatures. How can I choose which signature Mail adds automatically?
Follow steps **1** to **4** in the subsection "Create a Signature Block" to display the Signatures preferences and choose an account. Click the **Choose Signature** ◊ and then click the signature you want to insert automatically into each message. If you prefer to add a signature manually, click **None**.

Can I format my signature text?
Yes. Follow steps **1** to **4** in the subsection "Create a Signature Block" to display the Signatures preferences and choose an account. Click the signature you want to modify and then use the commands on the Format menu to format your signature.

Receive and Read Email Messages

When another person sends you an email, that message ends up in your account mailbox on the incoming mail server maintained by your ISP or email provider. Therefore, you must connect to the incoming mail server to retrieve and read messages sent to you. You can do this using Mail, which takes care of the details behind the scenes. By default, Mail automatically checks for new messages while you are online, but you can also check for new messages at any time.

Receive and Read Email Messages

Receive Email Messages

1 Click **Get Mail** (✉).

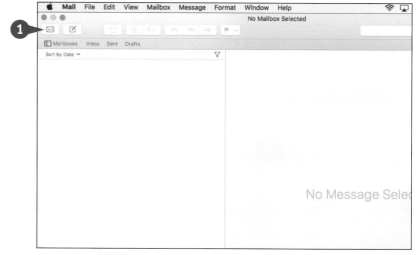

2 Click **Inbox**.

Ⓐ If you have new messages, they appear in your Inbox folder with a blue dot in this column.

Ⓑ The Inbox command and the Mail icon (📧) in the Dock show the number of unread messages in the Inbox folder.

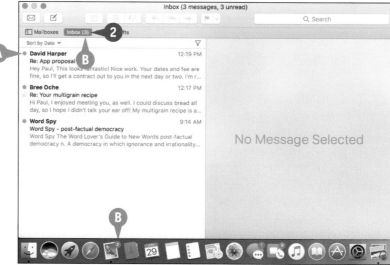

Read a Message

1 Click the message.

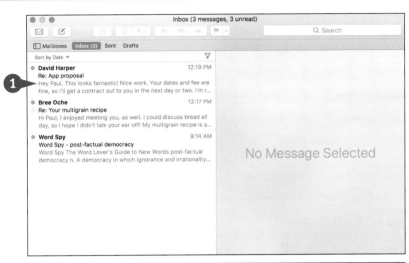

Mail displays the message text in the preview pane.

2 Read the message text in the preview pane.

Note: If you want to open the message in its own window, you can double-click the message.

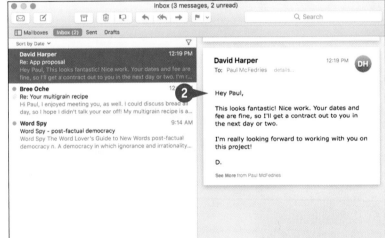

Can I change how often Mail automatically checks for messages?
Yes. Click **Mail** and then click **Preferences**. The Mail preferences appear. Click the **General** tab. Click the **Check for new messages** ⬦ and then click the time interval that you want Mail to use when checking for new messages automatically. If you do not want Mail to check for messages automatically, click **Manually** instead. Click **Close** (●) to close the Mail preferences.

Reply to a Message

When a message you receive requires a response — whether it is answering a question, supplying information, or providing comments — you can reply to that message. Most replies go only to the person who sent the original message. However, it is also possible to send the reply to all the people who were included in the original message's To and Cc lines. Mail includes the text of the original message in the reply, but you should edit the original message text to include only enough of the original message to put your reply into context.

Reply to a Message

1. Click the message to which you want to reply.

2. Click the reply type you want to use:

Ⓐ You can click **Reply** (↩) to respond only to the person who sent the message.

Ⓑ You can click **Reply All** (↩↩) to respond to all the addresses in the message's From, To, and Cc lines.

A message window appears.

Ⓒ Mail automatically inserts the recipient addresses.

Ⓓ Mail also inserts the subject line, preceded by *Re:*.

Ⓔ Mail includes the original message text at the bottom of the reply.

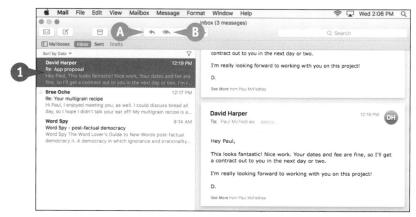

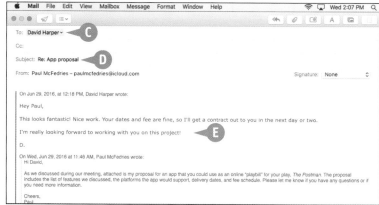

③ Edit the original message to include only the text relevant to your reply.

④ Click the area above the original message text.

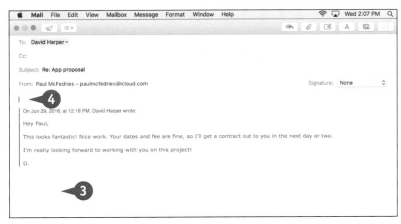

⑤ Type your reply.

⑥ Click **Send** (✈).

Mail sends your reply.

Note: Mail stores a copy of your reply in the Sent folder.

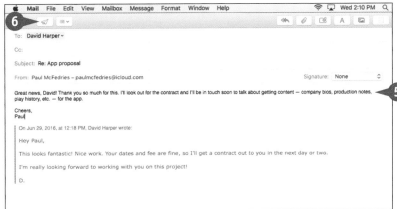

TIP

I received a message inadvertently. Is there a way that I can pass it along to the correct recipient?
Yes. Mail comes with a feature that enables you to pass along inadvertent messages to the correct recipient. Click the message that you received inadvertently, click **Message**, and then click **Redirect** (or press Shift + ⌘ + E). Type the recipient's address and then click **Send**. Replies to this message will be sent to the original sender, not to you.

Forward a Message

If a message has information relevant to or that concerns another person, you can forward a copy of the message to that person. You can also include your own comments in the forward.

In the body of the forward, Mail includes the original message's addresses, date, and subject line. Below this information Mail also includes the text of the original message. In most cases, you will leave the entire message intact so your recipient can see it. However, if only part of the message is relevant to the recipient, you should edit the original message accordingly.

Forward a Message

1 Click the message that you want to forward.

2 Click **Forward** (→).

Note: You can also press
Shift + ⌘ + F.

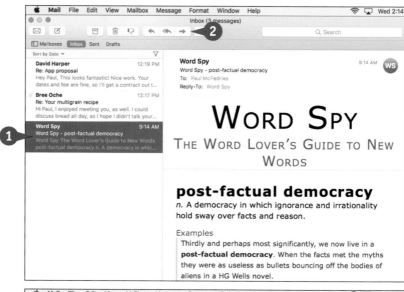

A message window appears.

A Mail inserts the subject line, preceded by *Fwd:*.

B The original message's addressees (To and From), date, subject, and text are included at the top of the forward.

3 Type the email address of the person to whom you are forwarding the message.

4 To send a copy of the forward to another person, type that person's email address in the Cc line.

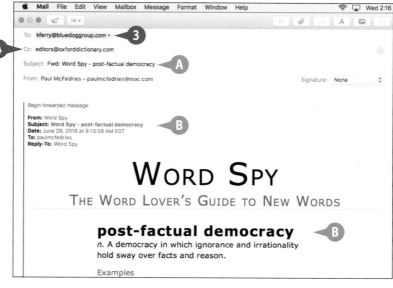

5 Edit the original message to include only the text relevant to your forward.

6 Click the area above the original message text.

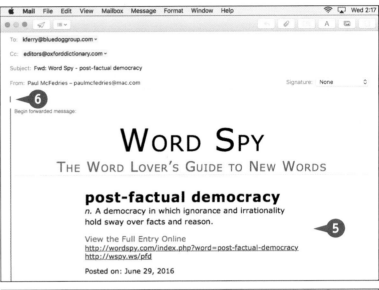

7 Type your comments.

8 Click **Send** (✈).

Mail sends your forward.

Note: Mail stores a copy of your forward in the Sent folder.

Note: You can forward someone a copy of the actual message rather than just a copy of the message text. Click the message, click **Message**, and then click **Forward As Attachment**. Mail creates a new message and includes the original message as an attachment.

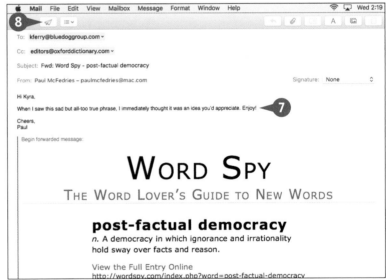

TIP

Mail always formats my replies as rich text, even when the original message is plain text. How can I fix this problem?

You can configure Mail to always reply using the same format as the original message. To do this, click **Mail** and then click **Preferences** to open the Mail preferences. Click the **Composing** tab. Click the **Use the same message format as the original message** check box (☐ changes to ☑) and then click **Close** (●) to close the Mail preferences.

Open and Save an Attachment

If you receive a message that has a file attached, you can open the attachment to view the contents of the file. However, although some attachments require only a quick viewing, other attachments may contain information that you want to keep. In this case, you should save these files to your Mac's hard drive so that you can open them later without having to launch Mail.

Be careful when dealing with attached files. Computer viruses are often transmitted by email attachments.

Open and Save an Attachment

Open an Attachment

1 Click the message that has the attachment, as indicated by the Attachment symbol (📎).

A An icon appears for each message attachment.

2 Double-click the attachment you want to open.

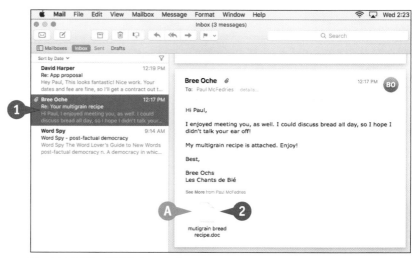

The file opens in the associated application.

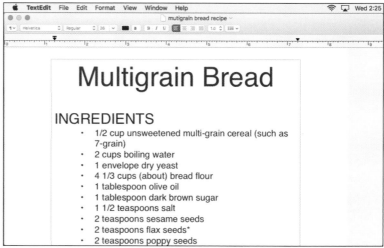

Save an Attachment

1 Click the message that has the attachment, as indicated by the Attachment symbol ( ).

2 Right-click the attachment you want to save.

3 Click **Save Attachment**.

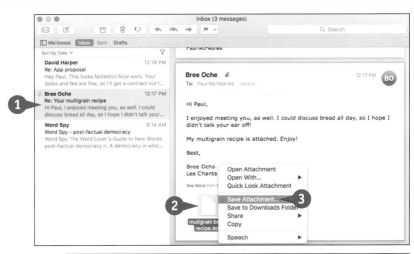

Mail prompts you to save the file.

4 Click in the Save As text box and edit the filename, if desired.

5 Click the **Where** and select the folder into which you want the file saved.

6 Click **Save**.

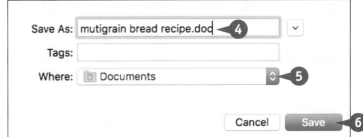

Can I open an attachment using a different application?
In most cases, yes. macOS usually has a default application that it uses when you double-click a file attachment. However, it also usually defines one or more other applications capable of opening the file. To check this out, right-click the icon of the attachment you want to open and then click **Open With**. In the menu that appears, click the application that you prefer to use to open the file.

Are viruses a big problem on the Mac?
No, not yet. Most viruses target Windows PCs and only a few malicious programs target the Mac. However, as the Mac becomes more popular, expect to see more Mac-targeted virus programs. Therefore, you should still exercise caution when opening email attachments.

Create a Mailbox for Saving Messages

After you have used Mail for a while, you may find that you have many messages in your Inbox. To keep the Inbox uncluttered, you can create new mailboxes and then move messages from the Inbox to the new mailboxes.

You should use each mailbox you create to save related messages. For example, you could create separate mailboxes for people you correspond with regularly, projects you are working on, different work departments, and so on.

Create a Mailbox for Saving Messages

Create a Mailbox

1 Click **Mailbox**.

2 Click **New Mailbox**.

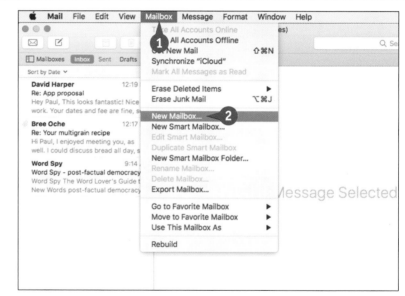

The New Mailbox dialog appears.

3 Click the **Location** and then click where you want the mailbox located.

Note: Click **On My Mac** to have the mailbox available only on your Mac; if you want to make the mailbox available on any computer that has iCloud access, click **iCloud** instead.

4 Type the name of the new mailbox.

5 Click **OK**.

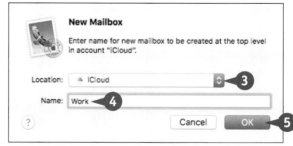

6 Click **Mailboxes**.

Mail displays your account's mailboxes.

A The new mailbox appears in the location you chose in step **3**, such as in the iCloud list shown here.

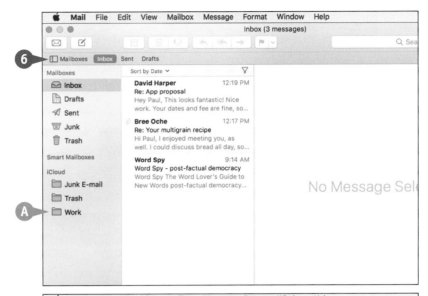

Move a Message to Another Mailbox

1 Position the mouse pointer (🔺) over the message you want to move.

2 Click and drag the message and drop it on the mailbox to which you want to move it.

Mail moves the message.

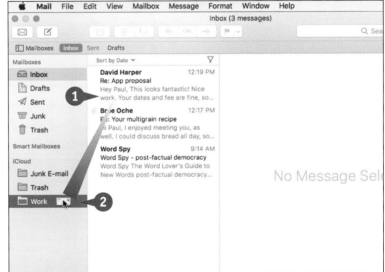

How do I rename a mailbox?

Right-click the mailbox and then click **Rename Mailbox**. Type the new name and then press Return. Note that Mail does not allow you to rename any of the built-in mailboxes, including Inbox, Drafts, and Trash.

How do I delete a mailbox?

Right-click the mailbox and then click **Delete Mailbox**. When Mail asks you to confirm the deletion, click **Delete**. Note that Mail does not allow you to delete any of the built-in mailboxes, including Inbox, Drafts, and Trash. Remember, too, that when you delete a mailbox, you also delete any messages stored in that mailbox.

Add Events and Contacts from a Message

You can save time and effort by adding items to Contacts and Calendar directly from Mail. As you learn in Chapter 6, you use the Contacts application to create new contacts, and you use the Calendar application to schedule new events. Quite often, however, you get the new information for a contact or an event from an email message you have received. Instead of using the cumbersome process of copying information from Mail to Contacts or Calendar, you can use Mail to add these new items directly.

Add Events and Contacts from a Message

1 Click the message that contains the event information or contact data.

A If Mail recognizes the data for either an event or a contact, it lets you know here.

2 Click **add** beside the data you want to enter.

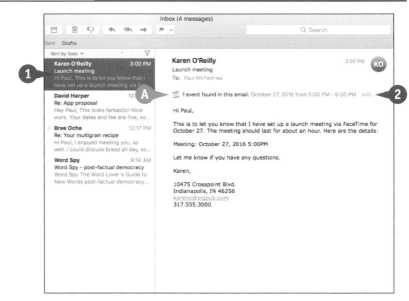

Mail displays the data.

3 If you are adding an event, click **Add To Calendar**.

Note: If you are adding a contact, click **Add To Contacts** instead.

Mail adds the event or the contact.

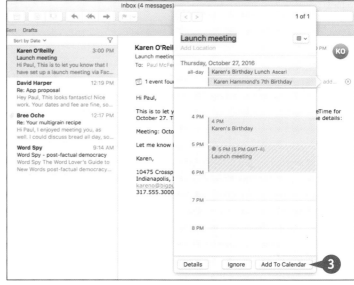

Process Messages Using Gestures

You can process your incoming Mail faster by using gestures to implement common tasks. With the Mail app on an iPhone or iPad, you can swipe right or left on a message to get quick access to a few message-related chores. That same convenience is also available in the macOS Mail application. Using a trackpad or a Mighty Mouse, you can swipe right on a message to mark it as unread, and you can swipe left on a message to delete it.

Process Messages Using Gestures

Mark a Message as Unread

1 Swipe to the right on the message.

Note: If you are using a trackpad, use two fingers to swipe; if you are using a Mighty Mouse, use one finger to swipe.

2 Tap **Mark as Unread**.

Mail changes the message status to unread.

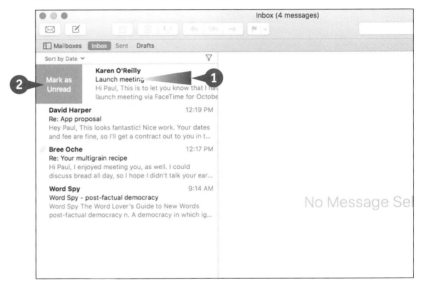

Delete a Message

1 Swipe to the left on the message.

2 Tap **Trash**.

Mail moves the message to the Trash folder.

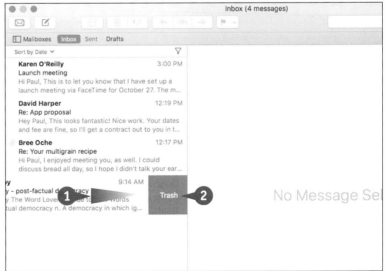

CHAPTER 4

Enhancing Online Privacy

This chapter helps you stay secure online by showing you a number of tasks designed to make your Internet sessions as safe and as private as possible. You learn how to delete your browsing history, prevent ad sites from tracking you online, browse the web privately, control junk email, and more.

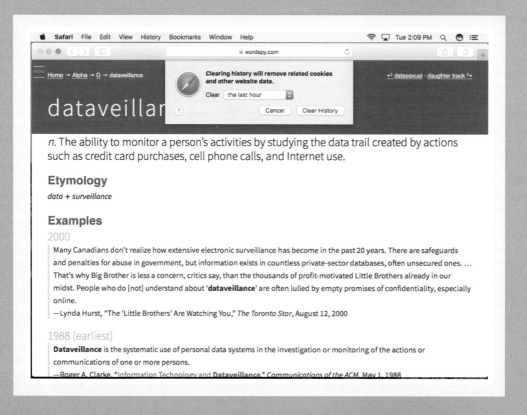

Delete a Site from Your Browsing History

You can enhance your privacy as well as the safety of other people who use your Mac by removing a private or dangerous site from your browsing history. Safari maintains your *browsing history*, which is a list of the sites you have visited. If you share your Mac with others, you might not want them to access certain private sites in your history. Similarly, if you accidentally stumble upon a dangerous or inappropriate site, you likely do not want others to see it. To help prevent both scenarios, you can delete the site from your browsing history.

Delete a Site from Your Browsing History

Delete a Single Site

1. Click **History**.

2. Click **Show All History**.

   You can also run the Show All History command by pressing ⌘+Y.

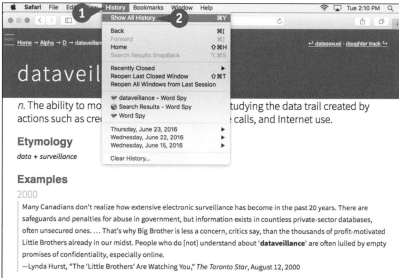

The History list appears.

3. Right-click the site you want to remove.

4. Click **Remove**.

Note: You can also click the site and then press Delete.

Safari deletes the site from your browsing history.

Note: To return to Safari, either click **History** and then click **Hide History**, or press ⌘+Y.

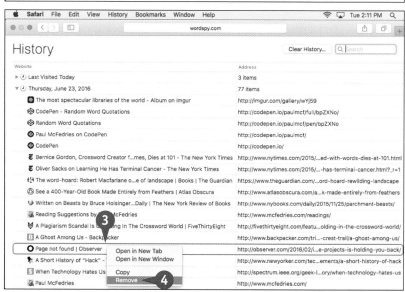

Delete an Entire Day

1 Click **History**.

2 Click **Show All History**.

You can also run the Show All History command by pressing ⌘+Y.

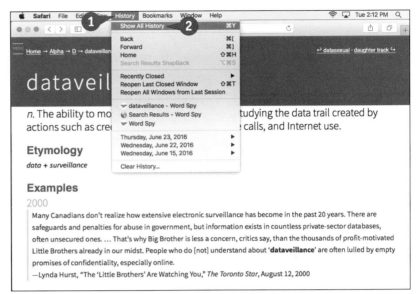

The History list appears.

3 Right-click the date you want to remove.

4 Click **Remove**.

Safari deletes the date from your browsing history.

Note: To return to Safari, either click **History** and then click **Hide History**, or press ⌘+Y.

Note: To learn about the Clear History command, see section "Remove Saved Website Data," later in this chapter.

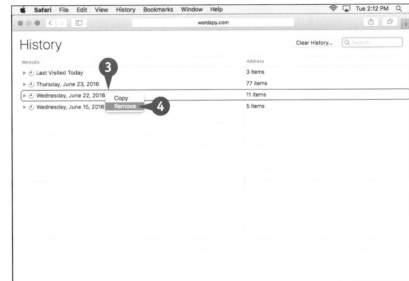

Is there a way to clear my browsing history automatically?

Yes. If you regularly delete all your browsing history, constantly running the Clear History command can become tiresome. Fortunately, you can configure Safari to make this chore automatic. Click **Safari** and then click **Preferences** to display the Safari preferences. Click the **General** tab. Click the **Remove history items** ⬦ and then click the length of time after which you want Safari to automatically remove an item from your browsing history. For example, if you click **After one day**, Safari clears out your browsing history daily.

Prevent Websites from Tracking You

You can often prevent advertising sites from tracking your online movements by blocking the tracking files (called *cookies*) that they store on your Mac, as well as other mechanisms that they use for tracking users. Advertisers want to track the sites that you visit in order to deliver ads targeted to your likes and preferences. However, you cannot be sure how these sites are using the information they store about you. Therefore, many people prefer to configure Safari to request that websites not use their tracking features. Note, however, that there is no guarantee as yet that websites will honor a so-called *Do Not Track* request.

Prevent Websites from Tracking You

1 Click **Safari**.

2 Click **Preferences**.

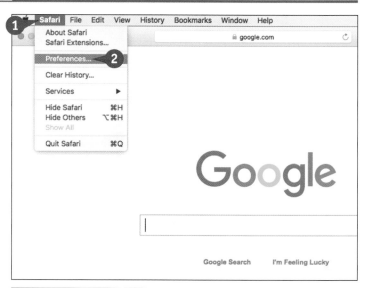

The Safari preferences appear.

3 Click the **Privacy** tab.

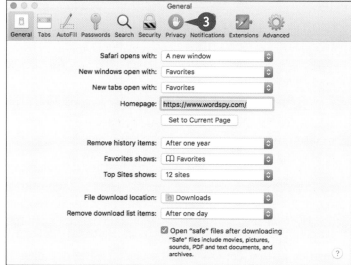

④ Click the **Allow from websites I visit** option (○ changes to ⦿).

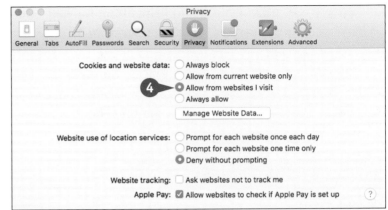

⑤ Click the **Ask websites not to track me** check box (☐ changes to ☑).

⑥ Click **Close** (⬤).

Safari no longer accepts cookies from third-party sites and sends all websites a Do Not Track request.

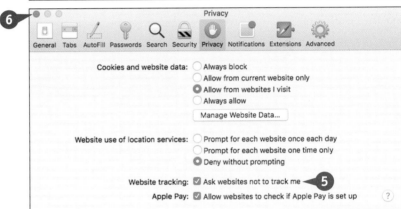

How can a website track me online?

Usually by using a *cookie*, a small text file that the website stores on your Mac. Cookies are used routinely by any website that needs to "remember" information about your session at that site, such as shopping cart and logon data.

A *third-party cookie* is set by a site other than the one you are viewing. An advertising site might store information about you in a third-party cookie and then use it to track your online activities. This works because the advertiser has ads on dozens or hundreds of websites, and that ad is the mechanism that enables the advertiser to set and read its cookie.

Remove Saved Website Data

To ensure that other people who have access to your Mac cannot view information from sites you have visited, you can delete Safari's saved website data.

Saving website data is useful because it enables you to quickly revisit a site. However, it is also dangerous because other people who use your Mac can just as easily visit or view information about those sites. This can be a problem if you visit financial sites, private corporate sites, or some other page that you would not want another person to visit. You reduce this risk by deleting your saved website data.

Remove Saved Website Data

1 Click **Safari**.

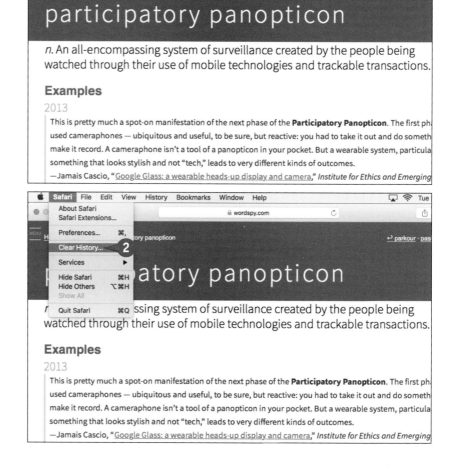

2 Click **Clear History**.

The Clear History dialog appears.

Note: Despite its name, the Clear History command removes not only your website history, but *all* your saved website data.

3 Click the **Clear** 🔽 and then click the history interval you want to remove.

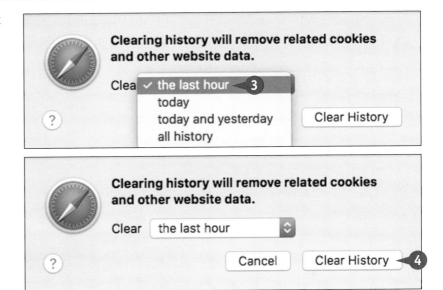

4 Click **Clear History**.

Safari deletes the website data from the time interval you specified.

What types of website data does Safari save?

Besides your browsing history, the website data that Safari stores includes copies of page text, images, and other content so that sites load faster the next time you view them. Safari also tracks what sites you visit most often and uses that data to populate the Top Sites page that appears when you open a new tab or window.

Safari also saves the names of files you have downloaded, the names of websites that you have given permission to use your current location, and the names of websites that you have given permission to use the Notification Center.

Enable Private Browsing

If you regularly visit websites that contain sensitive or secret data, you can ensure that no one else sees any data for these sites by deleting Safari's saved website data, as described in the previous section, "Remove Saved Website Data." However, if these sites represent only a small percentage of the places you visit on the web, deleting all your website data is overkill. A better solution is to turn on Safari's Private Browsing feature before you visit private sites. This tells Safari to temporarily stop saving any website data. When you are ready to surf regular websites again, you can turn off Private Browsing to resume saving your website data.

Enable Private Browsing

1 Click **File**.

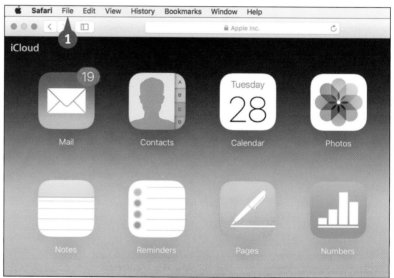

2 Click **New Private Window**.

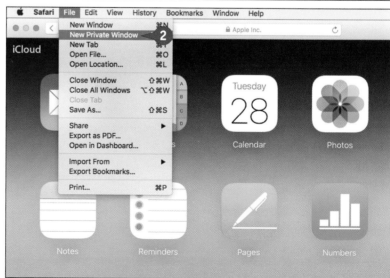

Safari creates a new window and activates the Private Browsing feature.

Ⓐ The address bar's dark background tells you that Private Browsing is turned on.

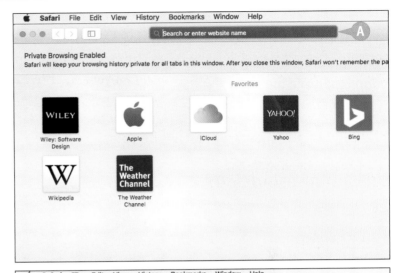

❸ Visit the sites you want to see during your private browsing session.

❹ When you are done, close the Private Browsing window.

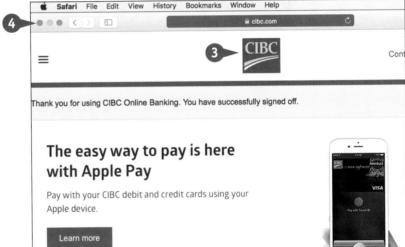

Can I prevent websites from requesting my location without having to activate Private Browsing?
Yes. Click **Safari** and then click **Preferences** to open the Safari preferences. Click the **Privacy** tab. In the Website Use of Location Services section, click the **Deny without prompting** option (◯ changes to ◉) and then click **Close** (●).

Safari's Search box displays suggestions based on my previous entries. Can I prevent this?
Yes. Click **Safari** and then click **Preferences** to open the Safari preferences. Click the **Search** tab. Click the **Include search engine suggestions** check box (☑ changes to ☐), click the **Include Safari Suggestions** check box (☑ changes to ☐), and then click **Close** (●).

Delete a Saved Website Password

You can avoid unauthorized access to a website by removing the site's password that you saved earlier using Safari.

Many websites require a password, along with a username or email address. When you fill in this information and log on to the site, Safari offers to save the password so that you do not have to type it again when you visit the same page in the future. This is convenient, but it has a downside: Anyone who uses your Mac can also access the password-protected content. If you do not want this to happen, you can tell Safari to remove the saved password.

Delete a Saved Website Password

1 Click **Safari**.

2 Click **Preferences**.

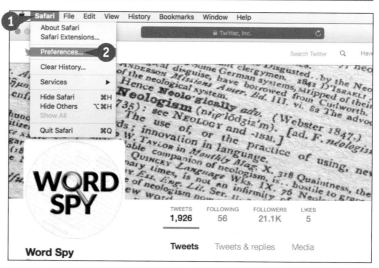

The Safari preferences appear.

3 Click the **Passwords** tab.

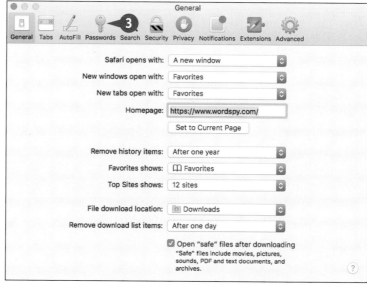

④ Click the web password you want to remove.

⑤ Click **Remove**.

Ⓐ If you no longer want Safari to save your website passwords, you can click the **AutoFill user names and passwords** check box (☑ changes to ☐).

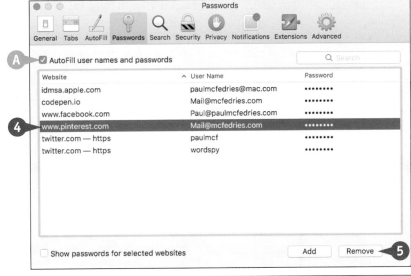

Safari asks you to confirm.

⑥ Click **Remove**.

Safari removes the password.

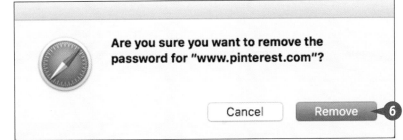

TIP

Are there any other website password security risks that I should know about?

Yes. Many websites offer to "remember" your login information. They do this by placing your username and password in a cookie stored on your Mac. Although convenient, it may lead to a problem: Other people who use your Mac to surf to the same sites can also access the password-protected content. To avoid this, be sure to click the website option (Ⓐ) that asks if you want to save your login data (☑ changes to ☐). Alternatively, you can set up separate user accounts for each person who uses your Mac, as described in Chapter 12.

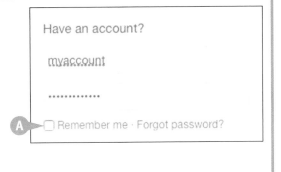

Delete Saved Credit Card Data

You can avoid unauthorized use of your credit card by deleting card data that you saved earlier using Safari.

Most online purchases require a credit card, which means entering the number, expiration date, and CVV (card verification value) at checkout. To avoid the effort this requires, you can save your card number and expiration date (but not the CVV) and have Safari enter them automatically during checkout. However, anyone who uses your Mac can also use your card information, provided they also know your card's CVV. To prevent this, you can delete the saved credit card data.

Delete Saved Credit Card Data

1 Click **Safari**.

2 Click **Preferences**.

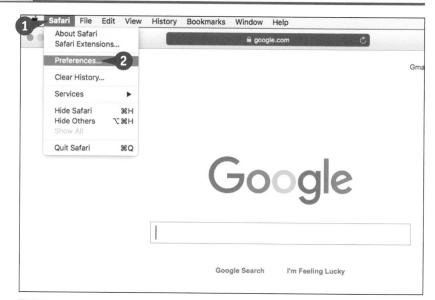

The Safari preferences appear.

3 Click the **AutoFill** tab.

4 To the right of the Credit Cards check box, click **Edit**.

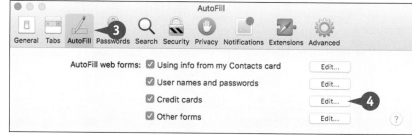

Safari displays the list of your saved credit cards.

5 Click the credit card data you want to remove.

6 Click **Remove**.

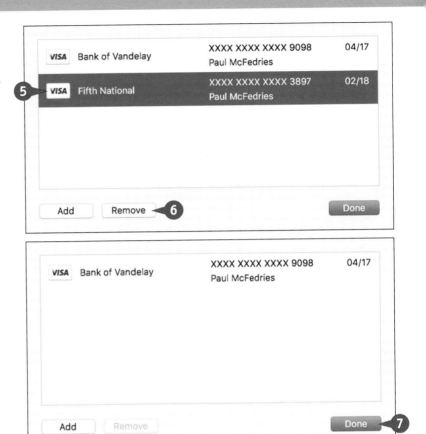

Safari removes the saved credit card data.

7 Click **Done**.

What can I do if Safari does not offer to save credit card data that I enter into a web form?
You can enter your credit card data by hand. To do this, click **Safari**, click **Preferences**, and then click the **AutoFill** tab. Click **Edit** to the right of the Credit Cards check box to display the credit card list. Click **Add** to create a new credit card entry. Type the credit card description, number, and expiry date, pressing `Tab` after you fill in each field. Type the name that appears on the credit card and then click **Done**.

Move Spam to the Junk Mailbox Automatically

Junk email — or *spam* — refers to unsolicited, commercial email messages that advertise anything from baldness cures to cheap printer cartridges. Many spams advertise deals that are simply fraudulent, and others feature such unsavory practices as linking to adult-oriented sites and sites that install spyware. Mail enables *junk mail filtering*, which looks for spam as it arrives in your Inbox and then marks each such message as junk. This enables you to quickly recognize junk mail and either delete it or move it to the Junk mailbox. However, you can customize Mail to automatically move all junk messages to the Junk mailbox.

Move Spam to the Junk Mailbox Automatically

1 Click **Mail**.

2 Click **Preferences**.

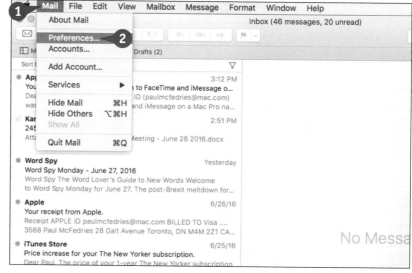

The Mail preferences appear.

3 Click the **Junk Mail** tab.

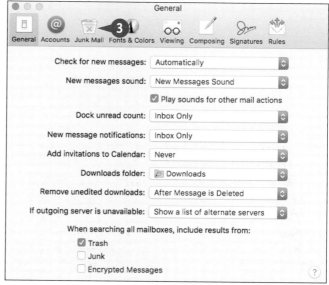

4 Click the **Move it to the Junk mailbox** option (◯ changes to ◉).

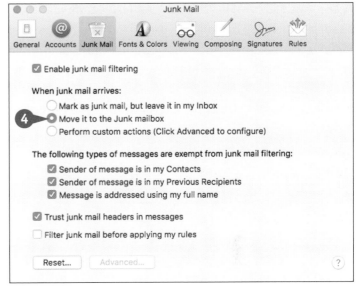

5 Click **Close** (⬤).

Mail closes the preferences and puts the new setting into effect.

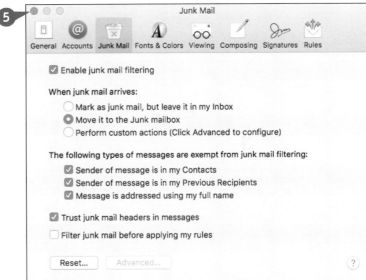

Why does Mail not mark some spam messages as junk?

Mail does not mark as junk any message addressed using your full name. To override this, click **Mail**, click **Preferences**, and then click the **Junk Mail** tab. Click the **Message is addressed using my full name** check box (☑ changes to ☐).

Is there a downside to automatically moving spam to the Junk mailbox?

Yes. Mail occasionally marks legitimate messages as junk. These are called *false positives*, and you should check for them by periodically opening the Junk mailbox. If you see one, click the message, click **Not Junk** in the preview pane, and then move the message to the Inbox.

Configure Advanced Junk Mail Filtering

You can gain greater control over Mail's junk mail filtering by configuring the advanced filtering options. These options are organized as a set of conditions that each message must meet before Mail marks it as junk, such as the sender not being in your contacts and the message containing spam content. The filtering options also specify a set of actions to perform on any message marked as junk, such as formatting the message with a special text color and moving it to the Junk mailbox. You can customize these options by deleting those you do not need and by adding new conditions and actions.

Configure Advanced Junk Mail Filtering

1 Click **Mail**.

2 Click **Preferences**.

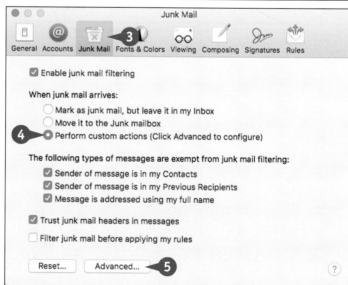

The Mail preferences appear.

3 Click the **Junk Mail** tab.

4 Click the **Perform custom actions** option (○ changes to ◉).

5 Click **Advanced**.

Safari displays the advanced junk mail filtering dialog.

Ⓐ Mail marks a message as junk if it meets all these conditions.

6 Click a condition's **Remove** icon (−) to delete it.

7 Click an **Add** icon (+) to create a new condition.

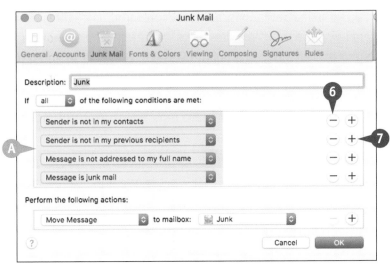

8 If you added a condition, use the pop-up menus and text box to define it.

9 Remove or add actions, as required.

10 Click **OK**.

Mail closes the dialog and puts the new filtering rules into effect.

11 Click **Close** (●).

Mail closes the preferences.

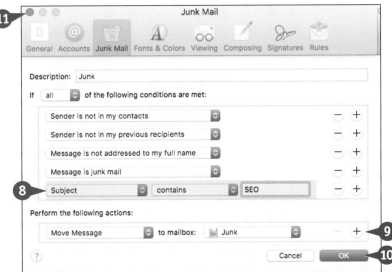

TIP

Almost all the spam I receive contains particular words in the subject or the message text. Can I set up junk mail filtering to handle this?

Yes. Click **Remove** (−) beside each existing condition. In the list of conditions, click **Add** (+). Click the first ⬦ and then click either **Subject** or **Message** content. In the second ⬦, click **contains**. In the text box, type the spam word. Repeat this procedure for each spam word you want to include in your filter. Click the **If** ⬦ and then click **any** in the pop-up menu. Click **OK**.

Disable Remote Images

You can make your email address more private by thwarting the remote images inserted into some email messages. A *remote image* is an image that resides on an Internet server computer instead of being embedded in the email message. A special code in the message tells the server to display the image when you open the message. This is usually benign, but the same code can also alert the sender of the message that your email address is working. If the sender is a spammer, then this usually results in you receiving even more junk email. You can prevent this by disabling remote images.

Disable Remote Images

Disable Remote Images

1 Click **Mail**.

2 Click **Preferences**.

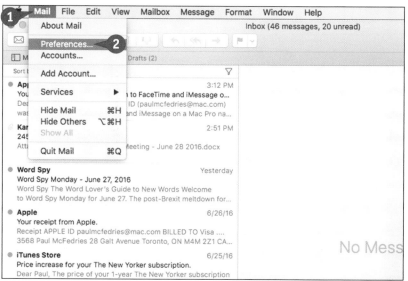

The Mail preferences appear.

3 Click the **Viewing** tab.

4 Click the **Load remote content in messages** check box (☑ changes to ☐).

5 Click **Close** (●).

Mail blocks remote images in your messages.

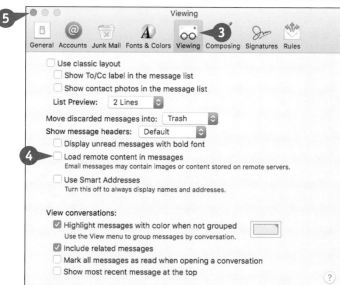

Display Remote Images in a Message

1 Click a message.

A Mail displays a placeholder for each remote image.

2 Click **Load Remote Content**.

B Mail displays the message's remote images.

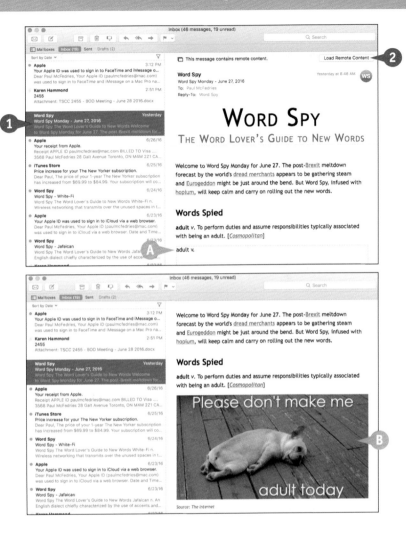

TIP

How do remote images cause me to receive more spam?

Many spammers include in their messages a *web bug*, which is a small and usually invisible image, the code for which is inserted into the email message. That code specifies a remote address from which to download the web bug when you display the message. However, the code also includes a reference to your email address. The remote server notes that you received the message, which means your address is a working one and is therefore a good target for further spam messages. By blocking remote images, you also block web bugs, which means you undermine this confirmation and so receive less spam.

CHAPTER 5

Talking via Messages and FaceTime

macOS comes with the Messages application, which you use to exchange instant messages with other macOS users, as well as anyone with an iPhone, iPad, or iPod touch. You can use FaceTime to make video calls.

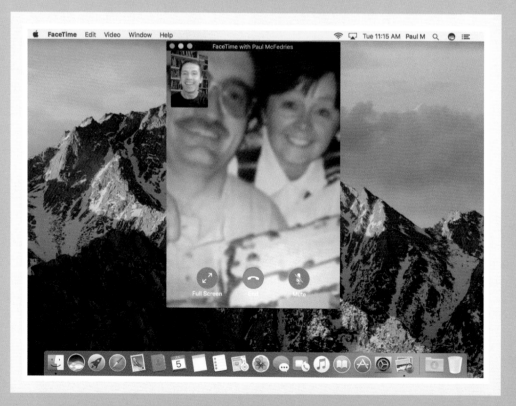

Sign In to Messages

macOS includes the Messages application to enable you to use the iMessage technology to exchange instant messages with other people who are online. The first time you open Messages, you might be required to sign in with your Apple ID. Note that signing in is optional. You can still use Messages with other instant messaging services such as AIM, Google, or Yahoo!, even if either you do not have an Apple ID or you have an Apple ID but are not signed in.

Sign In to Messages

1 Click **Messages** (💬).

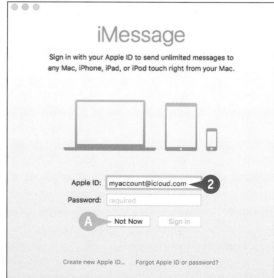

The iMessage dialog appears.

Ⓐ If you do not have or do not want to use an Apple ID with Messages, you can click **Not Now** and skip the rest of the steps in this section.

2 Type your Apple ID.

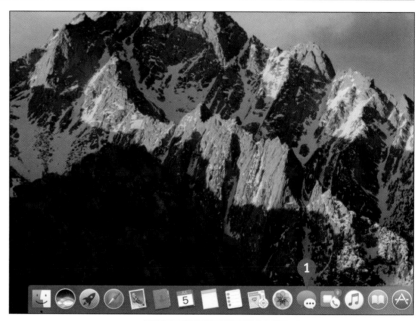

③ Type your Apple ID password.

④ Click **Sign in**.

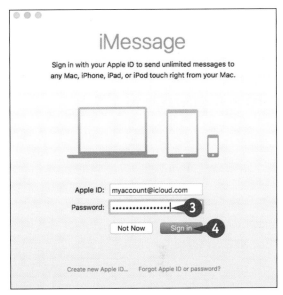

The Messages window appears.

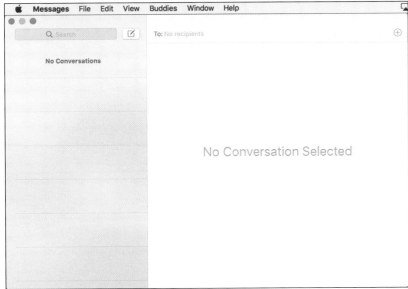

What if I do not have an Apple ID?
You can create a new Apple ID during the sign-in process. After you click **Messages** (💬) and the iMessage dialog appears, click **Create new Apple ID**. macOS opens Safari, which takes you to the Create an Apple ID page. Type your name, the email address you want to use as your Apple ID, and the password you want to use. You must also choose several security questions, specify your birthday and address, and provide a rescue email address. Click **Create Apple ID** to complete the operation.

Send a Message

In the Messages application, an instant messaging conversation is most often the exchange of text messages between two or more people who are online and available to chat.

An instant messaging conversation begins with one person inviting another person to exchange messages. In Messages, this means sending an initial instant message, and the recipient either accepts or rejects the invitation.

Send a Message

1 Click **Compose new message** ( ).

Note: You can also click **File** and then click **New Message**, or press ⌘+N.

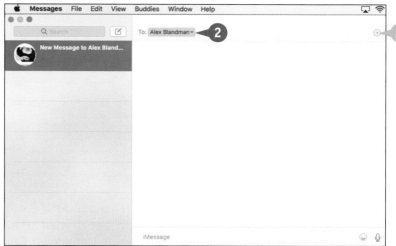

Messages begins a new conversation.

2 In the To field, type the message recipient using one of the following:

The person's email address.

The person's mobile phone number.

The person's name, if that person is in your Contacts list.

A You can also click **Add Contact** ( ) to select a name from your Contacts list.

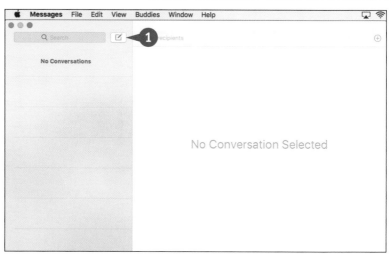

3 Type your message.

B You can also click 😊 if you want to insert an emoji symbol into your message.

4 Press Return.

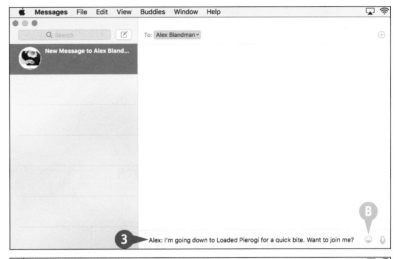

Messages sends the text to the recipient.

C The recipient's response appears in the transcript window.

D You see the ellipsis symbol (⋯) when the other person is typing.

5 Repeat steps **3** and **4** to continue the conversation.

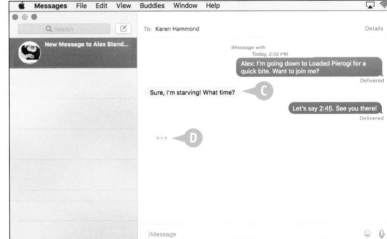

What is an emoji?
An *emoji* is a pictograph similar to a smiley or emoticon. Many emojis represent an emotional state, such as happy, sad, or angry. There are also many emojis that show symbols such as flowers or animals that you can use to add a bit of visual interest to your messages.

How do I make the Messages text a bit bigger?
To change the size of the text that appears in the Messages window, click **Messages** and then click **Preferences**. In the Messages preferences, click the **General** tab. Drag the **Text size** slider to the right to make the text bigger, or to the left to make the text smaller.

Send a File in a Message

I f, during an instant messaging conversation, you realize you need to send someone a file, you can save time by sending the file directly from the Messages application.

When you need to send a file to another person, your first thought might be to attach that file to an email message. However, if you happen to be in the middle of an instant messaging conversation with that person, it is easier and faster to use Messages to send the file. Note that not all instant message services support sending files.

Send a File in a Message

1 Start the conversation with the person to whom you want to send the file.

2 Click **Buddies**.

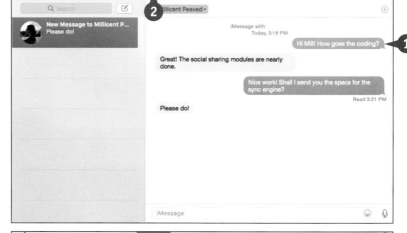

3 Click **Send File**.

Note: You can also press Option + ⌘ + F.

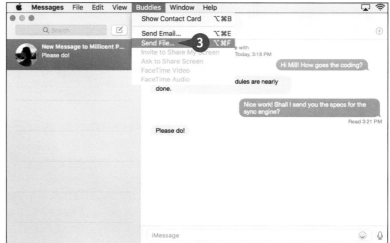

Messages displays a file selection dialog.

4 Click the file you want to send.

5 Click **Send**.

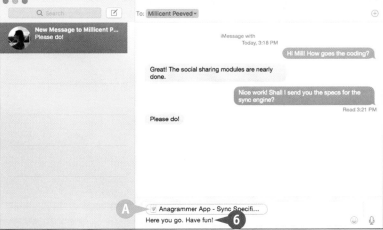

A Messages adds an icon for the file to the message box.

6 Type your message.

7 Press **Return**.

Messages sends the message and adds the file as an attachment.

TIP

How do I save a file that I receive during a conversation?
When you receive a message that has a file attachment, the message shows the name of the file, with the file's type icon to the left. Right-click the file attachment and then click **Save to Downloads** to save the file to your Downloads folder. Messages saves the file and then displays the Downloads folder.

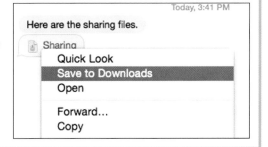

Sign In to FaceTime

FaceTime is a video and audio chat feature that enables you to see and speak to another person over the Internet. To use FaceTime to conduct video chats with your friends, you must each first sign in using your Apple ID. This could be an iCloud account that uses the Apple icloud.com address, or it could be your existing email address.

After you create your Apple ID, you can use it to sign in to FaceTime. Note that you only have to do this once. In subsequent sessions, FaceTime automatically signs you in.

Sign In to FaceTime

1 In the Dock, click **FaceTime** (▣).

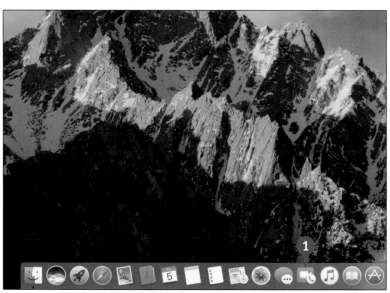

The FaceTime window appears.

2 Type your Apple ID email address.

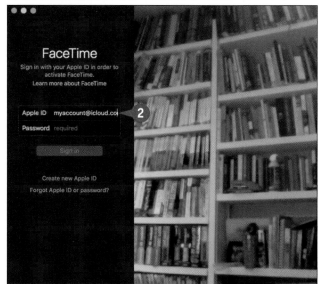

③ Type your Apple ID password.

④ Click **Sign in**.

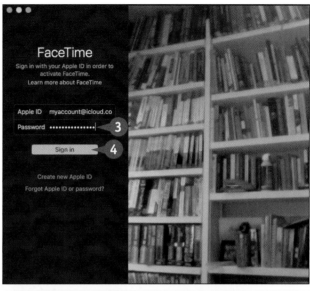

FaceTime verifies your Apple ID and then displays the regular FaceTime window.

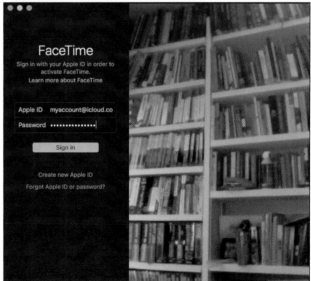

What equipment do I and the person I am calling need to use FaceTime?

For video calls, your Mac must have a web camera, such as the iSight camera that comes with many Macs. For both video and audio calls, your Mac must have a microphone, such as the microphone that is part of the iSight camera.

Which devices support FaceTime?

You can use FaceTime on any Mac running macOS or OS X or later. In all recent versions of OS X or macOS, FaceTime is installed by default. FaceTime is also an app that runs on the iPhone 4 and later, the iPad 2 and later, and the iPod touch fourth generation and later.

Connect Through FaceTime

O nce you sign in with your Apple ID, you can use the FaceTime application to connect with another person and conduct a video or audio chat. You connect using whatever email address or phone number the person has associated with his or her FaceTime account. FaceTime will attempt to connect to that person on any of his or her devices, which can include a Mac, an iPhone, an iPad touch, or an iPad.

Connect Through FaceTime

1 Begin typing the name of the contact or the phone number you want to call.

A Contacts that support FaceTime calling appear with the FaceTime icon (◼️◣).

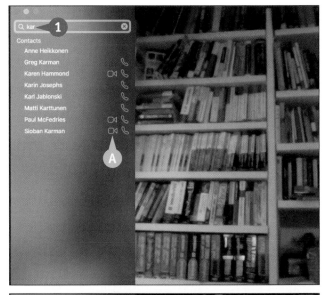

2 If you are calling a contact, click the contact's **FaceTime** icon (◼️◣).

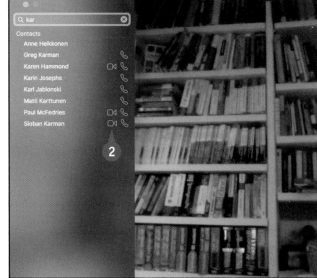

FaceTime sends a message to the contact asking if he or she would like a FaceTime connection.

③ The other person must click or tap **Accept** to complete the connection.

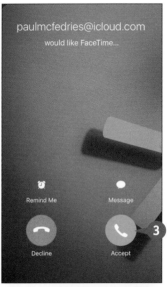

FaceTime connects with the other person.

Ⓑ The other person's video takes up the bulk of the FaceTime screen.

Ⓒ Your video appears in the picture-in-picture (PiP) window.

Note: You can click and drag the PiP to a different location within the FaceTime window.

④ When you finish your FaceTime call, click **End**.

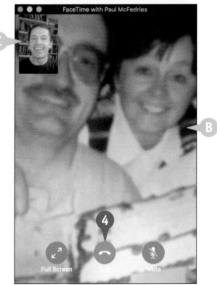

TIP

Can I use FaceTime to call a person without using video?
Yes, FaceTime also supports audio calls, which is useful if the other person does not have a device that supports FaceTime, or if you feel you do not know the other person well enough to place a video call. Use FaceTime to start typing the person's name and then click the **Audio** icon (📞) that appears to the right of the person's name. If you have an iPhone running iOS 8 or later nearby, then you can click the phone number that appears below the Call Using iPhone text; otherwise, click **FaceTime Audio**.

CHAPTER 6

Tracking Contacts and Events

In macOS, you use the Contacts application to manage your contacts by storing information such as phone numbers, email addresses, street addresses, and much more. You also use the Calendar application to enter and track events and to-do items.

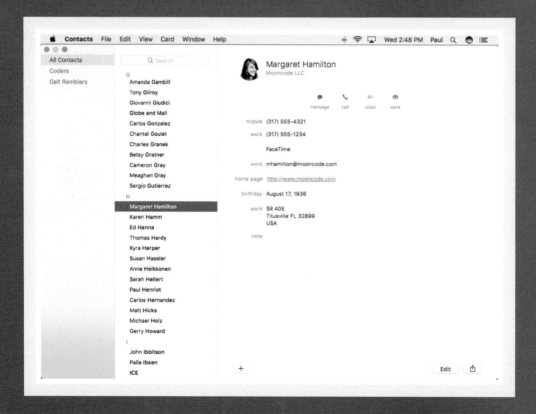

Add a New Contact

macOS includes the Contacts application for managing information about the people you know, whether they are colleagues, friends, or family members. The Contacts app refers to these people as *contacts*, and you store each person's data in an object called a *card*. Each card can store a wide variety of information. For example, you can store a person's name, company name, phone numbers, email address, instant messaging data, street address, notes, and much more. Although you will mostly use Contacts cards to store data about people, you can also use a card to keep information about companies.

Add a New Contact

1 In the Dock, click **Contacts** ( ).

2 Click **File**.

3 Click **New Card**.

Ⓐ You can also begin a new contact by clicking **Add** (+) and then clicking **New Contact**.

Note: You can also run the New Card command by pressing ⌘+Ⓝ.

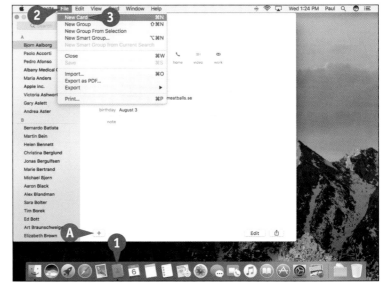

Ⓑ Contacts adds a new card.

4 In the First field, type the contact's first name.

5 In the Last field, type the contact's last name.

6 In the Company field, type the contact's company name.

7 If the contact is a company, click the **Company** check box (changes to ✓).

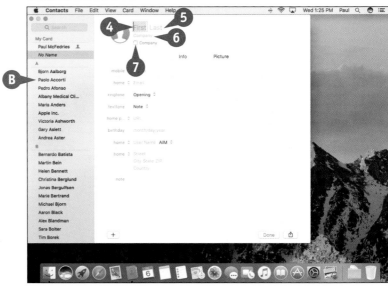

8 In the first Phone field, click ⟳ and then click the category you want to use.

9 Type the phone number.

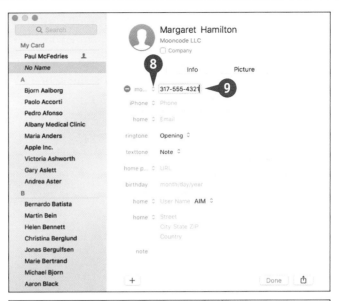

10 Repeat steps **8** and **9** to enter data in some or all of the other fields.

Note: To learn how to add more fields to the card, see the next section, "Edit a Contact."

11 Click **Done**.

Contacts saves the new card.

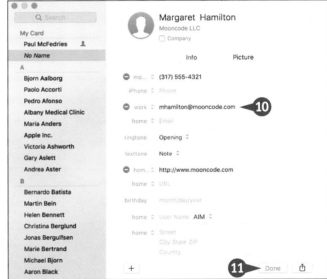

TIP

If I include a contact's email address, is there a way to send that person a message without having to type the address?

Yes. Click the contact's card, click the email address category (such as **work** or **home**), and then click **Send Email**. Mail displays a new email message with the contact already added in the To field. Fill in the rest of the message as required and then click **Send** (✈).

Edit a Contact

If you need to make changes to the information already in a contact's card, or if you need to add new information to a card, you can edit the card from within Contacts. The default fields you see in a card are not the only types of data you can store for a contact. Contacts offers a large number of extra fields. These include useful fields such as Middle Name, Nickname, Job Title, Department, URL (web address), and Birthday. You can also add extra fields for common data items such as phone numbers, email addresses, and dates.

Edit a Contact

1 Click the card you want to edit.

2 Click **Edit**.

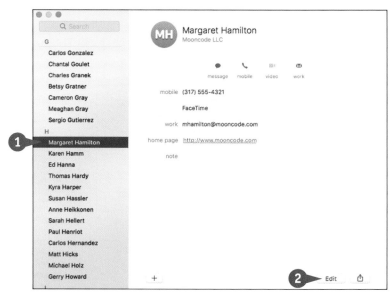

A Contacts makes the card's fields available for editing.

3 Edit the existing fields as required.

4 To add a field, click an empty placeholder and then type the field data.

5 To remove a field, click **Delete** (➖).

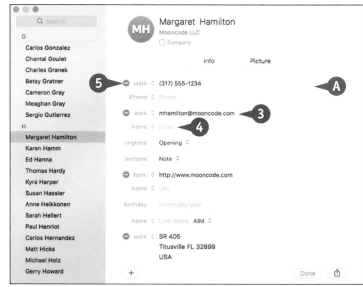

6 To add a new field type, click **Card**.

7 Click **Add Field**.

8 Click the type of field you want.

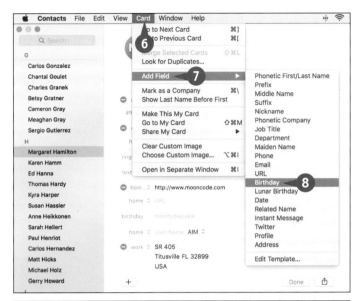

B Contacts adds the field to the card.

9 When you complete your edits, click **Done**.

Contacts saves the edited card.

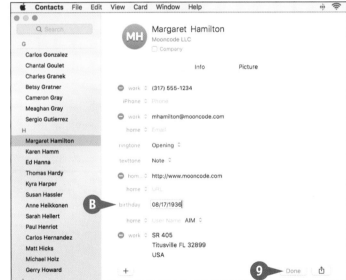

Create a Contact Group

Y ou can organize your contacts into one or more groups, which is useful for viewing just a subset of your contacts. For example, you could create separate groups for friends, family, work colleagues, or business clients. Groups are handy if you have many contacts in your address book. By creating and maintaining groups, you can navigate your contacts more easily. You can also perform groupwide tasks, such as sending a single email message to everyone in the group. You can create a group first and then add members, or you can select members in advance and then create the group.

Create a Contact Group

Create a Contact Group

1 Click **File**.

2 Click **New Group**.

Note: You can also run the New Group command by pressing Shift + ⌘ + N.

A Contacts displays the lists of groups and adds a new group.

3 Type a name for the group.

4 Press Return.

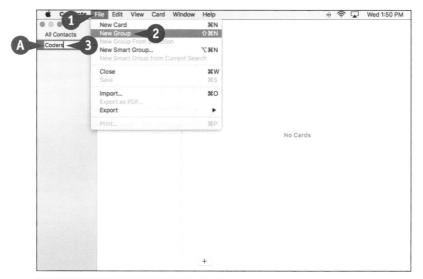

5 Click **All Contacts**.

6 Click and drag a contact to the group.

Contacts adds the contact to the group.

7 Repeat step **6** for the other contacts you want to add to the group.

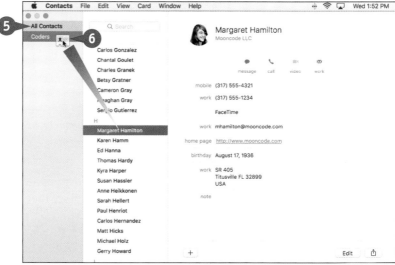

Create a Group of Selected Contacts

1 Select the contacts you want to include in the new group.

Note: To select multiple contacts, press and hold ⌘ and click each card.

2 Click **File**.

3 Click **New Group From Selection**.

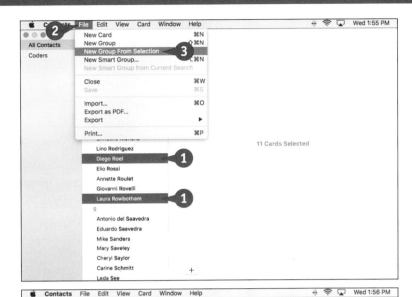

B Contacts adds a new group.

C Contacts adds the selected contacts as group members.

4 Type a name for the group.

5 Press Return.

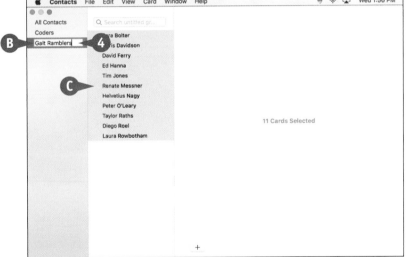

TIPS

Can I send an email message to the group?
Yes. With a group, you send a single message to the group, and Mail automatically sends a copy to each member. Right-click the group and then click **Send Email to "*Group*,"** where *Group* is the name of the group.

What is a Smart Group?
It is a group where each member has one or more fields in common, such as the company name or city. When you create the Smart Group, you specify one or more criteria, and then Contacts automatically adds members to the group who meet those criteria. Click **File**, click **New Smart Group**, and then enter your group criteria.

Navigate the Calendar

Calendar enables you to create and work with events, which are either scheduled appointments or activities such as meetings and lunches, or all-day activities such as birthdays or vacations. Before you create an event, you must first select the date on which the event occurs. You can do this in Calendar by navigating the built-in calendar or by specifying the date that you want.

Calendar also lets you change the calendar view to suit your needs. For example, you can show just a single day's worth of events or a week's worth of events.

Navigate the Calendar

Using the Calendar

1 In the Dock, click **Calendar** (🗓).

2 Click **Month**.

3 Click **Next Month** (**>**) until the month of your event appears.

A If you go too far, you can click **Previous Month** (**<**) to move back to the month you want.

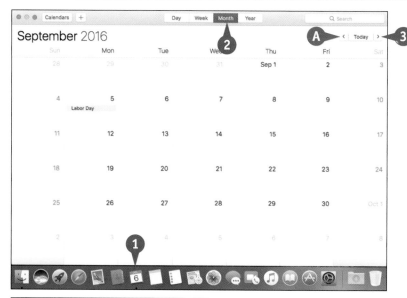

B To see a specific date, you can click the day and then click **Day** (or press ⌘+1).

C To see a specific week, you can click any day within the week and then click **Week** (or press ⌘+2).

D To return to viewing the entire month, you can click **Month** (or press ⌘+3).

E If you want to return to today's date, you can click **Today** (or press ⌘+T).

Go to a Specific Date

1 Click **View**.

2 Click **Go to Date**.

Note: You can also run the Go to Date command by pressing Shift + ⌘ + T.

The Go to Date dialog appears.

3 In the Date text box, type the date you want using the format mm/dd/yyyy.

F You can also click the month, day, or year and then click ⟡ to increase or decrease the value.

4 Click **Show**.

5 Click **Day**.

G Calendar displays the date.

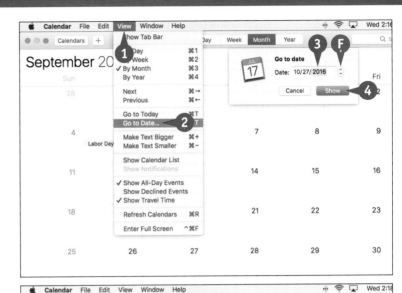

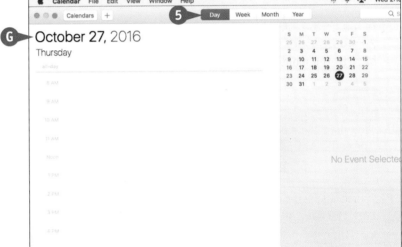

TIP

In the Week view, the week begins on Sunday. How can I change this to Monday?

Calendar's default Week view has Sunday on the left and Saturday on the right. To display the weekend days together, with Monday on the left signaling the start of the week, follow these steps: Click **Calendar** in the menu bar and then click **Preferences**; the Calendar preferences appear. Click the **General** tab. Click the **Start week on** ⟡, select **Monday** from the pop-up menu, and then click **Close** (⬤).

Create an Event

You can help organize your life by using Calendar to record your events — such as appointments, meetings, phone calls, and dates — on the date and time they occur.

If the event has a set time and duration — for example, a meeting or a lunch date — you add the event directly to the calendar as a regular appointment. If the event has no set time — for example, a birthday, anniversary, or multiple-day event such as a convention or vacation — you can create an all-day event.

Create an Event

Create a Regular Event

1 Navigate to the date when the event occurs.

2 Click **Calendars**.

3 Click the calendar you want to use.

4 Double-click the time when the event starts.

Note: If the event is less than or more than an hour, you can also click and drag the mouse pointer (▶) over the full event period.

A Calendar adds a one-hour event.

5 Type the name of the event.

6 Press Return.

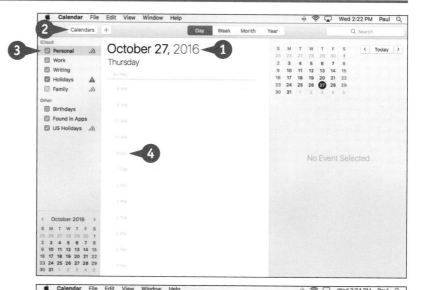

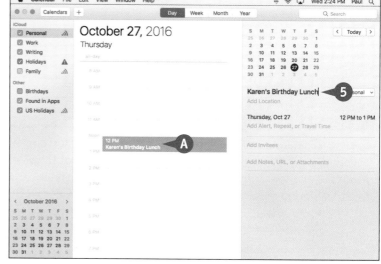

Create an All-Day Event

1 Click **Week**.

2 Navigate to the week that includes the date when the event occurs.

3 Click **Calendars**.

4 Click the calendar you want to use.

5 Double-click anywhere inside the event date's all-day section.

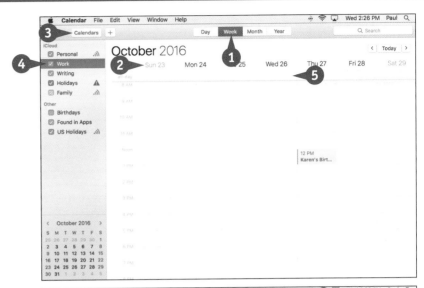

B Calendar adds a new all-day event.

6 Type the name of the event.

7 Press **Return**.

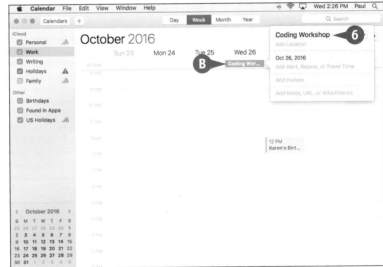

How can I specify event details such as the location and a reminder message?

Follow the steps in this section to create an event and then double-click the event. Type the location of the event in the Add Location text box. (Note that if you type an address, Calendar displays the location on a map.) Click the event's date or time, click **alert**, and then click the amount of time before the event that you want to receive the reminder. To add notes, attach a file, or add a web address, click **Add Notes, URL, or Attachments** and then click the type of information you want to add. Click outside the event. Calendar saves the new event configuration.

Create a Repeating Event

I f you have an activity or event that recurs at a regular interval, you can create an event and configure it to repeat in Calendar automatically. This saves you from having to add the future events repeatedly yourself because Calendar adds them for you.

You can repeat an event daily, weekly, monthly, or yearly. For even greater flexibility, you can set up a custom interval. For example, you could have an event repeat every five days, every second Friday, on the first Monday of every month, and so on.

Create a Repeating Event

1 Create an event.

Note: To create an event, follow the steps in the previous section, "Create an Event."

2 Double-click the event.

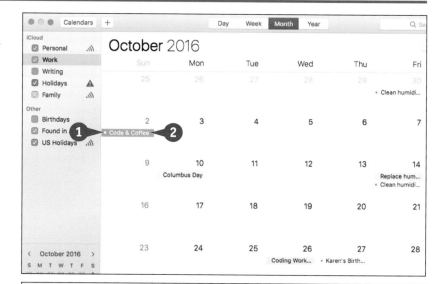

Calendar displays information for the event.

3 Click the event's date and time.

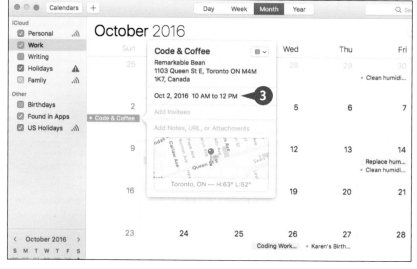

Calendar opens the event for editing.

4 Click the **repeat** ⌃.

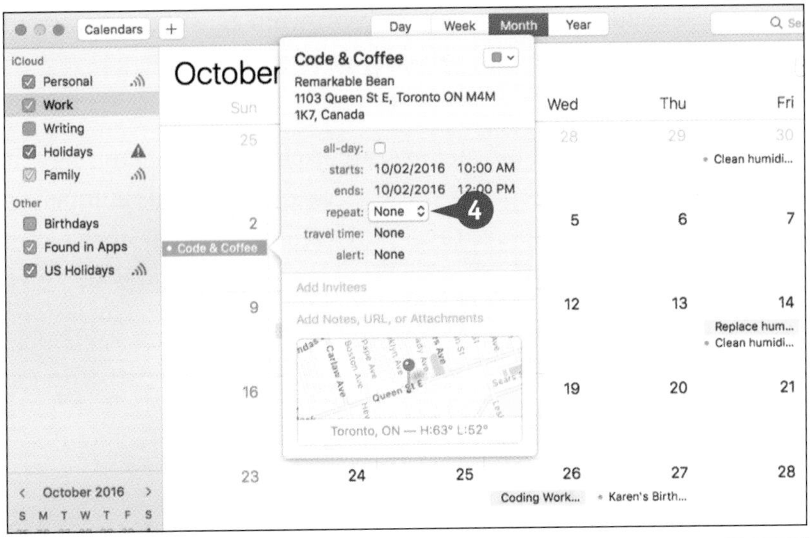

5 Click the interval you want to use.

A If you want to specify a custom interval such as every two weeks or the first Monday of every month, you can click **Custom** and configure your interval in the dialog that appears.

6 Press Return.

B Calendar adds the repeating events to the calendar.

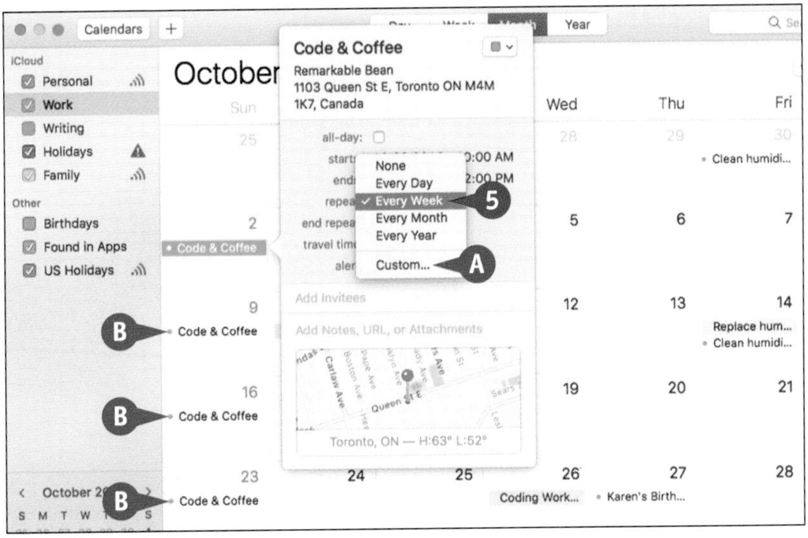

TIPS

How do I configure an event to stop after a certain number of occurrences?

Follow steps **1** to **5** to select a recurrence interval. Click the **end repeat** ⌃ and then select **After** from the pop-up menu. Type the number of occurrences you want. Click outside the event.

Can I delete a single occurrence from a recurring series of events?

Yes, you can delete one occurrence from the calendar without affecting the rest of the series. Click the occurrence you want to delete, and then press Delete. Calendar asks whether you want to delete all the occurrences or just the selected occurrence. Click **Delete Only This Event**.

Send or Respond to an Event Invitation

Y̲ou can include other people in your event by sending them invitations to attend. If you receive an event invitation yourself, you can respond to it to let the person organizing the event know whether you will attend.

If you have an event that requires other people, Calendar has a feature that enables you to send invitations to other people who use a compatible email program. The advantage of this approach is that when other people respond to the invitation, Calendar automatically updates the event. If you receive an event invitation yourself, the email message contains buttons that enable you to respond quickly.

Send or Respond to an Event Invitation

Send an Event Invitation

1 Create an event.

Note: To create an event, follow the steps in the section "Create an Event."

2 Double-click the event.

3 Click **Add Invitees**.

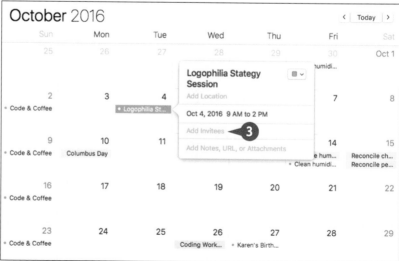

4 Begin typing the name of a person you want to invite.

5 Click the person you want to invite.

6 Repeat steps **4** and **5** to add more invitees.

7 Click **Send**.

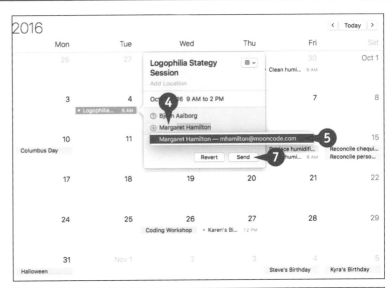

Handle an Event Invitation

A The Invitation button shows the number of pending invitations you have received.

B The event appears tentatively in your calendar.

1 Click **Invitation** (⬇).

2 Click the button that represents your reply to the invitation:

C You can click **Accept** if you can attend the event.

D You can click **Decline** if you cannot attend the event.

E You can click **Maybe** if you are currently not sure whether you can attend.

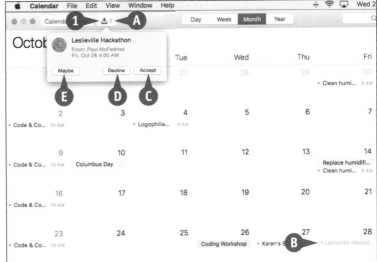

TIPS

Is it possible to see emailed invitations in Calendar before I decide whether to accept them?

Yes. Open Mail, click **Mail** in the menu bar, click **Preferences**, click **General**, click the **Add invitations to Calendar** ⬦, and then click **Automatically**. Events you have not responded to appear in gray in the calendar.

How do I know when a person has accepted or declined an invitation?

Double-click the event. In the list of invitees, you see a check mark beside each person who has accepted the invitation; you see a question mark beside each person who has not made a choice or who has selected Maybe; and you see a red Not symbol beside each person who has declined the invitation.

CHAPTER 7

Playing and Organizing Music

You can use iTunes to create a library of music and use that library to play songs, albums, and collections of songs called playlists. You can also purchase music from the iTunes Store and more.

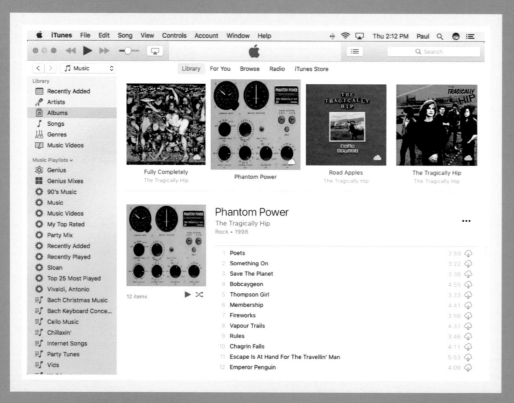

Understanding the iTunes Library

macOS includes iTunes to enable you to play back and manage various types of audio files. iTunes also includes features for organizing and playing videos, watching movies and TV shows, and organizing apps, but iTunes is mostly concerned with audio-related media and content.

Most of your iTunes time will be spent in the library, so you need to understand the various categories — such as music and audiobooks — that iTunes uses to organize the library's audio content. You also need to know how to configure the library to show only the categories you will be working with.

The iTunes Library

The iTunes library is where your Mac stores the files that you can play and work with in the iTunes application. Although iTunes has some video components, its focus is on audio features, so most of the library sections are audio-related. Besides music, you can also switch the library to work with podcasts, audiobooks, ringtones, and more.

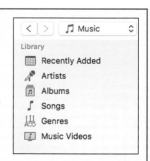

Understanding Library Categories

The Media menu just above the Library pane displays the various media types available in the iTunes library. The audio-related types include Music, Podcasts, Audiobooks, Tones, and Internet Radio.

When you select a media type, the Library pane shows you the contents of that type and the details for each item. For example, in the Music category, you can see details such as the name of each album and the artist who recorded it.

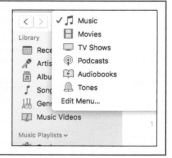

Configure the Library

You can configure which categories of the iTunes library appear in the Media menu. Click the **Media** ⌄ and then click **Edit Menu**. Click the check box for each type of media you want to work with (☐ changes to ☑) and then click **Done**.

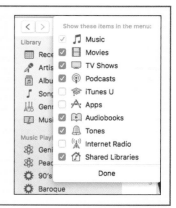

Navigate the iTunes Window

Familiarizing yourself with the various elements of the iTunes window is a good idea so that you can easily navigate and activate elements when you are ready to play audio files, music CDs, or podcasts; import and burn audio CDs; create your own playlists; or listen to Internet radio. In particular, you need to learn the iTunes playback controls because you will use them to control the playback of almost all music you work with in iTunes.

Ⓐ Playback Controls

These buttons control media playback and enable you to adjust the volume.

Ⓑ Status Area

This area displays information about the item currently playing or the action that iTunes is currently performing.

Ⓒ Media

Click an item in this menu to select the type of content you want to view.

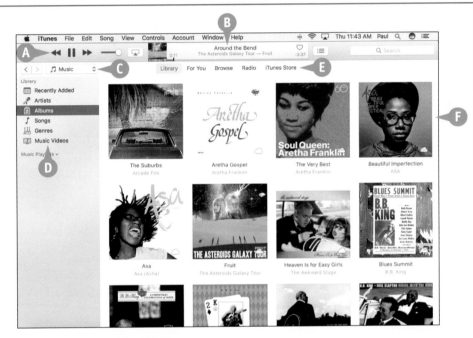

Ⓓ Group

The commands in this pane group the contents of the current iTunes media type.

Ⓔ iTunes Store

Click this command to access the iTunes Store, which enables you to purchase songs and albums, subscribe to podcasts, and more.

Ⓕ Contents

The contents of the current iTunes library source appear here.

Play a Song

Y̶ou use the Music category of the iTunes library to play a song that is stored on your computer. Although iTunes offers several methods to locate the song you want to play, the easiest method is to display the albums you have in your iTunes library, and then open the album that contains the song you want to play. While the song is playing, you can control the volume to suit the music or your current location. If you need to leave the room or take a call, you can pause the song currently playing.

Play a Song

1 Click the **Media** ⬍ and then click **Music**.

2 Click **Albums**.

You can also click a grouping option such as **Songs**, **Artists**, or **Genres**.

Note: To sort the current grouping, click **View**, click **Sort By**, and then click a sort option, such as **Title** or **Artist**.

3 Click the album that contains the song you want to play.

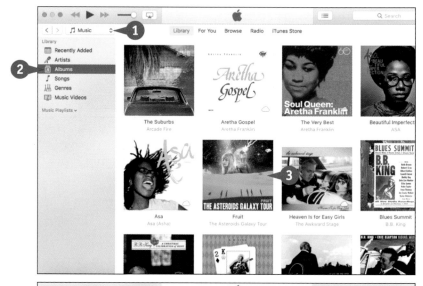

Ⓐ If you want to play the entire album, you can click **Play** (▶).

4 Double-click the song you want to play.

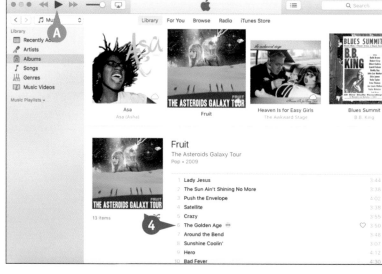

122

iTunes begins playing the song.

B Information about the song playback appears here.

C iTunes displays a speaker icon (🔊) beside the currently playing song.

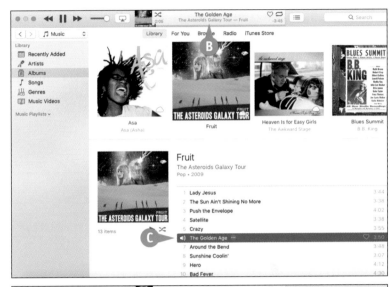

D If you need to stop the song temporarily, you can click **Pause** (❚❚).

Note: You can also pause and restart a song by pressing the Spacebar.

E You can use the Volume slider to adjust the volume (see the first Tip).

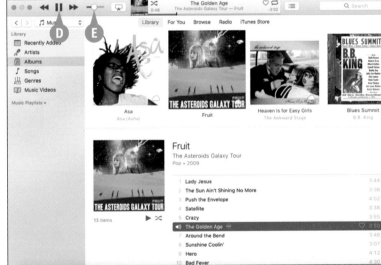

How do I adjust the volume?

To turn the volume up or down, click and drag the **Volume** slider to the left (to reduce the volume) or to the right (to increase the volume). You can also press ⌘+⬇ to reduce the volume, or ⌘+⬆ to increase the volume.

Can I share my music with my family?

Yes, you can activate Home Sharing, which enables you to share your iTunes library with other people on your network as long as you are all logged in to Home Sharing with the same Apple ID. Click **File**, click **Home Sharing**, and then click **Turn On Home Sharing.** Type your (or a family member's) Apple password and click **Turn On Home Sharing.**

Create a Playlist

A *playlist* is a collection of songs that are related in some way. Using your iTunes library, you can create customized playlists that include only the songs that you want to hear. For example, you might want to create a playlist of upbeat or festive songs to play during a party or celebration. Similarly, you might want to create a playlist of your current favorite songs to burn to a CD. Whatever the reason, once you create the playlist you can populate it with songs using a simple drag-and-drop technique.

Create a Playlist

Create the Playlist

1 Click **File**.

2 Click **New**.

3 Click **Playlist**.

Note: You can also create a new playlist by pressing ⌘+N.

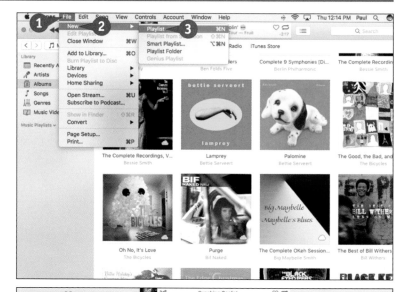

A iTunes creates a new playlist.

4 Type a name for the new playlist.

5 Press Return.

6 Click **Edit Playlist**.

iTunes opens the playlist for editing so that you can add your songs.

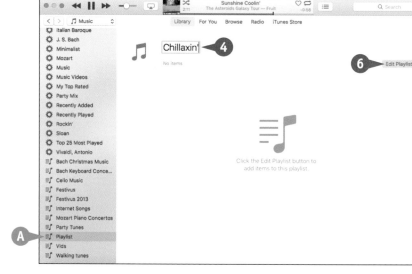

Add Songs to the Playlist

1 Open an album that has one or more songs you want to add to the playlist.

2 Click a song that you want to add to the playlist.

Note: If you want more than one song from the album's playlist, press and hold ⌘ and click each of the songs you want to add.

3 Drag the selected track and drop it on your playlist.

4 Repeat steps **2** and **3** to add more songs to the playlist.

5 Click **Done**.

B To access your playlists, you can use the **Music Playlists** pane.

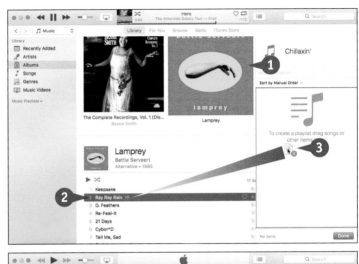

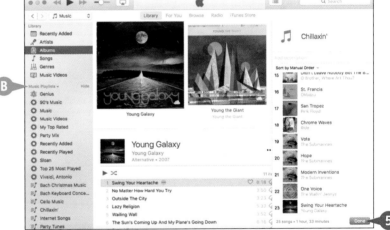

Is there a faster way to create and populate a playlist?
Yes. Press and hold ⌘ and then click each song you want to include in your playlist. Click **File**, click **New**, and then click **Playlist from Selection** (you can also press Shift+⌘+N). Type the playlist name and then press Return.

Can iTunes add songs to a playlist automatically?
Yes, you can create a *Smart Playlist* where the songs have one or more properties in common, such as the genre or text in the song title. Click **File**, click **New**, and then click **Smart Playlist** (you can also press Option+⌘+N). Use the Smart Playlist dialog to create rules that define what songs appear in the playlist.

Purchase Music from the iTunes Store

You can add music to your iTunes library by purchasing songs or albums from the iTunes Store. iTunes downloads the song or album to your computer and then adds it to both the Music category and the Purchased playlist. You can then play and manage the song or album just like any other content in the iTunes library. To purchase music from the iTunes Store, you must have an Apple ID, which you can obtain from https://appleid.apple.com.

Purchase Music from the iTunes Store

1 Click **iTunes Store**.

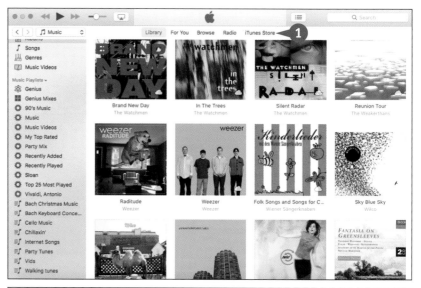

The iTunes Store appears.

2 Click **Music**.

3 Locate the music you want to purchase:

A You can use the Search box to search for an artist, album, or song.

B You can click **All Genres** to select a music genre.

C You can scroll down to view music in various categories.

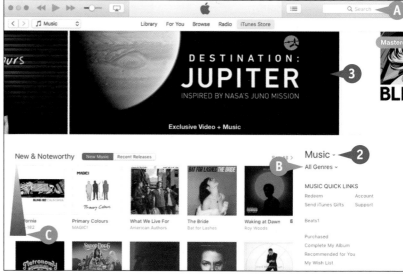

4 Click **Buy**.

D If you want to purchase just a song, you can click the song's price button instead.

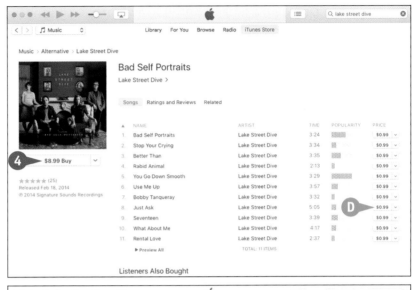

iTunes asks you to sign in to your iTunes Store account.

5 If you have not signed in to your account, you must type your Apple ID.

6 Type your password.

7 Click **Buy**.

iTunes charges your credit card and begins downloading the music to your Mac.

E To return to the iTunes library, you can click **Library**.

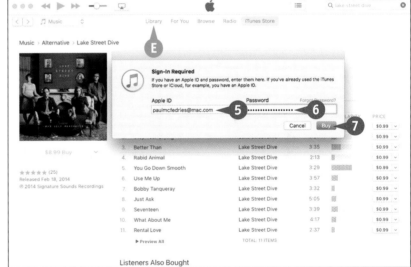

TIPS

Can I use my purchased music on other computers and devices?

Yes. When you purchase music through iTunes, you are given a license to play that music on any device (such as an iPod, iPad, or iPhone), as long as that device is signed in to iCloud using the same Apple ID that you used to purchase the music. You can also burn your music to CDs.

How do I redeem an iTunes gift card?

Scratch off the sticker that covers the card's redeem code. Access the iTunes Store, click **Redeem**, and then enter your account password. In the Redeem Code screen, type the redemption code and then click **Redeem**.

Apply Parental Controls

If you are setting up a user account in Mac Pro for a child, you can use iTunes' parental controls to ensure the child does not have access to music that has been marked as having explicit content. You can also disable certain content types — such as podcasts, the iTunes Store, and Internet radio stations — that could offer content not suitable for the child. Finally, you can also disable access to shared iTunes libraries, which might contain unsuitable music.

Apply Parental Controls

1 Log in to macOS using the child's user account.

2 Click **iTunes**.

3 Click **Preferences**.

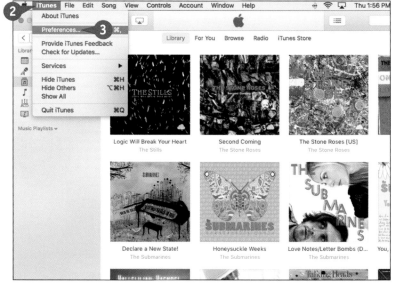

The iTunes preferences appear.

4 Click the **Restrictions** tab.

5 In the Disable section, click the check box beside each type of content you do not want the user to access (☐ changes to ✅).

6 Click the **Ratings for** ⬍ and then click the country ratings you want to use.

7 To ensure the user cannot access explicit musical content, click the **Music with explicit content** check box (☐ changes to ✅).

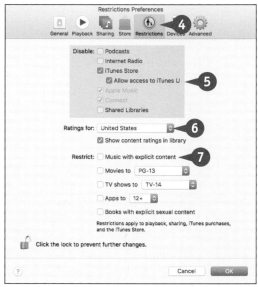

iTunes displays an overview of what it means to restrict explicit content.

8 Click **Restrict Explicit Content**.

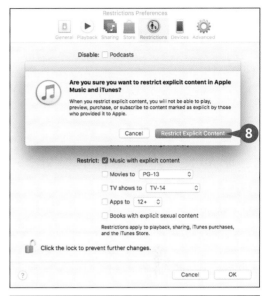

9 Click **OK**.

iTunes puts the parental controls into effect.

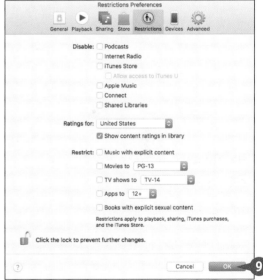

Is it not possible for the child to open the iTunes preferences and disable the parent controls?
Yes, although this is not likely to be a concern for young children. However, for older children who know their way around macOS, you should lock the parental controls to avoid having them changed. Follow steps **1** to **4** to open the child's user account and display the Restrictions tab. Click the lock icon (🔓), type your macOS administrator password, and then click **OK**. 🔓 changes to 🔒, indicating that the controls in the Restrictions tab are now locked and can be unlocked only with your administrator password. Click **OK**.

Subscribe to a Podcast

You can use iTunes to locate, subscribe, manage, and listen to your favorite podcasts. A *podcast* is an audio feed — or sometimes a feed that combines both audio and video — that a publisher updates regularly with new episodes. The easiest way to get each episode is to subscribe to the podcast. This ensures that iTunes automatically downloads each new episode to your iTunes library. You can subscribe to podcasts via either the publisher's website or the iTunes Store.

Subscribe to a Podcast

1 Click **iTunes Store**.

2 Click **Podcasts**.

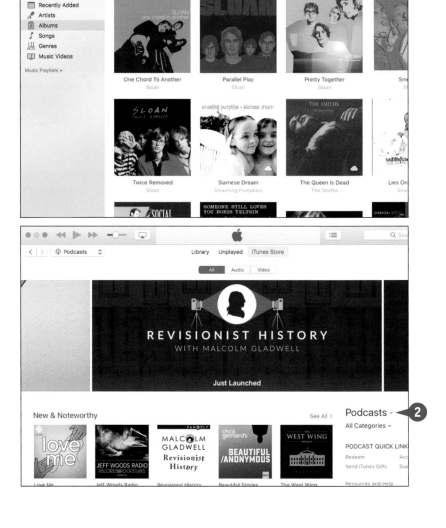

③ Locate the podcast to which you want to subscribe.

④ Click **Subscribe**.

Ⓐ If you want to listen to just one episode before subscribing, you can click the episode's **Get** button instead.

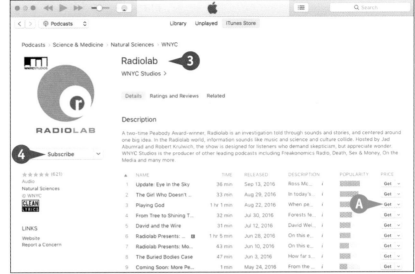

iTunes asks you to confirm.

⑤ Click **Subscribe**.

iTunes begins downloading the podcast.

To listen to the podcast, click the subscription in the Podcasts category of the library.

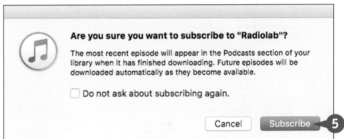

TIP

How do I subscribe to a podcast via the web?

Use your web browser to navigate to the podcast's home page, click the **iTunes** link to open a preview of the podcast, click **View in iTunes**, and then follow steps 4 and 5.

If the podcast does not have an iTunes link, copy the address of the podcast feed, switch to iTunes, click **File**, and then click **Subscribe to Podcast**. In the Subscribe to Podcast dialog, paste the address of the podcast feed into the URL text box and then click **OK**.

CHAPTER 8

Learning Useful macOS Tasks

macOS comes with many tools that help you accomplish everyday tasks. In this chapter, you learn how to integrate your Mac with an iPhone or iPad; create notes and reminders; work with notifications, tags, and maps; install fonts; and access special characters.

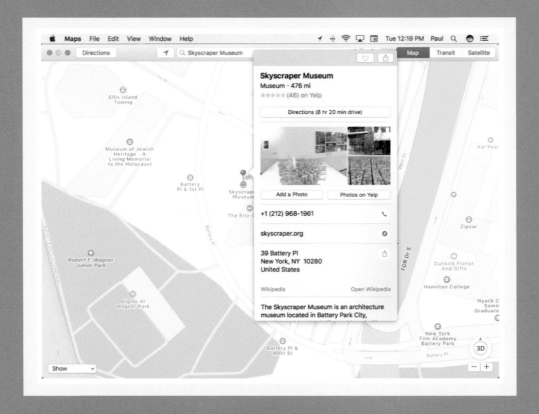

Integrate macOS and Your iPhone or iPad

*C*ontinuity is a set of features that enable you to integrate your Mac and your iPhone or iPad (as well as your iPod touch), and it includes the following: Handoff, for continuing tasks on one device that you started on another; taking phone calls on your Mac or sending Mac calls to your iPhone; Personal Hotspot for sharing your device's Internet connection with your Mac; accessing your macOS desktop and documents on any device; copying and pasting between devices; and unlocking macOS with Apple Watch.

For the Continuity features to work, your Mac must be running OS X Yosemite or later and your iPhone or iPad must be running iOS 8 or later. Also, your Mac and your device must be signed in to the same iCloud account.

Handoff

The Handoff feature enables you to begin certain tasks on your iPhone or iPad and then continue those tasks on your Mac. For example, if you are using Safari on your iPhone, an icon (Ⓐ) appears beside the macOS Dock, and clicking that icon opens the same web page in macOS Safari. Other Handoff-compatible tasks include composing an email, writing a text message, and working with apps such as Maps, Reminders, Calendar, and Contacts. Handoff works both ways, so if you start a task on your Mac, you can continue it on your iPhone or iPad.

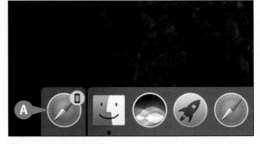

Phone Calls

Continuity enables you to initiate iPhone calls from your Mac. For example, if you come across a phone number while using Safari on your Mac, select the number, click the arrow that appears, and then click **Call "*Number*" Using iPhone** (where *Number* is the selected phone number). You can also initiate calls from Contacts or Calendar.

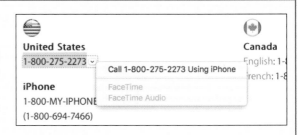

If your iPhone receives an incoming call, your Mac displays a notification that you can click to answer the call on your Mac.

Personal Hotspot

If your Mac cannot connect to a Wi-Fi network for Internet access, you can still get your Mac online by using your iPhone's (or iPad's) cellular connection as a temporary wireless network. When you enable the device's Personal Hotspot (tap **Settings** and then tap **Personal Hotspot**), your device appears in your Mac's list of nearby Wi-Fi networks (Ⓐ). Select the device and type the password to connect.

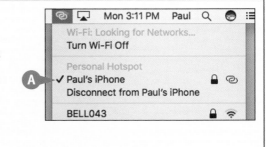

Desktop and Documents

You can synchronize the contents of your Mac user account's Desktop and Documents folders and access those contents from another Mac or from an iPhone or iPad. Continuity uses iCloud Drive to store your Desktop and Documents folders in iCloud. This means that any other Mac, a Windows PC, or any iPhone or iPad that is logged in to iCloud using the same user account can also access those files.

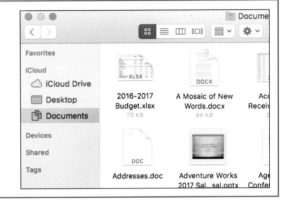

Universal Clipboard

A *clipboard* is a section of memory on your Mac or your iPhone or iPad that is used to store data that you copy or cut. When you open another

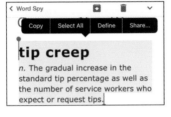
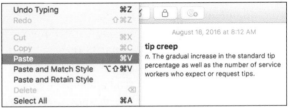

app or document and paste the data, macOS (or iOS) retrieves the data from the clipboard. The Universal Clipboard feature enables you copy or cut data on your iPhone or iPad and then paste it into an app on your Mac (and vice versa).

Unlock Your Mac with Apple Watch

If you have an Apple Watch and you have your iCloud account set up to use *two-factor authentication* — which sends you a confirmation message whenever you try to log in to iCloud using a new device — then you can configure your Mac to unlock automatically whenever your Apple Watch is within range (**A**).

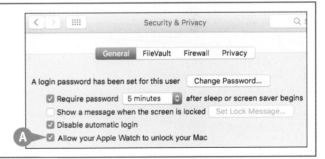

135

Using Handoff to Switch Between a Device and macOS

The Handoff feature enables you to use macOS to continue a task begun on your iPhone or iPad. Handoff requires that your iPhone or iPad is running iOS 8 or later, is close to your Mac (within about 30 feet), and has Bluetooth activated. Also, your Mac must be running OS X Yosemite or later, it must be relatively new (three or four years old at most), and it must have Bluetooth activated. Finally, as shown in this section, you must configure macOS to accept Handoff connections between your device and your Mac.

Using Handoff to Switch Between a Device and macOS

Enable Handoff

1 Click **System Preferences**.

2 Click **General**.

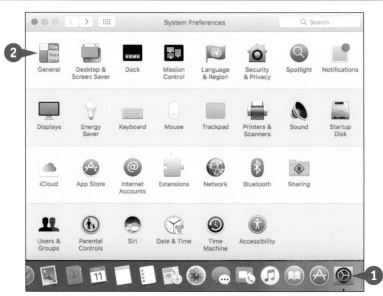

The General preferences appear.

3 Click the **Allow Handoff between this Mac and your iCloud devices** check box (☐ changes to ✓).

4 Click **Close** (⬤).

macOS now accepts Handoff connections between your Mac and your iPhone or iPad.

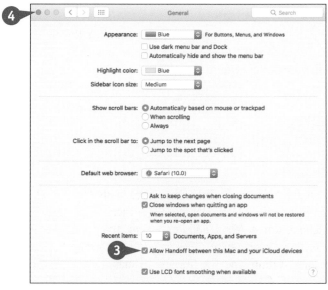

Using Handoff

1. On your iPhone or iPad, open an app that supports Handoff, such as Safari shown here.

2. Bring your iPhone or iPad within range (about 30 feet or less) of your Mac.

3. On your Mac, click the icon that appears to the left of the Dock.

   macOS retrieves the data from the iOS app and displays it in the macOS version of the app.

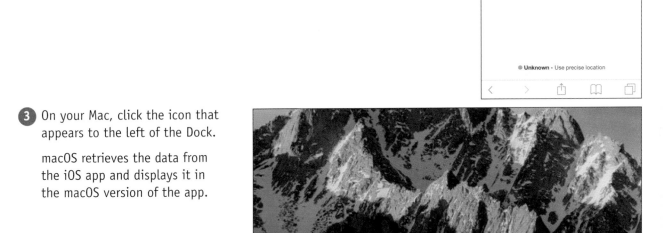

TIPS

Which iOS apps are compatible with Handoff?

Examples of Handoff-compatible apps made by Apple are Safari, Mail, Messages, Contacts, Calendar, Notes, Maps, and Reminders. Many third-party apps can also use Handoff, including Chrome, Airbnb, and The New York Times.

Can I also use Handoff to go from macOS to my iPhone or iPad?

Yes. On your Mac, open an app that supports Handoff. Bring your iPhone or iPad within range of your Mac, and then turn on, but do not unlock, the device. Tap the icon that appears in the lower-left corner of the Lock screen to load the app with the data from your Mac.

Install a Program Using the App Store

Y ou can enhance and extend macOS by installing new programs from the App Store. macOS comes with an impressive collection of applications — or *apps*. However, macOS does not offer a complete collection of apps. For example, macOS lacks apps in categories such as productivity, personal finance, and business tools. To fill in these gaps, you can use the App Store to locate, purchase, and install new programs, or look for apps that go beyond what the default macOS programs can do.

Install a Program Using the App Store

1 In the Dock, click **App Store** (🅐).

The App Store window appears.

2 Locate the app you want to install.

3 Click the price button or, if the app is free, as shown here, click the **Get** button instead.

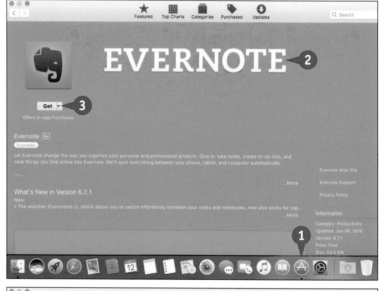

The price button changes to a Buy App button, or the Get button changes to an Install App button.

4 Click **Buy App** (or **Install App**).

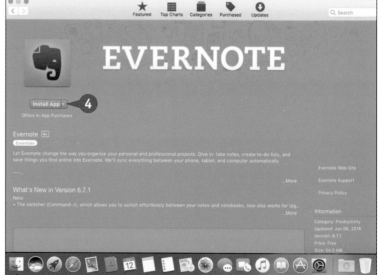

The App Store prompts you to log in with your Apple ID.

⑤ Type your Apple ID.

⑥ Type your password.

⑦ Click **Buy**.

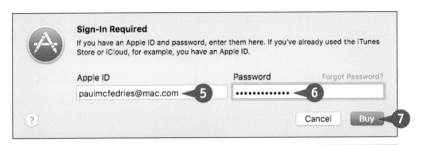

Ⓐ The App Store begins downloading the app. The download is indicated by a progress meter under the Launchpad icon. When you click **Launchpad** (🚀), you see the app's icon, which also shows the progress meter.

When the progress meter disappears, your app is installed. You can click **Launchpad** (🚀) and then click the app to run it.

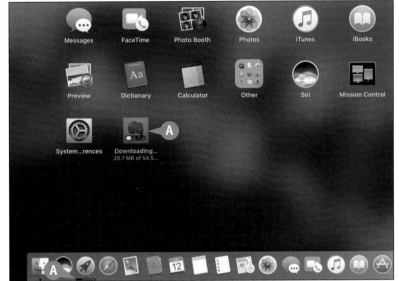

How do I use an App Store gift card to purchase apps?

If you have an App Store or iTunes gift card, you can redeem the card to give yourself store credit in the amount shown on the card. Scratch off the sticker on the back to reveal the code. Click **App Store** (Ⓐ) to open the App Store, click **Featured**, click **Redeem**, type the code, and then click **Redeem**. In the App Store window, the Account item shows your current store credit balance. Be sure to redeem the card before you make a purchase; you cannot apply the credit after the purchase is made.

Write a Note

You can use the Notes app to create simple text documents for things such as to-do lists and meeting notes. Word processing programs such as Word and Pages are useful for creating complex and lengthy documents. However, these powerful tools feel like overkill when all you want to do is jot down a few notes. For these simpler text tasks, the Notes app that comes with macOS is perfect because it offers a simple interface that keeps all your notes together. As you see in the next section, you can also pin a note to the macOS desktop for easy access.

Write a Note

Create a New Note

1 In the Dock, click **Notes** (⬜).

The first time you start Notes, it displays an overview of the app.

2 Click **Continue**.

The Notes window appears.

3 Click **File**.

4 Click **New Note**.

Ⓐ You can also click **New Note** (✏️), or press ⌘+N.

Ⓑ Notes creates the new note.

5 Click inside the note pane.

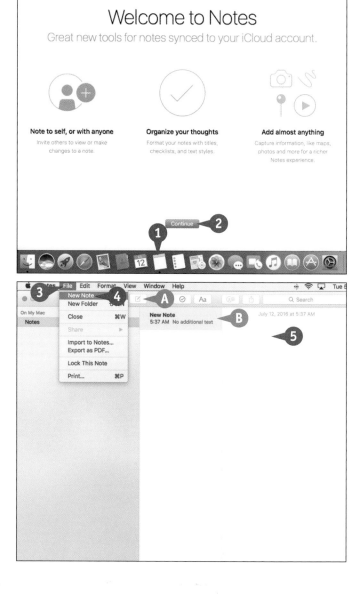

6 Type your note text.

C Notes uses the first line as the note title.

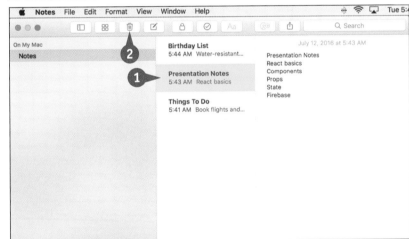

Delete a Note

1 Click the note you want to delete.

2 Click **Delete** (🗑).

The Notes app deletes the note.

TIPS

Can I synchronize my notes with my iPhone or iPad?

Yes, as long as you have an iCloud account set up in macOS, as described in Chapter 14, and you are syncing notes between your Mac and iCloud. To create a new note using iCloud, click **Notes** under the iCloud folder and then follow the steps in this section.

Can I create a bulleted or numbered list?

No, but you can create a checklist, which is a list of items with check boxes to the left of each item. When an item is complete, click its check box (☐ changes to ✅). To create a checklist, click **Format**, and then click **Checklist**.

Enhance Notes with Attachments

Y̶ou can enhance your notes by adding links to websites and by attaching files such as photos and documents. Most of your notes will contain only text, but you might need to augment a note with extra data, such as a link to a website that contains related content. Similarly, you can enhance your notes with related files such as photos, videos, maps, audio files, and documents.

Besides enhancing existing notes, you can also create notes that consist only of external links and files. For example, you could create a note that has links to websites on a particular topic.

Enhance Notes with Attachments

Add an Attachment to a Note

1 Open the application that contains the item you want to attach.

2 Select or display the item, such as a web page, as in this example.

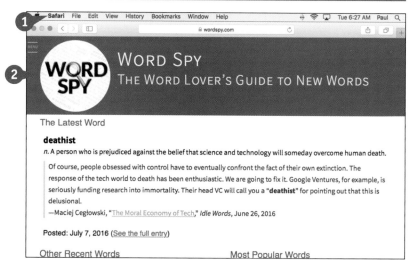

3 Click **Share** (⬆).

4 Click **Notes**.

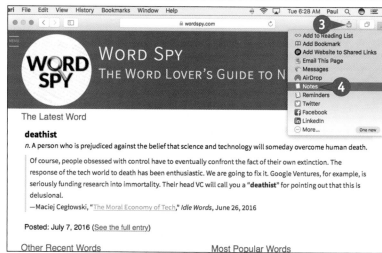

The Notes dialog appears.

Ⓐ The item appears in the note.

⑤ Type an optional description of the item.

⑥ Click the **Choose Note** ⬍ and then click the note to which you want to attach the item.

Note: To attach the item to a new note, you can click **New Note** in the Choose Note list.

⑦ Click **Save**.

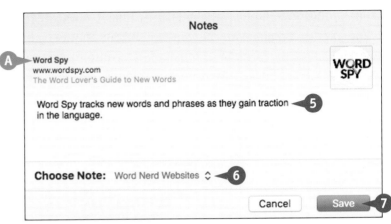

View Note Attachments

① In the Notes app, click **Browse attachments** (⊞).

Notes displays the Attachment Browser.

② Click an attachment category, such as **Websites** as in this example.

Ⓑ Notes displays the items in the category from all your notes.

③ Click **Browse attachments** (⊞) to return to your notes.

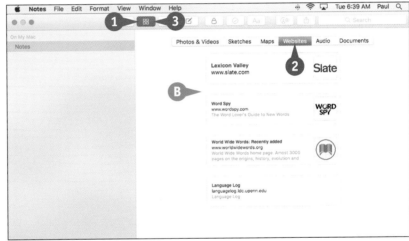

I have a lot of notes. Is there an easy way to see the note to which an item is attached?

Yes. Follow steps **1** and **2** in the subsection "View Note Attachments" to display the category of the attachment you want to view. Right-click the attachment and then click **Show in Note**. Notes exits the Attachment Browser and displays the note that contains the attachment.

How do I open an attachment in its original application?

Follow steps **1** and **2** in the subsection "View Note Attachments" to display the category of the attachment you want to open. Right-click the attachment and then click **Open Attachment** (you can also double-click the attachment).

Create a Reminder

You can use Reminders to have macOS display a notification when you need to perform a task. You can use Calendar to schedule important events, but you likely have many tasks during the day that cannot be considered full-fledged events: returning a call, taking clothes out of the dryer, turning off the sprinkler. If you need to be reminded to perform such tasks, Calendar is overkill, but macOS offers a better solution: Reminders. You use this app to create reminders, which are notifications that tell you to do something or to be somewhere.

Create a Reminder

1 In the Dock, click **Reminders** (▦).

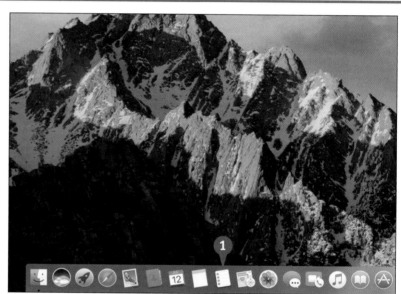

The Reminders app appears.

2 Click **New Reminder** (+).

A You can also click the next available line in the Reminders list.

Note: You can also click **File** and then click **New Reminder**, or press ⌘+N.

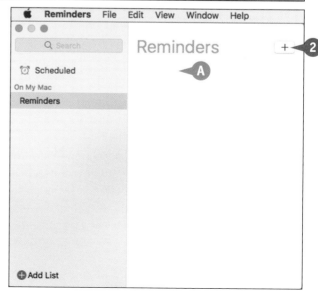

③ Type the reminder title.

④ Click **Show Info** (ⓘ).

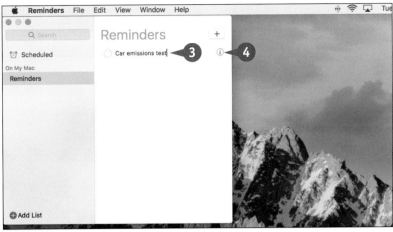

The Reminders app displays the reminder details.

⑤ Click the **On a Day** check box (☐ changes to ☑).

⑥ Specify the date and time you want to be reminded.

⑦ Click **Done**.

The Reminders app adds the reminder to the list.

Ⓑ When you have completed the reminder, click its radio button (◯ changes to ◉).

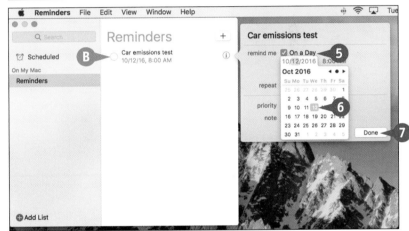

What does the At a Location option do?

The At a Location option allows the Reminders app to display a notification for a task when you arrive at or leave a location and you have your Mac notebook with you. To set this up, follow steps **1** to **4**, click the **At a Location** check box (☐ changes to ☑), and then type the address or choose a contact that has a defined address. Click either the **Leaving** or the **Arriving** option (◯ changes to ◉) and then click **Done**.

Create a New Reminder List

You can organize your reminders and make them easier to locate by creating new reminder lists. By default, Reminders comes with a single list called Reminders. However, if you use reminders frequently, the Reminders list can become cluttered, making it difficult to locate reminders. To solve this problem, you can organize your reminders by creating new lists. For example, you could have one list for personal tasks and another for business tasks. After you create one or more new lists, you can move some or all of your existing reminders to the appropriate lists.

Create a New Reminder List

Create a Reminder List

1 Click **Add List**.

Note: You can also click **File** and then click **New List**, or press ⌘+L.

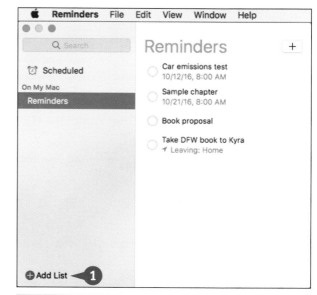

A The Reminders app adds the new list to the sidebar.

2 Type the list name.

3 Press Return.

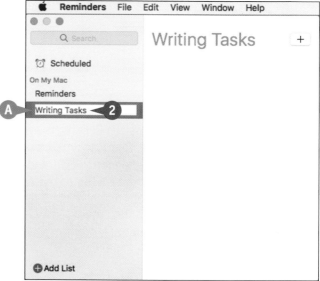

Move a Reminder to a Different List

1 Click the list that contains the reminder you want to move.

2 Click and drag the reminder and drop it on the destination list.

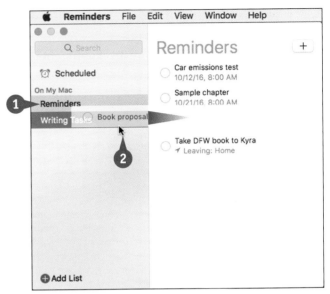

3 Click the destination list.

B The reminder now appears in the destination list.

Note: You can also right-click the reminder, click **Move to List**, and then click the destination list.

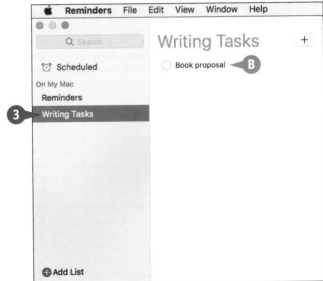

Why does my Reminders app not have a Completed list?

The Reminders app does not show the Completed list when you first start using the program. When you mark a reminder as complete (⬭ changes to ⬤), Reminders creates the Completed list and moves the task to that list.

Can I change the order of the lists in the sidebar?

Yes. By default, the Reminders app displays the new lists in the order you create them. To move a list to a new position, click and drag the list up or down in the sidebar. When the horizontal blue bar shows the list to be in the position you want, release the mouse button.

Work with the Notification Center

You can keep on top of what is happening while you are using your Mac by taking advantage of the Notification Center. Several apps take advantage of a feature called *notifications*, which enables them to send messages to macOS about events that are happening on your Mac. For example, the App Store uses the Notification Center to let you know when macOS updates are available. There are two types of notifications: a banner that appears temporarily and an alert that stays on-screen until you dismiss it. You can also open the Notification Center to view recent notifications.

Work with the Notification Center

Handle Alert Notifications

Ⓐ An alert notification displays one or more buttons.

❶ Click a button to dismiss the notification.

Note: In a notification about new macOS updates, you can click **Update** to open the App Store and see the updates. For details about the updates, click **Details**.

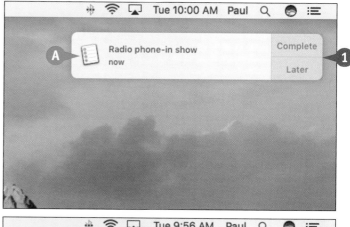

Handle Banner Notifications

Ⓑ A banner notification does not display any buttons.

Note: The banner notification stays on-screen for about 5 seconds and then disappears.

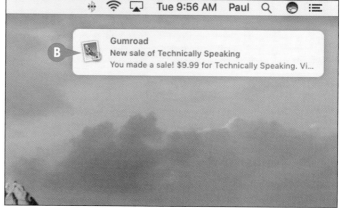

View Recent Notifications

1 Click **Notification Center** (≡).

Note: If your Mac has a trackpad, you can also open the Notification Center by using two fingers to swipe left from the right edge of the trackpad.

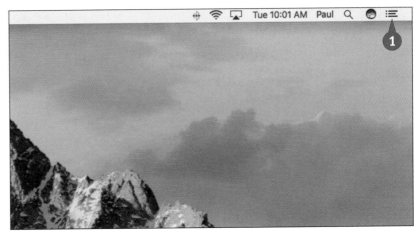

2 Click **Notifications**.

C macOS displays your recent notifications.

3 Click a notification to view the item in the original application.

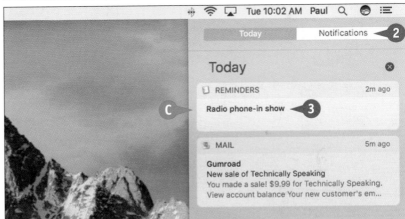

Can I control which apps use the Notification Center and how they use it?
Yes. Click **System Preferences** (⚙) in the Dock and then click **Notifications**. Click an app on the left side of the window and then click a notification style: None, Banners, or Alerts. To control the number of items the app can display in the Notification Center, click the **Show in Notification Center** option menu and select a number. To remove an app from the Notification Center, click the **Show in Notification Center** check box (☑ changes to ☐).

Organize Files with Tags

You can describe many of your files to macOS by adding one or more tags that indicate the content or subject matter of the file. A *tag* is a word or short phrase that describes some aspect of a file. You can add as many tags as you need. Adding tags to files makes it easier to search and organize your documents.

For an existing file, you can add one or more tags within Finder. If you are working with a new file, you can add tags when you save the file.

Organize Files with Tags

Add Tags with Finder

1. Click **Finder** ( ) in the Dock.

2. Open the folder that contains the file you want to tag.

3. Click the file.

4. Click **Edit Tags** ( ).

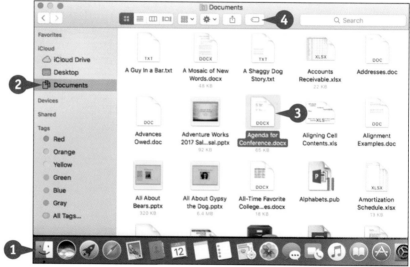

macOS displays the Tags sheet.

5. Type the tag.

Note: To assign multiple tags, you can separate each one with a comma.

6. Press **Return**.

macOS assigns the tag or tags.

7. Press **Return** again.

macOS closes the Tags sheet.

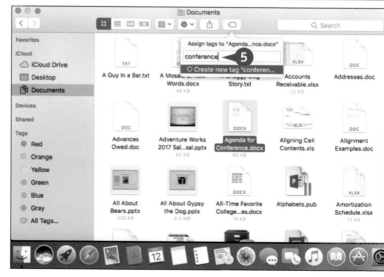

Add Tags When Saving

1 In the application, click the command that saves the new file.

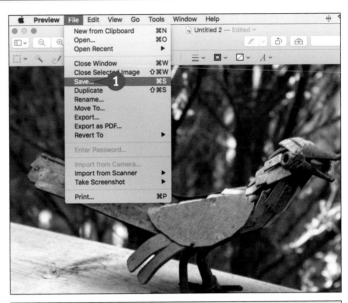

The application displays the Save sheet.

2 Type the tag into the Tags text box.

Note: To assign multiple tags, you can separate each one with a comma.

3 Choose the other save options, such as the filename, as needed.

4 Click **Save**.

The application saves the file and assigns that tag or tags.

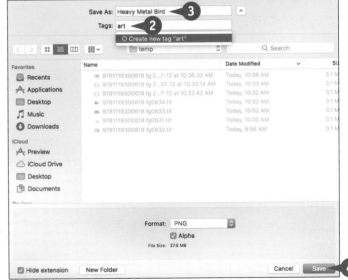

TIPS

Is there an easier method I can use to assign an existing tag to another file?

Yes. macOS keeps a list of your tags, and it displays that list each time you display the Tags sheet. You can assign the same tag to another file by displaying the Tags sheet and clicking the tag in the list that appears.

Can I assign the same tag or tags to multiple files?

Yes. First, use Finder to select all the files in advance. Click **Edit Tags** (⬭), type the tag, and macOS automatically assigns the tag to all the selected files.

Search Files with Tags

After you assign tags to your files, you can take advantage of those tags to make it easier to find and group related files.

Although keeping related files together in the same folder is good practice, that is not always possible. It can make locating and working with related files difficult. However, if you assign the same tag or tags to those files, you can use those tags to quickly and easily search for the files. No matter where the files are located, Finder shows them all together in a single window for easy access.

Search Files with Tags

Search for a Tag

1 Type the first few letters of the tag in Finder's Search box.

2 When the tag appears, click it.

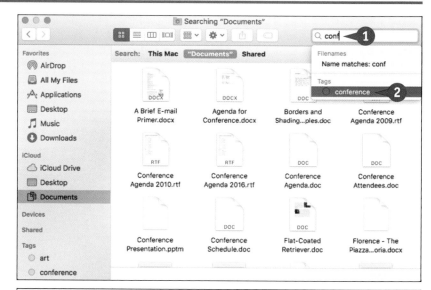

A Finder displays the files assigned that tag.

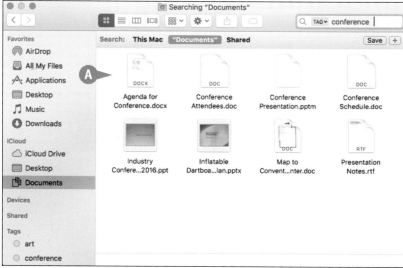

152

Select a Tag

1 In the Finder sidebar, click the tag.

B If you do not see the tag you want, you can click **All Tags** to display the complete list.

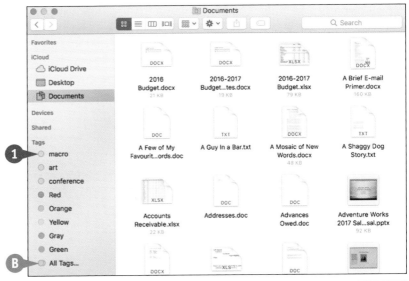

C Finder displays the files assigned that tag.

Note: With the tag folder displayed, you can automatically assign that tag to other files by dragging the files from another Finder window and dropping them within the tag folder.

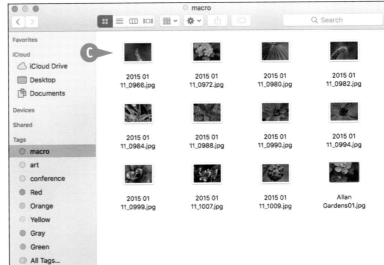

TIP

Can I control what tags appear in Finder's sidebar?
Yes, by following these steps:

1 Open Finder.

2 Click **Finder**.

3 Click **Preferences**.

4 Click the **Tags** tab.

5 For each tag you do not want to appear in the sidebar, click the check box to the right of the tag (☑ changes to ☐).

6 Click **Close** (●).

Search for a Location

You can use the Maps app to display a location on a map. Maps is a macOS app that displays digital maps that you can use to view just about any location by searching for an address or place name.

Maps comes with a Search box that enables you to search for locations by address or by name. If Maps finds the place, it zooms in and drops a pin on the digital map to show you the exact location. For many public locations, Maps also offers an info screen that shows you the location's address, phone number, and more.

Search for a Location

1 Click **Maps** ( ).

The first time you start Maps, macOS asks if the app can use your location.

Note: If you see the message "Maps is not authorized to access your location" instead, then you need to activate location services, as described in Chapter 11.

2 Click **Allow**.

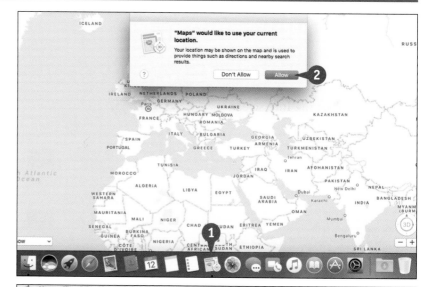

macOS starts the Maps app.

3 Type the address or name of the location into the Search box.

4 Press Return.

A If Maps displays the name of the location as you type, you can click the location instead.

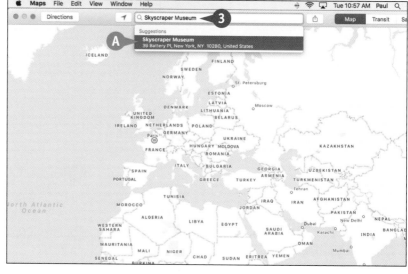

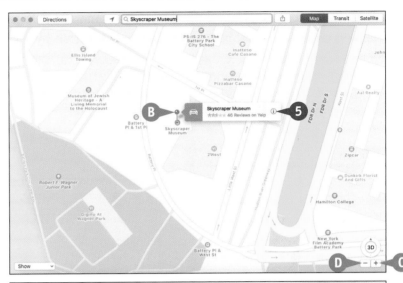

Ⓑ Maps drops a pin on the location.

Ⓒ You can click **Zoom In** (✚) or press ⌘ + ＋ to get a closer look.

Ⓓ You can click **Zoom Out** (—) or press ⌘ + － to see more of the map.

⑤ If Maps offers more data about the location, click **Show Info** (ⓘ).

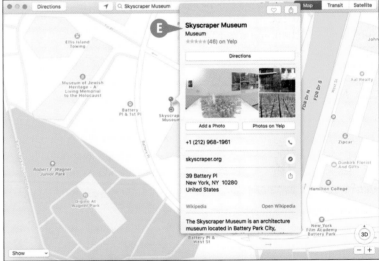

Ⓔ Maps displays the Info screen for the location.

Can I use Maps to show my current location?
Yes. Maps can use surrounding electronic infrastructure, particularly nearby wireless networks, to come up with a reasonably accurate calculation of your current location. Click **Current Location** (⌖), or click **View** and then click **Go to Current Location** (or press ⌘ + Ⓛ).

How do I save a location for future use?
You can save it as a favorite, which means you do not have to type the location's address or name each time. Display the location, click **Show Info** (ⓘ), click **Share** (⬆), and then click **Add to Favorites**. You can also click **Edit** and then click **Add to Favorites** (or press ⌘ + Ⓓ).

Get Directions to a Location

esides displaying locations, Maps also understands the roads and highways found in most cities, states, and countries. This means that you can use the Maps app to get specific directions for traveling from one location to another. You specify a starting point and destination for a trip, and Maps then provides you with directions for getting from one point to the other. Maps highlights the trip route on a digital map and also gives you specific details for negotiating each leg of the trip.

Get Directions to a Location

1 Add a pin to the map for your destination.

Note: See the previous section, "Search for a Location," to learn how to add a pin.

2 Click **Directions**.

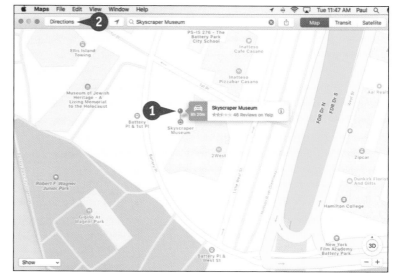

The Directions pane appears.

A Your pinned location appears in the End text box.

Maps assumes you want to start the route from your current location.

3 To start the route from another location, type the name or address in the Start text box.

4 Select how you intend to travel to the destination: Drive, Walk, or take Transit.

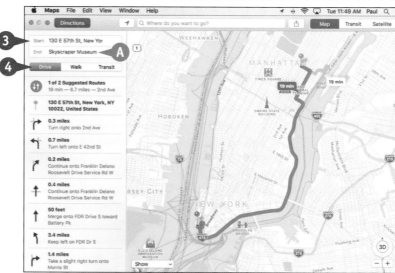

B Maps displays the suggested route for your journey.

C This area tells the distance and approximate traveling time.

D This area displays the various legs of the journey.

E If Maps displays alternate routes, you can click a banner to view the route.

5 Click the first leg of the trip.

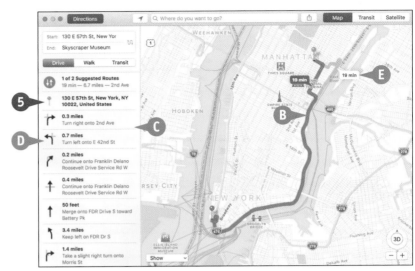

F Maps zooms in to show you just that leg of the trip.

6 As you complete each leg of the trip, click the next leg for further instructions.

Note: To learn how to send a map to your iPhone, iPad, or iPod touch, see the section "Share Information with Other People" in Chapter 9.

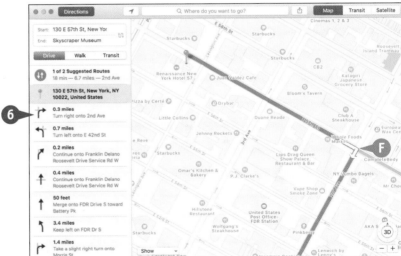

TIPS

Can I get traffic information?
Yes, Maps can display current traffic conditions for most major cities. Click **View** and then click **Show Traffic**. On the map, you see orange lines where traffic is slow and red lines where traffic is heavy.

Can I get directions even though I do not have an exact address?
Yes. You can give Maps the approximate location and it generates the appropriate directions. To specify a location without knowing its address, click **Edit** and then click **Drop Pin** (or press Shift + ⌘ + D). Maps drops a purple pin randomly on the map. Click and drag the pin to the location you want.

Install a Font

macOS ships with a large collection of fonts, but if you require a different font for a project, you can download the font files and then install them on your Mac.

Macs have always placed special emphasis on typography, so it is no surprise that macOS ships with nearly 300 fonts. However, typography is a personal, exacting art form, so your Mac might not have a particular font that would be just right for a newsletter, greeting card, or similar project. In that case, you can download the font you need and then install it.

Install a Font

1 Click **Finder** ( ).

The Finder window appears.

2 Open the folder that contains the font files.

3 Select the font files you want to install.

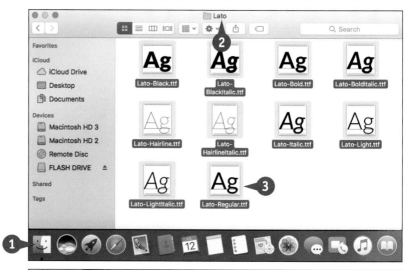

4 Click **File**.

5 Click **Open**.

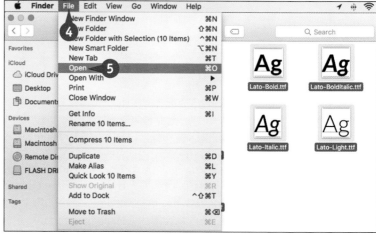

macOS launches the Font Book application.

6 Click **Install Font**.

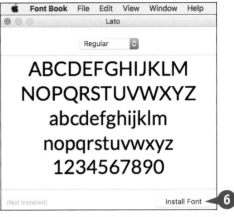

Font Book installs the font.

A The typeface name appears in the Fonts list.

7 Click ▶ to open the typeface and see its individual fonts (▶ changes to ▼).

8 Click a font.

B A preview of the font appears here.

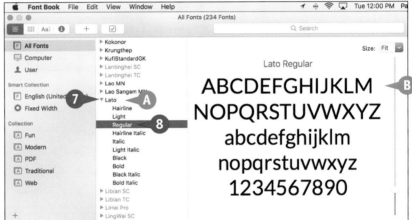

TIPS

What is the difference between a font and a typeface?

A *typeface* is a unique design applied to each letter, number, and symbol. A *font* is a particular style of a typeface, such as regular, bold, or italic. However, in everyday parlance, most people use the terms *typeface* and *font* interchangeably.

What is a font collection?

A *collection* is a group of related fonts. For example, the Fun collection contains fonts normally used with informal designs. To add your font to an existing collection, drag it from the Fonts list and drop it on the collection. To create a collection, click **File** and then click **New Collection** (or press ⌘+N).

Access Non-Keyboard Characters

You can make your documents more readable and more useful by inserting special symbols not available via your keyboard. The keyboard is home to a large number of letters, numbers, and symbols. However, the keyboard is missing some useful characters. For example, it is missing the foreign characters in words such as café and Köln. Similarly, your writing might require mathematical symbols such as ÷ and ½, financial symbols such as ¢ and ¥, or commercial symbols such as © and ®. These and many more symbols and emoji icons are available in macOS via the Emoji & Symbols Viewer.

Access Non-Keyboard Characters

Display the Character Viewer

1. Click **System Preferences** (⚙).

   The System Preferences appear.

2. Click **Keyboard**.

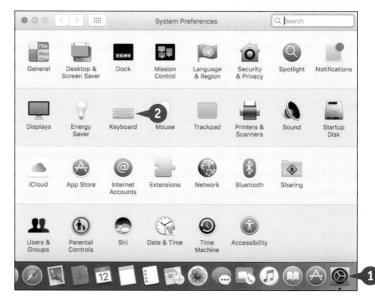

The Keyboard preferences appear.

3. Click the **Keyboard** tab.

4. Click the **Show viewers for keyboard, emoji, and symbols in menu bar** check box (☐ changes to ✓).

5. Click **Show Viewers for Keyboard, Emoji, and Symbols** (⌨).

6. Click **Show Emoji & Symbols**.

   The Emoji & Symbols viewer appears.

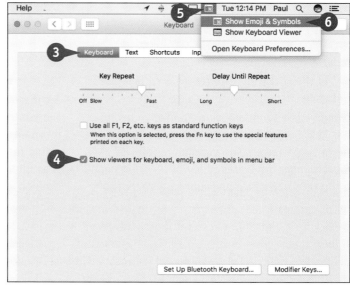

Insert a Character

1 In the document, position the insertion point where you want the character to appear.

2 In the Emoji & Symbols viewer, select a category.

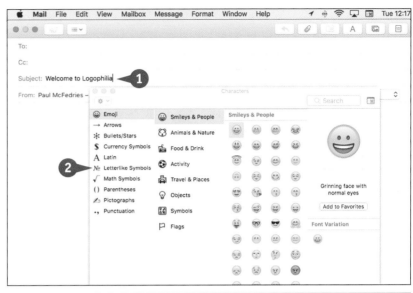

3 Double-click the character you want to use.

A The character appears in the document at the insertion point.

4 Click **Close** (●).

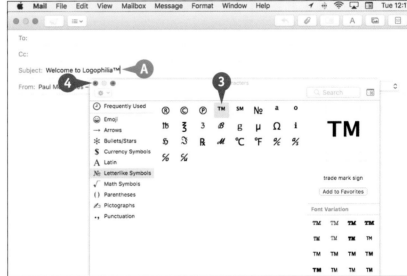

Can I access the Character Viewer if I choose not to display the menu bar icon?

Yes, in some applications you can access the Emoji & Symbols viewer directly. For example, in TextEdit, you can click **Edit** and then click **Emoji & Symbols**, or you can press **Control** + **⌘** + **Spacebar**. This command is also available in Calendar, Contacts, Mail, Messages, and Notes.

Is there an easier way to access characters that I often use?

Yes, you can add those characters to the Emoji & Symbol viewer's Favorites section. To add a character to the Favorites section, display the Emoji & Symbols viewer, click the character, and then click **Add to Favorites**.

CHAPTER 9

Connecting to Social Networks

In this age of ubiquitous social connection, macOS makes everything easier by enabling you to connect and post content to a number of social networks, including Facebook, Twitter, LinkedIn, Flickr, and Vimeo.

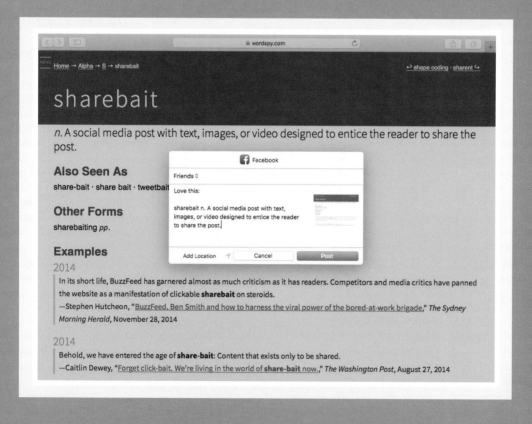

Sign In to Your Facebook Account

If you have a Facebook account, you can use it to share information with your friends directly from macOS because macOS has built-in support for Facebook accounts. This enables you to post status updates and other data directly from many macOS apps. For example, you can send a link to a web page from Safari or post a photo from Photos. macOS also displays notifications when your Facebook friends post to your News Feed. Before you can post or see Facebook notifications, you must sign in to your Facebook account.

Sign In to Your Facebook Account

1 Click **System Preferences** (⚙).

Note: You can also click **Apple** (🍎) and then click **System Preferences**.

The System Preferences appear.

2 Click **Internet Accounts**.

The Internet Accounts preferences appear.

3 Click **Facebook**.

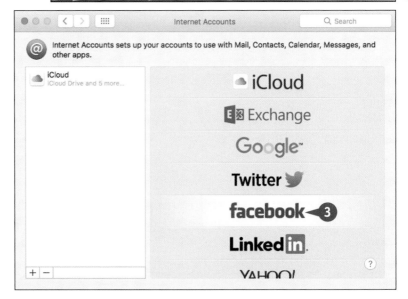

System Preferences prompts you for your Facebook username and password.

④ Type your Facebook username.

⑤ Type your Facebook password.

⑥ Click **Next**.

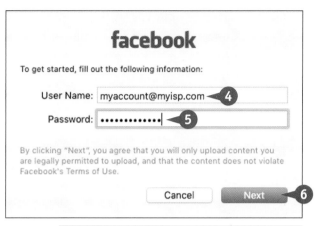

System Preferences displays information detailing what signing in to Facebook entails.

⑦ Click **Sign In**.

macOS signs in to your Facebook account.

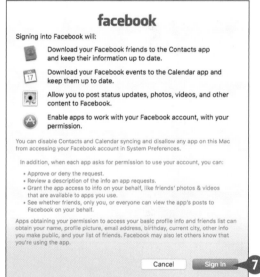

Is there an easy way to add my Facebook friends' profile pictures to the Contacts app?

Yes. Follow steps **1** and **2** to open the Internet Accounts window, click your Facebook account, and then click **Update Contacts**. When System Preferences asks you to confirm, click **Update Contacts**.

Can I prevent Facebook friends and events from appearing in the Contacts and Calendar apps?

Yes. Follow steps **1** and **2** to open the Internet Accounts window and then click your Facebook account. To remove your Facebook friends from Contacts, click the **Contacts** check box (☑ changes to ☐). To remove your Facebook events or friends' birthdays from Calendar, click the **Calendars** check box (☑ changes to ☐).

Post to Facebook

Once you sign in to your Facebook account, you begin seeing notifications whenever your friends post to your News Feed. However, macOS's Facebook support also enables you to use various macOS apps to post information to your Facebook News Feed. For example, if you surf to a web page that you want to share, you can post a link to that page. You can also post a photo to your News Feed.

Post to Facebook

Post a Web Page

1. Use Safari to navigate to the web page you want to share.

2. Click **Share** (⬆).

3. Click **Facebook**.

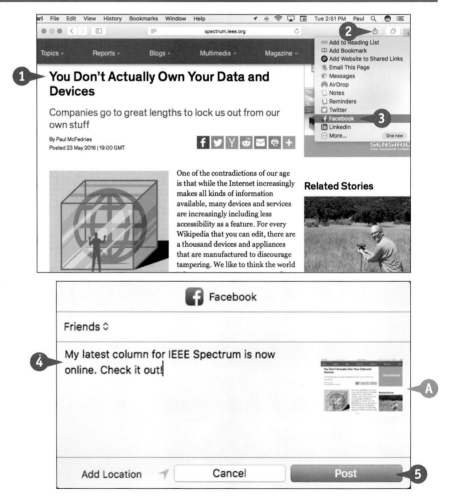

macOS displays the Facebook share sheet.

A. The web page appears as an attachment inside the post.

4. Type your post text.

5. Click **Post**.

Post a Photo

1 In Finder, open the folder that contains the photo you want to share.

2 Click the photo.

3 Click **Share** (⬆).

4 Click **Facebook**.

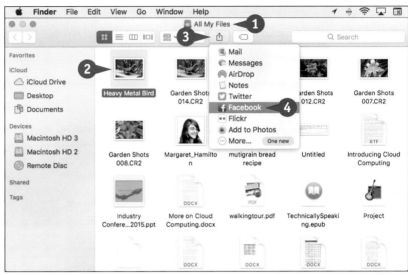

macOS displays the Facebook share sheet.

B The photo appears as an attachment inside the post.

5 Type some text to accompany the photo.

6 Click **Post**.

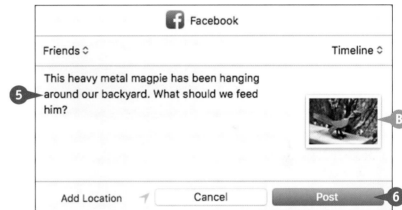

TIPS

How do I control who sees the links and photos that I post to Facebook?

In the Facebook share sheet, click **Friends** to open a pop-up menu that lists your sharing choices, including your Facebook groups and three predefined choices: Public (anyone can view the post), Friends (only your Facebook friends can view the post), and Only Me (only you can view the post).

Can I add a location to my Facebook posts?

Yes, in the Facebook share sheet, click **Add Location**. Note that when you first click this link, macOS asks if Facebook is allowed to use your location, so be sure to click **Allow**.

Publish a Photos Album to Facebook

If you have connected macOS to your Facebook account, you can use that connection to publish a collection of Photos pictures to a new album in your Facebook profile. The easiest way to do this is to upload an album that you have created in Photos. However, you can also upload a selection of photos from the Photos library, or an item in the Faces or Places categories.

Publish a Photos Album to Facebook

1 In Photos, click the album you want to publish to Facebook.

Note: To learn how to use the Photos app, see Chapter 10.

If you want to upload a different collection of photos, select the photos.

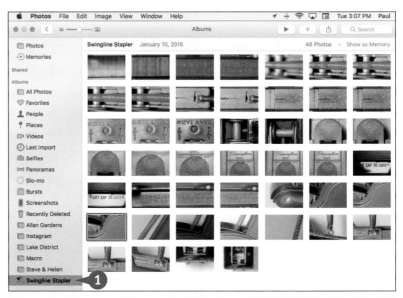

2 Click **Share** (⬆).

3 Click **Facebook**.

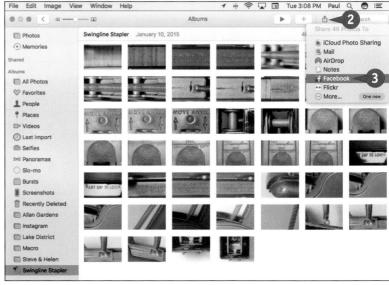

Photos displays the Facebook photo-sharing options.

④ Type a description of the photos.

⑤ Click **Timeline**.

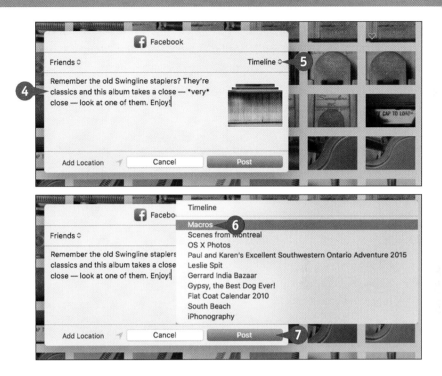

Photos displays a list of your Facebook albums.

⑥ Click the album to which you want to add the photos.

⑦ Click **Post**.

TIP

Can I upload a folder of photos as a Facebook album?
No, not directly. That is, you cannot do this from Finder. Instead, you need to import the folder into Photos and then share the folder. In Photos, click **File** and then click **Import** (or press Shift + ⌘ + I). In the Import Photos dialog, click the folder you want to use and then click **Review for Import**. Click **Import All New Photos**. Photos imports the folder. Click **Albums**, click **Last Import**, and then share the photos to Facebook by following steps **2** to **7**.

Sign In to Your Twitter Account

If you have a Twitter account, you can use it to share information with your followers directly from macOS, which comes with built-in support for Twitter. This enables you to send tweets directly from many macOS apps. For example, you can send a link to a web page from Safari or tweet a photo from Photos. macOS also displays notifications if you are mentioned on Twitter or if a Twitter user sends you a direct message. Before you can tweet or see Twitter notifications, you must sign in to your Twitter account.

Sign In to Your Twitter Account

1 Click **System Preferences** (⚙).

Note: You can also click **Apple** () and then click **System Preferences**.

The System Preferences appear.

2 Click **Internet Accounts**.

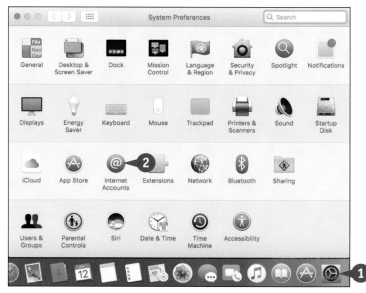

The Internet Accounts preferences appear.

3 Click **Twitter**.

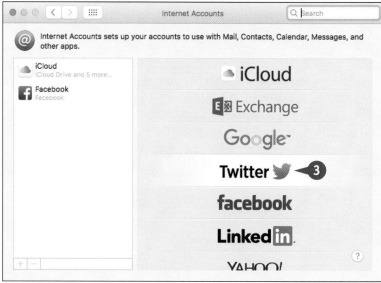

System Preferences prompts you for your Twitter username and password.

④ Type your Twitter username.

⑤ Type your Twitter password.

⑥ Click **Next**.

System Preferences displays information detailing what signing in to Twitter entails.

⑦ Click **Sign In**.

macOS signs in to your Twitter account.

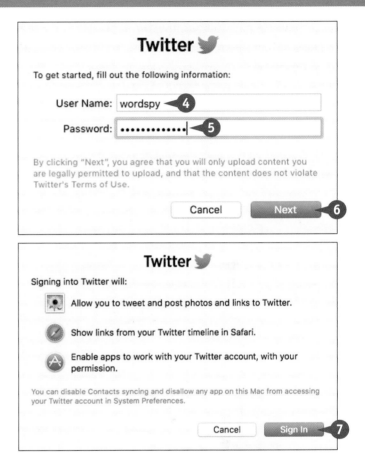

TIP

Some of the people in my contacts list are on Twitter. Is there an easy way to add their Twitter usernames to the Contacts app?
Yes, macOS has a feature that enables you to give permission for Twitter to update your contacts. Twitter examines the email addresses in the Contacts app, and if it finds any that match Twitter users, it updates Contacts with each person's username and account photo.

Follow steps **1** and **2** to open the Internet Accounts window, click your Twitter account, and then click **Update Contacts**. When macOS asks you to confirm, click **Update Contacts**.

Send a Tweet

After you sign in to your Twitter account, you can send tweets from various macOS apps. Although signing in to your Twitter account is useful for seeing notifications that tell you about mentions and direct messages, you will mostly use it for sending tweets to your followers. For example, if you come across a web page that you want to share, you can tweet a link to that page. You can also take a picture using Photo Booth and tweet that picture to your followers.

Send a Tweet

Tweet a Web Page

1. Use Safari to navigate to the web page you want to share.

2. Click **Share** (⬆).

3. Click **Twitter**.

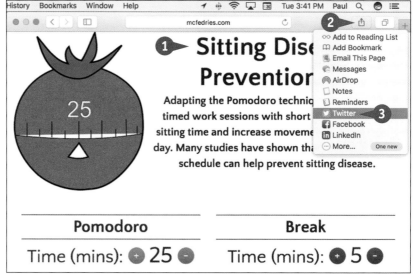

macOS displays the Tweet share sheet.

Ⓐ The attachment appears as a link inside the tweet.

4. Type your tweet text.

Ⓑ This value tells you how many characters you have remaining.

5. Click **Post**.

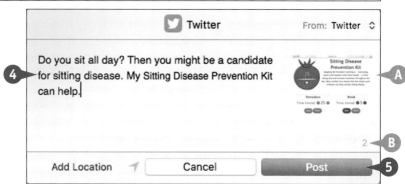

Tweet a Photo Booth Photo

1 Use Photo Booth to take a picture.

Note: To learn how to use the Photo Booth app, see Chapter 10.

2 Click the picture you want to share.

3 Click **Share** (⬆️).

4 Click **Twitter**.

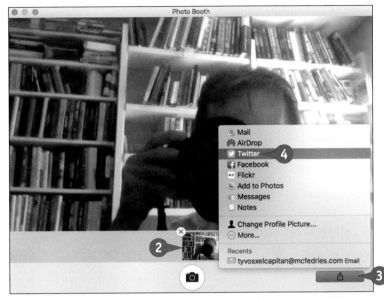

macOS displays the Twitter share sheet.

C The attachment appears as a link inside the tweet.

5 Type your tweet text.

D This value tells you how many characters you have remaining.

6 Click **Post**.

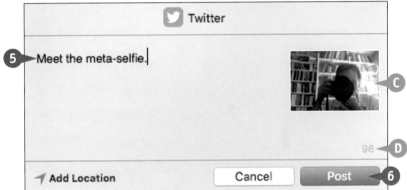

Are there other apps I can use to send tweets?

Yes. If you open a photo using Quick Look (click the photo in Finder and then press Spacebar), you can click **Share** (⬆️) and then click **Twitter**. Similarly, you can open a photo in Preview, click **Share** (⬆️), and then click **Twitter**. Also, with your permission, many third-party apps can use your sign-in information to send tweets without requiring separate Twitter logins for each app.

Can I add a location to my tweets?

Yes, but you must enable location services on macOS, as described in Chapter 11. In the Twitter share sheet, click **Add Location** to insert your current location.

Connect to Your LinkedIn Account

You can use your LinkedIn account to share information with your connections directly from macOS, because macOS comes with built-in support for LinkedIn. This enables you to use Safari to send web page links to your connections and to display the links that your connections share. macOS also displays notifications if one of your connections endorses you or sends you a message. Before you can post updates or see LinkedIn notifications, you must sign in to your LinkedIn account.

Connect to Your LinkedIn Account

1 Click **System Preferences** (⚙).

Note: You can also click **Apple** () and then click **System Preferences**.

The System Preferences appear.

2 Click **Internet Accounts**.

The Internet Accounts preferences appear.

3 Click **LinkedIn**.

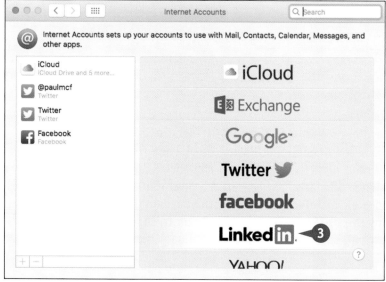

System Preferences prompts you for your LinkedIn username and password.

④ Type your LinkedIn username.

⑤ Type your LinkedIn password.

⑥ Click **Next**.

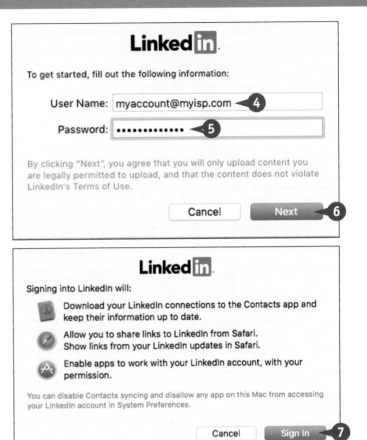

System Preferences displays information detailing what signing in to LinkedIn entails.

⑦ Click **Sign In**.

macOS signs in to your LinkedIn account.

Is there an easy way to add my LinkedIn connections' profile pictures to the Contacts app?

Yes. Follow steps 1 and 2 to open the Internet Accounts window, click your LinkedIn account, and then click **Update Contacts**. When System Preferences asks you to confirm, click **Update Contacts**.

Can I prevent my LinkedIn connections from appearing in the Contacts app?

Yes. Follow steps 1 and 2 to open the Internet Accounts window and then click your LinkedIn account. To remove your LinkedIn connections from the Contacts app, click the **Contacts** check box (☑ changes to ☐).

Post to LinkedIn

After you sign in to your LinkedIn account in macOS, you can send updates to your connections. Although signing in to your LinkedIn account is useful for seeing notifications that tell you about endorsements and other messages, you will mostly use it for sending updates to your followers. For example, if you come across a web page that you want to share, you can post a link to that page. You can share the link with just your connections or with the entire LinkedIn community.

Post to LinkedIn

1. Use Safari to navigate to the web page you want to share.

2. Click **Share** (⬆).

3. Click **LinkedIn**.

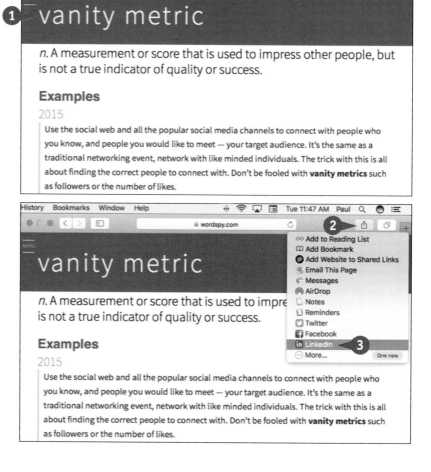

macOS displays the LinkedIn share sheet.

Ⓐ The attachment appears as a link inside the post.

④ Type your update text.

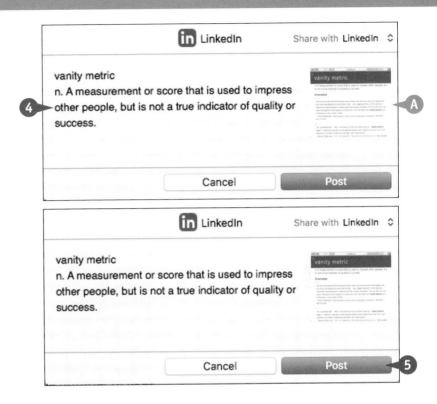

⑤ Click **Post**.

macOS sends the update to LinkedIn.

TIPS

How do I control who sees the updates that I post to LinkedIn?
In the LinkedIn share sheet, click the **Share with ⬍** in the upper-right corner and then click either **LinkedIn** (all of LinkedIn can view the update) or **Connections** (only your LinkedIn connections can view the post).

Are there other apps I can use to send updates?
None of the other default macOS apps support LinkedIn. However, with your permission, many third-party apps are able to use your sign-in information to send updates from the apps without requiring separate LinkedIn logins for each program.

Update Your Social Network Profile Picture

You can use macOS social network connections to easily and quickly update the profile picture for one or more of your accounts. All supported social networks identify you with a photo, which is part of your account profile. Updating this picture for just a single social network is usually a convoluted task, and it is only made worse if you want to use the same photo across multiple social networks. macOS enables you to take a single Photo Booth picture and use it to update your profile picture for Facebook, Twitter, and LinkedIn.

Update Your Social Network Profile Picture

1 Use Photo Booth to take a picture.

Note: To learn how to use the Photo Booth app, see Chapter 10.

2 Click the picture you want to use.

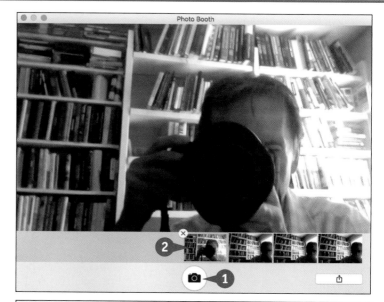

3 Click **Share** (⬆).

4 Click **Change Profile Picture**.

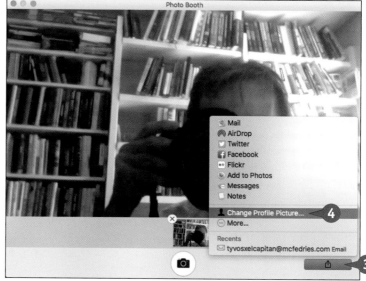

5 Drag the photo to the position you want.

6 Use this slider to set the magnification you want.

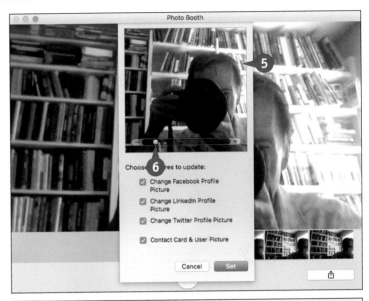

Photo Booth asks which profile you want to update.

7 Click to deselect the profile pictures you do not want to update (☑ changes to ☐).

8 Click **Set**.

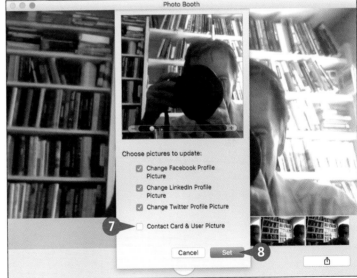

TIP

Can I update my Facebook profile picture from Photos?

Not directly, but you can use Photos to share an image to a Facebook album, and then use Facebook to set that image as your profile picture. In Photos, click the photo you want to use for your Facebook profile picture, click **Share** (□), and then click **Facebook**. In the Facebook share sheet, select **Only Me** in the left pop-up and choose an album in the right pop-up. Click **Post**. Log in to Facebook, click the photo you shared, hover the mouse pointer (↖) over the photo, and then click **Make Profile Picture**. Facebook updates your profile picture.

Connect to Your Flickr Account

Tens of millions of people use Flickr to share their photos with the world. If you have a Flickr account, you can use it to share photos directly from macOS, which comes with built-in support for Flickr. This enables you to send photos from many macOS apps, including Finder, Preview, Photos, and Photo Booth. Before you can send photos, you must sign in to your Flickr account.

Connect to Your Flickr Account

1 Click **System Preferences** (⚙).

Note: You can also click **Apple** (🍎) and then click **System Preferences**.

The System Preferences appear.

2 Click **Internet Accounts**.

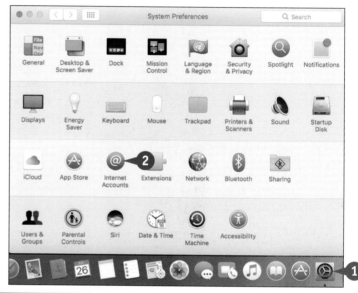

The Internet Accounts preferences appear.

3 Click **Flickr**.

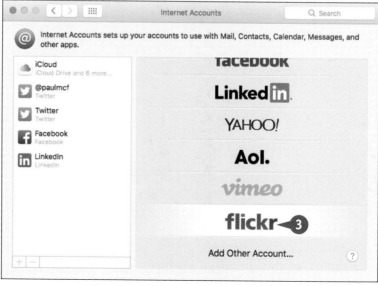

System Preferences prompts you for your Yahoo! ID and password.

④ Type your Yahoo! ID.

Note: Your Yahoo! ID is the email address associated with your Yahoo! account.

⑤ Type your Flickr password.

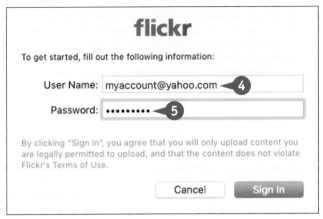

⑥ Click **Sign In**.

macOS signs in to your Flickr account.

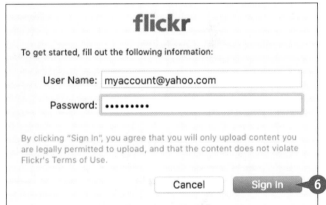

TIP

Can I temporarily disable my Flickr account?
Yes. This is a useful technique if you know you will not be using your Flickr account for a while because it reduces clutter in the macOS sharing menus. To disable Flickr, follow steps **1** and **2** to open the Internet Accounts window. Click your Flickr account and then click the **Enable This Account** check box (☑ changes to ☐). Note that you can also use this technique to disable your Facebook, LinkedIn, and Vimeo accounts, if needed.

Send Photos to Flickr

Flickr is all about sharing your photos, so once you have connected macOS to your Flickr account, you can begin using that connection to upload photos. You can upload individual photos to Flickr using Finder, Quick Look, Preview, or Photo Booth, and those photos appear as part of your Flickr Photostream or an album. Similarly, you can upload multiple photos or an album from the Photos app, and you can add those photos to an existing Flickr album.

Send Photos to Flickr

1. In Finder, Quick Look, Preview, or Photo Booth, select or open the photo or photos you want to upload. In Photos, you can also select an album to upload.

2. Click **Share** (📤).

3. Click **Flickr**.

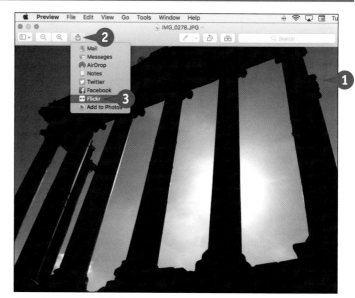

macOS displays the Flickr share sheet.

Ⓐ The photo appears inside the post.

4. Type a title.

5. Type a description.

6. Type one or more tags, separated by commas.

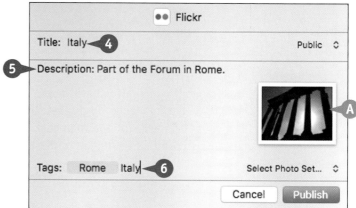

7 Click the **Access** ⭍ and then click who can see the photo.

8 To add the photo to an album (also called a photo set), click the **Select Photo Set** ⭍ and then click an album.

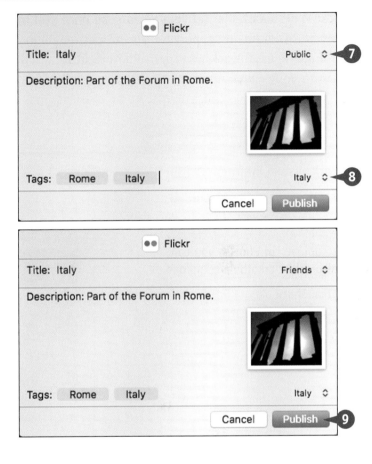

9 Click **Publish**.

macOS sends the photo to Flickr.

Do I have to specify a Flickr album for my photo?
No. If you do not want the photo to appear in an album, or if you do not have a suitable album for the photo, do not choose anything from the Select Photo Set list. This tells Flickr to post the photo to your Photostream.

How can I upload my photos to a new Flickr album?
Unfortunately, you cannot do this within macOS. Instead, you need to sign in to your Flickr account on the web using Safari or another browser. Once you are signed in, open your albums and then click **Create new album**.

Set Up Your Vimeo Account

If you have a Vimeo account, you can use it to post videos online directly from macOS, which comes with built-in support for Vimeo. This enables you to send videos from many macOS apps, including Finder, QuickTime Player, Photo Booth, and iMovie. Before you can send videos, you must sign in to your Vimeo account.

Set Up Your Vimeo Account

1 Click **System Preferences** ().

Note: You can also click **Apple** (🍎) and then click **System Preferences**.

The System Preferences appear.

2 Click **Internet Accounts**.

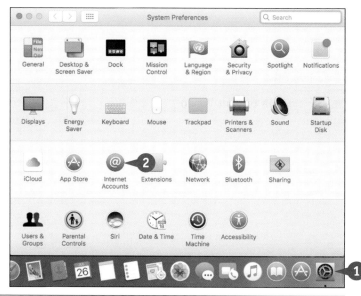

The Internet Accounts preferences appear.

3 Click **Vimeo**.

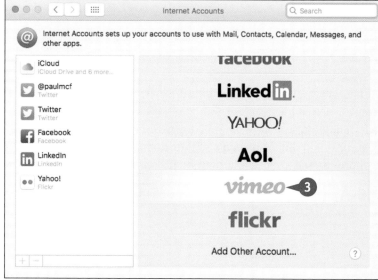

System Preferences prompts you for your Vimeo login data.

4 Type the email address associated with your Vimeo account.

5 Type your Vimeo password.

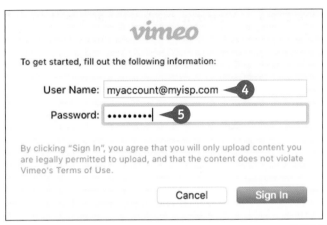

6 Click **Sign In**.

macOS signs in to your Vimeo account.

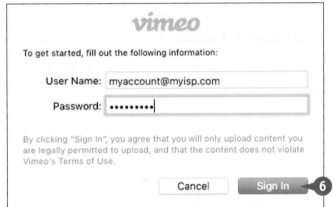

TIP

How do I delete my Vimeo account?

If you no longer use your Vimeo account, you should delete it from macOS. This not only reduces clutter in the macOS sharing menus, but also makes the Internet Accounts window easier to navigate.

To delete your Vimeo account, follow steps **1** and **2** to open the Internet Accounts window. Click your Vimeo account and then click **Remove** (—). When macOS asks you to confirm, click **OK**. Note that you can also use this technique to delete any other account that you no longer use.

Send a Video to Vimeo

Vimeo is one of the web's most popular video-sharing services, so once you have connected macOS to your Vimeo account, you can begin using that connection to upload videos. You have two ways to publish photos from macOS to Vimeo. First, you can use a macOS share sheet to upload a video to Vimeo using Finder, QuickTime Player, or Photo Booth. Second, you can upload a video to Vimeo from an iMovie project, which gives you many more options for publishing the video.

Send a Video to Vimeo

Send a Video Using a Share Sheet

1. In Finder, QuickTime Player, or Photo Booth, select or open the video you want to upload.

2. Click **Share** (⬆).

3. Click **Vimeo**.

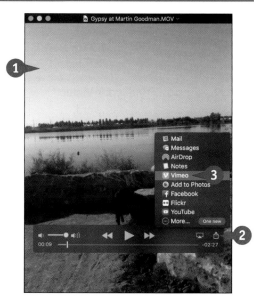

macOS displays the Vimeo share sheet.

Ⓐ The attachment appears as a link inside the post.

4. Type a title.

5. Type a description.

6. Type one or more tags, separating each with a comma.

7. If you want anyone to be able to view the video, click the **Make this movie personal** check box (☑ changes to ☐).

8. Click **Publish**.

macOS sends the video to your Vimeo account.

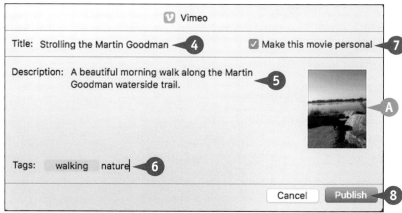

186

Send a Video from an iMovie Project

1. In iMovie, open the project you want to publish to Vimeo.

2. Click **Share**.

3. Click **Vimeo**.

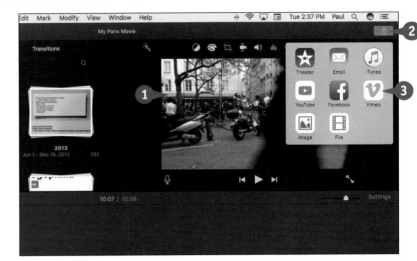

iMovie displays the Vimeo dialog.

4. Click **Sign In**, type your Vimeo email address and password, and then click **OK**.

5. Type a title.

6. Type a description.

7. Type one or more tags, separating each with a comma.

8. Click the **Resolution** ⬦ and then **click** the movie size you want to use.

9. Click the **Viewable By** ⬦ and then click with whom you want to share the video.

10. Click **Next**.

11. Click **Publish** (not shown).

iMovie uploads the video.

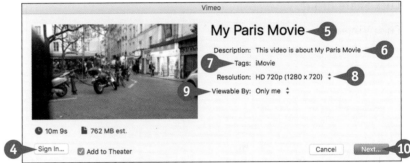

TIP

Do I have to sign in to Vimeo every time I want to upload a video using iMovie?
No, you can tell iMovie to save your sign-in data so that you do not have to enter it each time. In iMovie, click **Share** (📤) and then click **Vimeo** to open the Vimeo dialog. Click **Sign In**, type your Vimeo email address and password, and then click to activate the **Remember this password in my keychain** check box (☐ changes to ☑). Click **OK**. The next time you click **Share** and then **Vimeo**, iMovie enters your Vimeo email address and password automatically.

Share Information with Other People

You can use macOS to share information with other people, including web pages, notes, pictures, videos, photos, and maps. macOS was built with sharing in mind. It comes with a feature called the *share sheet*, which not only enables you to easily share data via Facebook and Twitter, as you have seen in this chapter, but also via multiple other methods such as email and instant messaging.

Share Information with Other People

Share a Web Page

1. Use Safari to navigate to the web page you want to share.

2. Click **Share** (⬆).

3. Click the method you want to use to share the web page.

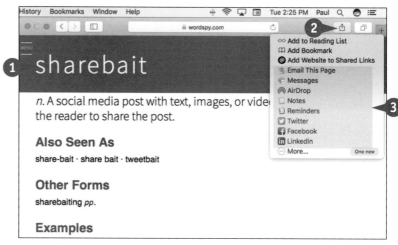

Share a Note

1. In the Notes app, click the note you want to share.

2. Click **Share** (⬆).

3. Click the method you want to use to share the note.

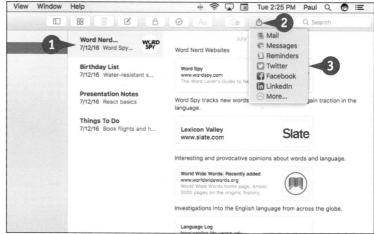

Share a Photos Picture

1 In Photos, click the picture you want to share.

2 Click **Share** (📤).

3 Click the method you want to use to share the picture.

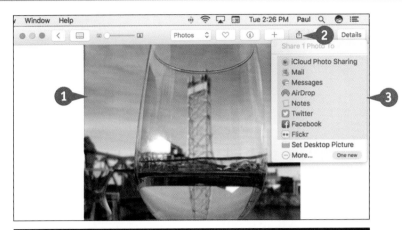

Share a Video

1 In QuickTime Player, open the video you want to share.

2 Click **Share** (📤).

3 Click the method you want to use to share the video.

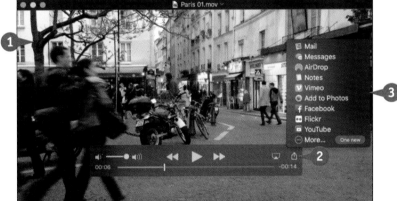

TIPS

Can I share a map or directions with my iPhone or iPad?
Yes. Maps and directions are usually much easier to use on a handheld device such as an iPhone or iPad. First, use the Maps app to display the map or the directions to a location. Click **Share** (📤) and then click **Send to** *Device*, where *Device* is the name of the device you want to use.

How do I share a Photo Booth photo?
Use Photo Booth (see Chapter 10) to snap the photo using your Mac's attached camera. Click the photo, click **Share** (📤), and then click the method you want to use to share the photo.

Viewing and Editing Photos and Videos

Whether you want to look at your photos, or you want to edit them to fix problems, macOS comes with a number of useful tools for viewing and editing photos. It also offers tools for viewing digital videos.

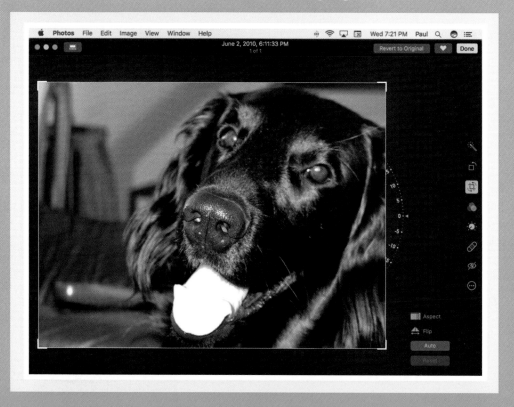

View a Preview of a Photo

macOS offers several tools you can use to see a preview of any photo on your Mac. The Finder application has a number of methods you can use to view your photos, but here you learn about the two easiest methods. First, you can preview any saved image file using the macOS Quick Look feature. Second, you can see photo previews by switching to the Cover Flow view. You can also preview photos using the Preview application.

View a Preview of a Photo

View a Preview with Quick Look

1. In Finder, open the folder that contains the photo you want to preview.

2. Click the photo.

3. Click **File**.

4. Click **Quick Look** "*file*," where *file* is the filename of the photo.

Note: You can also launch Quick Look by pressing Spacebar.

Ⓐ Finder displays a preview of the photo.

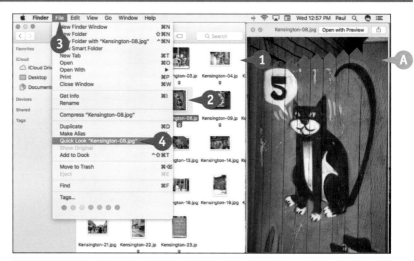

View a Preview with Cover Flow

1. In Finder, open the folder that contains the photo you want to preview.

2. Click the photo.

3. Click **Cover Flow** (⊞).

Ⓑ Finder displays a preview of the photo.

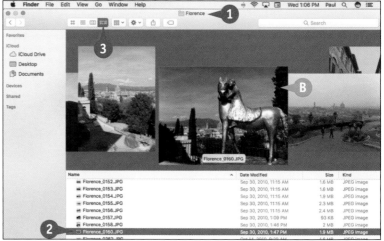

View a Preview in the Preview Application

1 In Finder, open the folder that contains the photo you want to preview.

2 Click the photo.

3 Click **File**.

4 Click **Open With**.

5 Click **Preview**.

Note: In many cases, you can also simply double-click the photo to open it in the Preview application.

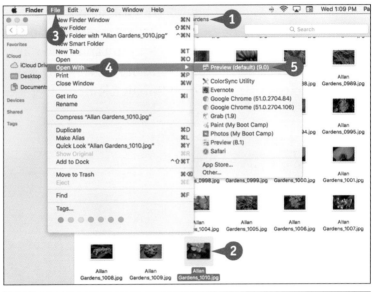

The Preview application opens and displays the photo.

6 Use the toolbar buttons to change how the photo appears in the Preview window.

C More commands are available on the View menu.

7 When you finish viewing the photo, click **Close** (⬤).

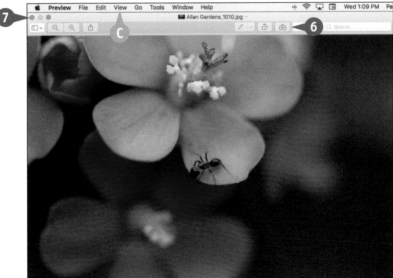

TIPS

Is there an easier way to preview multiple photos using the Preview application?

Yes. In Finder, navigate to the folder that contains the photos and then select each file that you want to preview. Either click and drag the mouse pointer (⬆) over the photos, or press and hold ⌘ and click each one. In Preview, press Option + ⬇ and Option + ⬆ to navigate the photos.

Is there a way that I can zoom in on just a portion of a photo?

Yes. In Preview, click and drag your mouse pointer (⬆) to select the portion of the photo that you want to magnify. Click **View** and then click **Zoom to Selection** (or press ⌘ + *).

View a Slideshow of Your Photos

Instead of viewing your photos one at a time, you can easily view multiple photos by running them in a slideshow. You can run the slideshow using the Preview application or Quick Look. The slideshow displays each photo for a few seconds and then Preview automatically displays the next photo. Quick Look also offers several on-screen controls that you can use to control the slideshow playback. You can also configure Quick Look to display the images full screen.

View a Slideshow of Your Photos

1 In Finder, open the folder that contains the photos you want to view in the slideshow.

2 Select the photos you want to view.

3 Click **File**.

4 Click **Open With**.

5 Click **Preview**.

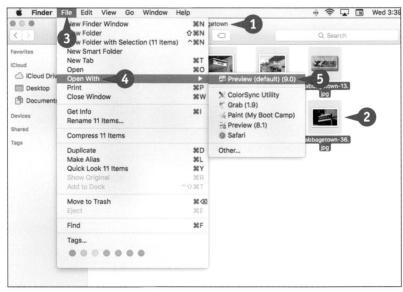

The Preview window appears.

6 Click **View**.

7 Click **Slideshow**.

You can also select Slideshow by pressing Shift + ⌘ + F.

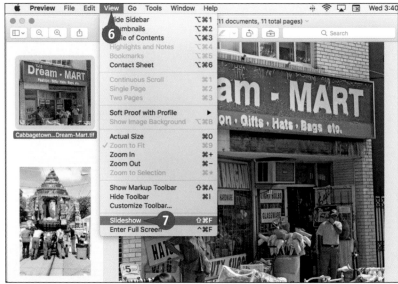

194

Preview opens the slideshow window.

8 Move the mouse pointer (+).

A Preview displays the slideshow controls.

9 Click **Play** (▶). Play (▶) changes to Pause (❚❚).

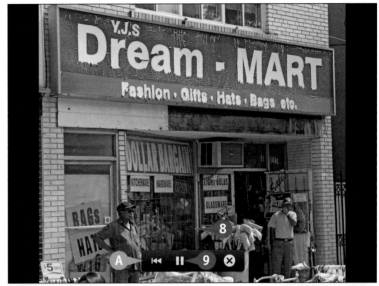

Preview begins the slideshow.

B You can click **Next** (▶▶) to move to the next photo.

C You can click **Back** (◀◀) to move to the previous photo.

D You can click **Pause** (❚❚) to suspend the slideshow.

10 When the slideshow is over or when you want to return to Finder, click **Close** (✕) or press Esc.

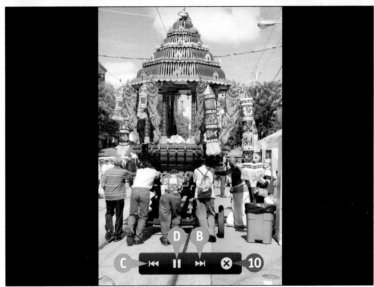

TIPS

Can I jump to a specific photo during the slideshow?
Yes. With the slideshow running, press Spacebar to stop the show. Use the arrow keys to select the photo that you want to view in the slideshow. Click **Play** to resume the slideshow.

What keyboard shortcuts can I use when viewing a slideshow?
Press → or ↑ to display the next photo, and press ← or ↓ to display the previous photo. Press Esc to end the slideshow.

Import Photos from a Digital Camera

You can import photos from a digital camera and save them on your Mac. You can use the Photos application to handle importing photos. Photos enables you to add a name and a description to each import, which helps you to find your photos after the import is complete. To perform the import, you need a cable to connect your digital camera to your Mac. Most digital cameras come with a USB cable. Note that the steps in this section also apply to importing photos from an iPhone or iPad.

Import Photos from a Digital Camera

Import Photos from a Digital Camera

1 Connect one end of the cable to the digital camera.

2 Connect the other end of the cable to a free USB port on your Mac.

3 Turn the camera on and put it in either playback or computer mode.

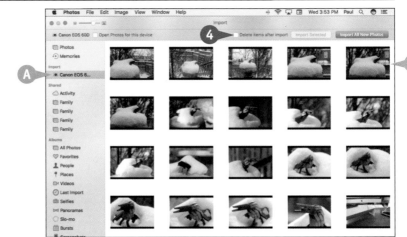

Your Mac launches the Photos application.

Note: You can also launch the application by clicking **Photos** (🌸) in the Dock.

Ⓐ Your digital camera appears in the Import section.

Ⓑ Photos displays previews of the camera's photos.

4 If you want Photos to remove the images from your camera after the import, click the **Delete items after import** check box (☐ changes to ☑).

⑤ Click and drag the mouse pointer (🖎) around the photos you want, or press and hold ⌘ and click each photo you want to select.

⑥ Click **Import X Selected**, where X is the number of photos you selected in step **5**.

Ⓒ To import all the photos from the digital camera, you can click **Import All New Photos**.

Photos imports the photos from the digital camera.

View the Imported Photos

① Under Albums, click **Last Import**.

Ⓓ The imported photos appear.

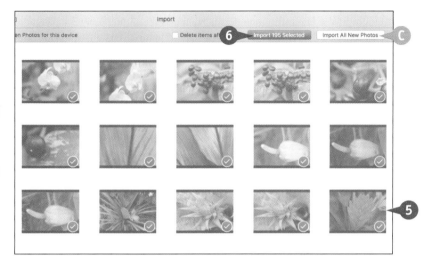

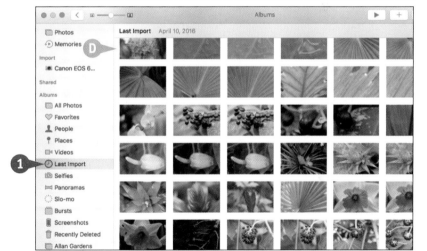

TIP

When I connect my digital camera, why do I see Image Capture instead of Photos?
Your Image Capture app is not configured to open Photos when you connect your camera. To fix this, connect your digital camera to your Mac; the Image Capture application opens. (If the Image Capture application did not open, click **Finder** [🙂] in the Dock, click **Applications**, and then double-click **Image Capture**.) Click the **Connecting** 🔷 and then click **Photos**. Click **Image Capture** in the menu bar and then click **Quit Image Capture**.

View Your Photos

If you want to look at several photos, you can use the Photos application. Photos offers a single-image view, which hides everything else and displays each photo using the entire height of the window. Once you activate the single-image view, Photos offers on-screen controls that you can use to navigate backward and forward through the photos. You can also configure single-image view to show thumbnail images of each photo, so you can quickly jump to any photo you want to view.

View Your Photos

1 In the Photos application, click **Photos** or press ⌘+**1**.

Ⓐ The Photos view organizes your photos by *moments* — that is, by the date they were taken.

2 Locate the date that contains the photos you want to view.

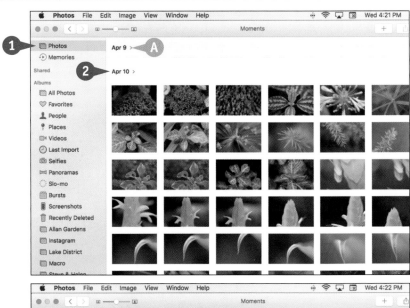

3 Double-click the first photo you want to view.

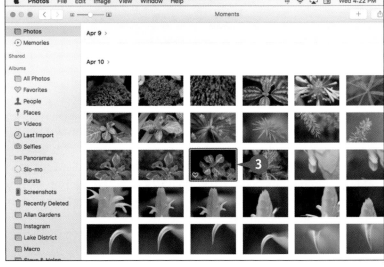

Photos displays the photo.

④ Click **Next** (>) to view the next photo.

Ⓑ You can also click **Previous** (<) to see the previous photo.

Note: You can also navigate photos by pressing ➡ and ⬅.

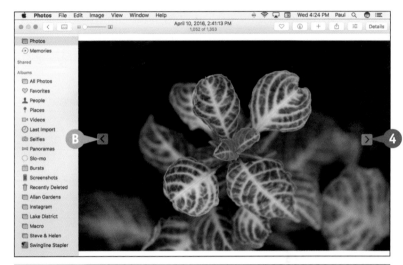

⑤ When you are done, click **Photos** or press ⌘+1 to return to the Photos view.

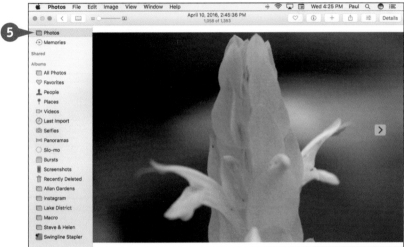

TIP

Is there a way that I can jump quickly to a particular photo in full-screen mode?
Yes. Click **View** and then click **Show Split View** (or press Option + S). Photos uses the left side of the window to show thumbnails of the photos in the current date. Use the vertical scroll bar to bring the thumbnail of the photo you want into view. Click the photo's thumbnail. Photos displays the photo in full-screen mode.

Create an Album

You can use Photos to organize your photos into albums. In Photos, an *album* is a collection of photos that are usually related in some way. For example, you might create an album for a series of vacation photos, for photos taken at a party or other special event, or for photos that include a particular person, pet, or place. Using your Photos library, you can create customized albums that include only the photos that you want to view.

Create an Album

1 Click **New** (**+**).

A To add an entire moment to a new album, you can move the mouse pointer (**↖**) over the moment and then click **New** (**+**) beside the moment.

2 Click **Album**.

Note: You can also start a new album by pressing **⌘**+**N**.

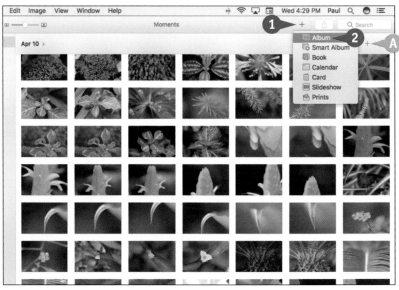

The Create New Album dialog appears.

3 Type a name for the new album.

4 Click **OK**.

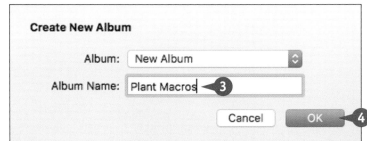

Photos prompts you to add items to the new album.

5 Click each photo you want to add to the album.

6 Click **Add**.

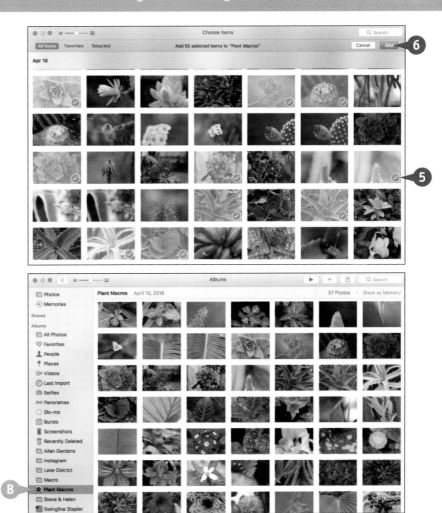

B The new album appears in the Albums section.

Is there any way to make Photos add photos to an album automatically?

Yes, you can create a *Smart Album* where the photos that appear in the album have one or more properties in common, such as the description, rating, date, or text in the photo title. Click **File** and then click **New Smart Album** (you can also press Option + ⌘ + N). Use the Smart Album dialog to create one or more rules that define what photos you want to appear in the album.

Crop a Photo

If you have a photo containing elements that you do not want to see, you can often cut out those elements. This is called *cropping*, and you can do this with the Photos app. When you crop a photo, you specify a rectangular area of the photo that you want to keep. Photos discards everything outside of the rectangle. Cropping is a useful feature because it can help give focus to the true subject of a photo. Cropping is also useful for removing extraneous elements that appear near the edges of a photo.

Crop a Photo

1 Open the photo you want to crop.

2 Click **Edit Photo** (≋).

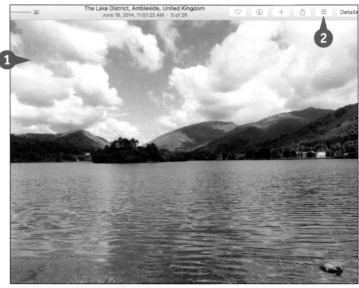

Photos displays its editing tools.

3 Click **Crop**.

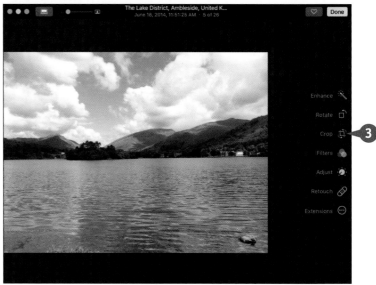

Photos displays a cropping rectangle on the photo.

④ Click and drag a corner or side to define the area you want to keep.

Note: Remember that Photos keeps the area inside the rectangle.

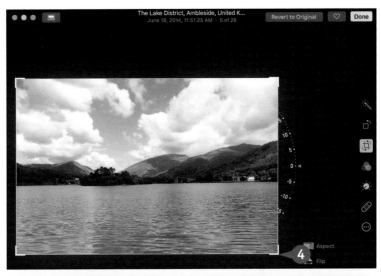

⑤ Click **Done**.

Photos saves the cropped photo and exits edit mode.

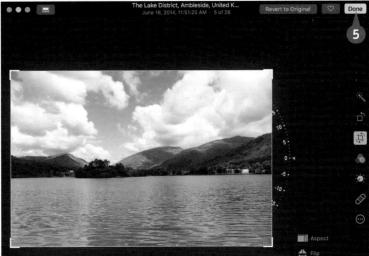

Is there a quick way to crop a photo to a certain size?
Yes, Photos enables you to specify either a specific shape, such as square, or a specific ratio, such as 4 x 3 or 16 x 9. Follow steps **1** to **3** to display the Crop tool. Click **Aspect** (Ⓐ) and then click the size or ratio you want to use. You can also click **Custom** (Ⓑ) to specify a custom ratio.

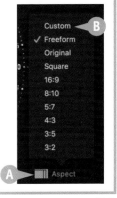

Rotate a Photo

You can rotate a photo using the Photos app. Depending on how you held your camera when you took a shot, the resulting photo might show the subject sideways or upside down. This may be the effect you want, but more likely this is a problem. To fix this problem, you can use Photos to rotate the photo so that the subject appears right-side up. You can rotate a photo either clockwise or counterclockwise.

Rotate a Photo

1 Open the photo you want to rotate.

Note: A quick way to rotate a photo is to right-click the photo and then click **Rotate Clockwise**.

2 Click **Edit Photo** (≋).

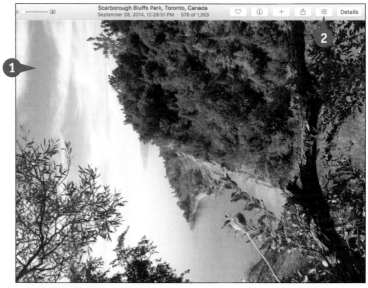

Photos displays its editing tools.

3 Click **Rotate**.

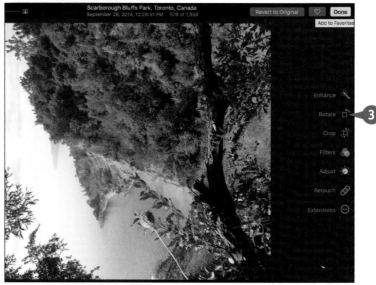

Ⓐ Photos rotates the photo 90 degrees counterclockwise.

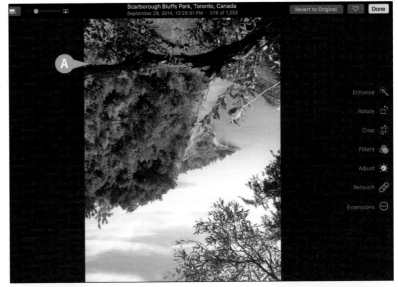

④ Repeat step **3** until the subject of the photo is right-side up.

⑤ Click **Done**.

Photos saves your changes and exits edit mode.

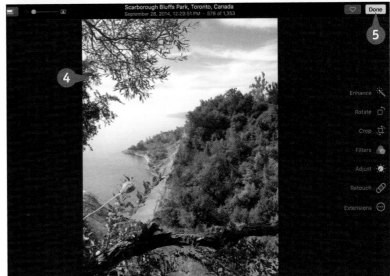

TIP

Can I rotate a photo clockwise instead?

Yes. With the editing tools displayed, press and hold Option. The Rotate icon changes from 🔁 to 🔁. Press and hold Option and then click **Rotate** to rotate the photo clockwise by 90 degrees. You can also right-click the photo and then click **Rotate Clockwise**.

Straighten a Photo

Yiou can straighten a crooked photo using the Photos app. If you do not use a tripod when taking
pictures, getting your camera perfectly level when you take a shot is very difficult and requires
a lot of practice and a steady hand. Despite your best efforts, you might end up with a photo
that is not quite level. To fix this problem, you can use Photos to nudge the photo clockwise or
counterclockwise so that the subject appears straight.

Straighten a Photo

1 Open the photo you want to
straighten.

2 Click **Edit Photo** (≋).

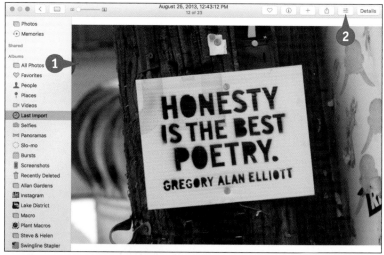

Photos displays its editing
tools.

3 Click **Crop**.

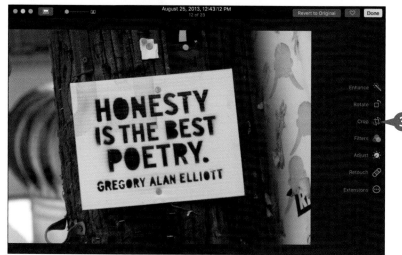

Photos displays its cropping and straightening tools.

4 Click and drag the **Angle** slider.

Drag the slider up to angle the photo counterclockwise.

Drag the slider down to angle the photo clockwise.

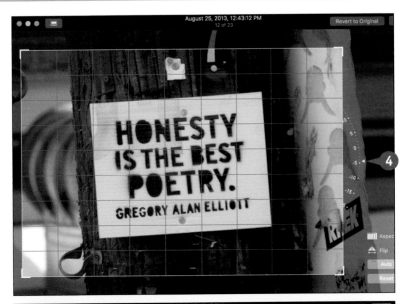

5 Click **Done**.

Photos saves your changes and exits edit mode.

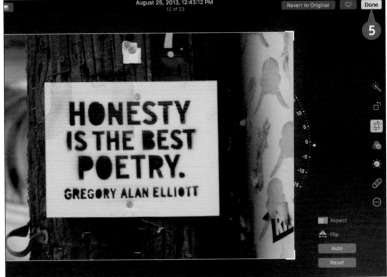

TIP

How do I know when my photo is level?
Use the gridlines that Photos places over the photo while you drag the **Angle** slider. Locate a horizontal line in your photo and then rotate the photo so that this line is parallel to the nearest horizontal line in the grid. You can also match a vertical line in the photo with a vertical line in the grid.

Remove Red Eye from a Photo

You can remove red eye from a photo using the Photos app. When you use a flash to take a picture of one or more people or animals, in some cases the flash may reflect off the subjects' retinas. The result is the common phenomenon of *red eye*, where each pupil appears red instead of black. If you have a photo where one or more subjects have red eyes due to the camera flash, you can use Photos to remove the red eye and give your subjects a more natural look.

Remove Red Eye from a Photo

1 Open the photo that contains the red eye.

2 Click **Edit Photo** (⊜).

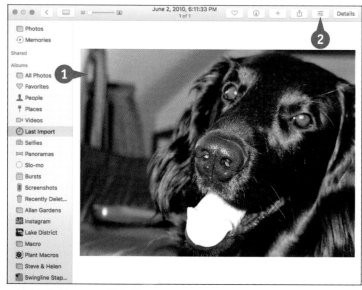

Photos displays its editing tools.

3 Click **Red-eye**.

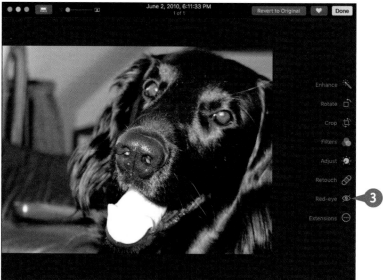

Photos displays its Red-eye controls.

A You may be able to fix the red eye automatically by clicking **Auto**. If that does not work, continue with the rest of these steps.

B If needed, you can click and drag this slider to the right to zoom in on the picture.

4 Move the Red-Eye pointer over a red eye in the photo.

5 Click the red eye.

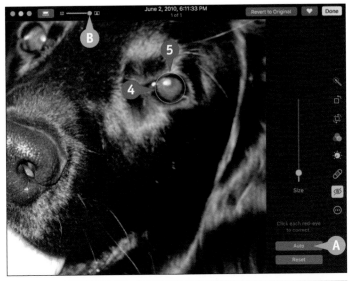

C Photos removes the red eye.

6 Repeat steps 4 and 5 to fix any other instances of red eye in the photo.

7 Click **Done**.

Photos saves your changes and exits edit mode.

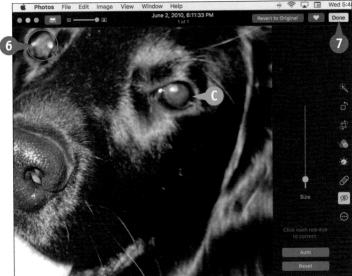

Why does Photos remove only part of the red eye in my photo?
The Red-Eye pointer may not be set to a large enough size. The tool should be approximately the same size as the subject's eye. If it is not, as shown here (A), follow steps 1 to 3 to display the Red-eye controls. Click and drag the **Size** slider until the Red-Eye pointer is the size of the red-eye area. Use your mouse to move the circle over the red eye and then click.

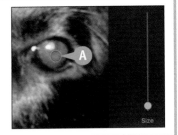

Add Names to Faces in Your Photos

Y̶ou can make your photos easier to manage and navigate by adding names to the faces that appear in each photo. This is sometimes called *tagging*, and it enables you to navigate your photos by name.

Specifically, Photos includes a special Faces section in its library, which organizes your faces according to the names you assign when you tag your photos. This makes it easy to view all your photos in which a certain person appears.

Add Names to Faces in Your Photos

1 Open the photo that you want to tag.

2 Click **Show Info** (ⓘ).

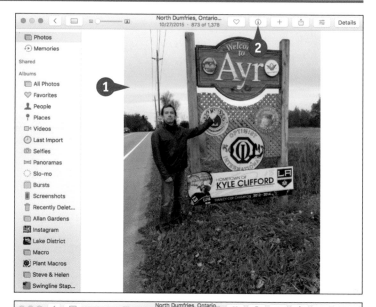

Photos displays information about the photo.

A Photos displays an icon for each face in the photo.

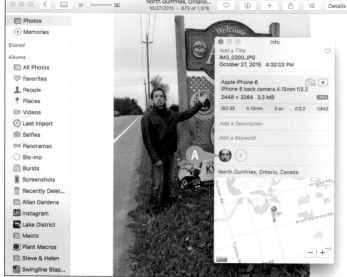

3 Click the icon for the face you want to work with Faces.

B Photos displays its naming tools around the face.

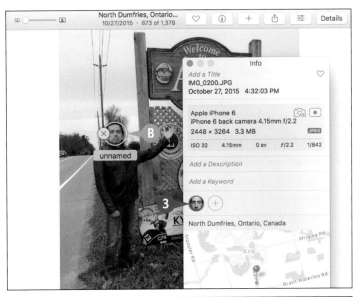

4 Type the person's name.

5 Press Return.

6 Repeat steps 3 to 5 to name each person in the photo.

7 Click **Close** (●).

Photos saves the changes and exits naming mode.

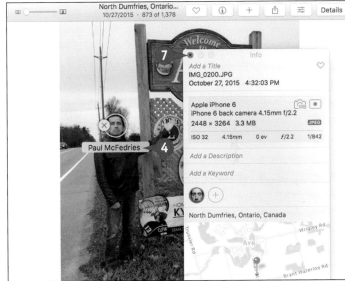

TIP

How do I view all the photos that contain a particular person?
You can open a photo, click **Show Info** (ⓘ), and then double-click the person's face. You can also click the **People** album. Photos displays the names and sample photos of each person you have named. Double-click the person you want to view. Photos displays all the photos that contain the person.

Mark Your Favorite Photos

You can make it easier and faster to find the photos you like best by marking those photos as favorites. If you take photos regularly, you can easily end up with hundreds or even thousands of images in your Photos library, and you might end up creating dozens of albums. Locating a cherished photo quickly becomes a time-consuming and frustrating chore. You can greatly speed up the task of locating such photos by marking them as favorites. Photos stores all your favorites in a special album, so it takes only a few clicks to view them.

Mark Your Favorite Photos

Mark a Single Photo

1. Open the photo that you want to mark as a favorite.

2. Click **Add to Favorites** (♡).

   Photos marks the photo as a favorite.

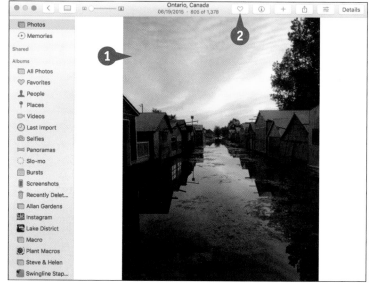

Mark Multiple Photos

1. Open the album that contains the photos you want to mark as favorites.

2. Press and hold ⌘ and click each photo you want to mark.

3. Click **Add to Favorites** (♡) in one of the selected photos.

   Photos marks all the selected photos as favorites.

Note: To view your favorites, you can click **Albums** and double-click the **Favorites** album.

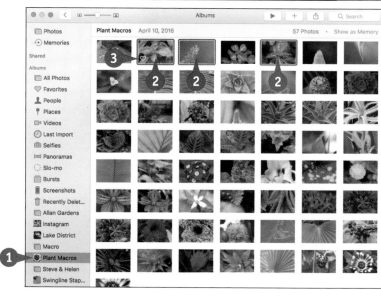

Set an Album's Key Photo

You can make it easier to navigate your albums and to understand the content of your albums by setting the key photo for each album. The *key photo* is the image that appears in the Albums view as the thumbnail used to display the album. As such, the key photo acts as a representative of all the photos in the album, so it should therefore either reflect the content of that album or contain text or an image that help you to identify the album.

Set an Album's Key Photo

1 Open the album you want to work with.

2 Double-click the image that you want to set as the album's key photo.

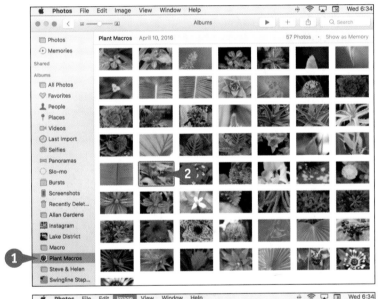

Photos opens the image.

3 Click **Image**.

4 Click **Make Key Photo**.

You can also press Shift + ⌘ + K.

Photos sets the image as the album's key photo.

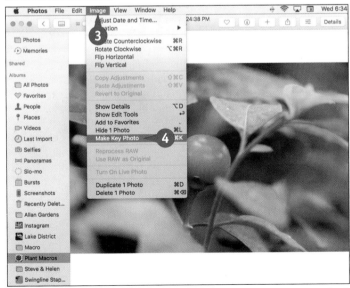

Email a Photo

If you have a photo that you want to share with someone, and you know that person's email address, you can send the photo in an email message. Using Photos, you can specify what photo you want to send, and Photos creates a new message. Even if a photo is very large, you can still send it via email because you can use Photos to shrink the copy of the photo that appears in the message.

Email a Photo

1 Open the photo you want to send.

2 Click **Share** (□).

3 Click **Mail**.

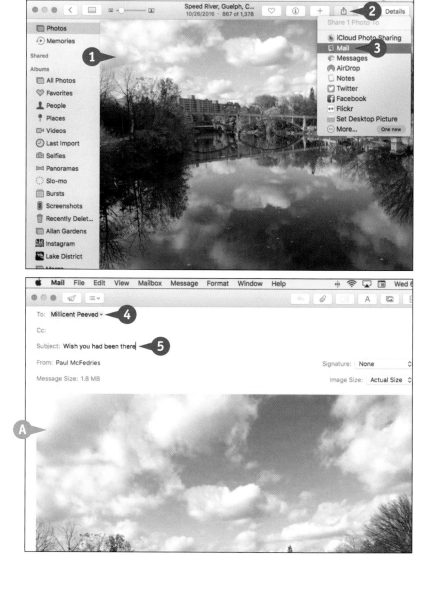

A Photos creates a new message and adds the photo to the message body.

4 Type the address of the message recipient.

5 Type the message subject.

⑥ Click to the left of the image.

⑦ Press **Return** once or twice to move the image down.

⑧ Click here and then type your message text.

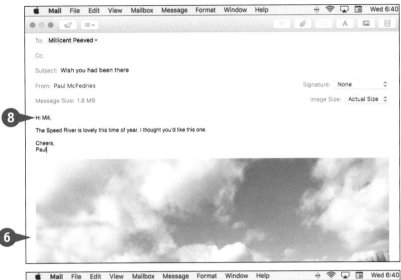

⑨ Click **Send**.

Photos sends the message with the photo.

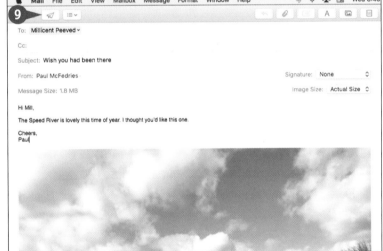

TIP

How do I change the size of the photo?
You need to be careful when sending photos because a single image can be several megabytes in size. If your recipient's email system places restrictions on the size of messages it can receive, your message might not go through.

To change the size of the photo, click the **Image Size** ⬍ and then click the size you want to use for the sent photo, such as Small or Medium. Note that this does not affect the size of the original photo, just the copy that is sent with the message.

Take Your Picture

You can use your Mac to take a picture of yourself. If your Mac comes with a built-in iSight or FaceTime HD camera, or if you have an external camera attached to your Mac, you can use the camera to take a picture of yourself using the Photo Booth application. After you take your picture, you can email that picture, add it to Photos, or set it as your user account or Messages buddy picture.

Take Your Picture

Take Your Picture with Photo Booth

1. Click **Spotlight** (🔍).

2. Type **photo booth**.

3. Click **Photo Booth**.

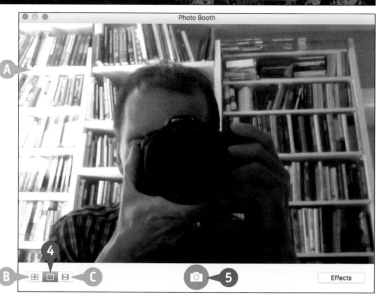

The Photo Booth window appears.

Ⓐ The live feed from the camera appears here.

4. Click **Take a still picture** (▢).

Ⓑ You can click **Take four quick pictures** (⊞) to snap four successive photos, each about 1 second apart.

Ⓒ You can click **Take a movie clip** (▤) to capture the camera feed as a movie.

5. Click **Take Photo** (📷).

Photo Booth counts down 3 seconds and then takes the photo.

Work with Your Photo Booth Picture

D Photo Booth displays the picture.

1 Click the picture.

2 Click **Share** (⬆).

E You can click **Add to Photos** to add the image to the Photos app.

F You can click **Change Profile Picture** to set the photo as your user account picture.

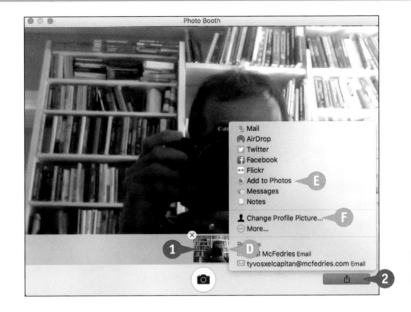

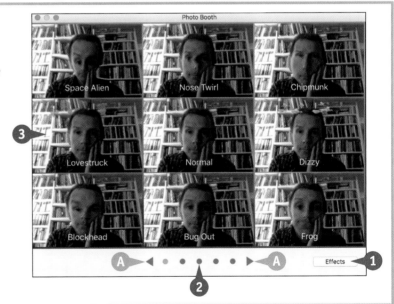

TIP

Can I make my photos more interesting?

Definitely. Photo Booth comes with around two dozen special effects. Follow these steps:

1 Click **Effects**.

2 Click an icon to select a different page of effects.

A You can also use the arrows (◀ and ▶) to change pages.

3 Click the effect you want to use.

217

Play Digital Video with QuickTime Player

macOS comes with an application called QuickTime Player that can play digital video files in various formats. You will mostly use QuickTime Player to play digital video files stored on your Mac, but you can also use the application to play digital video from the web.

QuickTime Player enables you to open video files, navigate the digital video playback, and control the digital video volume. Although you learn only how to play digital video files in this section, the version of QuickTime that comes with macOS comes with many extra features, including the capability to record movies and audio and to cut and paste scenes.

Play Digital Video with QuickTime Player

1 Click **Spotlight** (🔍).

2 Type **quick**.

3 Click **QuickTime Player**.

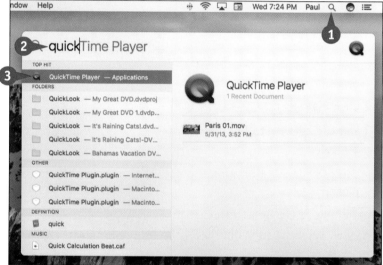

The QuickTime Player application appears. If you see the Open dialog, skip to step **6**.

4 Click **File**.

5 Click **Open File**.

Note: You can also press ⌘+O.

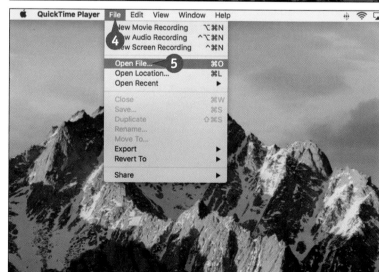

The Open dialog appears.

6 Locate and click the video file you want to play.

7 Click **Open**.

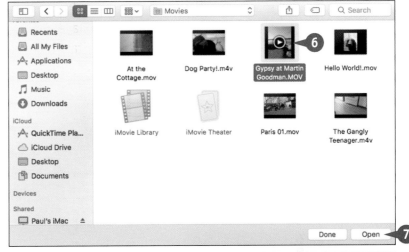

QuickTime opens a new player window.

8 Click **Play** (▶).

Ⓐ You can click ▶▶ to fast-forward the video.

Ⓑ You can click ◀◀ to rewind the video.

Ⓒ You can click and drag this slider to adjust the volume.

If you want to view the video in full-screen mode, press ⌘+F.

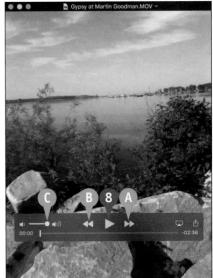

TIP

Can I use QuickTime Player to play a video from the web?
Yes. As long as you know the Internet address of the video, QuickTime Player can play most video formats available on the web. In QuickTime Player, click **File** and then click **Open Location** (or press ⌘+U). In the Open URL dialog, type or paste the video address in the Movie Location text box and then click **Open**.

CHAPTER 11

Securing macOS

Threats to your computing-related security and privacy often come from the Internet and from someone simply using your Mac while you are not around. To protect yourself and your family, you need to understand these threats and know what you can do to thwart them.

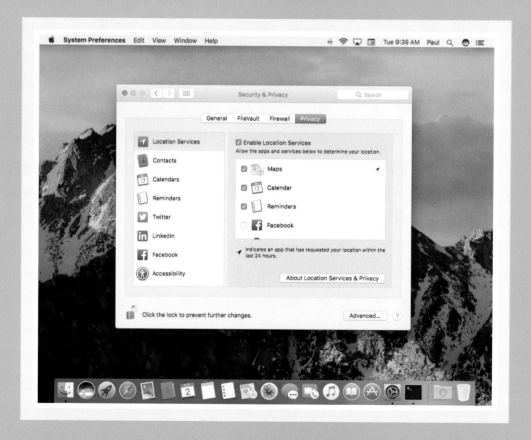

Change Your Password

You can make macOS more secure by changing your password. For example, if you turn on file sharing, as described in Chapter 15, you can configure each shared folder so that only someone who knows your password can get full access to that folder. Similarly, you should change your password if other network users know your current password and you no longer want them to have access to your shared folders. Finally, you should also change your password if you feel that your current password is too easy to guess. See the Tip to learn how to create a secure password.

Change Your Password

1 Click **System Preferences** (⚙).

The System Preferences appear.

2 Click **Users & Groups**.

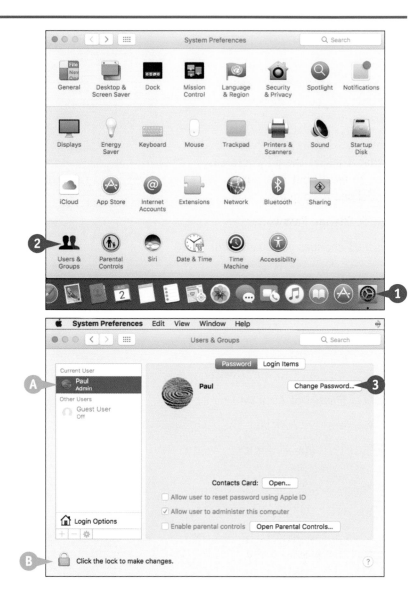

The Users & Groups preferences appear.

Ⓐ Your user account is selected automatically.

Ⓑ If you want to work with a different user account, you must click the lock icon (🔒), type your administrator password (🔒 changes to 🔓), and then click the account.

3 Click **Change Password**.

The Change Password dialog appears.

④ Type your current password.

⑤ Type your new password.

⑥ Retype the new password.

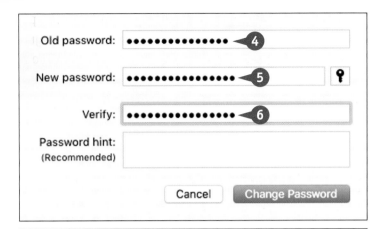

⑦ Type a hint that macOS will display if you forget the password.

Note: Construct the hint in such a way that it makes the password easy for you to recall, but hard for a potential snoop to guess.

⑧ Click **Change Password**.

macOS changes your password.

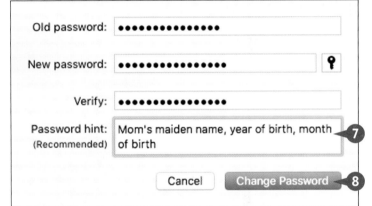

TIP

How do I create a secure password?
Follow these steps:

① Follow steps 1 to 4 in this section.

② Click **Password Assistant** (🔑).

The Password Assistant dialog appears.

③ Click the **Type** ⬍ and then click a password type.

④ Click and drag the **Length** slider to set the password length you want to use.

⑤ Click the **Suggestion** ⌄ and then click the password you want to use.

⑥ Click **Close** (⬤).

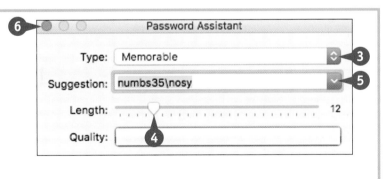

You can enhance your Mac's security by configuring macOS to ask for your user account password when the system wakes up from either the screen saver or sleep mode. Protecting your account with a password prevents someone from logging on to your account, but what happens when you leave your Mac unattended? If you remain logged on to the system, any person who sits down at your computer can use it to view and change files.

To prevent this, activate the screen saver or sleep mode before you leave your Mac unattended, and configure macOS to require a password on waking.

Require a Password on Waking

1 Click **Apple** (🍎).

2 Click **System Preferences**.

You can also click **System Preferences** (🕐) in the Dock.

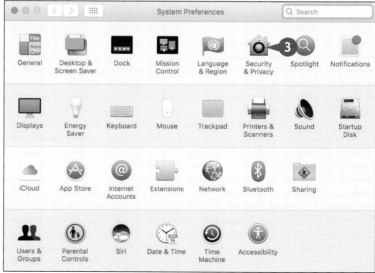

The System Preferences appear.

3 Click **Security & Privacy**.

The Security & Privacy preferences appear.

④ Click the **General** tab.

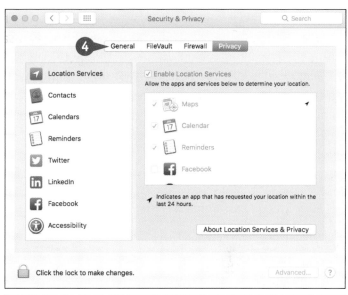

⑤ Click the **Require password** check box (☐ changes to ☑).

⑥ Click **Close** (●).

macOS puts the new setting into effect.

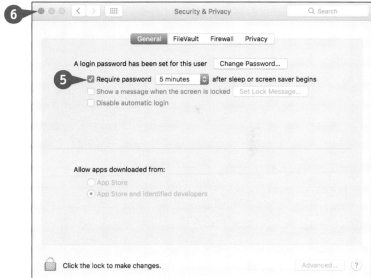

TIPS

How do I activate the screen saver or sleep mode before I leave my Mac unattended?

To put your Mac display to sleep, press `Control` + `Shift` and then press the eject key (⏏). To engage full sleep mode, click **Apple** ( ) and then click **Sleep**.

If I engage the screen saver or sleep mode accidentally, entering my password is a hassle. Is there a workaround for this?

Yes, you can tell macOS to not require the password as soon as the screen saver or sleep mode is activated. Follow steps **1** to **5**, click the **Require password** , and then click the amount of time you want macOS to wait.

Disable Automatic Logins

You can enhance your Mac's security by preventing macOS from logging in to your user account automatically. If you are the only person who uses your Mac, you can configure macOS to automatically log in to your account. This saves time at startup by avoiding the login screen, but it opens a security hole. If a snoop or other malicious user has access to your Mac, that person can start the computer and gain access to your documents, settings, web browsing history, and network. To prevent this, configure macOS to disable the automatic login.

Disable Automatic Logins

① Click **Apple** (⚫).

② Click **System Preferences**.

You can also click **System Preferences** (⚙) in the Dock.

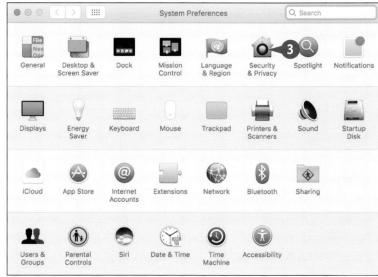

The System Preferences appear.

③ Click **Security & Privacy**.

The Security & Privacy preferences appear.

4 Click the lock icon (🔒).

macOS prompts you for your administrator password.

5 Type the administrator password.

6 Click **Unlock**.

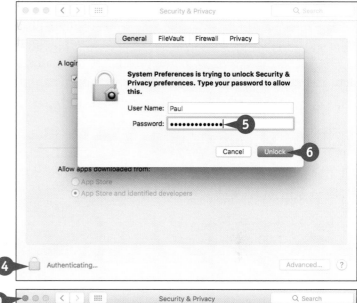

macOS unlocks the preferences (🔒 changes to 🔓).

7 Click the **General** tab.

8 Click the **Disable automatic login** check box (☐ changes to ☑).

9 Click **Close** (⬤).

macOS puts the new setting into effect.

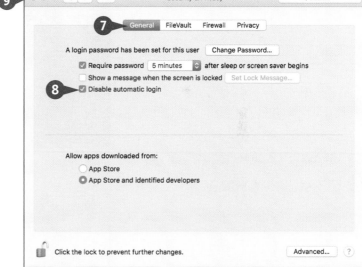

TIP

Is there a way to get macOS to log out of my account automatically?
Yes, you can configure the system to log you out of your account when macOS has been idle for a specified amount of time. Follow steps **1** to **7** to unlock and display the General tab and then click **Advanced**. In the dialog that appears, click the **Log out after *X* minutes of inactivity** check box (☐ changes to ☑) and then use the spin box to set the amount of idle time after which macOS logs you out automatically. You can select a time as short as 5 minutes and as long as 960 minutes.

Configure App Downloads

You can ensure that malware cannot be installed on your Mac by configuring the system to allow only app downloads from the Mac App Store. By default, macOS allows downloads from the App Store and from so-called *identified developers*. The reason for this heightened security is that malware developers are starting to target Macs now that they have become so popular. The extra security is a response to that and is designed to prevent users from accidentally installing malware. However, you can configure this feature to be even more secure, which is useful if you are setting up a user account for a child.

Configure App Downloads

1 Click **Apple** (🍎).

2 Click **System Preferences**.

You can also click **System Preferences** (⚙) in the Dock.

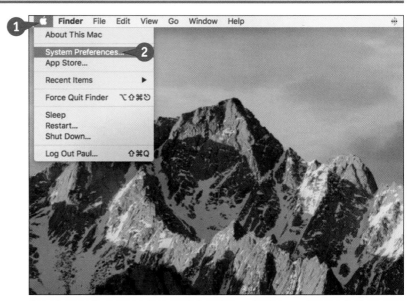

The System Preferences appear.

3 Click **Security & Privacy**.

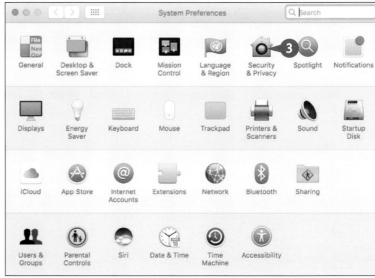

The Security & Privacy preferences appear.

④ Click the lock icon (🔒).

macOS prompts you for your administrator password.

⑤ Type the administrator password.

⑥ Click **Unlock**.

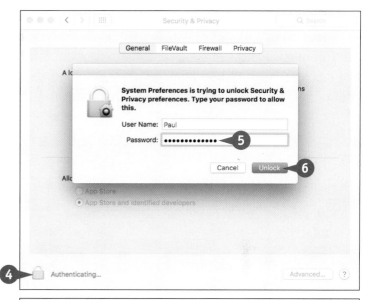

macOS unlocks the preferences (🔒 changes to 🔓).

⑦ Click the **General** tab.

⑧ Click the **App Store** option (○ changes to ◉).

⑨ Click **Close** (●).

macOS puts the new setting into effect.

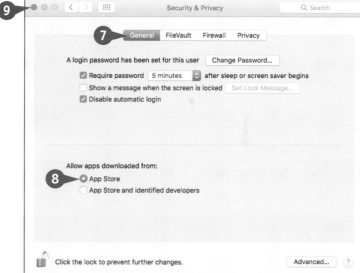

What is an identified developer?

An *identified developer* has registered with Apple and has a security certificate for digitally signing apps, thus certifying where the apps came from. It is possible a malicious developer could spoof a digitally signed app, so allowing only App Store apps is the safest option.

How can I install an app that I downloaded from the web?

If you are certain the app is legitimate — it was created by a reputable developer and purchased from a reputable dealer — double-click the downloaded file to open the disk image. Right-click (or Control-click) the installer, click **Open**, and then click **Open** when macOS asks you to confirm.

Turn On the Firewall

You can make your Mac's Internet connection much more secure by turning on the macOS firewall. A *firewall* is a tool designed to prevent malicious users from accessing a computer connected to the Internet. Chances are your network router already implements a hardware firewall, but you can add an extra layer of protection by also activating the macOS software firewall. This will not affect your normal Internet activities, such as web browsing, emailing, and instant messaging.

Turn On the Firewall

1 Click **Apple** ().

2 Click **System Preferences**.

You can also click **System Preferences** () in the Dock.

The System Preferences appear.

3 Click **Security & Privacy**.

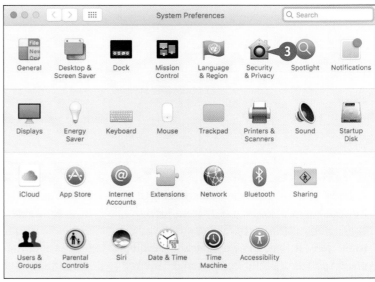

The Security & Privacy preferences appear.

④ Click the lock icon (🔒).

macOS prompts you for your administrator password.

⑤ Type the administrator password.

⑥ Click **Unlock**.

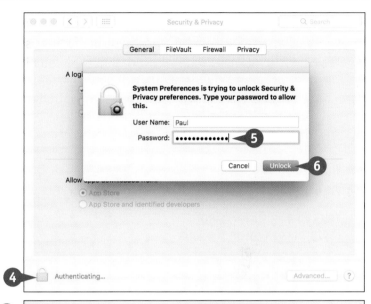

macOS unlocks the preferences (🔒 changes to 🔓).

⑦ Click the **Firewall** tab.

⑧ Click **Turn On Firewall**.

⑨ Click **Close** (⬤).

macOS puts the new setting into effect.

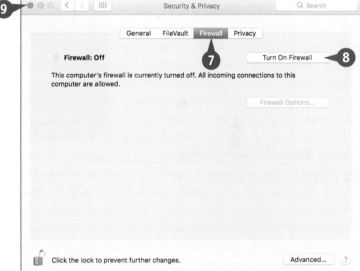

TIPS

Can I prevent online malicious users from finding my Mac?

Yes. Malicious users often probe connected machines for vulnerabilities, so put macOS into *stealth mode*, which hides it from these probes. Follow steps **1** to **7**, click **Firewall Options**, click the **Enable stealth mode** check box (☐ changes to ☑), and then click **OK**.

Can I use Internet apps such as my FTP program through the firewall?

macOS allows digitally signed apps to receive connections, but to use an Internet app that is not digitally signed you must add it as an exception. Follow steps **1** to **7**, click **Firewall Options**, click **Add** (+), click the application you want to use, and then click **Add**.

Configure Location Services

*L*ocation services refers to the features and technologies that provide apps and system tools with access to location data, particularly the current location of your Mac. This is a handy and useful thing, but it is also something that you need to keep under your control because your location data, especially your current location, is fundamentally private and should not be given to applications thoughtlessly. Fortunately, macOS comes with a few tools for controlling and configuring location services.

Configure Location Services

1 Click **Apple** (🍎).

2 Click **System Preferences**.

You can also click **System Preferences** (⚙) in the Dock.

The System Preferences appear.

3 Click **Security & Privacy**.

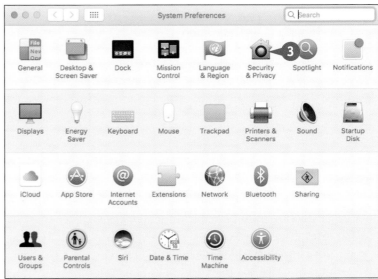

The Security & Privacy preferences appear.

④ Click the lock icon (🔒).

macOS prompts you for your administrator password.

⑤ Type the administrator password.

⑥ Click **Unlock**.

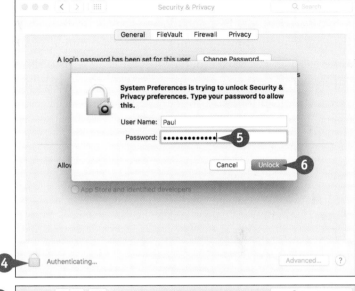

macOS unlocks the preferences (🔒 changes to 🔓).

⑦ Click the **Privacy** tab.

⑧ Click **Location Services**.

⑨ Click the check box beside each app that you do not want to determine your location (✓ changes to ☐).

Note: This list will be empty if none of your apps have requested to use location services.

⑩ Click **Close** (●).

macOS puts the new setting into effect.

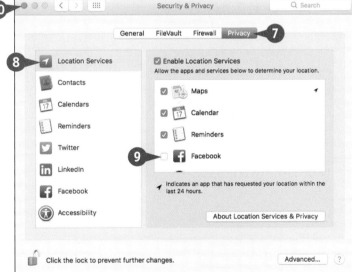

How does the location services feature know my location?

Location services uses several bits of data to determine your location. First, it looks for known Wi-Fi networks that are near your location. Second, if you are connected to the Internet, it uses the location information embedded in your unique Internet Protocol (IP) address.

Can I turn off location services?

Yes. Follow steps **1** to **7** to unlock and display the Privacy tab. Click **Location Services** and then click the **Enable Location Services** check box (✓ changes to ☐). Note, however, that by turning off location services, you disable many features in apps such as Reminders and Maps.

Enable the Guest User Account

You can give a family member, friend, or other visitor temporary and secure access to your Mac or your network by letting that person log in using the built-in Guest User account. This account is given only limited privileges, so anyone logged in under that account cannot access or edit your data, change macOS settings, or install apps. Also, any files created by the Guest User account are deleted when that account logs out. The Guest User account is disabled by default, so to allow your visitor to log in under that account, you must first enable it.

Enable the Guest User Account

1. Click **System Preferences** (⚙).

   The System Preferences appear.

2. Click **Users & Groups**.

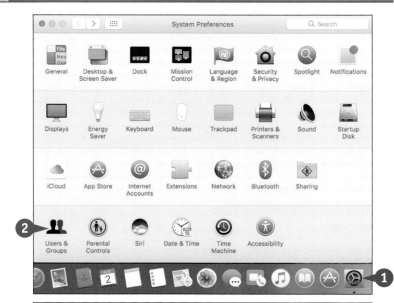

The Users & Groups preferences appear.

3. Click the lock icon (🔒).

   macOS prompts you for your administrator password.

4. Type the administrator password.

5. Click **Unlock**.

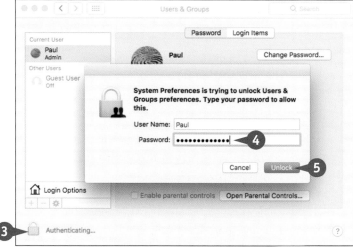

macOS unlocks the preferences
(🔒 changes to 🔓).

6 Click **Guest User**.

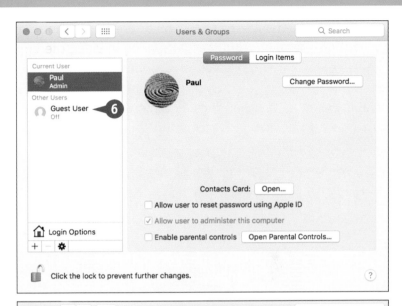

7 Click the **Allow guests to log in to this computer** check box
(☐ changes to ☑).

Visitors can now log in to your Mac using the Guest User account.

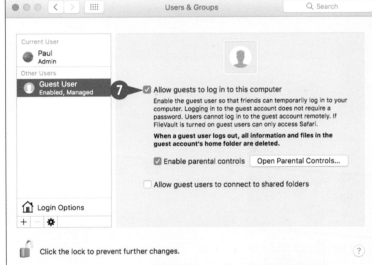

How do visitors log in using the Guest User account?
Once you have activated the Guest User account, follow these steps to log in to your Mac with the Guest User account:

1 Click your user name in the menu bar.

2 Click **Guest User**.

Alternatively, you can click **Apple** (🍎), click **Log Out** *User*, where *User* is your user name, and then click **Log Out**. In the login window, click **Guest User**.

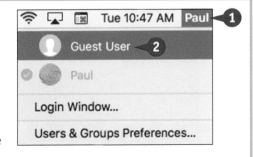

Customizing macOS

macOS comes with a number of features that enable you to customize your Mac. For example, you might not like the default desktop background or the layout of the Dock. Not only can you change the appearance of macOS to suit your taste, but you can also change the way macOS works to make it easier and more efficient for you to use.

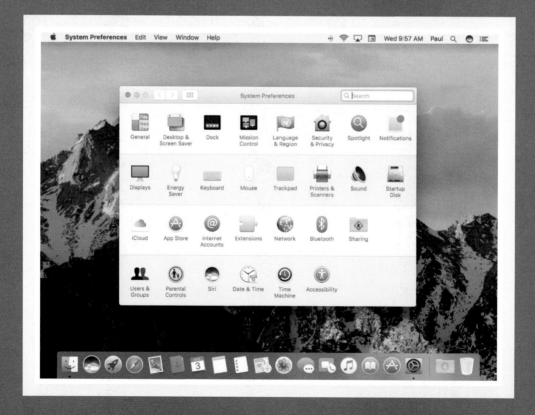

Display System Preferences

You can find many of the macOS customization features in System Preferences, a collection of settings and options that control the overall look and operation of macOS. You can use System Preferences to change the desktop background, specify a screen saver, set your Mac's sleep options, add user accounts, and customize the Dock, to name some of the tasks that you learn about in this chapter. To use these settings, you must know how to display the System Preferences.

Display System Preferences

Open System Preferences

① In the Dock, click **System Preferences** (⚙).

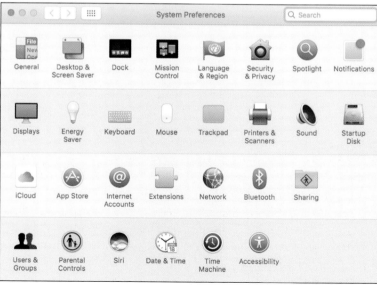

The System Preferences appear.

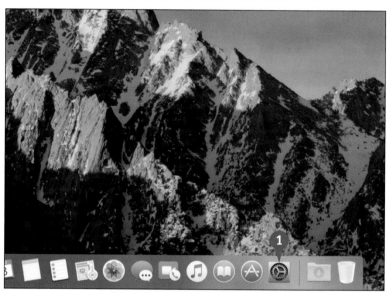

Close System Preferences

1 Click **System Preferences**.

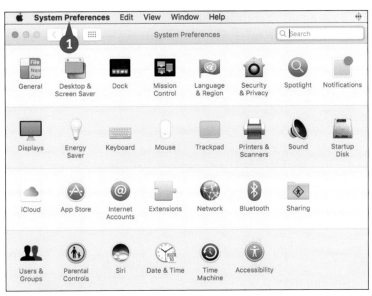

2 Click **Quit System Preferences**.

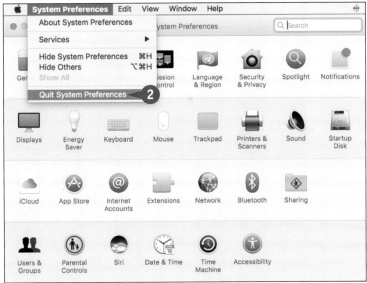

TIPS

Are there other methods I can use to open System Preferences?

If you have hidden the Dock (see the section "Hide the Dock") or removed the System Preferences icon from the Dock, you can click **Apple** (🍎) and then click **System Preferences**.

Sometimes when I open System Preferences, I do not see all the icons. How can I restore the original icons?

When you click an icon in System Preferences, the window changes to show just the options and settings associated with that icon. To return to the main System Preferences window, click ⟨ until the window appears. You can also click **Show All** (▦) or press ⌘+🅛.

Change the Desktop Background

To give macOS a different look, you can change the default desktop background. macOS offers a wide variety of desktop background options. For example, macOS comes with several dozen images you can use, from abstract patterns to photos of plants and other natural images. You can also choose a solid color as the desktop background, or you can use one of your own photos. You can change the desktop background to show either a fixed image or a series of images that change periodically.

Change the Desktop Background

Set a Fixed Background Image

1 In the Dock, click **System Preferences** (⚙) (not shown).

2 In the System Preferences, click **Desktop & Screen Saver**.

Note: You can also right-click (or `Control`-click) the desktop and then click **Change Desktop Background**.

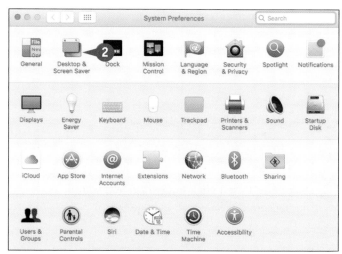

The Desktop & Screen Saver preferences appear.

3 Click **Desktop**.

4 Click the image category you want to use.

A To add a folder, you can click **Add** (➕), open the folder, and then click **Choose**.

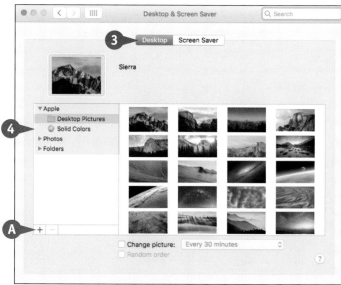

5 Click the image you want to use as the desktop background.

Your Mac changes the desktop background.

6 If you chose a photo in step **5**, click ⬍ and then click an option to determine how your Mac displays the photo.

Note: Another way to set a fixed background image is to select a photo in the Photos app, click **Share** (📤), and then click **Set Desktop**.

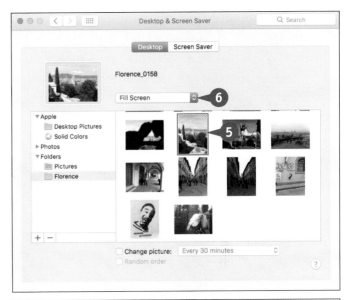

Set a Changing Background Image

1 Click the **Change picture** check box (☐ changes to ☑).

2 Click ⬍ and then click how often you want the background image to change.

3 If you want your Mac to choose the periodic image randomly, click the **Random order** check box (☐ changes to ☑).

Your Mac changes the desktop background periodically based on your chosen interval.

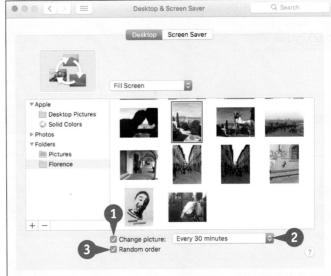

TIP

How do the various options differ for displaying a photo?

Your Mac gives you five options: **Fill Screen** expands the photo proportionally in all four directions until it fills the entire desktop. **Fit to Screen** expands the photo proportionally in all four directions until the photo is either the same height as the desktop or the same width as the desktop. **Stretch to Fill Screen** expands the photo in all four directions until it fills the entire desktop; the resulting image may no longer be proportional as a result. **Center** displays the photo at its actual size and places the photo in the center of the desktop. **Tile** repeats your photo multiple times to fill the entire desktop.

Set Your Mac's Sleep Options

You can make macOS more energy-efficient by configuring parts of your Mac to go into sleep mode automatically when you are not using them. *Sleep mode* means that your display or your Mac is in a temporary low-power mode. This saves energy on all Macs, and saves battery power on a notebook Mac. For example, you can set up macOS to put the display to sleep automatically after a period of inactivity. Similarly, you can configure macOS to put your entire Mac to sleep after you have not used it for a specified amount of time.

Set Your Mac's Sleep Options

Open the Energy Saver Preferences

1 In the Dock, click **System Preferences** (icon) (not shown).

2 In the System Preferences, click **Energy Saver**.

The Energy Saver preferences appear.

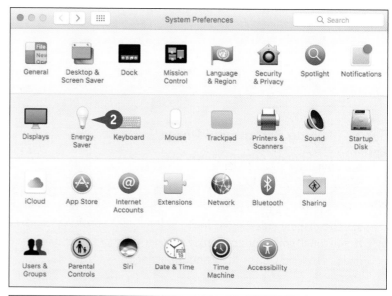

Set Sleep Options for a Desktop Mac

1 Click and drag the slider to set the display sleep timer.

This specifies the period of inactivity after which your display goes to sleep.

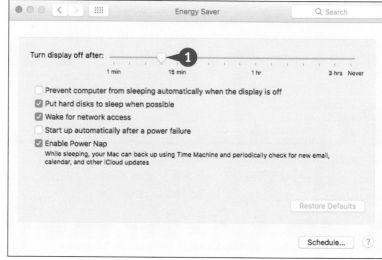

Set Sleep Options for a Notebook Mac

1 Click **Battery**.

2 Click and drag the slider to set the computer sleep timer for when your Mac is on battery power.

3 Click and drag the slider to set the display sleep timer for when your Mac is on battery power.

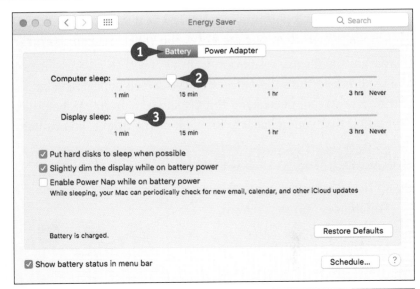

4 Click **Power Adapter**.

5 Click and drag the slider to set the computer sleep timer for when your Mac is plugged in.

6 Click and drag the slider to set the display sleep timer for when your Mac is plugged in.

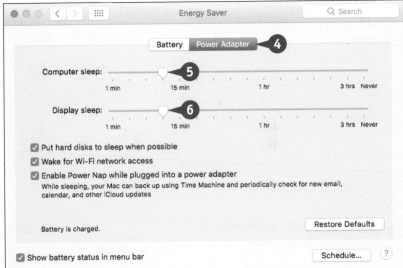

TIPS

How do I wake a sleeping display or computer?

If your Mac's display is in sleep mode, you can wake it by moving your mouse pointer (▶) or sliding your finger on the trackpad. You can also wake up the display or your entire Mac by pressing any key.

I changed the display sleep timer, and now I never see my screen saver. Why?

You set the display sleep timer to less than your screen saver timer. For example, if you configured the screen saver timer to 15 minutes and the display sleep timer to 10 minutes, macOS always puts the display to sleep before the screen saver appears.

Change the Display Resolution and Brightness

You can change the resolution and the brightness of the macOS display. This enables you to adjust the display for best viewing or for maximum compatibility with whatever application you are using.

Increasing the display resolution is an easy way to create more space on the screen for applications and windows because the objects on the screen appear smaller. Conversely, if you have trouble reading text on the screen, decreasing the display resolution can help because the screen objects appear larger. If you find that your display is too dark or too bright, you can adjust the brightness for best viewing.

Change the Display Resolution and Brightness

1 In the Dock, click **System Preferences** (🔘) (not shown).

2 In the System Preferences, click **Displays**.

The Displays preferences appear.

3 Click **Display**.

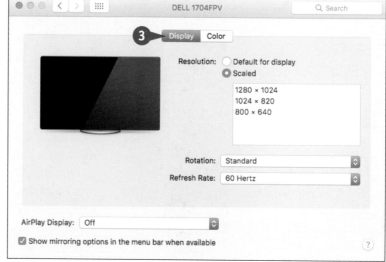

4 Select the resolution:

Ⓐ To have macOS set the resolution based on your display, you can click the **Default for display** option (◯ changes to ◉).

Ⓑ To set the resolution yourself, you can click the **Scaled** option (◯ changes to ◉) and then click the resolution you want to use.

macOS adjusts the screen to the new resolution.

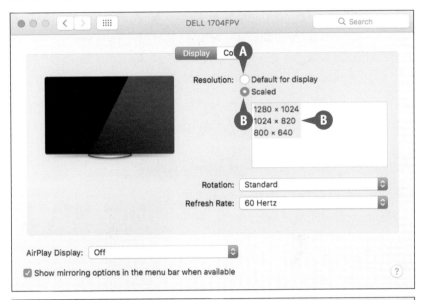

5 For some screens, you can click and drag the **Brightness** slider to set the display brightness.

macOS adjusts the screen to the new brightness.

Ⓒ If you do not want macOS to adjust the notebook screen brightness based on the ambient light, you can click the **Ambient light compensation** check box (☑ changes to ☐).

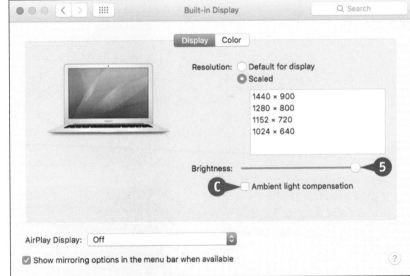

TIPS

What do the resolution numbers mean?
These numbers are expressed in *pixels*, which are the individual dots that make up what you see on your Mac's screen, arranged in rows and columns. So a resolution of 1440 x 900 means that the display is using 1,440-pixel rows and 900-pixel columns.

Why do some resolutions also include the word "stretched"?
Most older displays use an aspect ratio (width to the height) of 4:3. However, most new displays use a *widescreen* aspect ratio of either 16:9 or 16:10. Resolutions designed for 4:3 displays use only part of a widescreen display. To make them use the entire display, choose the *stretched* version of the resolution, although in some cases this may distort screen text and images.

245

Create an App Folder in Launchpad

You can make Launchpad easier to use by combining multiple icons into a single storage area called an *app folder*. Normally, Launchpad displays icons in up to five rows per screen, with at least seven icons in each row, so you can have at least 35 icons in each screen. Also, if you have configured your Mac with a relatively low display resolution, you might see only partial app names in Launchpad.

All this can make it difficult to locate your apps. However, app folders can help you organize similar apps and reduce the clutter on the Launchpad screens.

Create an App Folder in Launchpad

1 Click **Launchpad** (📍).

Ⓐ Launchpad displays icons for each installed application.

2 Click the dot for the Launchpad screen you want to work with.

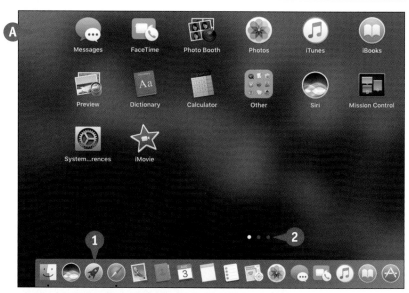

3 Click and drag an icon that you want to include in the folder, and drop it on another icon that you want to include in the same folder.

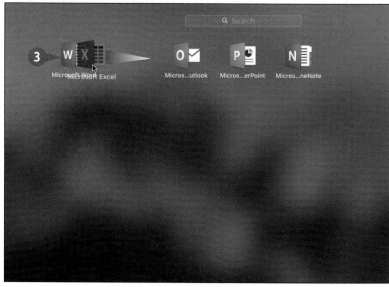

Launchpad creates the app folder.

B Launchpad applies a name to the folder based on the type of applications in the folder.

C Launchpad adds the icons to the app folder.

D To specify a different name, you can click the name and then type the one you prefer.

4 Click the Launchpad screen, outside of the app folder.

E Launchpad displays the app folder.

5 To add more icons to the new app folder, click and drag each icon and drop it on the folder.

Note: To launch a program from an app folder, you can click **Launchpad** (✈), click the app folder to open it, and then click the program's icon.

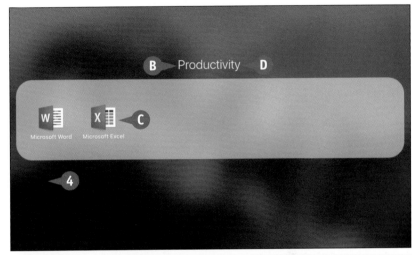

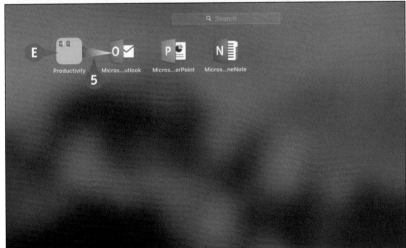

How do I make changes to an app folder?
Open Launchpad and then click the app folder. To rename the folder, click the current name, type the new name, and then press `Return`. To rearrange the icons, drag and drop the apps within the folder. When you are done, click outside the app folder.

How do I remove an icon from an app folder?
Open Launchpad and then click the app folder. To remove an app, click and drag the app out of the folder. Launchpad closes the folder, and you can then drop the icon within the Launchpad screen.

Add a User Account

You can share your Mac with another person by creating a user account for that person. This enables the person to log in to macOS and use the system. The new user account is completely separate from your own account. This means that the other person can change settings, create documents, and perform other macOS tasks without interfering with your own settings or data. For maximum privacy for all users, you should set up each user account with a password.

Add a User Account

1 In the Dock, click **System Preferences** (⊚) (not shown).

2 In the System Preferences, click **Users & Groups**.

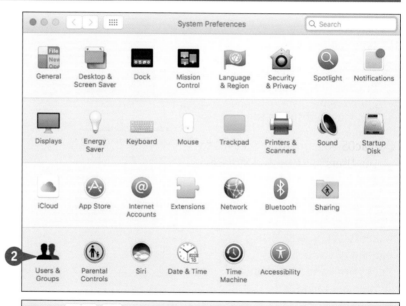

Ⓐ To modify accounts, you must click the lock icon (🔒) and then type your administrator password (🔒 changes to 🔓).

3 Click **Add** (+).

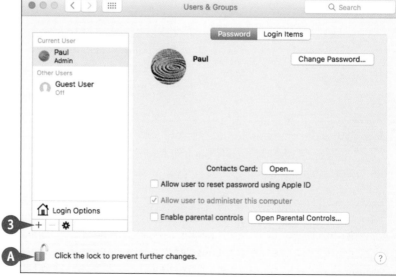

The New Account dialog appears.

④ Click the **New Account** ◆ and then click an account type.

⑤ Type the user's name.

⑥ Edit the short username that macOS creates.

⑦ Type and retype the user's password.

⑧ Type a hint that macOS will display if the user forgets the password.

⑨ Click **Create User**.

Ⓑ macOS adds the user account to the Users & Groups preferences.

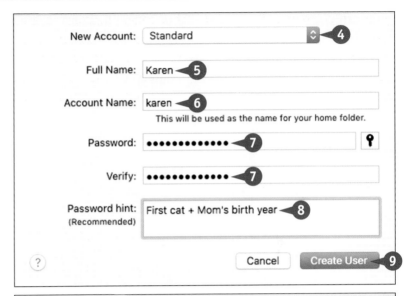

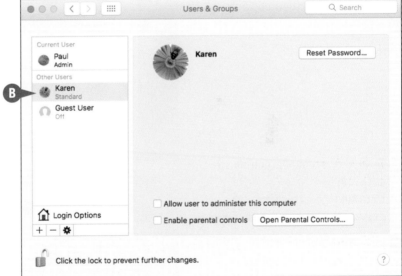

TIPS

Which account type should I use for the new account?

The Standard type is a good choice because it can make changes only to its own account settings. Avoid the Administrator type because it enables the user to make major changes to the system. Consider the Managed with Parental Controls account type for children.

How do I change the user's picture?

Click the user and then click the picture. macOS displays a list of the available images. If you see one you like, click it. If your Mac has a camera attached and the user is nearby, you can click **Camera** and then click **Camera** (📷) to take the user's picture.

Customize the Dock

You can customize various aspects of the Dock by using System Preferences to modify a few Dock options. For example, you can make the Dock take up less room on the screen by adjusting the size of the Dock. You can also make the Dock a bit easier to use by turning on the Magnification feature, which enlarges Dock icons when you position the mouse pointer (▶) over them. You can also make the Dock easier to access and use by moving it to either side of the screen.

Customize the Dock

1 In the Dock, click **System Preferences** (⚙).

2 In the System Preferences, click **Dock**.

Note: You can also open the Dock preferences by clicking **Apple** (), clicking **Dock**, and then clicking **Dock Preferences**.

The Dock preferences appear.

3 Click and drag the **Size** slider to make the Dock smaller or larger.

A You can also click and drag the Dock divider: Drag up to increase the Dock size, and drag down to decrease the Dock size.

B System Preferences adjusts the size of the Dock.

Note: If your Dock is already as wide as the screen, dragging the Size slider to the right (toward the Large value) has no effect.

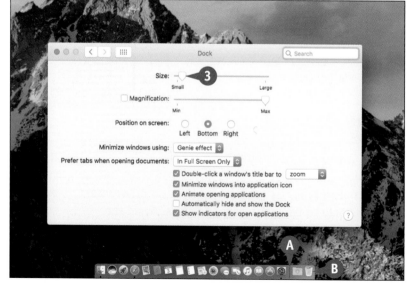

④ Click the **Magnification** check box (☐ changes to ☑).

⑤ Click and drag the **Magnification** slider to set the magnification level.

ⓒ When you position the mouse pointer (▶) over a Dock icon, your Mac magnifies the icon.

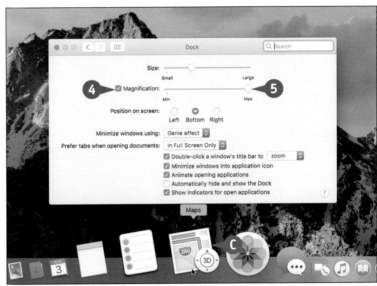

⑥ Use the **Position on screen** options to click where you want the Dock to appear, such as the **Left** side of the screen (◯ changes to ◉).

ⓓ Your Mac moves the Dock to the new position.

⑦ Click the **Minimize windows using** ⬍ and then click the effect you want your Mac to use when you minimize a window by clicking ⬤ in the window's toolbar: **Genie effect** or **Scale effect**.

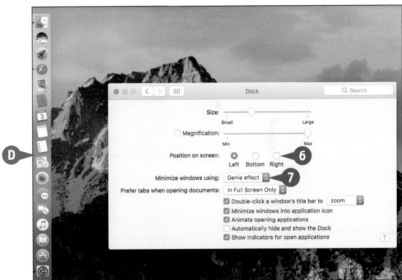

TIP

Is there an easier method I can use to control some of these preferences?
Yes, you can control these preferences directly from the Dock. To set the Dock size, click and drag the Dock divider left or right. For the other preferences, right-click (or **Control**-click) the Dock divider. Click **Turn Magnification On** to enable the magnification feature; click **Turn Magnification Off** to disable this feature. To change the Dock position, click **Position on Screen** and then click **Left**, **Bottom**, or **Right**. To set the minimize effect, click **Minimize Using** and then click either **Genie Effect** or **Scale Effect**.

Add an Icon to the Dock

The icons on the Dock are convenient because you can open them with just a single click. You can enhance the convenience of the Dock by adding an icon for an application you use frequently.

The icon remains in the Dock even when the application is closed, so you can always open the application with a single click. You can add an icon to the Dock even if the program is not currently running.

Add an Icon to the Dock

Add an Icon for a Nonrunning Application

1 Click **Finder** (🙂).

2 Click **Applications**.

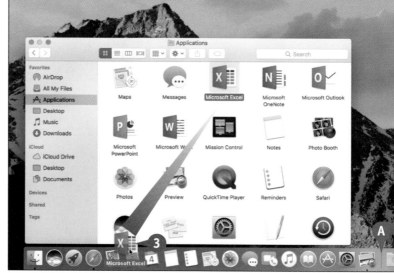

3 Click and drag the application icon, and then drop it inside the Dock.

A Be sure to drop the icon anywhere to the left of the Dock divider.

B macOS adds the application's icon to the Dock.

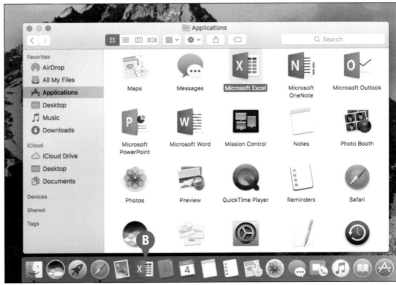

Add an Icon for a Running Application

1 Right-click (or **Control**-click) the application icon in the Dock.

2 Click **Options**.

3 Click **Keep in Dock**.

The application's icon remains in the Dock even after you close the program.

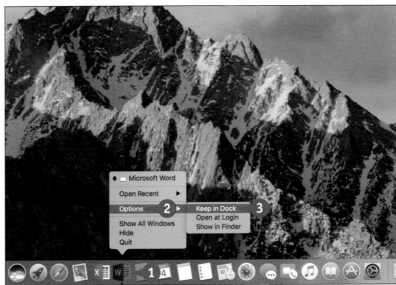

TIPS

Can my Mac start the application automatically each time I log in?

Yes. You can configure your application as a *login item*, which is a program or similar item that runs automatically after you log in. Right-click (or **Control**-click) the application's Dock icon, click **Options**, and then click **Open at Login**.

How do I remove an icon from the Dock?

Drag it off the Dock, or right-click (or **Control**-click) the application's Dock icon, click **Options**, and then click **Remove from Dock**. If the application is running, macOS removes the icon from the Dock when you quit the program. You can remove any application icon except Finder (　).

Hide the Dock

When you are working in an application, you might find that you need to maximize the amount of vertical space the application window takes up on-screen. This might come up, for example, when you are reading or editing a long document or viewing a large photo. In such cases, you can size the window to maximum height, but macOS will not let you go past the Dock. You can work around this by hiding the Dock. When the Dock is hidden, it is still easily accessible whenever you need to use it.

Hide the Dock

Turn On Dock Hiding

1 Right-click (or **Control**-click) the Dock divider.

2 Click **Turn Hiding On**.

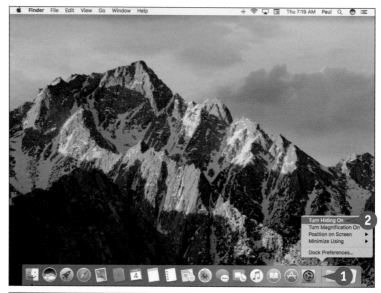

A macOS removes the Dock from the desktop.

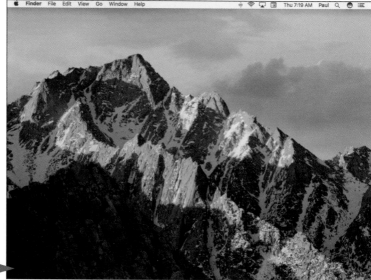

Display the Dock Temporarily

1 Move the mouse pointer (🖰) to the bottom of the screen.

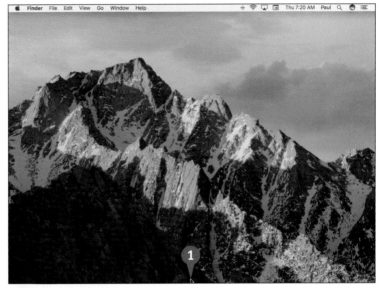

B macOS temporarily displays the Dock.

Note: To hide the Dock again, you can move the mouse pointer (🖰) away from the bottom of the screen.

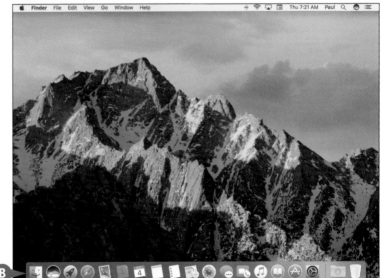

TIPS

Is there a faster way to hide the Dock?
Yes. You can quickly hide the Dock by pressing `Option`+`⌘`+`D`. This keyboard shortcut is a toggle, which means that you can also turn off Dock hiding by pressing `Option`+`⌘`+`D`. When the Dock is hidden, you can display it temporarily by pressing `Control`+`F3` (on some keyboards you must press `Fn`+`Control`+`F3`).

How do I bring the Dock back into view?
When you no longer need the extra screen space for your applications, you can turn off Dock hiding to bring the Dock back into view. Display the Dock, right-click (or `Control`-click) the Dock divider, and then click **Turn Hiding Off**.

Add a Widget to the Notification Center

The Notification Center is a macOS application that you use not only to view your latest notifications, but also to display widgets. A widget is a mini-application, particularly one designed to perform a single task, such as displaying the weather, showing stock data, or working with reminders. You can customize the Notification Center to include any widgets that you find useful or informative. macOS comes with several widgets, and there are also many widgets available via the App Store.

Add a Widget to the Notification Center

1 Click **Notification Center** (☰).

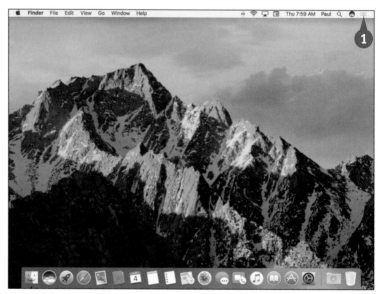

2 Click **Today**.

macOS displays the Notification Center and its current set of widgets.

3 Click **Edit**.

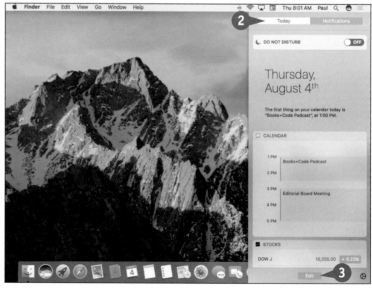

macOS displays its collection of widgets.

4 Click **Add** (⊕) beside the widget you want to add.

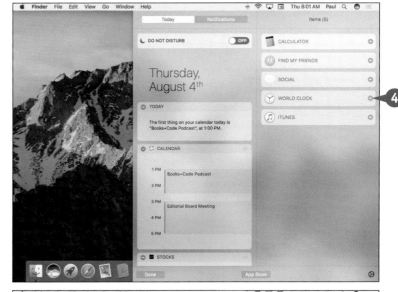

A macOS adds the widget to the Notification Center.

5 Click and drag the widget to the position you prefer.

6 Click **Done**.

macOS updates the Notification Center.

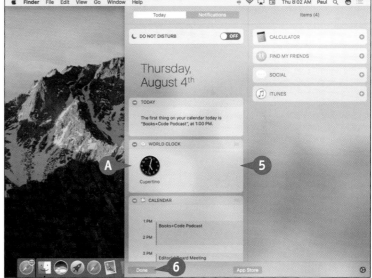

TIPS

Can I get more widgets?
Yes, the App Store has a section dedicated to Notification Center widgets, some of which are free. To see what is available, follow steps **1** to **3** to open the widgets list for editing and then click **App Store**.

How do I remove a widget from the Notification Center?
To remove a widget, follow steps **1** to **3** to open the widgets list for editing, and then click **Remove** (⊖) that appears to the left of the widget. macOS removes the widget and adds it to the Items list, just in case you want to use it again later. Click **Done**.

Extend the Desktop Across Multiple Displays

You can improve your productivity and efficiency by connecting a second monitor to your Mac. To work with an extra display, your Mac must have a video output port — such as a Thunderbolt port or Mini DisplayPort — that matches a corresponding port on the second display. If you do not have such a port, check with Apple or the display manufacturer to see if an adapter is available that enables your Mac to connect with the second display. After you connect your Mac to the display, you can extend the macOS desktop across both monitors.

Extend the Desktop Across Multiple Displays

1 Connect the second monitor to your Mac.

2 Open System Preferences.

Note: See the section "Display System Preferences," earlier in this chapter.

3 Click **Displays**.

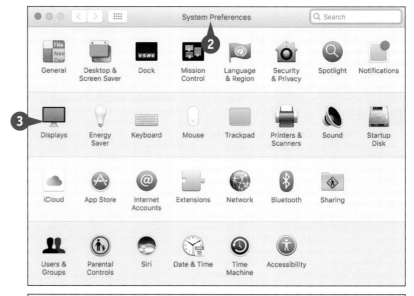

The Displays preferences appear.

4 Click **Arrangement**.

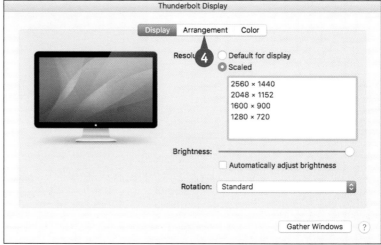

A This window represents your Mac's main display.

B This window represents the second display.

C This white strip represents the macOS menu bar.

5 Click and drag the windows to set the relative arrangement of the two displays.

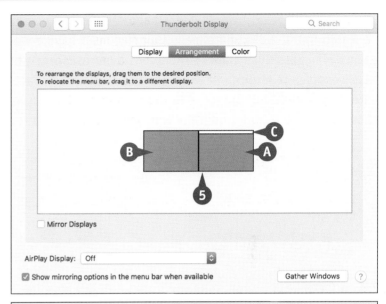

6 To move the menu bar and Dock to the second display, click and drag the menu bar and drop it on the second display.

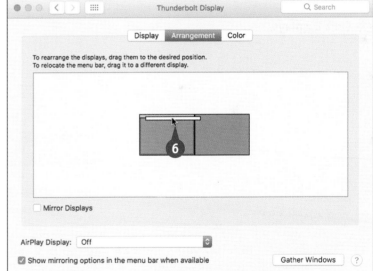

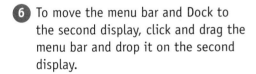
TIPS

Can I use a different desktop background in each display?

Yes. To set the desktop background on the second display, open System Preferences and click **Desktop & Screen Saver**. On the second display, use the Secondary Desktop dialog to set the desktop picture or color, as described in the section "Change the Desktop Background."

Can I just use the second display to show my main macOS desktop?

Yes. This is called *mirroring* the main display because the second display shows exactly what appears on your Mac's main monitor, including the mouse pointer (⬉). Follow steps 1 to 4 to display the Arrangement tab and then click the **Mirror Displays** check box (☐ changes to ☑).

Customize the Share Menu

The Share menu appears in many macOS applications, including Finder, Safari, Preview, Maps, and Notes. You use the Share menu's extensions to perform actions on the application's content. For example, in Safari you can use the Share menu to create a bookmark; send the page URL via email, text message, or AirDrop; or share the page on Twitter, Facebook, or LinkedIn. If you find that extensions are on the Share menu that you never use, you can reduce clutter on the menu by removing those items. You can also reorder the menu to put the items you use most often near the top.

Customize the Share Menu

Display the Share Menu Extensions

1 In the Dock, click **System Preferences** (⚙).

2 In the System Preferences, click **Extensions**.

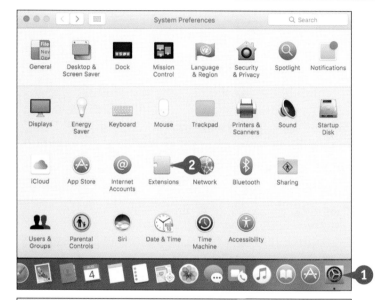

The Extensions preferences appear.

3 Click **Share Menu**.

A macOS displays the extensions available for the Share menu.

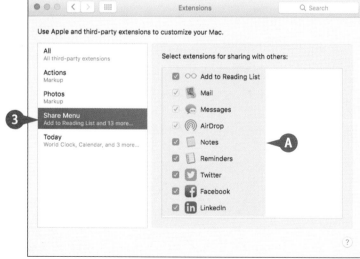

260

Remove a Share Menu Extension

1 To temporarily remove an extension from the Share menu, click its check box (✓ changes to ☐).

The next time you open the Share menu, you will no longer see the extension.

Note: macOS moves the disabled extension to the bottom of the list. To enable the extension later on, you can scroll to the bottom of the list and click the extension's check box (☐ changes to ✓).

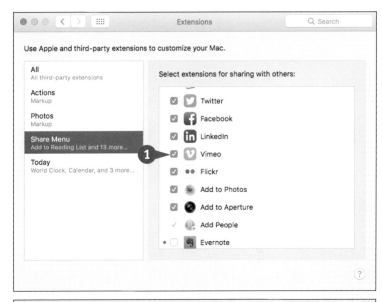

Move a Share Menu Extension

1 Position the mouse pointer (↖) over the name of the icon of the extension you want to move.

2 Click and drag the extension up or down to the new menu position and then release the extension.

The next time you open the Share menu, you will see the extension in its new position.

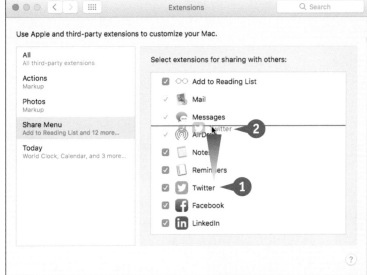

TIPS

Is there a quicker method I can use to customize the Share menu?

Yes, if you are working in an application that includes the Share menu. If so, click **Share** (⬆) and then click **More**. macOS automatically runs System Preferences, opens the Extensions preferences, and selects the Share Menu item.

What is the difference between the Share menu and a share sheet?

The Share menu is a list of macOS extensions that let you share your data. When you select some Share menu items, such as Facebook or Twitter (see Chapter 9), macOS displays a *share sheet*, which enables you to add extras such as text and location before you share the data.

CHAPTER 13

Maintaining macOS

To keep macOS running smoothly, maintain top performance, and reduce the risk of computer problems, you need to perform some routine maintenance chores. This chapter shows you how to empty the Trash, delete unnecessary files, uninstall applications, back up and restore your files, recondition your notebook battery, and more.

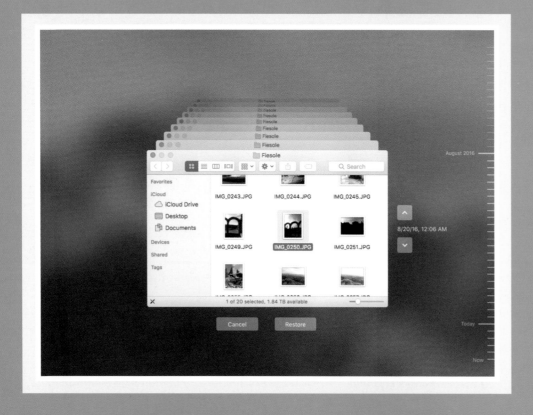

Empty the Trash

You can free up disk space on your Mac by periodically emptying the Trash. When you delete a file or folder, macOS does not immediately remove the file from your Mac's hard drive. Instead, macOS moves the file or folder to the Trash. This is useful if you accidentally delete an item because it means you can open the Trash and restore the item. However, all those deleted files and folders take up disk space, so you need to empty the Trash periodically to regain that space. You should empty the Trash at least once a week.

Empty the Trash

1 Click the desktop.

2 Click **Finder** from the menu.

3 Click **Empty Trash**.

Ⓐ You can also right-click **Trash** (🗑) and then click **Empty Trash**.

Note: Another way you can select the Empty Trash command is to press Shift + ⌘ + Delete.

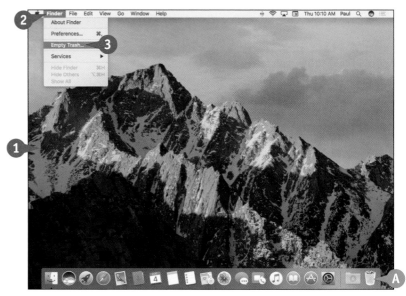

macOS asks you to confirm the deletion.

4 Click **Empty Trash**.

macOS empties the Trash (🗑 changes to 🗑).

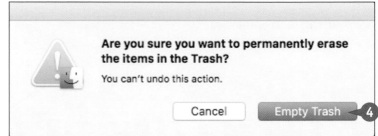

Are you sure you want to permanently erase the items in the Trash?

You can't undo this action.

Cancel   Empty Trash

Organize Your Desktop

You can make your macOS desktop easier to scan and navigate by organizing the icons. The macOS desktop automatically displays icons for objects such as your external hard drives, inserted CDs and DVDs, disk images, and attached iPods. The desktop is also a handy place to store files, file aliases, copies of documents, and more. However, the more you use your desktop as a storage area, the harder it is to find the icon you want. You can fix this by organizing the icons.

Organize Your Desktop

1 Click the desktop.

2 Click **View**.

3 Click **Clean Up By**.

4 Click **Name**.

You can also right-click the desktop, click **Clean Up By**, and then click **Name**, or press Option + ⌘ + 1.

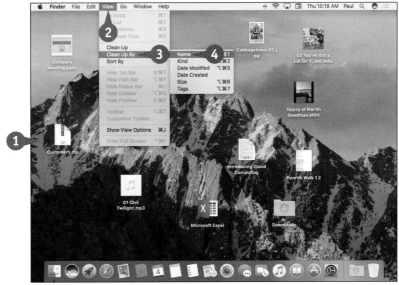

A Your Mac organizes the icons alphabetically and arranges them in columns from right to left.

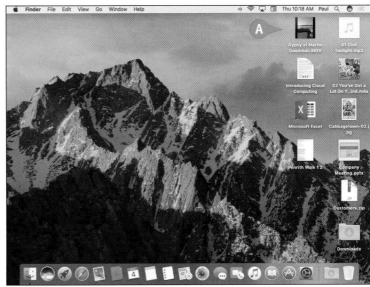

Check Hard Drive Free Space

To ensure that your Mac's hard drive does not become full, you should periodically check how much free space it has left. If you run out of room on your Mac's hard drive, you will not be able to install more applications or create more documents, and your Mac's performance will suffer. To ensure your free space does not become too low — say, less than about 50GB — you can check how much free space your hard drive has left. You should check your Mac's hard drive free space about once a month.

Check Hard Drive Free Space

Check Free Space Using Finder

1 Click **Finder** ( ).

2 Click any folder on your Mac's hard drive, such as **Downloads**, as shown here.

Note: Do not click Desktop, because that might only show you how much free space you have on your iCloud account.

3 In the status bar, read the available value, which tells you the amount of free space left on the hard drive.

If you do not see the status bar, press ⌘+⁄.

Display Free Space on the Desktop

1 Display your Mac's HD (hard drive) icon on the desktop, as described in the first Tip.

2 Click the desktop.

3 Click **View**.

4 Click **Show View Options**.

Note: You can also run the Show View Options command by pressing ⌘+J.

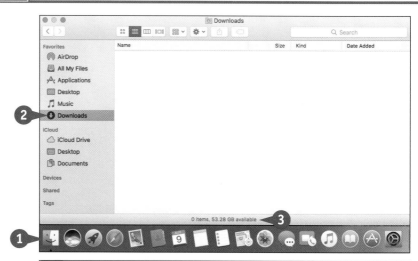

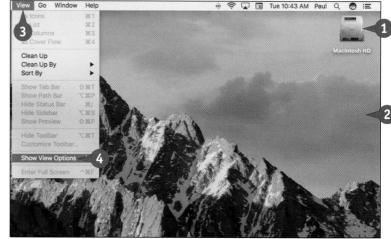

The Desktop dialog appears.

5 Click the **Show item info** check box (☐ changes to ☑).

A Your Mac displays the amount of free hard drive space under the Macintosh HD icon.

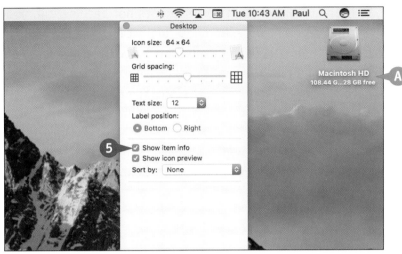

6 Drag the **Icon size** slider until you can read all the icon text.

7 If you still cannot read all the text, click the **Text size** ⬦ and then click a larger size.

8 Click **Close** (⬤).

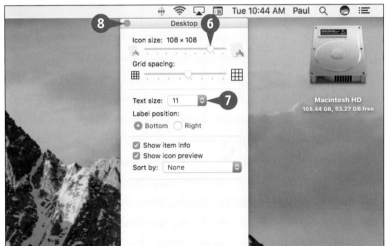

TIPS

My Mac's hard drive icon does not appear on the desktop. How do I display it?
Click the desktop, click **Finder** in the menu bar, and then click **Preferences**. Click the **General** tab, click the **Hard disks** check box (☐ changes to ☑), and then click **Close** (⬤).

What should I do if my Mac's hard drive space is getting low?
First, empty the Trash, as described earlier in this chapter. Next, uninstall applications you no longer use, as described in the next section. If you have large documents you no longer need, either move them to an external hard drive or flash drive, or delete them and then empty the Trash.

Uninstall Unused Applications

If you have an application that you no longer use, you can free up some disk space and reduce clutter in the Applications folder by uninstalling that application. When you install an application, the program stores its files on your Mac's hard drive, and although most programs are quite small, many require hundreds of megabytes of space. Uninstalling applications you do not need frees up the disk space they use and removes their icons or folders from the Applications folder. In most cases, you must be logged on to macOS with an administrator account to uninstall applications.

Uninstall Unused Applications

1 Click **Finder** ( ).

2 Click **Applications**.

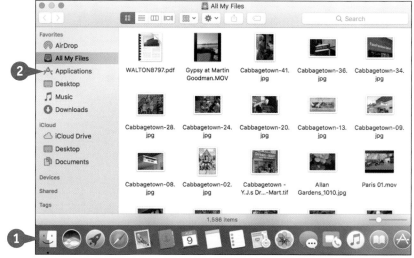

3 Click and drag the application or its folder and drop it on **Trash** ( ).

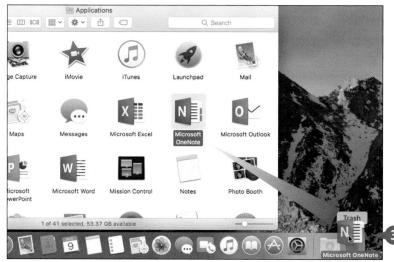

macOS prompts you for an administrator password.

④ Type the password.

⑤ Click **OK**.

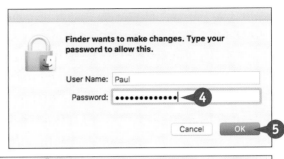

Ⓐ macOS uninstalls the application.

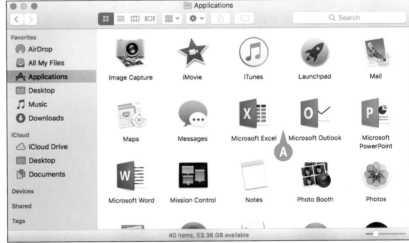

TIP

Is there another way to uninstall an application?
Yes, in some cases. A few Mac applications come with a separate program for uninstalling the application:

① Follow steps **1** and **2**.

② Open the application's folder, if it has one.

Note: Some programs store their uninstallers in Utilities, which is a subfolder of Applications.

③ Double-click the **Uninstall** (or **Uninstaller**) icon and then follow the instructions on-screen.

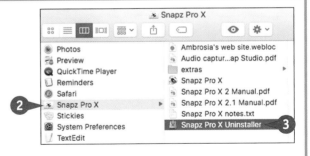

Force a Stuck Application to Close

When you are working with an application, you may find that it becomes unresponsive and you cannot interact with the application or even quit the application normally. In that case, you can use a macOS feature called Force Quit to force a stuck or unresponsive application to close, which enables you to restart the application or restart your Mac.

Unfortunately, when you force an application to quit, you lose any unsaved changes in that application's open documents. Therefore, you should make sure the application really is stuck before forcing it to quit. See the second Tip for more information.

Force a Stuck Application to Close

1 Click **Apple** (🍎).

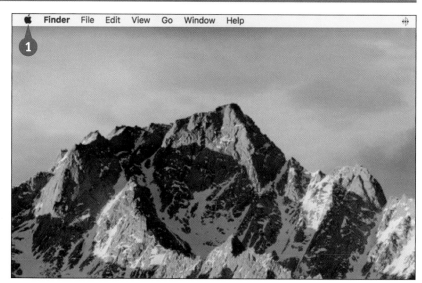

2 Click **Force Quit**.

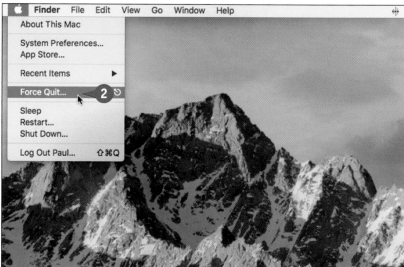

The Force Quit Applications window appears.

3 Click the application you want to shut down.

4 Click **Force Quit**.

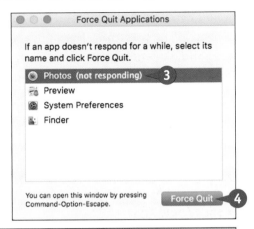

Your Mac asks you to confirm that you want to force the application to quit.

5 Click **Force Quit**.

Your Mac shuts down the application.

6 Click **Close** (⬤) to close the Force Quit Applications window.

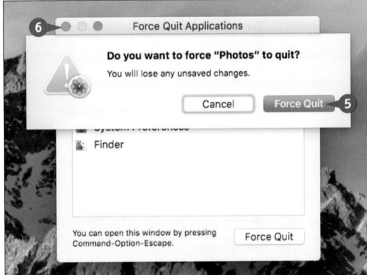

TIPS

Are there easier ways to run the Force Quit command?

Yes. From the keyboard, you can run the Force Quit command by pressing `Option` + `⌘` + `Esc`. If the application has a Dock icon, press and hold `Control` + `Option`, click the application's Dock icon, and then click **Force Quit**.

If an application is not responding, does that always mean the application is stuck?

Not necessarily. Some operations — such as recalculating a large spreadsheet or rendering a 3-D image — can take a few minutes, and the application can appear stuck. Low memory can also cause an application to seem stuck. In this case, try shutting down applications to free some memory.

Configure Time Machine Backups

One of the most crucial macOS maintenance chores is to configure your system to make regular backups of your files. Macs are reliable machines, but they can crash and all hard drives eventually die, so at some point your data will be at risk. To avoid losing that data forever, you need to configure Time Machine to perform regular backups.

To use Time Machine, your Mac requires a second hard drive. This can be a second internal drive on a Mac mini, but on most Macs the easiest course is to connect an external hard drive.

Configure Time Machine Backups

① Connect an external USB or Thunderbolt hard drive to your Mac.

If macOS asks if you want to use the hard drive as your backup disk, click **Use as Backup Disk** and then skip the rest of these steps.

② Click **System Preferences** (⚙).

The System Preferences appear.

③ Click **Time Machine**.

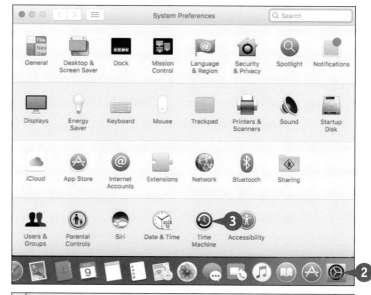

The Time Machine preferences appear.

④ Click **Select Backup Disk**.

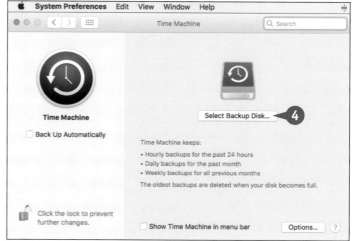

Time Machine displays a list of available backup devices.

⑤ Click the external hard drive.

⑥ Click **Use Disk**.

Note: If the drive contains data, Time Machine will ask you to confirm that you want the drive's data erased. If you are sure the drive contains no valuable information, you can click **Erase**. Otherwise, click **Don't Erase**, check the drive's contents, and then repeat these steps.

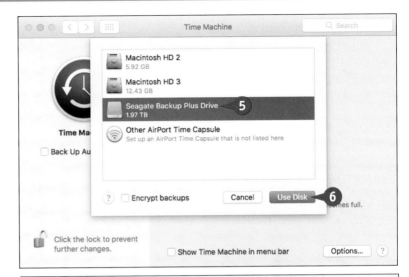

Ⓐ Time Machine enables backups and prepares to run the first backup automatically in 2 minutes.

⑦ Click **Close** (●).

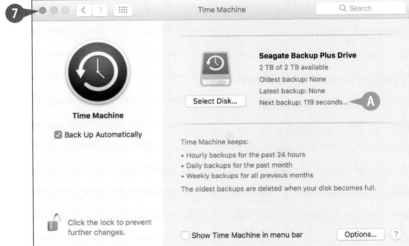

TIP

How do Time Machine backups work?
Time Machine backups are handled automatically as follows:

- The initial backup occurs 2 minutes after you configure Time Machine for the first time. This backup includes your entire Mac.

- Another backup runs every hour. These hourly backups include files and folders you have changed or created since the most recent hourly backup.

- Time Machine runs a daily backup that includes only those files and folders that you have changed or created since the most recent daily backup.

- Time Machine runs a weekly backup that includes only those files and folders that you have changed or created since the most recent weekly backup.

Restore an Earlier Version of a File

If you improperly edit or accidentally overwrite a file, some apps enable you to revert to an earlier version of the file. Why would you want to revert to an earlier version of a file? One reason is that you might improperly edit the file by deleting or changing important data. In some cases, you may be able to restore that data by going back to a previous version of the file. Similarly, if you overwrite the file with a different file, you can fix the problem by restoring an earlier version of the file.

Restore an Earlier Version of a File

1 Open the file you want to restore.

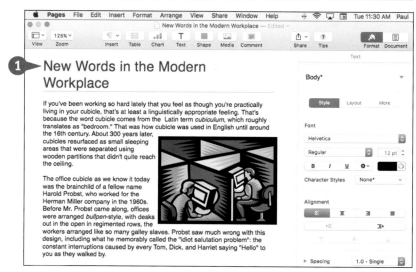

2 Click **File**.

3 Click **Revert To**.

Note: If you do not see the Revert To command, it means the application does not support this feature.

A To restore the most recently saved version, you can click **Last Saved**.

B To restore the most recently opened version, you can click **Last Opened**.

4 Click **Browse All Versions**.

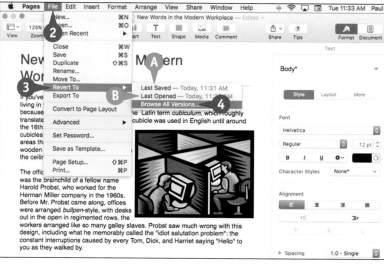

The restore interface appears.

C This window represents the current version of the file.

D Each of these windows represents an earlier version of the file.

E This area tells you when the displayed version of the file was saved.

F You can use this timeline to navigate the earlier versions.

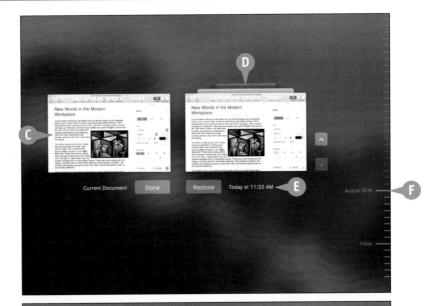

5 Navigate to the date that contains the version of the file you want to restore.

Note: See the first Tip to learn how to navigate the Time Machine backups.

6 Click **Restore**.

macOS reverts the file to the earlier version.

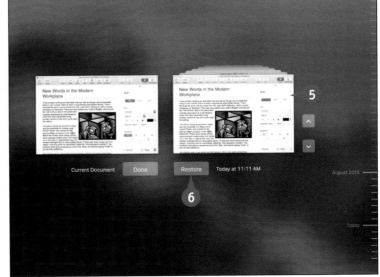

How do I navigate the previous versions?

There are two methods you can use:

- Use the timeline on the right side of the window to click a specific version.
- Click the title bars of the version windows.

Can I restore a previous version without overwriting the current version of the file?

Yes, you can restore a copy of the file. This is useful if the current version has data you want to preserve, or if you want to compare the two versions. Follow steps **1** to **5** to navigate to the version you want to restore. Press and hold (Option), and then click **Restore a Copy**.

Restore Files Using Time Machine

If you have configured macOS to make regular Time Machine backups, you can use those backups to restore a lost file. If you accidentally delete a file, you can quickly restore it by opening the Trash folder. However, that does not help you if you have emptied the Trash folder. Similarly, if the program or macOS crashes, a file may become corrupted.

Because Time Machine makes hourly, daily, and weekly backups, it stores older copies of your data. You can use these backups to restore any file that you accidentally delete, has become corrupted, or you need an earlier version of.

Restore Files Using Time Machine

1 Click **Finder** (🙂).

2 Open the folder you want to restore, or the folder that contains the file you want to restore.

Note: If you have repaired or replaced your original hard drive, you can restore the entire drive by pressing ⇧ Shift + ⌘ + C and then double-clicking the drive (usually **Macintosh HD**).

3 Click **Spotlight** (🔍).

4 Type **time machine**.

5 Double-click **Time Machine**.

The Time Machine interface appears.

A Each window represents a backed-up version of the folder.

B This area tells you when the displayed version of the folder was backed up.

C You can use this timeline to navigate the backed-up versions.

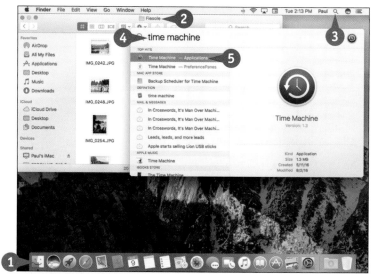

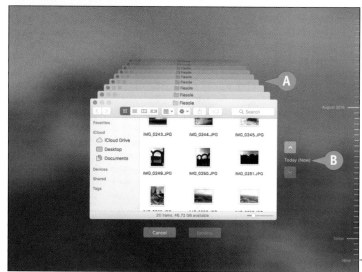

6 Navigate to the date that contains the backed-up version of the folder or file.

Note: See the Tip to learn how to navigate the Time Machine backups.

7 If you are restoring a file, click the file.

8 Click **Restore**.

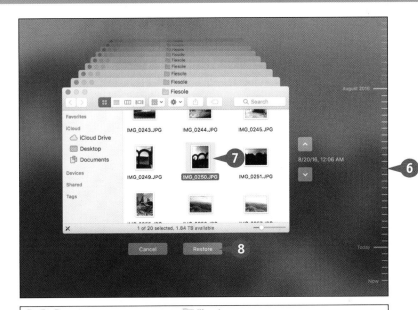

If another version of the folder or file already exists, Time Machine asks if you want to keep it or replace it.

9 Click **Replace**.

Time Machine restores the folder or file.

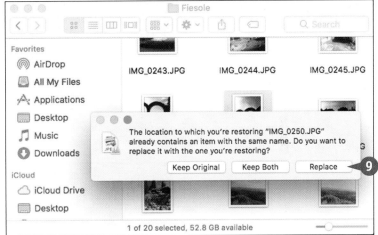

TIP

How do I navigate the backups in the Time Machine interface?
Here are the most useful techniques:

- Click the top arrow to jump to the earliest version; click the bottom arrow to return to the most recent version.
- Press and hold ⌘ and click the arrows to navigate through the backups one version at a time.
- Use the timeline to click a specific version.
- Click the version windows.

Recondition Your Mac Notebook Battery

To get the most performance out of your Mac notebook's battery, you need to recondition the battery by cycling it. *Cycling* a battery means letting it completely discharge and then fully recharging it again. Most Mac notebook batteries slowly lose their charging capacity over time. For example, if you can use your Mac notebook on batteries for 4 hours today, later on you will only be able to run the computer for 3 hours on a full charge. You cannot stop this process, but you can delay it significantly by cycling the battery once a month or so.

Recondition Your Mac Notebook Battery

Display the Battery Status Percentage

1 Click **Battery Status** (🔋).

2 Click **Show Percentage**.

Your Mac shows the percentage of available battery power remaining.

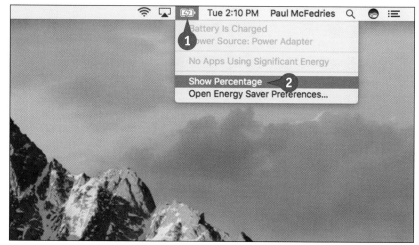

Cycle the Battery

1 Disconnect your Mac notebook's power cord.

Ⓐ The Battery Status icon changes from 🔋 to 🔋.

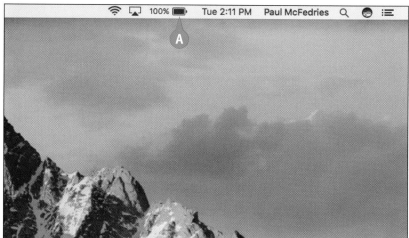

2 Operate your Mac notebook normally by running applications, working with documents, and so on.

3 As you work, keep your eye on the battery status percentage.

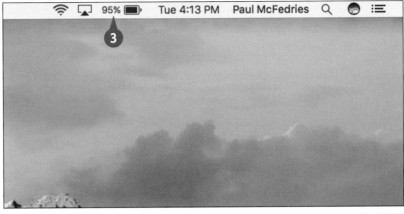

When the battery status reaches 8% the meter turns red, and when the status reaches 5%, macOS warns you that the system will soon go into sleep mode.

4 Click **Close**.

5 Reattach the power cord.

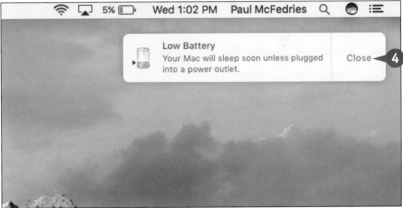

Your Mac restarts and the Battery Status icon changes from ▇ to ⚡.

6 Leave your Mac plugged in at least until the battery status shows 100%.

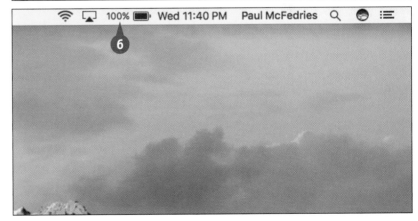

TIP

I do not see the battery status in my menu bar. How do I display it?
Click **System Preferences** (⚙) in the Dock to open System Preferences, and then click **Energy Saver**. In the Energy Saver window, click the **Show battery status in menu bar** check box (☐ changes to ✅). Click **Close** (⬤).

Restart Your Mac

If an application is behaving erratically or if a device attached to your Mac stops working, it often helps to restart your Mac. By rebooting the computer, you reload the entire system, which is often enough to solve many computer problems.

For a device that gets power from the Mac, such as some external hard drives, restarting your Mac might not resolve the problem because the device remains powered up the whole time. You can *power cycle* — shut down and then restart — such devices as a group by power cycling your Mac.

Restart Your Mac

Restart Your Mac

1 Click **Apple** (🍎).

2 Click **Restart**.

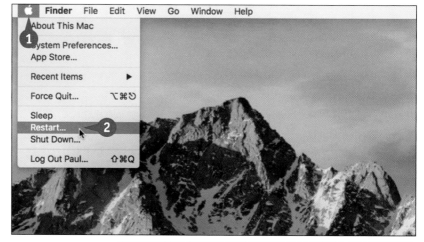

Your Mac asks you to confirm.

3 Click **Restart**.

Note: To bypass the confirmation dialog, you can press and hold **Option** when you click the **Restart** command.

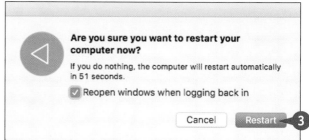

Power Cycle Your Mac

1 Click **Apple** ().

2 Click **Shut Down**.

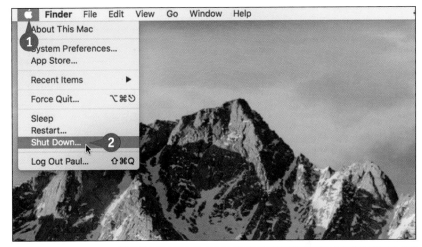

Your Mac asks you to confirm.

Note: To bypass the confirmation dialog, you can press and hold Option when you click **Shut Down**.

3 Click **Shut Down**.

4 Wait for 30 seconds to give all devices time to spin down.

5 Turn your Mac back on.

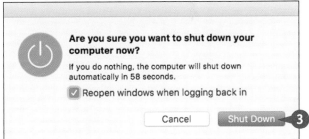

TIP

What other basic troubleshooting techniques can I use?

- Make sure that each device is turned on, that cable connections are secure, and that insertable devices (such as USB devices) are properly inserted.
- If a device is battery-powered, replace the batteries.
- If a device has an on/off switch, power cycle the device by turning it off, waiting a few seconds for it to stop spinning, and then turning it back on again.
- Close all running programs.
- Log out of your Mac — click **Apple** (); click **Log Out *User***, where *User* is your Mac username; and then click **Log Out** — and then log back in again.

CHAPTER 14

Working with iCloud

You can get a free iCloud account, which is an online service that lets you automatically synchronize data between iCloud and your Mac (as well as your iPhone, iPad, or iPod touch). You can also use iCloud to generate website passwords, store documents online, and locate a lost Mac.

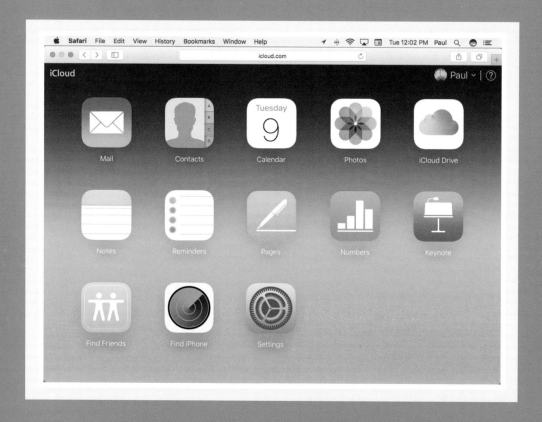

Create an Apple ID

To use iCloud, you need to create a free Apple ID, which you use to sign in to iCloud on the web and to synchronize your Mac and other devices. An Apple ID is an email address. You can use an existing email address for your Apple ID. When you use an existing email address, you are required to verify via email that the address is legitimate. Once you have created an Apple ID, you can use it to sign in to iCloud on the web, on your Mac, and on devices such as your iPhone or iPad.

Create an Apple ID

1 Click **System Preferences** (⚙).

The System Preferences appear.

2 Click **iCloud**.

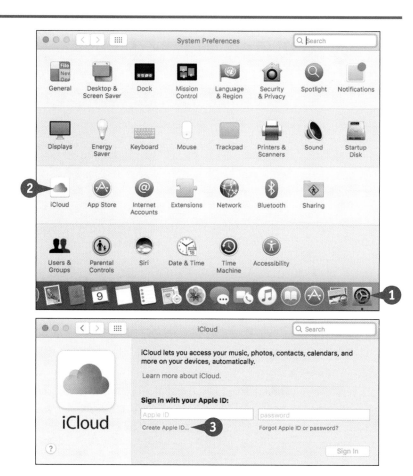

The iCloud preferences appear.

3 Click **Create Apple ID**.

The first dialog for creating an Apple ID appears.

4 Click the three **Birthday** pop-up menus to choose your month, day, and year of birth.

5 Click **Continue**.

6 Type your name.

7 Type the email address you want to use.

8 Type the password (twice).

9 Click **Next**.

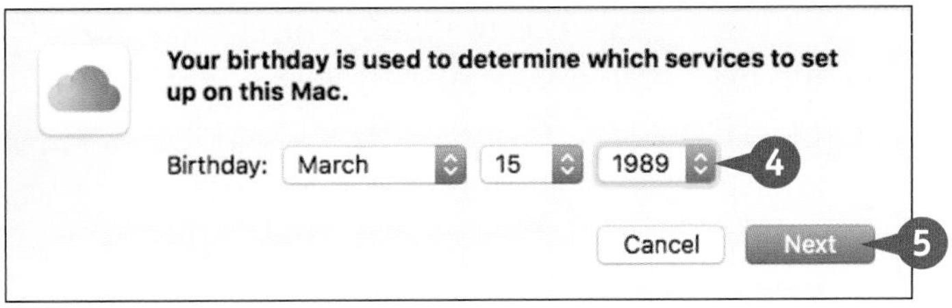
Your birthday is used to determine which services to set up on this Mac.
Birthday: March 15 1989
4
Cancel
Next
5

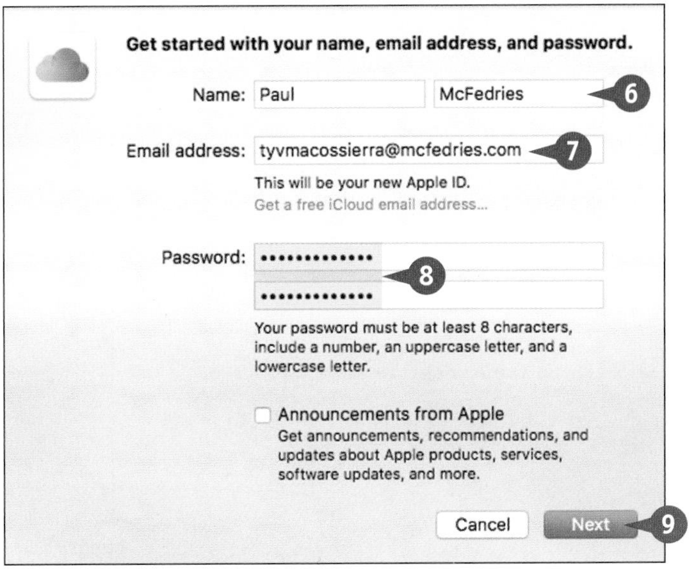
Get started with your name, email address, and password.
Name: Paul McFedries
6
Email address: tyvmacossierra@mcfedries.com
7
This will be your new Apple ID.
Get a free iCloud email address...
Password:
8
Your password must be at least 8 characters, include a number, an uppercase letter, and a lowercase letter.
Announcements from Apple
Get announcements, recommendations, and updates about Apple products, services, software updates, and more.
Cancel
Next
9

TIP

iCloud does not accept my password. Why?

Apple has fairly stringent requirements when it comes to the passwords used for iCloud accounts. First, the entire password must be at least eight characters long. Anything less and Apple rejects it. Also, the password must include at least one character from each of the following three sets: lowercase letters, uppercase letters, and numbers. If you do not use at least one character from each of those sets, Apple will reject your password. Finally, spaces are not allowed, so make sure you are not including any spaces in your password.

continued ▶

Although there is nothing to stop you from using any email address as your Apple ID, you really should use an address that belongs to you. Also, you need to be able to retrieve and read messages that are sent to that address, because this is part of the verification process. That is, once you give Apple your details and agree to the terms of service, Apple will send a verification message to the email address you provided. Before you can use your iCloud account, you must click a verification link in that message.

Create an Apple ID (continued)

10 For each security question, click ◘ to select a question and then type an answer.

11 Click **Next**.

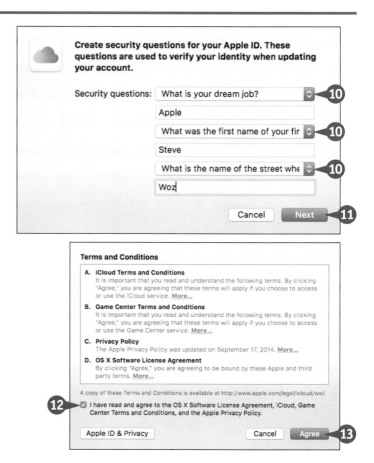

12 Click the check box (☐ changes to ☑).

13 Click **Agree**.

Apple sends an email message to the address you typed in step 7.

14 In your email program, open the message from Apple.

15 Click **Verify now**.

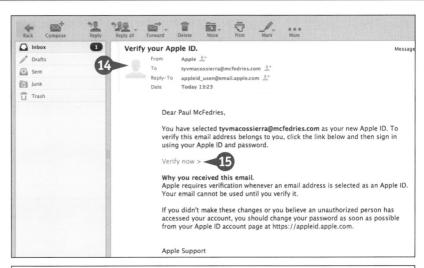

Apple prompts you to sign in to verify your email address.

16 Type your Apple ID (that is, the email address from step 7).

17 Type your password.

18 Click **Continue**.

Apple verifies your address and then macOS sets up your iCloud account on your Mac.

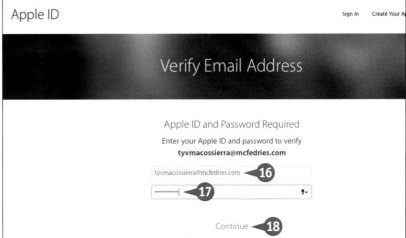

TIP

Why do I not see any iCloud data on my Mac?
At this point, you have verified your address and macOS has set up your new iCloud account on your Mac. However, macOS does not synchronize any iCloud data automatically. Instead, you need to sign in to iCloud on your Mac and then choose which services you want to synchronize between your Mac and iCloud. See the section "Set Up iCloud Synchronization," later in this chapter, for details.

Sign In to iCloud Online

Although you can access most iCloud features using your Mac, you can also sign in online using a web browser, which is useful if you need to access iCloud data when using someone else's Mac or Windows PC. Most modern browsers work well with iCloud, but Apple recommends that you use at least Safari 8, Firefox 22, Internet Explorer 10, or Chrome 28.

To sign in to iCloud using a Mac, you must be using at least OS X Lion 10.7.5, although Apple recommends OS X Yosemite (10.10.3) or later. To access iCloud using a Windows PC, the PC must be running Windows 7 or later.

Sign In to iCloud Online

1 In your web browser, type **www.icloud.com**.

2 Press **Return**.

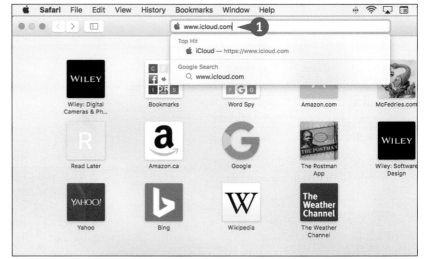

The iCloud Login page appears.

3 Type your Apple ID in the Apple ID text box.

4 Type the password for your Apple ID in the Password text box.

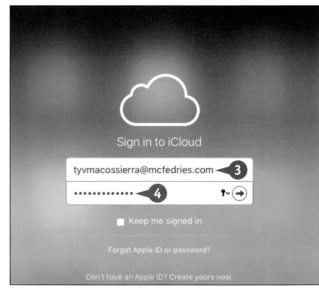

A If you want iCloud to sign you in automatically in the future, you can click the **Keep me signed in** check box (☐ changes to ☑).

5 Click **Sign In** (→).

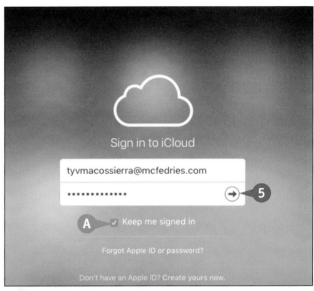

The first time you sign in, iCloud prompts you to configure some settings.

6 Click **Add Photo**, drop a photo on the dialog that appears, and then click **Done**.

7 Click **Start Using iCloud.**

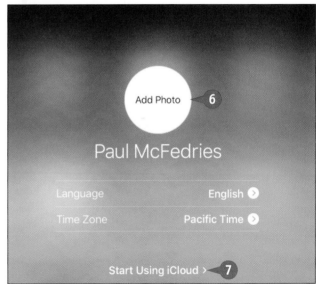

TIPS

Can I sign in from my Mac?
Yes. Click **System Preferences** (⚙) in the Dock (or click and then click **System Preferences**) and then click **iCloud**. Type your Apple ID and password and then click **Sign In**.

How do I sign out from iCloud?
When you are done working with your iCloud account, if you prefer not to remain signed in to your account, click your account name in the upper-right corner of the iCloud page and then click **Sign Out**.

Set Up iCloud Synchronization

You can ensure that your Mac and your iCloud account have the same data by synchronizing the two. The main items you will want to synchronize are email accounts, contacts, calendars, reminders, and notes. However, there are many other types of data you may want to synchronize to iCloud, including Safari bookmarks, photos, and documents. If you have a second Mac, a Windows PC, or an iPhone, iPad, or iPod touch, you can also synchronize it with the same iCloud account, which ensures that your Mac and the device use the same data.

Set Up iCloud Synchronization

1 Click **System Preferences** (⚙).

The System Preferences appear.

2 Click **iCloud**.

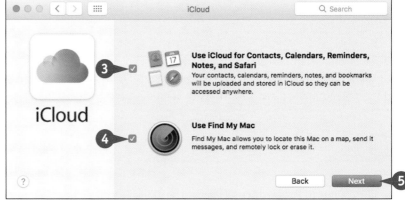

The first time you open iCloud, macOS prompts you to choose which iCloud services you want to use.

3 If you do not want to sync your data to iCloud, click the **Use iCloud for Contacts, Calendars, Reminders, Notes, and Safari** check box (☑ changes to ☐).

4 If you do not want to use iCloud to locate your Mac, click the **Use Find My Mac** check box (☑ changes to ☐).

5 Click **Next**.

If you elected to use Find My Mac, macOS asks you to confirm.

6 Click **Allow**.

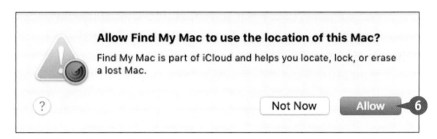

Allow Find My Mac to use the location of this Mac?

Find My Mac is part of iCloud and helps you locate, lock, or erase a lost Mac.

Not Now   Allow —6

The iCloud preferences appear.

7 Click the check box beside a type of data you want to sync (☐ changes to ☑).

Note: If you do not want to sync a type of data, click its check box (☑ changes to ☐). If macOS asks if you want to keep or delete the iCloud data that you are no longer syncing, click **Keep** or click **Delete from Mac**.

Your Mac synchronizes the data with your iCloud account.

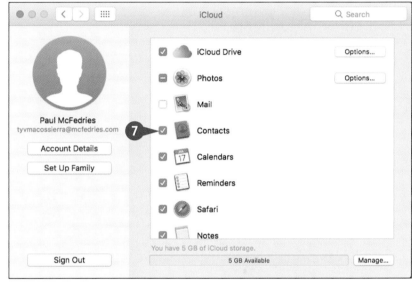

TIP

What happens if I modify an appointment, contact, bookmark, or other data in iCloud?
The synchronization process works both ways. That is, all the Mac data you selected to synchronize is sent to your iCloud account. However, the data on your iCloud account is also sent to your Mac. This means that if you modify, add, or delete data on your iCloud account, those changes are also reflected in your Mac's copies.

Set Up iCloud Keychain

You can make it easier to navigate secure websites by setting up iCloud Keychain. A *keychain* is a master list of usernames and passwords that a system stores for easy access by an authorized user. iCloud Keychain is a special type of keychain that stores website passwords auto-generated by Safari, as described in the next section, "Generate a Website Password." This means that you do not have to remember these passwords because Safari can automatically retrieve them from your iCloud account.

Set Up iCloud Keychain

1 Click **System Preferences** (⚙).

The System Preferences appear.

2 Click **iCloud**.

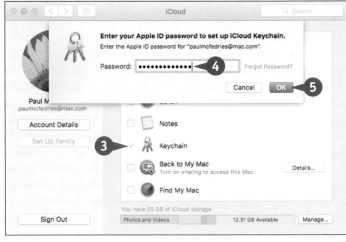

The iCloud preferences appear.

3 Click the **Keychain** check box (☐ changes to ☑).

Note: If macOS prompts you to create a password to unlock your screen, see Chapter 11.

macOS prompts you for your Apple ID password.

4 Type your password.

5 Click **OK**.

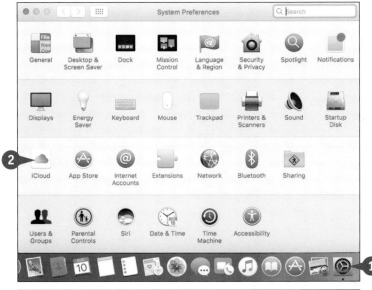

macOS prompts you to enter an iCloud security code.

6 Type a six-digit security code.

7 Click **Next**.

macOS prompts you to confirm the iCloud security code.

8 Repeat steps **6** and **7** to confirm the security code.

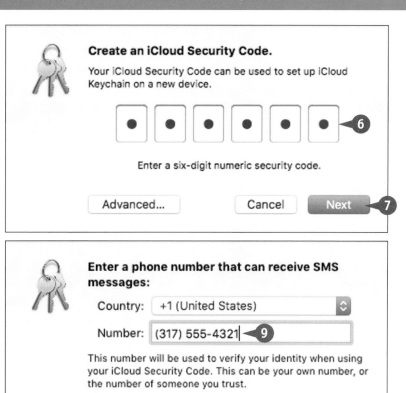

macOS prompts you to enter a phone number that can receive SMS (text) messages.

Note: If you have previously set up a phone number with iCloud, macOS sends a verification code to that number and then prompts you to enter the code.

9 Type the phone number.

10 Click **Done**.

macOS activates iCloud Keychain.

TIPS

Can I use iCloud Keychain only on my Mac?

No, *any* Mac or iOS device such as an iPhone or iPad that uses the same iCloud account has access to the same keychain, so your saved website passwords also work on those devices. On the downside, this sets up a possible security problem should you lose your iPhone or iPad. Therefore, be sure to configure your device with a passcode lock to prevent unauthorized access to your iCloud Keychain.

How do I change my security code or verification phone number?

If you want to use a different security code, or if the phone number you use for verification has changed, you should update these important security features as soon as possible. Display the iCloud preferences and then click **Options** beside Keychain.

Generate a Website Password

You can make it easier and faster to navigate many websites by using Safari to generate, and iCloud to store, passwords for those sites that require you to log in. Many websites require you to set up an account, which means you must log in with a username and password. Good security practices dictate using a unique and hard-to-guess password for each site, but this requires memorizing a large number of passwords. To enhance security and ease web navigation, you can use Safari to automatically generate for each site a unique and secure password stored safely with your iCloud account.

Generate a Website Password

Generate a Website Password

1 Turn on iCloud Keychain.

Note: See the previous section, "Set Up iCloud Keychain," to learn how to activate iCloud Keychain.

2 In Safari, navigate to a web page that requires a new password.

3 Click inside the password field.

A Safari displays its suggested password.

4 Click the password.

B iCloud enters the password. iCloud also enters the password in the confirmation field, if one exists.

5 Fill in the rest of the website form data as required.

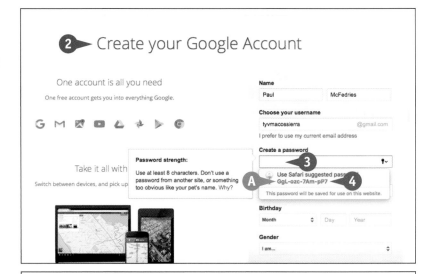

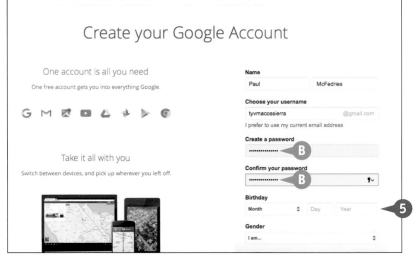

Using a Generated Website Password

1 In Safari, navigate to a web page that requires you to log in using a previously generated password.

2 Click inside the Password box.

3 Click **Keychain** (🔑⌄).

4 Click the saved website password.

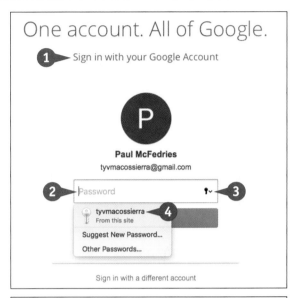

C Safari fills in the website password.

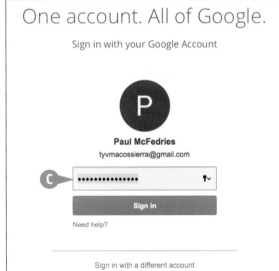

How do I get access to website passwords on another device?
You must activate iCloud Keychain on the other device and then authorize the other device to use the keychain. When you activate iCloud Keychain — see the previous section — iCloud gives you two ways to continue. As a first option, if a device that has previously been authorized to use your iCloud Keychain is available, click **Request Approval.** On the other device, click **Allow.** As a second option, if a device that has previously been authorized to use your iCloud Keychain is not available, click **Use Code**, type your six-digit iCloud security code, click **Next**, and then enter the verification code that iCloud sends via text message.

Activate and Configure iCloud Drive

You can use the iCloud Drive feature to store documents online. You can then access those documents either via the iCloud website or by using any other device — such as an iPhone or iPad — that is signed in to the same iCloud account. iCloud Drive works with all your Mac apps, so you can store any document in any iCloud Drive folder. If you have apps that you do not want to access your online storage, you can configure iCloud Drive to exclude those apps.

Activate and Configure iCloud Drive

1 Click **System Preferences** ( ).

The System Preferences appear.

2 Click **iCloud**.

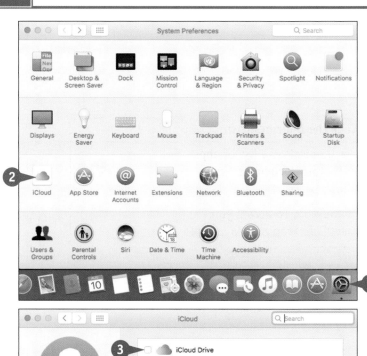

The iCloud preferences appear.

3 Click the **iCloud Drive** check box (changes to).

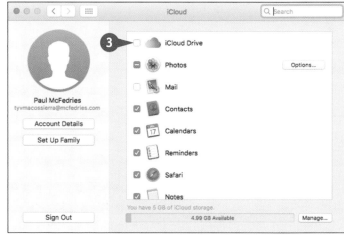

macOS activates iCloud Drive on your Mac.

4 Click **Options**.

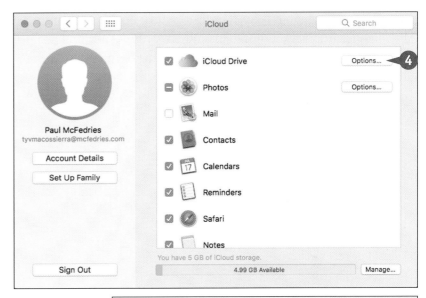

5 Click the **Documents** tab.

macOS displays a list of apps that store documents using iCloud Drive.

A If you want to access your macOS desktop and documents on other devices, leave this check box selected (☑).

6 Click the check box for each app that you do not want to access iCloud Drive (☑ changes to ☐).

7 Click **Done**.

macOS puts your iCloud Drive settings into effect.

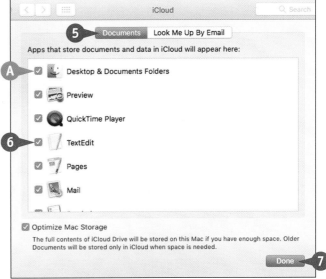

TIP

How do apps store documents using iCloud Drive?
It depends on the app. In some cases, an app is given its own iCloud Drive folder, which is a special storage area called an *application library*. Apps that get their own folders on iCloud Drive include TextEdit, Preview, Pages, Numbers, and Keynote. For all other apps, as well as apps that have their own libraries, you can store documents either in the main iCloud Drive folder or in a subfolder.

Access Your Desktop and Documents on Other Devices

By default, macOS configures iCloud Drive to store the contents of your macOS desktop and your Documents folder in iCloud. This enables you to access those files from other Macs and devices such as an iPhone, iPad, or iPod touch. This means in many cases that you only have to create a single copy of a document because you can now access that one copy on all your devices.

To access the same desktop and Documents folder on your devices, they must all be signed in to the same iCloud account.

Access Your Desktop and Documents on Other Devices

Access Your Desktop and Documents on Another Mac

1 Click **Finder** ( ).

2 In the iCloud Drive section of the sidebar, click either **Desktop** or **Documents**.

A The files stored on your desktop or your Documents folder appear.

3 Double-click the file you want to work with.

macOS opens the file in its associated app.

Note: If you have not yet configured iCloud Drive, see the next section, "Save and Open Documents Using iCloud Drive."

Access Your Desktop and Documents on an iOS Device

1 On the Home screen, tap **iCloud Drive**.

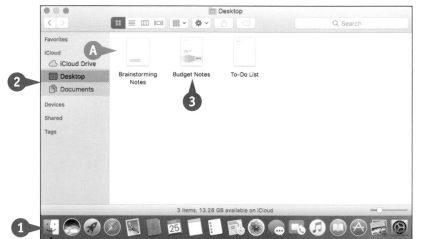

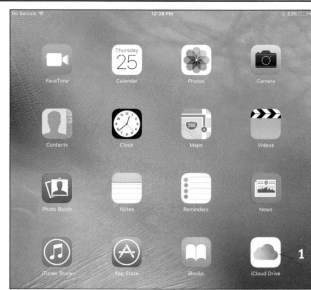

298

The iCloud Drive app opens.

2 Tap either **Desktop** or **Documents**.

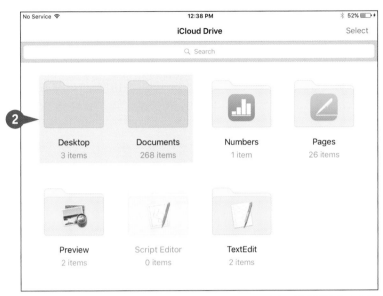

B iCloud Drive displays the files stored on your desktop or your Documents folder.

3 Tap the file you want to work with.

iOS opens the file in its associated app.

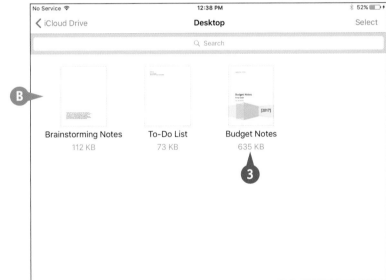

Save and Open Documents Using iCloud Drive

ow that you have activated iCloud Drive, you can use any macOS application to save your documents to iCloud Drive. If a program has its own iCloud Drive application library, you can use that folder to save your documents. Otherwise, you can save your documents in any iCloud Drive folder.

Once you have documents saved to iCloud Drive, you can use the associated macOS applications to open and work with those documents. You can also access iCloud Drive documents directly using Finder.

Save and Open Documents Using iCloud Drive

Save to an Application Library

1. Run the app's Save command.

Note: In most apps, you run the Save command by clicking **File** and then clicking **Save**, or by pressing ⌘+S.

2. Click the **Where** ⊕ and then click **App — iCloud**, where *App* is the name of the app, such as Pages, as shown here.

3. Fill in the other file details.

4. Click **Save**.

macOS saves the document to the program's application library.

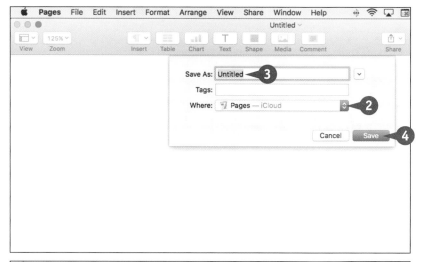

Save to Any iCloud Drive Folder

1. Run the app's Save command.

2. Click **Expand** (⌄).

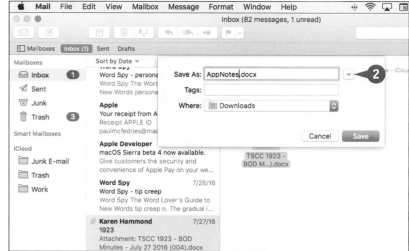

macOS expands the dialog.

③ In the Favorites section of the sidebar, click **iCloud Drive**.

macOS displays the contents of your main iCloud Drive folder.

④ Double-click the folder you want to use to store the document.

⑤ Fill in the other file details.

⑥ Click **Save**.

macOS saves the document to the iCloud Drive folder.

Open a Document Using Finder

① Click **Finder** (👤).

② In the sidebar's Favorites section, click **iCloud Drive**.

③ Open the folder than contains the document you want to open.

④ Double-click the document.

macOS opens the document in its associated application.

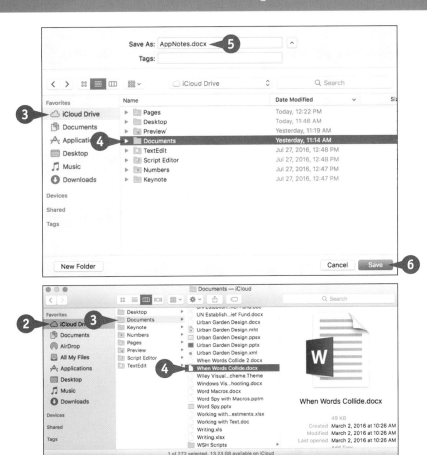

Can I create my own folders on iCloud Drive?

Yes, there are couple of methods you can use. The first method is to follow steps 1 to 3 in the subsection "Open a Document Using Finder" to open the folder where you want your new folder to appear. Click **File** and then click **New Folder** (or press Shift + ⌘ + N), type a name for the folder, and then press Return. Alternatively, sign in to iCloud as described in the section "Sign In to iCloud Online." Click **iCloud Drive**, double-click the folder where you want the new folder to appear, and then click **New Folder** (⊞). Type the folder name and then press Return.

Manage Your iCloud Storage

The iCloud preferences include a feature that enables you to manage your iCloud Drive storage. When you sign up for iCloud, Apple automatically gives you 5GB of free storage. Upgrading your storage, as described in the Tip at the end of this section, costs money, so if you do not want to spend anything for your iCloud Drive storage, then you need to manage your storage. This means deleting data that you no longer need from iCloud Drive. You can delete the backups stored for one or more devices, or you can delete the documents and data stored by one or more apps.

Manage Your iCloud Storage

1 Click **System Preferences** (⚙).

The System Preferences appear.

2 Click **iCloud**.

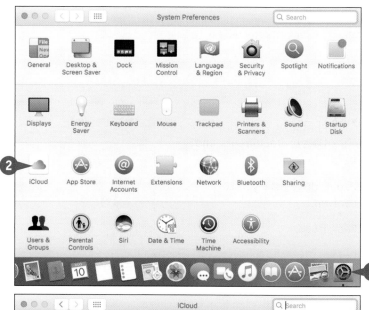

The iCloud preferences appear.

3 Click **Manage**.

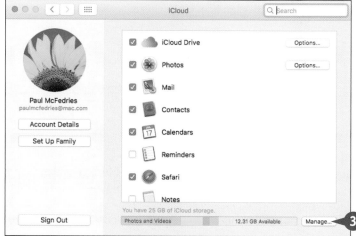

The Manage Storage dialog appears.

4 Click **Backups**.

5 Click the device backup you want to remove.

6 Click **Delete**.

iCloud Drive asks you to confirm.

7 Click **Delete**.

iCloud Drive removes the device backup.

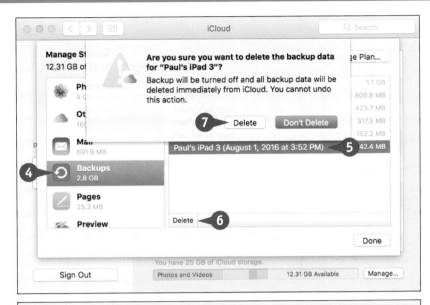

8 Click an app.

9 Click **Delete Documents and Data**.

iCloud Drive asks you to confirm.

10 Click **Delete**.

11 Repeat steps **8** to **10** to remove the data for other apps, as needed.

12 Click **Done**.

macOS puts your iCloud Drive settings into effect.

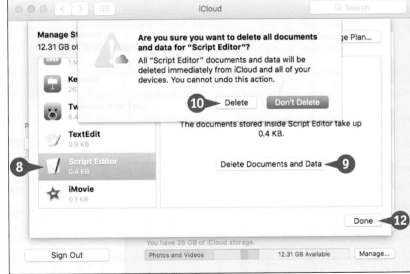

TIP

How do I change my iCloud storage plan?

iCloud Drive comes with 5GB of online file storage. If you are getting low on iCloud Drive storage space, then you should consider upgrading your storage plan to give yourself more room. You can get 50GB for $0.99 a month, 200GB for $2.99 a month, or 1TB for $9.99 a month. To upgrade your plan, follow steps **1** to **3** to open the Manage Storage dialog, and then click **Change Storage Plan**. The Upgrade iCloud Storage dialog appears. Click the storage plan you want to use, click **Next**, type your Apple ID password, and then click **Buy**.

Set Up Family Sharing

Not being able to see what other members of your family are sharing on iCloud has long been a major drawback of the service because the only way to work around it was to share an account. Now, however, iCloud offers a feature called Family Sharing, which lets up to six family members share each other's content, including photos, calendars, and reminders. And if purchases are made through the App Store, iTunes Store, or iBookstore using a single credit card, then each family member also gets access to the others' purchased apps, songs, movies, TV shows, and e-books, where the seller allows that sharing.

Set Up Family Sharing

Note: These steps assume you want to be the Family Sharing organizer, which means you are responsible for maintaining Family Sharing.

1. Click **System Preferences** (⚙) in the Dock (not shown).

2. Click **iCloud** (not shown).

   The iCloud preferences appear.

3. Click **Set Up Family**.

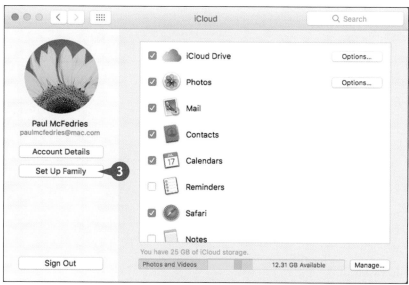

The Family Sharing preferences appear.

4. Click **Continue**.

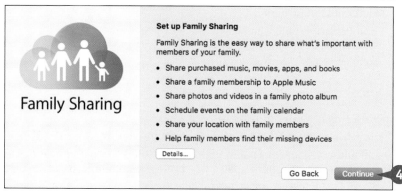

iCloud asks if you want to be the organizer.

5 Click **Continue**.

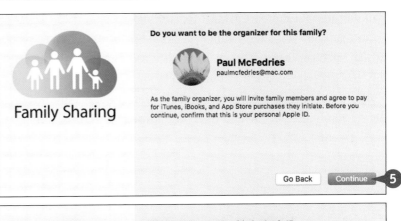

iCloud lets you know that purchases made through your account will be shared with your family.

6 Click **Continue**.

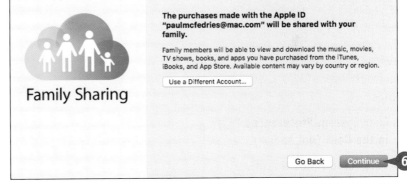

iCloud displays the payment method associated with your account.

7 Click **Continue**.

iCloud asks if you want to share your location with your family.

8 Click the **Share your location** option (○ changes to ●) (not shown).

9 Click **Continue** (not shown).

iCloud sets up Family Sharing.

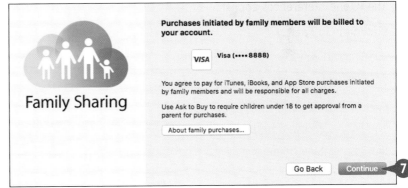

TIP

How do I add family members?
When you complete the Family Sharing setup, iCloud displays the Manage Family Sharing dialog. You can also display this dialog at any time by clicking **Manage Family** in the iCloud preferences. Click **Add Family Member** (+), enter the person's name or email address, and then click **Continue**. Click the **Ask this family member to enter the password** option (○ changes to ●) and then type the password for that person's iCloud account. If you do not know the password, click **Send *Name* an invitation** instead (where *Name* is the family member's name). Click **Continue**.

Locate and Lock a Lost Mac, iPod, iPhone, or iPad

You can use iCloud to locate a lost or stolen Mac, iPod touch, iPhone, or iPad. Depending on how you use your Mac, iPod touch, iPhone, or iPad, you can end up with many details of your life residing on the device. That is generally a good thing, but if you happen to lose your device, you have also lost those details, plus you have created a large privacy problem because anyone can now see your data. You can locate your device and even remotely lock the device using an iCloud feature called Find My iPhone, which also works for Macs, iPod touches, and iPads.

Locate and Lock a Lost Mac, iPod, iPhone, or iPad

1 Sign in to the iCloud website.

Note: See the section "Sign In to iCloud Online," earlier in this chapter.

2 Click **Find iPhone**.

Note: If iCloud asks you to sign in to your account, type your password and click **Sign In**.

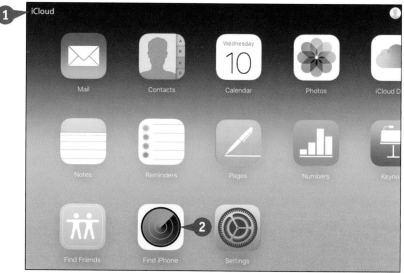

3 Click **All Devices**.

4 Click the device you want to locate.

A iCloud displays the device location on a map.

5 Click **Lost Mode**.

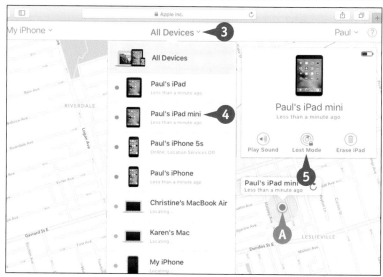

The Lost Mode dialog appears. If the device is not protected by a passcode, iCloud prompts you to enter one. If the device is protected by a passcode, you can skip to step **8**.

6 Type a six-digit lock code.

7 Type the lock code again to confirm (not shown).

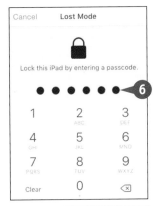

iCloud prompts you to enter a phone number where you can be contacted.

8 Type the phone number.

9 Click **Next**.

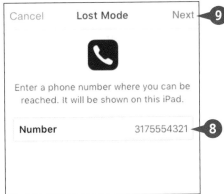

iCloud prompts you to enter a message to display on the device.

10 Type your message.

11 Click **Done**.

iCloud locks the device and sends the message, which then appears on the device screen.

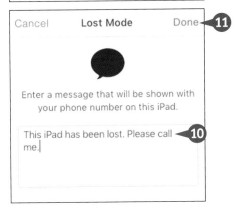

TIP

I tried to enable Find My Mac, but macOS would not allow it. How can I enable Find My Mac?
You first need to enable location services. To do this, click **System Preferences** (⚙) in the Dock. In the System Preferences, click **Security & Privacy**, click the lock icon (🔒), type your macOS administrator password, and then click **OK** (🔒 changes to 🔓). Click **Privacy**, click **Location Services**, and then click the **Enable Location Services** check box (☐ changes to ☑).

CHAPTER 15

Networking with macOS

If you have multiple computers in your home or office, you can set up these computers as a network to share information and equipment. This chapter gives an overview of networking concepts and shows you how to connect to a network, how to work with the other computers on your network, and how to share your Mac's resources with other network users.

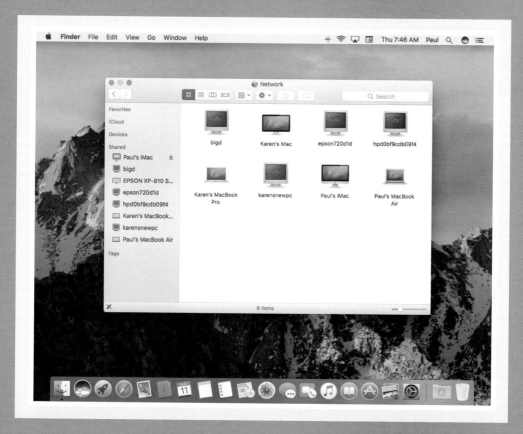

Wired Networking

Network Cable

A *network cable* is a special cable designed for exchanging information. One end of the cable plugs into the Mac's network port, if it has one. The other end plugs into a network connection point, which is usually the network's router (discussed next), but it could also be a switch, hub, or even another Mac. Information, shared files, and other network data travel through the network cables.

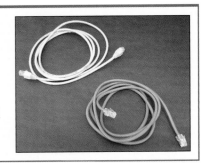

Router

A *router* is a central connection point for all the computers on the wired portion of the network. For each computer, you run a network cable from the Mac's network port to a port in the router. When network data travels from computer A to computer B, it first goes out through computer A's network port, along its network cable, and into the router. Then the router passes the data along computer B's network cable and into its network port.

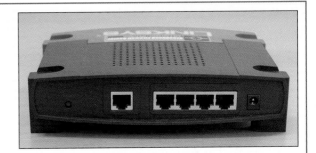

Wireless Networking

Wireless Connections

A *wireless network* is a collection of two or more computers that communicate with each other using radio signals instead of cable. The most common wireless technology is Wi-Fi (rhymes with hi-fi) or 802.11. Each of the four main types (802.11ac, 802.11b, 802.11g, and 802.11n) has its own range and speed limits. The other common wireless technology is Bluetooth, which enables devices to communicate directly with each other.

Wireless Router

A *wireless router* is a device that receives and transmits signals from wireless computers to form a wireless network. Many wireless routers also accept wired connections, which enables both wired and wireless computers to form a network. If your network has a broadband modem, you can connect the modem to your wireless router to extend Internet access to all the computers on the network.

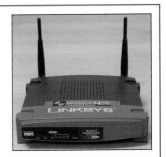

Connect a Bluetooth Device

You can make wireless connections to devices such as mice, keyboards, headsets, and cell phones by using the Bluetooth networking technology. The networking tasks that you learn about in the rest of this chapter require special equipment to connect your computers and devices. However, with Bluetooth devices, the networking is built in, so no extra equipment is needed. For Bluetooth connections to work, your device must be Bluetooth-enabled, and your Mac and the Bluetooth device must remain within about 30 feet of each other.

Connect a Bluetooth Device

Connect a Bluetooth Device Without a Passkey

1 Click **System Preferences** (⚙) in the Dock.

2 Click **Bluetooth**.

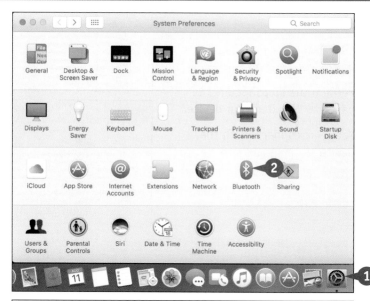

The Bluetooth preferences appear.

3 Click **Turn Bluetooth On**.

macOS activates Bluetooth and makes your Mac discoverable.

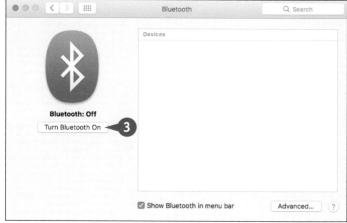

④ Perform whatever steps are necessary to make your Bluetooth device discoverable.

Note: For example, if you are connecting a Bluetooth mouse, the device often has a separate switch or button that makes the mouse discoverable, so you need to turn on that switch or press that button.

Ⓐ A list of the available Bluetooth devices appears here.

⑤ Click **Pair** beside the Bluetooth device you want to connect.

⑥ Perform the steps required to pair your Mac and your device.

Ⓑ Your Mac connects with the device.

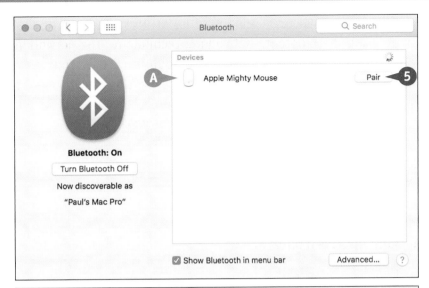

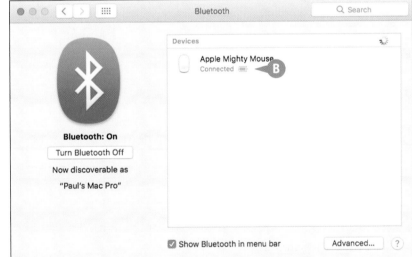

TIPS

What does it mean to make a device discoverable?

This means that you configure the device to broadcast that it is available for a Bluetooth connection. Controlling the broadcast is important because you usually want to use a Bluetooth device such as a mouse or keyboard with only a single computer.

What does pairing mean?

As a security precaution, many Bluetooth devices do not connect automatically to other devices. Otherwise, a stranger with a Bluetooth device could connect to your cell phone or even your Mac. To prevent this, most Bluetooth devices require you to type a password before the connection is made. This is known as *pairing* the two devices.

continued ▶

A Bluetooth mouse and a Bluetooth headset do not require any extra pairing steps, although with a headset you must configure macOS to use it for sound output. However, pairing devices such as a Bluetooth keyboard and a Bluetooth cell phone does require an extra step. In most cases, pairing is accomplished by your Mac generating a six- or eight-digit *passkey* that you must then type into the Bluetooth device (assuming that it has some kind of keypad). In other cases, the device comes with a default passkey that you must type into your Mac to set up the pairing.

Connect a Bluetooth Device (continued)

Connect a Bluetooth Device with a Passkey

1 Turn the device on, if required.

2 Turn on the switch that makes the device discoverable, if required.

3 Follow steps **1** and **2** in the subsection "Connect a Bluetooth Device Without a Passkey" to display a list of available Bluetooth devices.

4 Click **Pair** beside your Bluetooth device.

The Bluetooth Setup Assistant displays a passkey.

5 Use the Bluetooth device to type the displayed passkey.

6 Press **Return**.

macOS connects to the device. If you see the Keyboard Setup Assistant, follow the on-screen instructions to set up the keyboard for use with your Mac.

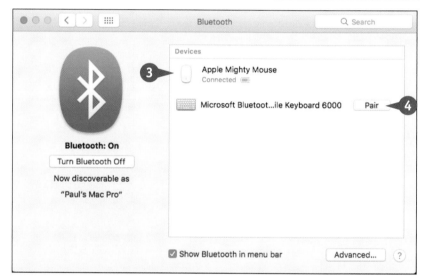

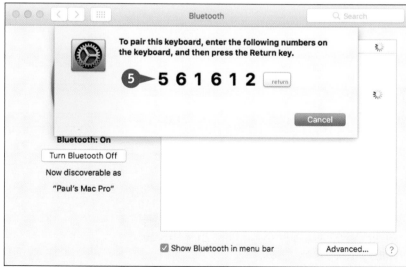

Listen to Audio Through Bluetooth Headphones

1. Click **System Preferences** (⊚) in the Dock.

2. Click **Sound**.

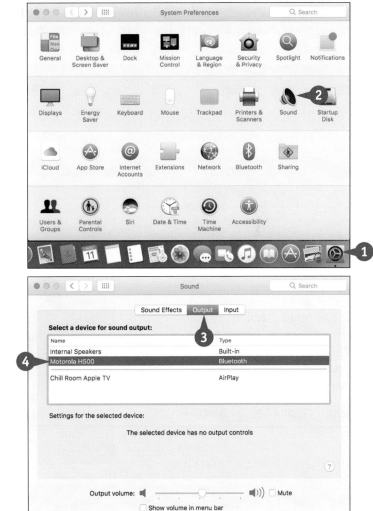

The Sound preferences appear.

3. Click the **Output** tab.

4. Click the Bluetooth headphones.

TIP

How do I remove a Bluetooth device?
To remove a Bluetooth device, first follow steps **1** and **2** in the subsection "Connect a Bluetooth Device Without a Passkey." Position the mouse pointer (▶) over the device you want to disconnect and then click **Disconnect** (✖) (Ⓐ). When macOS asks you to confirm, click **Remove**. macOS removes the device.

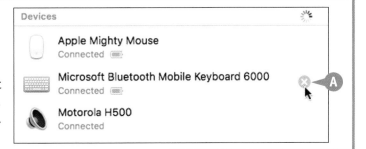

Connect to a Wireless Network

All the latest Macs have built-in wireless networking capability that you can use to connect to a wireless network that is within range. This could be a network in your home, your office, or a public location such as a coffee shop. In most cases, this also gives you access to the wireless network's Internet connection.

Most wireless networks have security turned on, which means you must know the correct password to connect to the network. However, after you connect to the network once, your Mac remembers the password and connects automatically the next time the network comes within range.

Connect to a Wireless Network

1 Click **Wi-Fi status** ( ) in the menu bar.

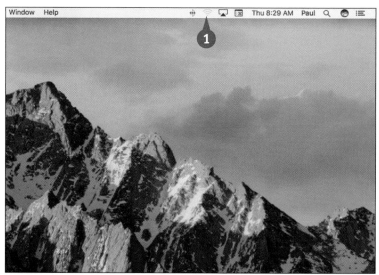

Your Mac locates the wireless networks within range of your Mac.

Ⓐ The available networks appear in the menu.

Ⓑ Networks with a lock icon ( ) require a password to join.

2 Click the wireless network you want to join.

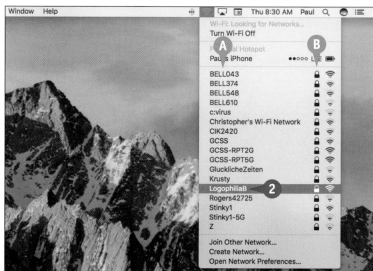

316

If the wireless network is secure, your Mac prompts you for the password.

③ Type the network password in the Password text box.

Ⓒ If the password is very long and you are sure no one can see your screen, you can click the **Show password** check box (☐ changes to ☑) to see the actual characters rather than dots. This helps to ensure you type the password correctly.

④ Click **Join**.

Your Mac connects to the wireless network.

Ⓓ The Wi-Fi status icon changes from 🛜 to 🛜 to indicate the connection.

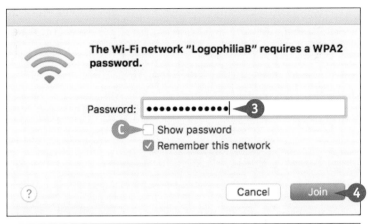

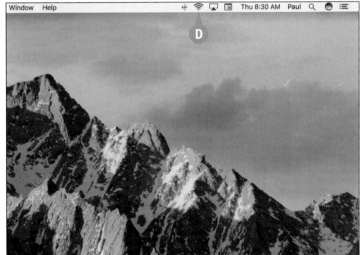

I know a particular network is within range, but I do not see it in the list. Why not?

As a security precaution, some wireless networks do not broadcast their availability. However, you can still connect to such a network, assuming you know its name and the password. Click **Wi-Fi status** (🛜) and then click **Join Other Network**.

I do not see the Wi-Fi status icon on my menu bar. How do I display the icon?

Click **System Preferences** (⚙) to open the System Preferences. Click **Network**, click **Wi-Fi**, and then click the **Show Wi-Fi status in menu bar** check box (☐ changes to ☑).

Connect to a Network Resource

To see what other network users have shared on the network, you can use the Network folder to view the other computers and then connect to them to see their shared resources. To get full access to a Mac's shared resources, you must connect with a username and password for an administrator account on that Mac. To get access to the resources that have been shared by a particular user, you must connect with that user's name and password. Note, too, that your Mac can also connect to the resources shared by Windows computers.

Connect to a Network Resource

1 Click the desktop.

2 Click **Go**.

3 Click **Network**.

Note: Another way to run the Network command is to press Shift + ⌘ + K.

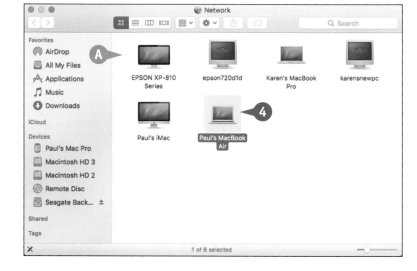

The Network folder appears.

A Each icon represents a computer on your local network.

4 Double-click the computer to which you want to connect.

macOS attempts to connect to the network computer. The attempt usually either fails or macOS logs on using the Guest account.

Note: The Guest account has only limited access to the network computer.

5 Click **Connect As**.

Your Mac prompts you to connect to the network computer.

6 Click the **Registered User** option (○ changes to ◉).

7 Type the username of an account on the network computer into the Name text box.

8 Type the password of the account into the Password text box.

9 To store the account data, click the **Remember this password in my keychain** check box (☐ changes to ☑).

10 Click **Connect**.

Ⓑ Your Mac connects to the computer and shows the shared resources that you can access.

11 When you are done, click **Disconnect**.

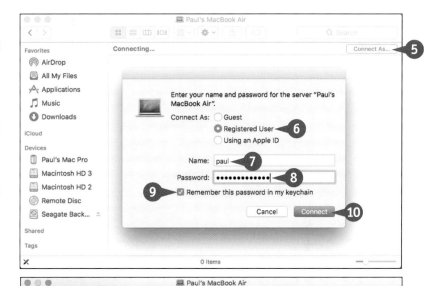

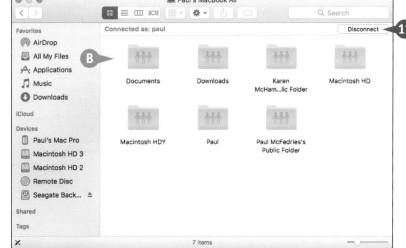

TIP

Is there a faster way to connect to a network computer?
Yes. In the Shared section of Finder's sidebar area, click the computer with which you want to connect (Ⓐ) and then follow steps **5** to **10** to connect as a registered user.

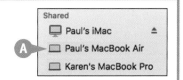

Turn On File and Printer Sharing

You can share your files with other network users. This enables those users to access your files over the network. Before you can share these resources, you must turn on your Mac's file-sharing feature. To learn how to share a particular folder, see the next section, "Share a Folder."

You can also share a printer that is connected directly to your Mac (such as via USB) with other network users. This enables those users to send print jobs to your printer over the network. Before this can happen, you must turn on your Mac's printer-sharing feature. To learn how to share a particular printer, see the section "Share a Printer," later in this chapter.

Turn On File and Printer Sharing

1. Click **Apple** (🍎).

2. Click **System Preferences**.

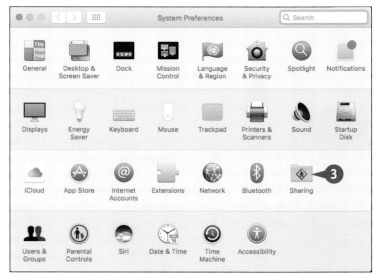

The System Preferences appear.

3. Click **Sharing**.

The Sharing preferences appear.

4 Click the **File Sharing** check box (☐ changes to ☑).

You can now share your folders, as described in the next section.

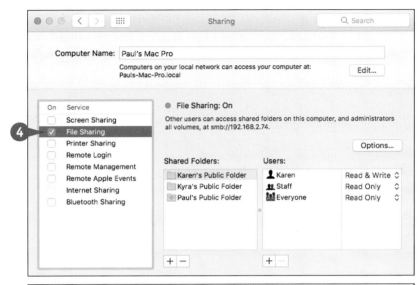

5 Click the **Printer Sharing** check box (☐ changes to ☑).

You can now share your printers, as described later in this chapter.

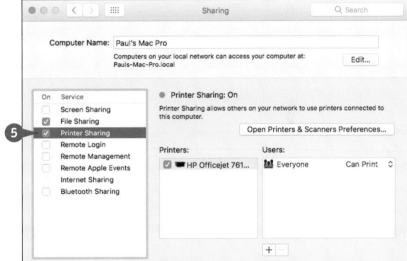

How do I look up my Mac IP address?
In System Preferences, click ❮ to return to the main window and then click **Network**. Click **Wi-Fi** if you have a wireless network connection, or click **Ethernet** if you have a wired connection. In the Status section, read the IP address value.

What is the Public folder and how do I access it?
The Public folder is a special folder for sharing files. Anyone who connects to your Mac using your username and password has full access to the Public folder. To access the folder, click **Finder** ( ), click **Go**, click **Home**, and then open the Public folder.

Share a Folder

You can share one of your folders on the network, enabling other network users to view and optionally edit the files you place in that folder. macOS automatically shares your user account's Public folder, but you can share other folders. Sharing a folder enables you to work on a file with other people without having to send them a copy of the file. macOS gives you complete control over how people access your shared folder. For example, you can allow users to make changes to the folder, or you can prevent changes.

Share a Folder

1 Open the Sharing preferences.

Note: See the previous section, "Turn On File and Printer Sharing," to learn how to display the Sharing preferences.

2 Click **File Sharing**.

Note: Be sure to click the **File Sharing** text, not the check box. This ensures that you do not accidentally uncheck the check box.

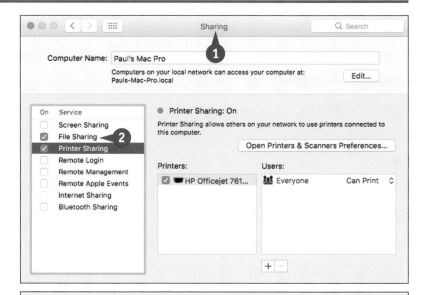

3 Under Shared Folders, click **Add** (+).

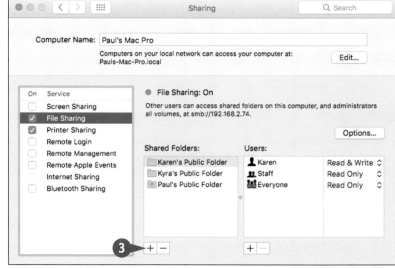

An Open dialog appears.

4 Click the folder you want to share.

5 Click **Add**.

Your Mac begins sharing the folder.

Note: You can also click and drag a folder from a Finder window and drop it on the list of shared folders.

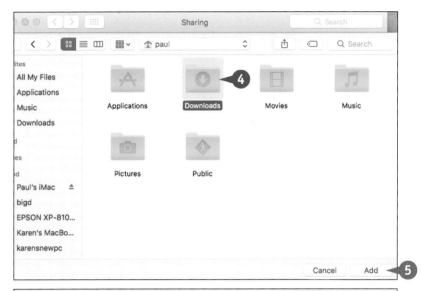

A The folder appears in the Shared Folders list.

6 Click the folder.

7 For the Everyone user, click the current permission and then click the permission you want to assign.

B The current permission is indicated with a check mark (☑).

macOS assigns the permission to the user.

C You can also click **Add** (**+**) under the Users list to add more users.

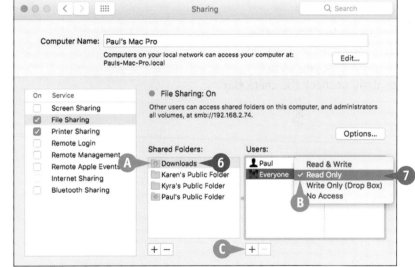

What are the differences between the permission types?
Read & Write means users can open files, add new files, rename or delete existing files, and edit file contents. Read Only means users can only open and read files, but cannot make changes to files. Write Only (Drop Box) means users can add files to the folder as a Drop Box, but cannot open the folder. No Access means users cannot see the folder.

Can I share folders with Windows users?
Yes. In the Sharing window, click **Options** and then click **Share files and folders using SMB** (☐ changes to ☑). Click your user account (☐ changes to ☑), type your password, click **OK**, and then click **Done**.

Share a Printer

If you have a printer connected directly to your Mac, you can share the printer with the network. This enables other network users to send their documents to your printer, as long as your Mac is running. Sharing a printer saves you money because you only have to purchase one printer for all the computers on your network. Sharing a printer also saves you time because you only have to install, configure, and maintain a single printer for everyone on your network. See the next section, "Add a Shared Printer," to learn how to configure macOS to use a shared network printer.

Share a Printer

1. Click **Apple** (🍎).

2. Click **System Preferences**.

Note: You can also click **System Preferences** (⚙️) in the Dock.

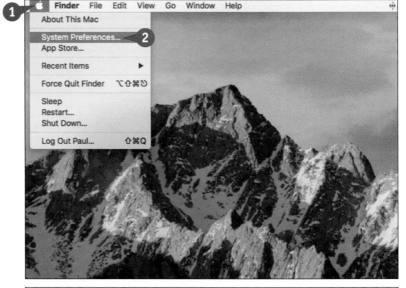

The System Preferences appear.

3. Click **Sharing**.

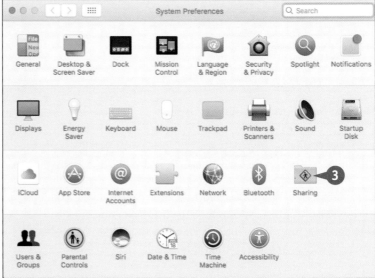

④ Click **Printer Sharing**.

Note: Be sure to click the **Printer Sharing** text, not the check box. This ensures that you do not accidentally uncheck the check box.

⑤ Click the check box beside the printer you want to share (☐ changes to ☑).

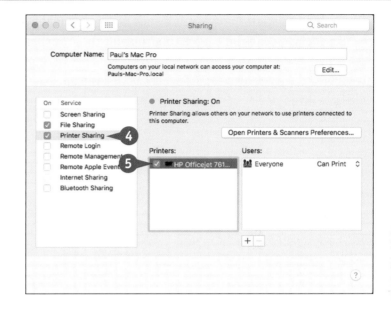

TIP

Is there another method I can use to share a printer?
Yes, you can follow these steps:

① Click **Apple** (🍎).

② Click **System Preferences**.

The System Preferences appear.

③ Click **Printers & Scanners**.

④ Click the printer you want to share.

⑤ Click the **Share this printer on the network** check box (☐ changes to ☑).

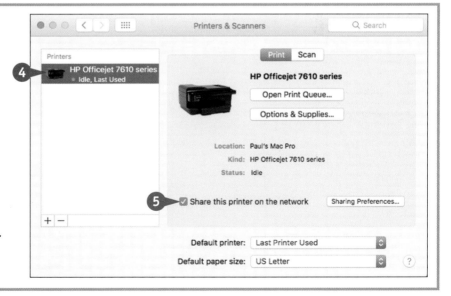

Add a Shared Printer

If another computer on your network has an attached printer that has been shared with the network, you can add that shared printer to your Mac. This enables you to send a document from your Mac to that shared printer, which means you can print your documents without having a printer attached directly to your Mac. Before you can print to a shared network printer, you must add the shared printer to macOS.

Add a Shared Printer

1 Click **System Preferences** (⚙) in the Dock.

The System Preferences appear.

2 Click **Printers & Scanners**.

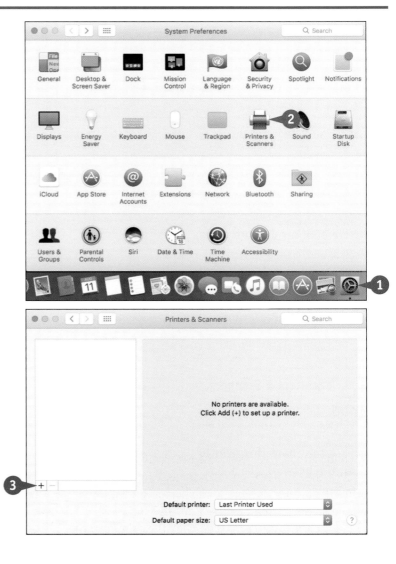

3 Click **Add** (+).

Note: If macOS displays a list of nearby printers, click the printer you want to add and skip the rest of these steps.

4 Click **Default**.

5 Click the shared printer.

Ⓐ Look for the word *Bonjour* or the word *Shared* in the printer description.

6 Click **Add**.

Note: If macOS alerts you that it must install software for the printer, click **Download & Install**.

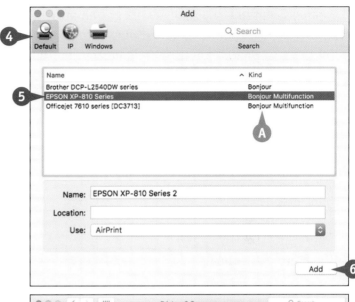

Ⓑ macOS adds the printer.

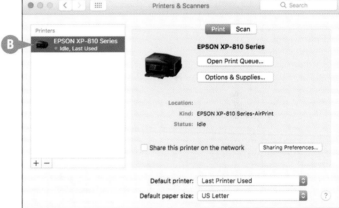

Can I add a shared Windows printer?
Yes. Follow steps **1** to **3** and then click the **Windows** tab. Click the Windows workgroup, click the computer sharing the printer, log on to the computer, and then click the shared printer. In the Print Using list, click **Add** (+), click **Other**, and then click the printer in the list. Click **Add**.

How do I print to the shared printer that I added?
In any application that supports printing, click **File** and then click **Print**. In the Print dialog, click the **Printer** 🔹, click **Add** (+), and then click the shared printer. Choose your other printing options and then click **Print**.

View macOS on Your TV

I f you have an Apple TV, you can use it to view your macOS screen on your TV. If you want to demonstrate something on your Mac to a group of people, it is difficult because most Mac screens are too small to see from a distance. However, if you have a TV or a projector nearby and you have an Apple TV device connected to that display, you can connect your Mac to the same wireless network and then send the macOS screen to the TV or projector. This is called *AirPlay mirroring*.

View macOS on Your TV

Mirror via System Preferences

1 Click **System Preferences** (🔘) in the Dock.

The System Preferences appear.

2 Click **Displays**.

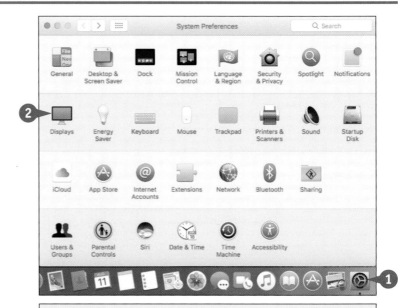

The display preferences appear.

3 Click the **AirPlay Display** ⬦ and then click your Apple TV.

macOS displays your Mac's screen on your TV.

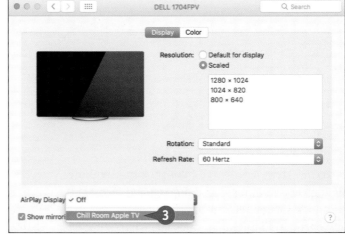

Mirror via the Menu Bar

① Follow steps **1** and **2** to open the display preferences.

② Click the **Show mirroring options in the menu bar when available** check box (☐ changes to ☑).

Ⓐ macOS adds the AirPlay Mirroring icon (🖵) to the menu bar.

③ Click **Close** (●).

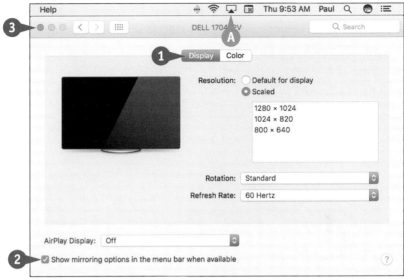

④ Click **AirPlay Mirroring** (🖵).

⑤ Click your Apple TV.

macOS displays your Mac's screen on your TV (🖵 changes to 🖵).

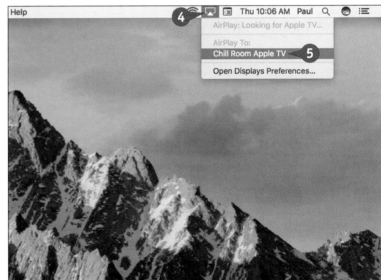

TIPS

How can I make my desktop fit my Mac's screen?
If you have a high-resolution TV, the macOS desktop might look small at that resolution. In System Preferences, click **Displays**, click the **Display** tab, click the **Optimize for** ⬍, and then click your Mac's screen.

Can I use my TV as a second monitor for the macOS desktop?
Yes. This is useful if you need extra screen room to display the desktop and applications. Click **AirPlay Mirroring On** (🖵) and then click **Use as Separate Display**.

Index

Index

Index

Index

Index